Integrated

Integrated Clinical Science

Other titles:

Cardiovascular Disease
Professor JR Hampton

Psychiatry
JL Gibbons

Haematology
JC Cawley

Neurology
RW Ross Russell
CM Wiles

Nephro-urology
Professor AW Asscher
Professor DB Moffat

Endocrinology
Professor CRW Edwards

Respiratory Disease
GM Sterling

Human Health and the Environment
Professor R Weir, C Smith

Musculoskeletal Disease
Professor RA Dickson
Professor V Wright

Projected:
Reproduction and Development

Integrated Clinical Science

Gastroenterology

Edited by

Peter F. Jones, MA, M.CHIR., FRCS Eng, FRCS Ed

Consultant Surgeon, Woodend General Hospital and Royal Aberdeen Children's Hospital
Clinical Professor of Surgery, University of Aberdeen
Surgeon to HM The Queen in Scotland

Peter W. Brunt, MD, FRCP

Consultant Physician/Gastroenterologist, Aberdeen Teaching Hospitals
Clinical Senior Lecturer in Medicine, University of Aberdeen
Physician to HM The Queen in Scotland
and

N. Ashley G. Mowat, FRCP

Consultant Physician/Gastroenterologist, Aberdeen Teaching Hospitals
Clinical Senior Lecturer in Medicine, University of Aberdeen

Series Editor

George P. McNicol, MD, PhD, FRSE, FRCP
(Lond, Edin, Glasg), FRCPath, Hon FACP

Principal and Vice Chancellor, University of Aberdeen. Lately Professor of Medicine, The University of Leeds, and Head, The University Department of Medicine, The General Infirmary, Leeds

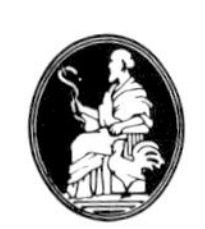

William Heinemann Medical Books Ltd
London

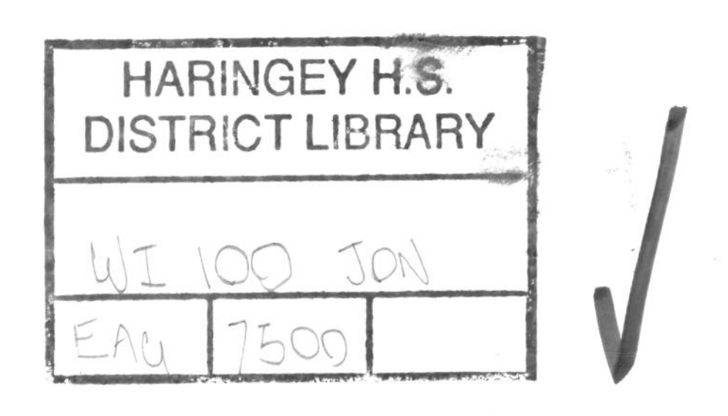

First Published 1985

ISBN 0-433-16608-8

Typesetting by Thomson Press (I) Ltd., New Delhi,
Printed and bound in Great Britain by the
Alden Press, Oxford

Contents

Preface

It is clearly desirable on educational grounds to adopt and teach a rational approach to the management of patients, whereby the basic scientific knowledge, the applied science and the art of clinical practice are brought together in an integrated way. Progress has been made in this direction, but after twenty-five years of good intentions, teaching in many medical schools is still split up into three large compartments, preclinical, paraclinical and clinical, and further subdivided on a disciplinary basis. Lip-service is paid to integration, but what emerges is often at best a coordinated rather than an integrated curriculum. Publication of the INTEGRATED CLINICAL SCIENCE series reflects the need felt in many quarters for a truly integrated textbook series, and is also intended as a stimulus to further reform of the curriculum.

The complete series will cover the core of clinical teaching, each volume dealing with a particular body system. Revision material in the basic sciences of anatomy, physiology, biochemistry and pharmacology is presented at the level of detail appropriate for Final MB examinations, and subsequently for rational clinical practice. Integration between the volumes ensures complete and consistent coverage of these areas, and similar principles govern the treatment of the clinical disciplines of medicine, surgery, pathology, microbiology, immunology and epidemiology.

The series is planned to give a reasoned rather than a purely descriptive account of clinical practice and its scientific basis. Clinical manifestations are described in relation to the disorders of structure and function which occur in a disease process. Illustrations are used extensively, and are an integral part of the text.

The editors for each volume, well-known as authorities and teachers in their fields, have been recruited from medical schools throughout the UK. Chapter contributors are even more widely distributed, and coordination between the volumes has been supervised by a distinguished team of specialists.

Each volume in the series represents a component in an overall plan of approach to clinical teaching. It is intended, nevertheless, that every volume should be self-sufficient as an account of its own subject area, and all the basic and clinical science with which an undergraduate could reasonably be expected to be familiar is presented in the appropriate volume. It is expected that, whether studied individually or as a series, the volume of INTEGRATED CLINICAL SCIENCE will meet a major need, assisting teachers and students to adopt a more rational and holistic approach in learning to care for the sick.

George P. McNicol
Series Editor

List of Contributors

Peter J Aggett
Senior Lecturer in Physiology
University of Aberdeen
Honorary Consultant Paediatrician
Royal Aberdeen Children's Hospital

Peter W Brunt
Consultant Physian/Gastroenterologist
Aberdeen Teaching Hospitals
Clinical Senior Lecturer in Medicine
University of Aberdeen

David N Clarke
Consultant Physician
Stirling Royal Infirmary

CW Imrie
Consultant Surgeon
Glasgow Royal Infirmary

Peter F Jones
Consultant Surgeon
Woodend General Hospital
and Royal Aberdeen Children's Hospital
Clinical Professor of Surgery
University of Aberdeen

Norman A Matheson
Consultant Surgeon
Aberdeen Royal Infirmary
Clinical Senior Lecturer in Surgery
University of Aberdeen.

N Ashley G Mowat
Consultant Physician/Gastroenterologist
Aberdeen Teaching Hospitals
Clinical Senior Lecturer in Medicine
University of Aberdeen

Alexander Munro
Consultant Surgeon
Raigmore Hospital
Inverness
Clinical Senior Lecturer in Surgery
University of Aberdeen

Christopher R Pennington
Consultant Physician
King's Cross Hospital
Dundee

Thomas S Sinclair
Senior Registrar in Medicine
Aberdeen Teaching Hospitals
Clinical Lecturer in Medicine
University of Aberdeen

John AR Smith
Senior Lecturer in Surgery
University of Sheffield
Honorary Consultant Surgeon
Hallamshire Hospital
Sheffield

Advisory Editors

Professor AS Douglas
Department of Medicine, University of Aberdeen

Pathology: Professor CC Bird
Institute of Pathology
University of Leeds

Physiology: Professor PH Fentem
Department of Physiology and Pharmacology
Nottingham University

Biochemistry: Dr RM Denton
Reader in Biochemisrty
University of Bristol

Anatomy: Professor RL Holmes
Department of Anatomy
University of Leeds

Pharmacology: Professor AM Breckenridge
Department of Clinical Pharmacology
Liverpool University

Editors' Foreword

Because of their diversity and scope and the rapid and continuing advances made in the past decade, the disorders of the alimentary tract present the writers of books with particular problems of presentation. Balance and emphasis are likely to reflect the preferences, interests and practice of the editors. However, we have endeavoured to cover this wide field in a reasonably comprehensive way, with extensive use of illustration. Our aim has been to include the material which the interested final year student might require for the Final MB examination. This should also provide core reading for the MRCP candidate, and offer a useful review of gastroenterology to the aspirant to the Final FRCS.

The first three chapters form a general introduction. The first contains a resumé of nutrition – which is the *raison d'etre* of the alimentary tract. The second chapter outlines the patterns and mechanisms of alimentary diseases, and their epidemiology, and the third deals with clinical method and investigation in gastroenterology.

Chapters 4 to 11 cover the organ systems from mouth to anus, and their principal diseases. The liver and biliary tract have been considered together.

In the remaining chapters we attempt to deal with various specific areas of gastroenterology which either affect more than one organ system (e.g. congenital malformations), or present particularly important aspects of management, e.g. gastrointestinal infections and the 'acute abdomen'.

Two chapters deserve special mention since they may appear to have been given disproportionately detailed treatment. The first concerns inflammatory bowel disease – a subject which displays particularly well the challenging problems of management seen in gastroenterology, and reflects the importance of the closest collaboration between general practitioner, physician and surgeon, together with their medical and paramedical colleagues such as radiologists, and dietitians. The second chapter deals with gastrointestinal haemorrhage, which can on occasion be the most urgent of all alimentary problems, and the area in which high standards of medical care and team management are vital and life saving. In addition, this is the chapter in the ICS series which deals with the vitally important topic of haemorrhagic shock.

We are deeply indebted to all our contributors who have so willingly provided material, and allowed us to weld it into a complete book. We have relied heavily on illustrations instead of description, and we are very appreciative of the skill with which Clare Little and her colleagues have interpreted our rough drawings. We have been greatly helped by the willing and accurate secretarial help provided by Miss Mary Grassick and Mrs Jan Amonoo.

Peter F. Jones
Peter W. Brunt
N. Ashley G. Mowat

Acknowledgements

We wish to thank the following for permission to redraw figures from their publications: Dr A.M. Dawson and Dr E.T. Swarbrick (Fig. 2.2), Dr Basil Morson (Fig. 9.14), and Professor H.L. Duthie (Fig. 11.3).

A number of figures have been drawn using material in tables in the following papers:

Fig. 3.15: Williams J.T., Thomson J.P.S. (1977). *Practitioner*. **219:** 327.
Fig. 9.18: Keddie N., Hargreaves A. (1968). *Lancet*. **2:** 749.
Fig. 10.2: Kyle J., Stark G. (1979). *Gut*. **20:** A441.
Fig. 10.3: Sinclair T.S. *et al*. (1983). *Gastroenterology*. **85:** 1.
Fig. 10.7: Mekhjian H.S. *et al*. (1979). *Gastroenterology*. **77:** 898.
Fig. 14.1: Johnston S.J. *et al*. (1973). *Brit. Med. J.* **3:** 655.
Fig. 15.1: Simon G.L., Gorbach S.L. (1984). *Gastroenterology*. **86:** 174.

We are very much indebted to the following colleagues who allowed us to copy radiographs and photomicrographs: Professor A.S. Douglas, Dr S.W.B. Ewen, Dr J.K. Hussey, Mr Z. Krukowski, Dr J. McPhie, Mr R.A. Morton and the Staff of the Department of Medical Illustration, Dr J. Porteous, Professor R. Postlethwaite, Dr T. Reid, Dr P. Ward and Dr J. Weir.

We thank the Trustees of the Tate Gallery for permission to reproduce *The Doctor* by Sir Luke Fildes.

Introduction

When, one hundred years ago, Luke Fildes created his famous painting, *The Doctor,* the only aids to diagnosis were the stethoscope and the patellar hammer, and useful drugs were limited to the opiates and digitalis. Although medical science has moved a long way since then, it is wise to remember that we know no more than *The Doctor* about the fundamental causes of the major gastro-enterological diseases – peptic ulcer, cancer of the alimentary tract, and inflammatory bowel disease. Although our ability to modify symptoms, to heal lesions and safely remove diseased tissues are enormously greater than they were one hundred years ago, our surgery remains basically excisional: oesophagectomy, gastrectomy, and intestinal resection are skilful and highly success-

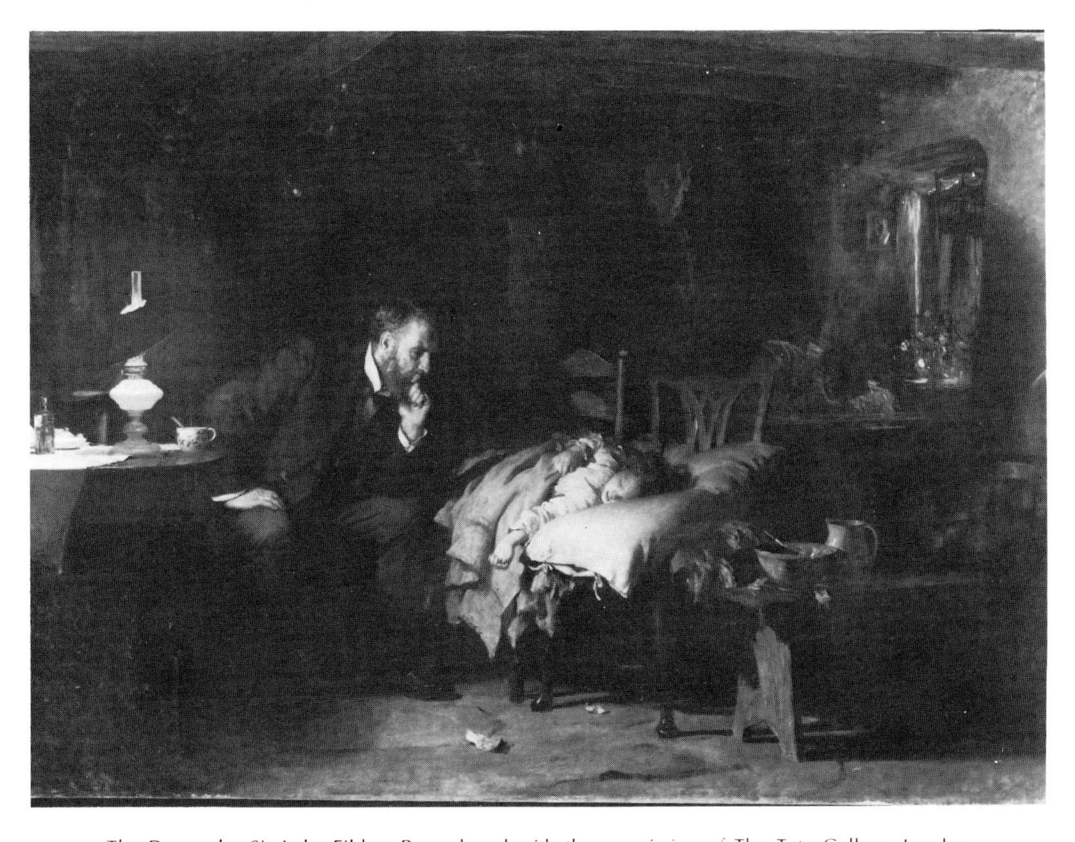

The Doctor by Sir Luke Fildes. Reproduced with the permission of The Tate Gallery, London.

ful procedures, but they still leave us in ignorance of the fundamental origins of the conditions treated.

Modern gastroenterology has grown over the last 40 years to become a meeting-ground for the skills of many specialists. The physiologist and biochemist are needed to understand the movements and secretions of the gut, the pathologist plays a vital role in mapping the behaviour and spread of gastrointestinal neoplasms, and the epidemiologist shows what wide differences there are in the geographic distribution of alimentary tract disease. In the clinical sphere, there are few patients who do not need investigation by the radiologist and the clinical chemist. There is certainly no department of medicine in which physician and surgeon have to work more closely to achieve the best care of their patients. Out of this partnership have grown departments of gastroenterology, led by a physician who can bring all these differing skills together. Such an individual needs a wide experience as a general physician because there are many diverse causes of abdominal symptoms. Moreover, disorders of alimentary function (such as the irritable bowel syndrome) are common and are often associated with social and emotional problems, whilst it is not surprising if these same problems arise in association with long-standing organic alimentary tract disease. For the correct treatment of many patients, the gastroenterologist also needs to be a physician who naturally thinks along surgical lines.

Gastroenterology began to emerge as a specialty in Britain in the 1930s and 40s, launched by such pioneers as Arthur Hurst and John Ryle at Guy's Hospital, London, and Sir Francis Avery Jones who, at the Central Middlesex Hospital, showed the advantages of a combined medical and surgical gastrointestinal unit, and the valuable epidemiological studies which can be made in a district general hospital. Gastroenterology is now a vigorous independent discipline which embraces many specialties and is still evaluating some remarkable technological developments. Little over a decade has seen the introduction of fibre-optic endoscopy and its more recent offshoots such as endoscopic catheterisation and incision of the ampulla of Vater, colonic polypectomy and coagulation of bleeding points in the stomach and duodenum. At the same time, the contribution of radiology has been remarkably enhanced, firstly by the ability to undertake mesenteric angiography and to embolise selectively the small arteries from which gastrointestinal haemorrhage has occurred, and secondly by the development of a remarkable range of scanning techniques – ultrasound, isotopic studies, and computerised axial tomography.

Because he could offer so little through medicines or surgery, Luke Fildes' Doctor was good at talking to his patients and their families, and his personal involvement played a vital part in the care of patients: most of this was conducted in their own homes, because Hospital was too often the place to which the patient went only to die. Today, with ready access to so many investigations, and the ability to initiate powerful drug therapy and major surgical procedures, the modern gastroenterologist still needs to preserve those same personal skills.

1

Human Nutrition

Eating is perhaps the only requirement in life which can be at the same time both a necessity and a pleasure. Normal human functioning – thought, physical activity, reproduction – and life itself, is fundamentally dependent on nutrition. The ingestion, processing and delivery of nutrients is the function of the gut, while the liver has a central role in metabolism and metabolic homeostasis. Starvation, loss of appetite and alimentary dysfunction will impair delivery, while liver failure leads to serious breakdown of metabolism and ultimately to death.

Within broad limits the nutritional requirements of man have been established. The composition of an 'average' man reflects the nature of the nutrients required in the diet. The continuous cellular turnover of proteins and lipids, the loss of desquamated epithelial cells and hair, and the loss of water and electrolytes in urine and sweat means that there is a daily obligate loss of nutrients to be replaced. Additionally, nutrients are required to meet the compositional and energy demands of growth and reproduction, thus these physiological stages are periods of increased susceptibility to malnutrition.

The body is able to synthesise many of the amino acids and fatty acids it needs for protein and lipid synthesis but is dependent upon an adequate supply of essential amino acids, fatty acids, minerals and vitamins. Whereas energy requirements may be met by the catabolism of fat stores and of some protein, this is only beneficial in the management of abnormal metabolic states such as obesity. Man otherwise requires a certain minimum daily energy and protein intake to maintain balance.

An individual's nutrient requirements cannot be predicted accurately; the metabolic and biochemical bases of nutrition and of nutrient interactions are defined too poorly for that, but the recommendations listed in Table 1.1 are designed to meet the requirements of 97% of a healthy population. Some of these recommended daily allowances may be too high; they are frequently revised and, whereas they provide a means of

Table 1.1

*Recommended and *Estimated Safe and Adequate Daily Allowance of Nutrients for Adults*

Nutrient	*Male*	*Female**
Energy (MJ)	10.1–12.2	7.6–8.8
Protein (g)	56	44
Vitamin A (μg)	1000	800
Vitamin D (μg)	5–10	5–10
Vitamin E (mg)	10	8
Vitamin K (μg)*	70–140	70–140
Vitamin C (mg)	60	60
Thiomen (mg)	1.2–1.5	1.0–1.1
Riboflavin (mg)	1.4–1.7	1.2–1.3
Niacin (mg)	16–19	13–15
Pyridoxine (mg)	2.2	2.0
Folic acid (μg)	400	400
Cobalamin (μg)	3.0	3.0
Calcium (mg)	800–1200	800–1200
Phosphorus (mg)	800–1200	800–1200
Magnesium (mg)	350–400	300
Iron (mg)	10–18	18
Zinc (mg)	15	15
Copper (mg)*	2–3	2–3
Iodine (μg)	150	150
Fluoride (mg)	1.5–4.0	1.5–4.0
Sodium (g)*	1.1–3.3	1.1–3.3
Potassium (g)*	1.9–5.6	1.9–5.6
Chloride (g)*	1.7–5.1	1.7–5.1

Data From: Food and Nutrition Board, National Research Council, National Academy of Sciences, 1980.
*Supplements are advised during pregnancy and lactation.

Table 1.2
Relative Nitrogen, Total Energy and Non-protein Energy Requirements for Nutritional Support. (After Woolfrom, A M J, 1979.)

Requirement	Clinical State		
	Non-catabolic	Inter-mediate	Hyper-catabolic
Nitrogen (g/24 hr)*	7.5	14	25
Total energy kJ/24 hr	9 600	14 400	19 200
Non-protein energy for adequate kJ/g metabolism of nitrogen	1200	960	648

4.2 kJ = 1 kcal.
*See text for calculation of nitrogen requirement – most patients are in the intermediate category.

assessing a patient's risk of nutritional deficiency, failure to meet these intakes does not necessarily constitute a deficiency state.

During states of increased catabolism, e.g. in severe inflammatory bowel disease or the badly burned patient, increased requirements for energy and protein are recognised (Table 1.2). Planned delivery of those nutritional requirements is an important element in the clinical management of such patients.

For most people, food is an important pleasure in life. Unfortunately vast numbers in the world lie at or below the minimum necessary nutritional intake for healthy life. Wide racial and cultural attitudes to food exist throughout the world and to some extent this influences the patterns of disease (see p. 12). Vegetarianism and veganism (total aversion to any food of animal origin) are common in Asia and, in veganism, specific nutritional deficiencies (such as vitamin B_{12}) may be seen. Overnutrition is a major problem of Western society and is associated with all the concomitants of obesity, such as ischaemic heart disease, hypertension, degenerative arthritis, venous thromboembolic disease, and increased risks of surgery. Some ethnic groups depend heavily upon animal protein and fat (e.g. Eskimos), whereas others (e.g. Bangladeshi) have very little meat in the diet. In some societies both the preparation and eating of food is treated as an art.

For the ill and undernourished patient, the cooking and presentation (sight and smell) of food is of increased importance. Unfortunately most hospitals fall down badly in this respect. The value of professional dieticians, not simply in advising and assessing patients but also in supervising preparation of diets, cannot be overemphasised.

ASSESSMENT OF NUTRITIONAL STATUS

A basic approach to every patient involves an assessment of the nutritional state. This may range from a simple observation that the patient has lost weight to a detailed laboratory examination of individual nutrients as noted below. In practice most assessments lie somewhere between these extremes and involve a search for the subtle signs of deficiencies (Figs 1.1–1.4). The observation and

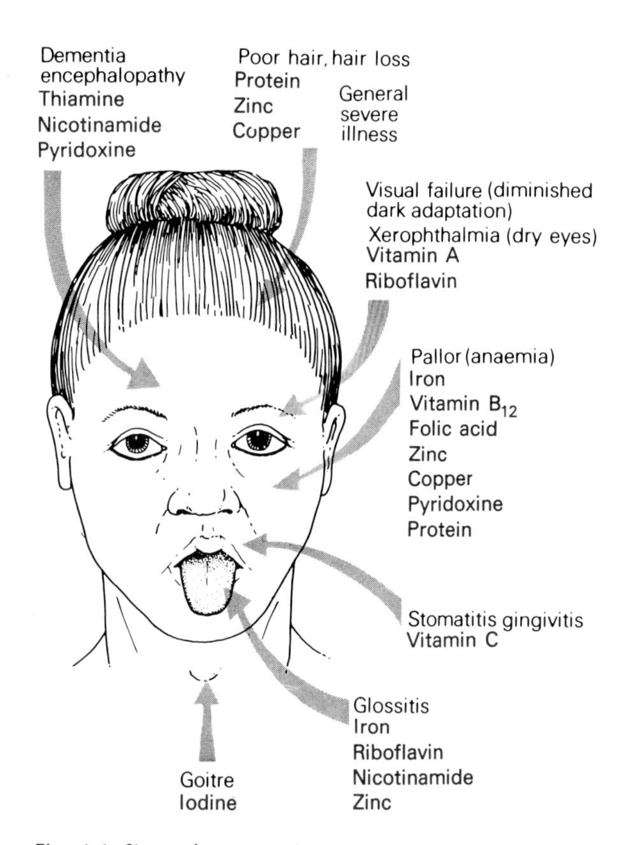

Fig. 1.1 *Signs of nutritional deficiency (deficient factors in red): the face.*

recording, over time, of body size and weight are important. 'Height for age' is an indication of stunting in growing children whereas 'weight for height' reflects adiposity or wasting from disease. In adults, weight and height can be related to optimal values (e.g. insurance company tables) and the 'body mass index' (weight in kg/height squared in m) correlates with body fat.

Biochemical investigations of 'nutrient status' can be performed, but some are not available routinely in most laboratories. Serum assays are available for the estimation of most of the fat- and water-soluble vitamins. Serum folate levels should be performed on plasma specimens taken after fasting, otherwise red-cell folate estimations are more reliable. Plasma or serum fatty acid profiles will enable estimation of the triene:tetraene ratio

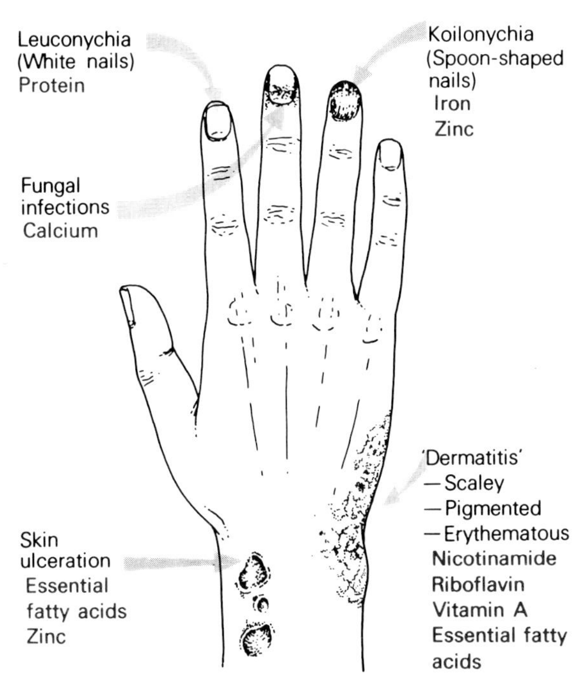

Fig. 1.2 *Signs of nutritional deficiency (deficient factors in red): the hands.*

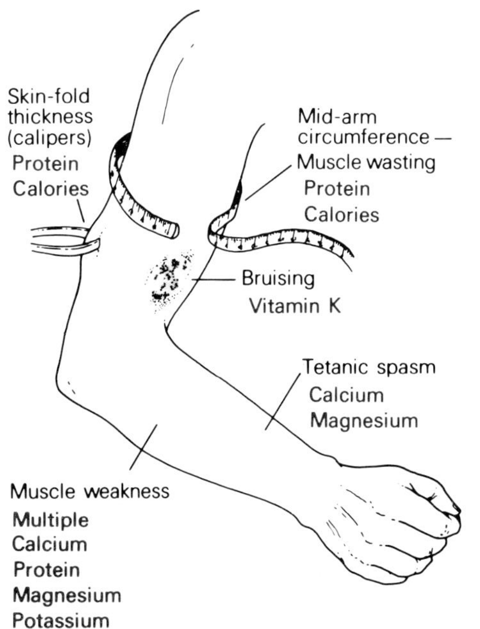

Fig. 1.3 *Signs of nutritional deficiency (deficient factors in red): the arms.*

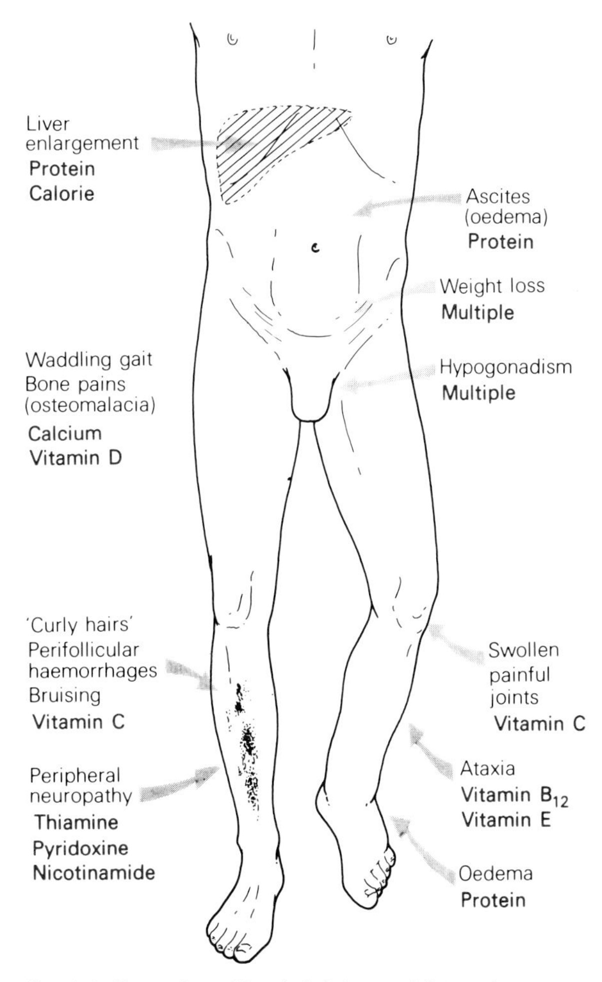

Fig. 1.4 *Signs of nutritional deficiency (deficient factors in red); the legs, and the abdomen.*

as an index of essential fatty acid deficiency. Vitamin K status is assessed by measurement of the prothrombin time, and vitamin C status can be determined by measuring its content in leucocytes. Plasma concentrations of zinc, copper and iron can be measured but are unreliable; leucocyte zinc concentrations may be a better criterion of tissue zinc depletion, and plasma iron-binding capacity, transferrin concentration, or ferritin levels are of value in measuring iron status. A reduced plasma transferrin level (<20 g/l) is also a sensitive index of protein malnutrition. A plasma albumin level below 35 g/l is suggestive of protein deficiency. Individual laboratories will have their own reference values to enable interpretation of these biochemical indices, but few can be interpreted reliably without reference to clinical features.

Deficiencies of most essential nutrients collectively and individually impair cell growth and division. This can readily be detected by assessing cell-mediated immunity. The peripheral lymphocyte count falls in malnutrition ($<1.2\times10^9$/l) and the in-vitro lymphoblast response to a mitogen such as phytohaemagglutinin is impaired. A simpler test is to measure the cutaneous hypersensitivity response to a range of antigens which the patient has previously been exposed to. Useful antigens, e.g. Candida, tuberculin (1 in 100 solution), streptokinase (5iu) and mumps (2 units), are injected on the anterior surface of the forearm and the area of induration is measured 24 or 48 hours later; normally the area exceeds 5 mm in diameter.

NUTRITIONAL SUPPORT

This aspect of clinical management is being increasingly appreciated; 20–50% of hospital patients are undernourished. In many cases, their nutrition deteriorates as a result of anorexia, iatrogenic starvation, and inadequate efforts at oral nutrition; this compromises recovery by predisposing patients to infections, poor wound healing, unresponsiveness to some drugs, and unnecessary loss of muscle mass which impairs mobilisation. Even so, the indications for clinical nutritional support are not well-established and it is not known whether the use of liquidised diets following simple surgery or fractures is truly beneficial. The need for such support in patients experiencing catabolic responses in association with major surgery, severe burns, intestinal resection or disease, or prolonged unconsciousness is more apparent. The metabolic rate is increased by 10% after simple surgery, by 20% after major surgery and multiple fractures, and by over 100% for severe burns. Septicaemias induce a 13% increase in energy requirements per degree celsius increase in core body temperature.

The endocrine response to trauma or sepsis involves increased secretion of cortisol, glucagon and catecholamines. Even though circulating insulin may be increased, the anabolic response of peripheral tissues to it is impaired. Unless the resultant nutrient demands of the increased catabolic state are met by exogenous support, body tissues become wasted. Fat stores and protein from muscle are used to provide energy, with the irretrievable loss of intracellular nutrients such as calcium, magnesium, phosphate and zinc in the urine. The potential benefit of nutritional support as an adjunct to cancer therapy is being investigated, as is its role in preoperative nutritional support.

It is not possible to accurately predict a patient's nutritional requirements. The increased nitrogen requirement can be assessed from the daily loss in urine, using the formula:

$$\text{nitrogen loss g/24 h} = (\text{urinary urea mmol/24 h} \times 0.028) + 2.$$

The last figure allows for obligatory loss of nitrogen in faeces and skin, but it is obviously unreliable if the patient has a protein-losing enteropathy or intestinal fistulae. An adequate non-protein energy supply is needed to achieve a positive nitrogen balance; an indication of the approximate requirements are shown in Table 1.2. The needs for water, electrolytes, fatty acids (linolenic acid), vitamins, minerals and trace elements are also higher than basal requirements in patients needing nutritional support, and these must be considered. Electrolyte balance can be determined by measuring electrolyte loss in urine, drainage fluids, gastric aspirates and intestinal effluent. The other nutrients are given on a more empirical basis.

Nutritional support can be given either enterally (i.e. via the intestine) or parenterally (intravenously).

Enteral Nutrition

If a patient has any gastrointestinal function, then an enteral route rather than a parenteral route should be preferred for nutritional support. It has the advantage of being physiological and it provides the luminal stimulus required to maintain intestinal function and, if necessary, to induce adaptation. If the patient can cooperate by swallowing, then the liquidised foods used for enteral nutrition can be given orally, as frequent sips; otherwise they can be administered continuously through a fine-bore polyvinyl catheter which is passed either nasogastrically or through a gastrostomy or jejunostomy. The continuous feeds can be dripped under gravity, and a pump is usually unnecessary. Nasogastric liquid feeding may continue during sleep, supplemented by oral feeding by day. Suitable feeds are available commercially or they can be prepared using blenderisers under sterile conditions.

If gastrointestinal function is normal, then whole protein sources can be used in feeds, but with defective intraluminal proteolysis or short bowel syndromes (where it would be wasteful to use the available lumen for intraluminal digestion), amino-acid absorption may be maximised by giving oligopeptide preparations. The major disadvantages of these are that they have a high osmolality and that they are expensive. Energy can be provided as glucose polymers, which have a low osmolality and can be hydrolysed by α-amylase and by mucosal maltase and α-dextrinase. A source of linolenic acid (or linolenic and arachidonic acids) should be added and, if lipolysis is impaired, medium-chain triacylglycerols can be used. Lipid (37 kJ/g) provides an alternative energy source to carbohydrate (17 kJ/g) and increases the palatability of the feeds for those taking them orally. Supplements of vitamins and essential minerals should be added routinely.

It used to be said that the most frequent complication of enteric feeding is osmotic diarrhoea with the attendant hazard of dehydration. This risk is reduced by continuous administration of the feeds and by using preparations with low osmolalities. Diarrhoea resulting from deficiencies of intestinal oligosaccharidases, bacterial overgrowth of the small intestine (often due to antibiotic use), and from enteric infections is also a potentially serious problem and there is a real risk of contamination of 'home-made' enteric feeds with the entero-pathogenic bacteria (*Klebsiella* spp., *E. coli* and *Salmonella* spp.).

A quarter of patients experience some abdominal distension and discomfort during the introduction of the regimen. The cause is not always clear; gastric distension with delayed emptying secondary to an excessive lipid content or to hypertonicity is a common cause, and this may also lead to vomiting with the risk of aspiration. Gastric emptying is improved, and the risk of aspiration is reduced, by nursing the patient in a semirecumbent position. The modern tubes do not produce nasopharyngeal and oesophageal erosions or strictures such as those seen with earlier types but they are displaced easily and it is wise to check their position frequently and certainly after the patient has been moved for any reason. Metabolic complications of nutritional support are considered below.

Enteral support has fewer complications and is less labour intensive than parenteral nutrition and, once established, it is much easier to maintain on an out-patient basis. Nevertheless, there are some patients in whom gastrointestinal function is so severely impaired that parenteral nutritional support is needed.

Parenteral Nutrition

The solutions used for intravenous feeding have high osmolalities and, if infused into peripheral veins, can cause thrombophlebitis. Preferably, these solutions should be administered via a silicon rubber catheter, the distal end of which is passed to the superior vena cava through a subclavian/cephalic or, less frequently, an internal jugular vein. This enables the venous return of 2–3 litres a minute to dilute the infused solution. To reduce the risk of infection, the catheter should be inserted with a strict aseptic technique and, as a further safeguard against infection, the percutaneous entry site should be separated from the venous entry site by tunnelling the catheter subcutaneously. The catheter should be used only for intravenous nutrition and not for giving blood or plasma. The use of the subclavian vein carries a definite risk of inducing pneumothorax, which is a serious additional hazard to an already severely ill patient. Therefore, a 'cut-down' upon a cephalic vein may be preferred.

The usual energy source for parenteral nutrition is glucose, given as hypertonic dextrose, but energy can be derived also from lipid, which has a higher energy density and is less sclerosant to the vasculature. In severe catabolic states (i.e. more than 18 g nitrogen loss in 24 h), however, glucose should be used because the uptake of plasma triacylglycerol by tissues is impaired. The potential value of ketone bodies as an alternative energy source is currently being explored. Nitrogen is provided as crystalline α amino acids, of which 40% should be essential amino acids. Lipid is administered as 10% or 20% Intralipid preparation, to which fat-soluble vitamin supplements can be added. Commercial supplements of trace elements and vitamins are available and these can be added to the infusates. A recent major practical advance has been the realisation that the nutrients are metabolised more efficiently if given simultaneously and that this reduces insulin requirements. Furthermore, the pre-mixing of the nutrient solutions reduces the risk of bacterial contamination. Ideally, the solutions are prepared daily, according to prescription, by a pharmacist and dispensed in sealed 'giving bags'. This procedure, with modern catheter techniques, has made home parenteral nutrition a possibility in the management of severe gastrointestinal failure.

Metabolic Complications of Nutritional Support

The progress of a patient receiving nutritional support should be monitored closely. It is valuable to keep a flow chart on which the patient's weight and other anthropomorphic data, the daily nutrient and energy uptake, and details of electrolyte, fluid and nitrogen balance can be recorded. The chart can also be used to collate the above data with daily or frequent determinations of haemoglobin, plasma electrolytes, urea, calcium, magnesium, inorganic phosphate, liver function tests and, if indicated, acid–base balance. Other biochemical tests of nutritional status (zinc, copper, selenium, prothrombin time) should be considered weekly or less frequently, depending on how stable the patient's condition is. With this approach, nutritional deficiencies can be avoided or anticipated, and the occasional problems of impaired liver function (e.g. cholestasis, and raised aminotransferases, γ-glutamyl transpeptidase and alkaline phosphatase activities) and hypophosphataemia will be detected.

The causes of abnormal liver function tests are not clear. Liver biopsies show widespread fatty infiltration with increased lymphocytes in the periportal areas; It is now recognised that cholestasis may occur. Fortunately these disorders are usually transient and mild; they resolve when nutritional support is withdrawn. Hypophosphataemia occurs more frequently with parenteral nutrition. An additional problem with enteral and parenteral nutritional support is the development of hyperglycaemia with the hazards of non-ketotic hyperosmolar coma and of dehydration secondary to glycosuria; this is due, in part, to the patient's catabolic state and relative insensitivity to insulin and it can be managed by giving, according to a sliding scale, additional insulin either subcutaneously or via an infusion.

The long-term complications of nutritional support are the development of deficiencies; these usually involve vitamins (e.g. D and E) and trace metals (zinc, copper and selenium).

2

An Introduction to Alimentary Disease

PATTERNS AND MECHANISMS OF DISEASE

Disease is the symptomatic expression of an interaction between the patient and some injury or stress. For the alimentary system, as for other systems, there is a relatively small variety of responses to a wide range of stimuli. Hence a given pattern of symptoms may reflect several possible aetiologies and considerable diagnostic effort may be expended to ensure correct treatment.

Infection

Of all infections and infestations to affect man those involving the liver and alimentary tract are the most common. Worldwide, they account for the greatest part of gastrointestinal disorders (see p. 24). By and large they reflect poor levels of nutrition, hygiene, water supplies and sewerage. It is significant that, notwithstanding development of vaccines (such as the new Hepatitis B vaccines), it is predominantly the biological sciences (elimination of vectors, e.g. insects) and social changes rather than medical advances that are eradicating gastrointestinal infections.

Host responses to infection and infestation depend upon a number of factors which include:

a. previous or concomitant infection
b. the nutritional state of the individual
c. immunocompetence
d. genetic predisposition

and no doubt other factors as yet unknown.

The possibility that infections, self-limiting in themselves, may trigger off both functional disturbances such as irritable bowel syndrome and organic disease such as idiopathic proctocolitis must be kept in mind.

Functional and Stress Disorders

In the 'developed' world, functional disorders account for the majority of alimentary symptoms. The gut, apart from the pharynx and anal canal, is entirely supplied by the autonomic nervous system, making it a very rich field for functional disorders. The association of the gut with emotion and feeling has been appreciated since Old Testament times, as expressions such as 'bowels of compassion' vividly attest. Phrases such as 'sick with fright' and 'examination runs' express experiences that are universal to the human race. Functional disorders begin at the extremes of these 'normal' physiological responses and may be associated with psychosocial stresses, neurotic illness, or personality disturbances. In many instances, however, they may imitate or accompany organic disease of the gut, and distinction can be difficult.

Several well defined patterns exist.

Anorexia

Loss of appetite is a common symptom of gastric and pancreatic malignancy and of hepatitis. However it frequently accompanies anxiety or tension and many general illnesses, and sometimes may be frankly psychological.

Anorexia nervosa is a not uncommon and potentially fatal illness affecting predominantly

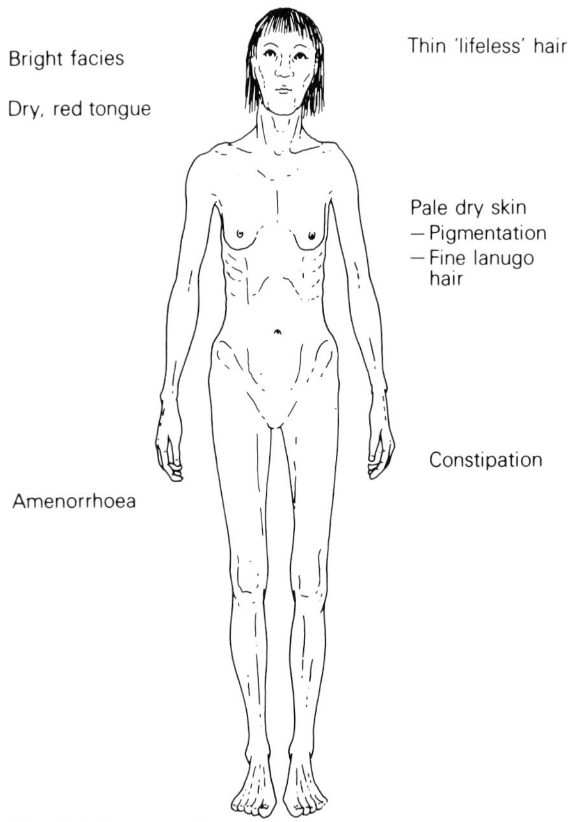

Fig. 2.1 *Features of anorexia nervosa.*

teenage and pre-menopausal adult females of the middle and upper classes. It may begin as a weight-reducing exercise, progress to bizarre food fads, and end with grossly distorted ideas of body image. Malnutrition is severe and the patient is thin, pale and, characteristically, inappropriately bright and cheerful. Amenorrhoea is usual. Repeated purgation and self-induced vomiting are common and the patient will go to extraordinary lengths to conceal food (and vomitus). Organic diseases causing malabsorption have to be carefully excluded (Fig. 2.1).

Treatment is difficult and requires long periods of hospital management with a patient, firm approach and gradual restoration of normal eating patterns. Failure is not uncommon and there is a considerable mortality.

Dysphagia (see also p. 59)

Only occasionally is a true severe difficulty in swallowing functional in origin. Minor degrees, however, are common especially in the aged, due to loss of normal peristalsis and irregular non-propulsive ('tertiary') contractions.

Globus hystericus is not a diagnosis but is a group name for a collection of symptoms whose cause is not yet known. Whilst there is often clear emotional stress, it must be remembered that this is also true of many patients with organic disease. Globus hystericus is thus a dangerous diagnostic label and, if it is to be used, should not be applied until full investigations have been completed and proved negative.

Vomiting

While it is sometimes due to gastric disease, pyloric obstruction or intestinal obstruction, vomiting is a very nonspecific symptom. It occurs also in severe pain of any cause, pancreatitis, liver failure, and non-alimentary causes such as raised intracranial pressure, glaucoma and drug toxicity.

Psychogenic vomiting (bulimia) and self-induced vomiting are often part of an 'anorexia nervosa' syndrome, as noted above, and may be cunningly concealed. Severe electrolyte disturbance and malnutrition may result.

Irritable gut syndrome (Irritable bowel syndrome)

This rather woolly diagnosis encompasses a vast number of patients displaying varying combinations of abdominal distension, discomfort, pain and alteration of bowel habit. The older synomyms, such as 'spastic colon' and 'mucous colitis', are too restrictive or frankly misleading. The functional defect may be widespread – from oesophagus to anus. A sense of distension and discomfort after food, often accompanied by flatulence and rumbling (borborygmi), is a common pattern and has been termed 'nervous dyspepsia', 'non-ulcer dyspepsia' or 'flatulent dyspepsia'. Peptic ulcer and gall-bladder disease and – less commonly – upper alimentary malignancy may present the same symptoms and will need to be excluded before a diagnosis of functional disorder can be established.

Pain is likewise common and can sometimes be severe. Manometric measurements, either with a radio-pill swallowed into the small bowel or with balloon sensors in the large bowel, confirm that this pain is associated with spasm and dysmotility in both small and large bowels. Pain can be reproduced in many sites by artificial bowel distension and the site of pain may show little relation to the area distended (Fig. 2.2). Very occasionally plain films taken during an attack may show gaseous distension of a segment of gut and this has led to the use of terminology such as the 'splenic flexure syndrome'. Indeed, in any case of recurring abdominal pain, plain (erect and supine) abdominal films taken during pain are invaluable to exclude organic obstruction.

Pain may or may not be associated with or relieved by eating or defaecation. It may occur in any quadrant of the abdomen, especially commonly the iliac fossae, and may even radiate into the back, chest, loins or front of thighs and can last for minutes or hours on end.

Constipation and diarrhoea or a combination of the two are very common functional symptoms of the irritable bowel syndrome. The stool may be pale, bulky or watery and contain mucus (but *not* blood) or may be like toothpaste or rabbit stools. An exaggerated gastrocolic reflex is common; pain before defaecation and explosive urgency are characteristic. A feeling of incomplete emptying may be complained of. Symptoms may often commence after an attack of 'gastroenteritis' or sometimes after the use of antibiotics. Stress may also be a trigger factor.

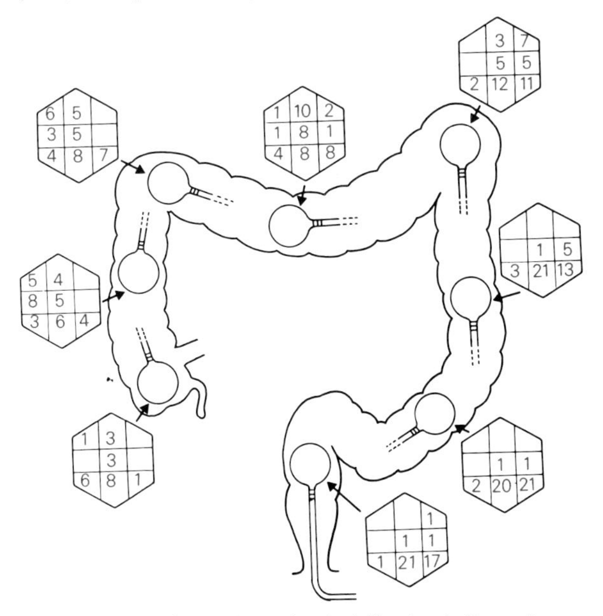

Fig. 2.2 *Sites of experienced pain following balloon distension of the colon in 48 patients (after Swarbrick et al., Lancet, 1980).*

As all these symptoms may also occur in organic disease such as diverticular disease, Crohn's disease and colonic cancer, a sigmoidoscopy and a barium enema examination are essential before making the diagnosis. In some cases malabsorption studies may have to be carried out.

These symptoms are among the commonest in gastroenterology and are the cause of a large proportion of the diagnostic work of gastrointestinal physicians and surgeons. Treatment can be difficult but, in mild cases, firm reassurance may be all that is necessary. Post-prandial epigastric discomfort and reflux can be treated with simple antacids (see p. 85); flatulence may be relieved by the addition of a defoaming agent, e.g. polymethylsiloxane (Simethicone). Where pain is prominent, antispasmodics (e.g. mebeverine) and anticholinergics (e.g. dicyclomine and propantheline) should be tried. Strong analgesics should be avoided. A high residue, high fibre diet is widely prescribed and may help. Empiric treatment of diarrhoea with codeine phosphate, loperamide or diphenoxylate may be helpful.

Recurrent abdominal pain in childhood

This term, along with 'periodic syndrome', 'abdominal migraine' and 'bilious attacks', refers to a group of ill-defined conditions with recurrent abdominal symptoms of no organic cause. According to Apley only about one in ten of children with recurring pain can be shown to have a physical basis for their symptoms. Emotional correlates are common, with behaviour disturbance, stress phenomena, enuresis, headaches and other features. Constipation may occur and many of these children without doubt have the paediatric equivalent of the irritable bowel syndrome.

Proctalgia fugax

This is an unpleasant, briefly disabling condition of unknown origin but believed to be due to spasm of the levator ani muscles. Severe lancinating pain deep in the rectum suddenly siezes the patient, frequently in bed at night, and lasts, mercifully, for only a few minutes. Sitting in a hot or an ice-cold bath and oral nitroglycerine may afford relief but there is no effective cure.

Stress as a factor in organic disease

Much has been written of the possible place of stress in causing structural diseases such as peptic ulcer and idiopathic proctocolitis – so much so that they have been called stress diseases. Much of this is exaggerated and the actual causal relationship is dubious. However, stressful events can certainly exacerbate such diseases and many others. One study compared measurable stress factors in normal subjects and in patients with irritable bowel and proctocolitis (ulcerative colitis); the colitis patients scored similarly to the normals, and only the irritable bowel patients had higher than normal scores.

Both Curling's ulcer and Cushing's ulcer (see p. 78) are examples of an organic condition that *does* seem to be directly related to stress in the form of burns and head injury respectively.

Disturbances of Gut Motility

Propulsive motility is central to gut function. The mechanisms include intrinsic myoelectrical activity, and both humoral and autonomic control. These are ill-understood but dysfunction may result from one or several of the following:

i. 'End organ' muscle dysfunction, as in scleroderma.
ii. Peripheral (autonomic) nervous system dysfunction, as occurs in diabetic autonomic neuropathy and surgical vagotomy.
iii. Central nervous system disturbance, as occurs in a wide variety of psychic stimuli (pain, fear, etc.) and stress disorders as already discussed above.
iv. Metabolic disturbances, as in atony due to hypokalaemia or hypercalcaemia.

Investigation

Gut dysmotility is still a difficult and unsatisfactory field to investigate except for the simple observations that can be made, for example, on x-ray screening. Intraluminal pressure recordings can be made by placing a small balloon attached to fine tubing in the oesophagus, or the anus and rectum, and attaching the tubing to a pressure transducer, which will allow tracings to be made. Alternatively, open-ended tubes perfused with saline can be used in the same way. The small bowel can be studied with a swallowed pressure-sensitive radio-pill. Gastric emptying can be studied by x-ray, radio-isotope scanning or dye dilution methods. In clinical practice those techniques have little application, with the exception of oesophageal manometry in achalasia and diffuse spasm.

Oesophageal motility (discussed in Chapter 4)

Gastric motility

This is essentially a phasic contraction through the body and antrum into the pylorus – about 3 cycles per minute after eating. Nausea and vomiting are associated with inhibition of gastric tone, delay in emptying, and retrograde duodenogastric contractions. The act of vomiting itself is complex and also involves strong visceral and somatic contractions forcing gastric content into the oesophagus. Duodenogastric regurgitation of bile may lead to gastritis and is probably important in the genesis of gastric ulcer (p. 78). Bile reflux in the oesophagus can cause a notably severe oesophagitis.

Small bowel motility

This consists of sequences of quiescence, irregular contractions, and regular bands of segmentation. Irregular contractile activity increases after eating and, with some retrograde motion, serves to mix bowel contents and also propels the chyme to the ileocaecal valve (a process normally taking about 4 hours). Bursts of irregular activity are associated with diarrhoea whereas increased segmentation follows opiate-like drugs and is associated with constipation. The role of endogenous opiates (enkephalins: p. 22) may well be important in gut motility but is as yet not understood.

Colonic motility

Predominantly segmental ring-like contractions actually slow colonic propulsion, and onward movement is achieved by occasional peristaltic activity and sudden rush (mass) movements. These latter are increased by cholinergic drugs and stimulant laxatives (and may also occur in inflammatory bowel disease). Patients with diverticular disease and irritable bowel syndrome have exaggerated contractility, mainly of the sigmoid, although in the latter condition there is usually a very widespread gut dysmotility.

In health the rectum is empty. Defaecation depends upon sensory stimuli on rectal filling (following mass movement), relaxation of the anal sphincters and puborectalis and accompanying abdominal wall contractions. Failure of this stimulation/relaxation phenomenon leads to faecal stasis (dyschezia) and is an important mechanism of constipation (see Table 2.1). Organic disease or absence of the myenteric plexuses occurs in Hirschsprung's disease (see p. 265).

Constipation

This is a condition characterised primarily by dysmotility but with a wide range of causative factors (Table 2.1). It is perhaps the commonest disease

Table 2.1
Causes of Constipation

1. *Simple 'idiopathic'*
   Loss of regular habit, e.g. travel, changes in food, lack of exercise, ignoring calls to stool, etc.
   Debility: Confinement to bed
2. *Primary colonic disease*
   Obstruction, e.g. carcinoma
   Painful anorectal disorders
   Aganglionosis (Hirschsprung's disease)
   Inflammatory disease (distal)
   Diverticular disease
   Scleroderma
3. *Neurological causes*
   Paralysis, e.g. injury, Multiple sclerosis
4. *Endocrine causes*
   Hypothyroidism
   Hypercalcaemia
5. *Metabolic causes*
   Dehydration
   Porphyria
   Lead poisoning
6. *'Functional' or primary disturbance of motility*
   Irritable bowel (spastic colon) syndrome
   Idiopathic megacolon and pseudo-obstruction
7. *Psychiatric causes*
   Depression
   Anorexia nervosa
8. *Iatrogenic causes*
   Drugs, e.g. many analgesic drugs
   (immobilisation, bed-pans)

known to man and absorbs vast amounts of anxious attention and unnecessary (even harmful) treatment. It is said that Louis XIV had no less than 2000 enemas in his lifetime and pressed the same treatment upon his courtiers! Stimulants of colonic activity such as polyphenolic compounds (senna, cascara) and castor oil are effective but suitable only for short-term use; their abuse is widespread and may lead to permanent failure of colonic motility (cathartic colon). Stool softeners (e.g. paraffin, poloxalkols) are also used in the short-term safely, but for long-term use only bulking agents (bran, celluloses, hydrophilic gums and colloids) are safe.

Treatment

Drugs affecting motility are also used widely in symptomatic relief of alimentary symptoms. Metoclopramide and domperidone relieve nausea and vomiting partly by improving gastric emptying. Spasmolytic drugs such as anticholinergics (e.g. dicyclomine) and mebeverine are used in relief of pain. Opiates (e.g. codeine phosphate) and other drugs increasing segmentation (e.g. diphenoxylate, loperamide) relieve diarrhoea; it is believed by some that their action could be dangerous in inflammatory bowel disease by inducing toxic dilatation.

Nutritional and Toxic Disease

Malnutrition or subnutrition is the commonest problem currently affecting the world; nearly two-thirds of the population fall below the minimum requirements set by the World Health Organisation. Malnutrition is a significant contributor to the high infant mortality of underdeveloped countries (Fig. 2.3).

Kwashiorkor is a common disease of weanlings in poor countries where the adequate protein of mothers' milk is replaced by carbohydrate foods. Wasting, growth retardation, oedema, irritability, anorexia and fatigue are common features. Marasmus implies not simply protein deficiency but multifactorial malnutrition. These states are complicated by infection and infestation.

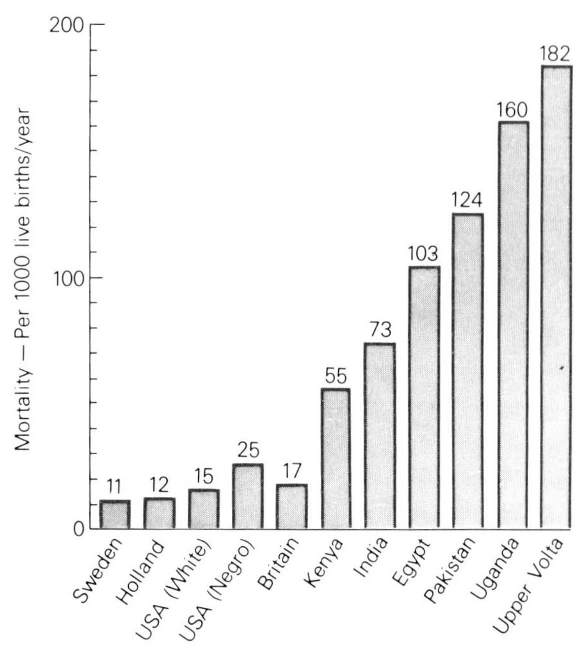

Fig. 2.3 *Infant mortality (per 1000 live births per year).*

Secondary effects on the gut are common in starvation states. Partial or subtotal villous atrophy (see p. 131) together with pancreatic atrophy lead to malabsorption and diarrhoea which further complicate the picture.

Overnutrition is a major problem of developed countries. The associated problems, such as obesity and ischaemic heart disease, have a real bearing on alimentary disease. One variant of this deserves more detailed comment: i.e. excessive alcohol intake.

Alcohol abuse is one of the major medicosocial problems of our time and affects most countries in the world, especially France, Germany, USA, Russia, Poland, Italy, and Portugal. In the USA in 1979 it was estimated that alcoholism cost the nation $113 000 million in medical costs, accidents, industrial losses, etc. The problem, while somewhat less serious in Britain, is still a vast drain on resources, to say nothing of the human misery it provokes. Alcohol consumption in Britain has been increasing steadily in the second half of this century (Fig. 2.4). Since there is a clear rela-

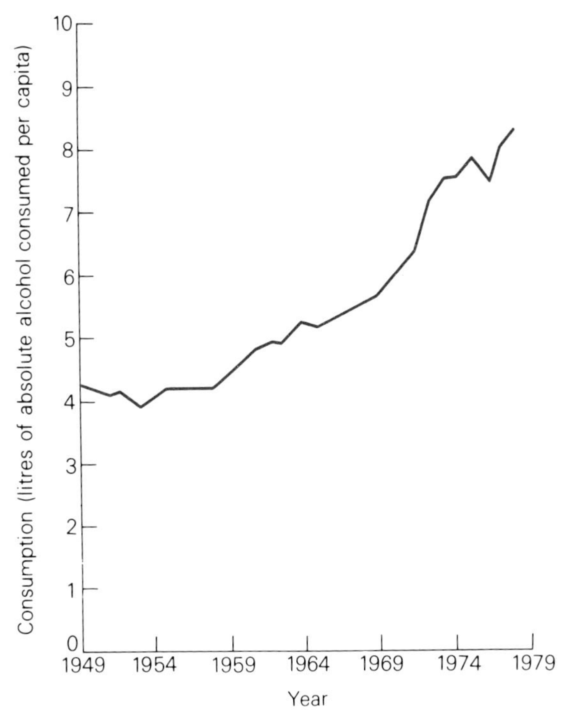

Fig. 2.4 *Increasing consumption of alcohol in UK (from British Journal on Alcohol and Alcoholism, Vol. 17, No. 4).*

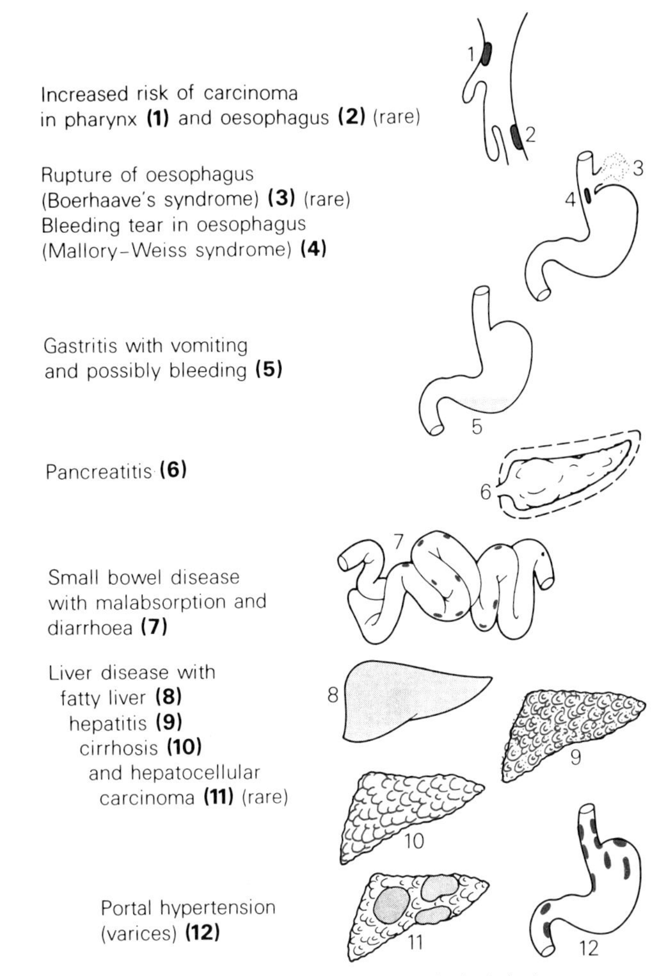

Fig. 2.5 *Gastrointestinal complications of alcohol abuse.*

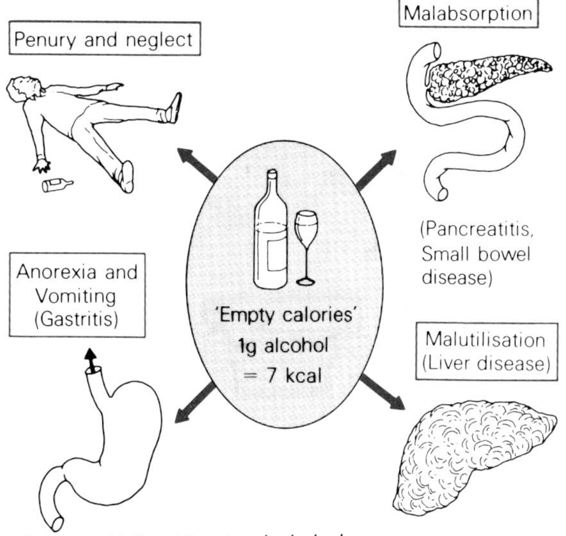

Fig. 2.6 *Malnutrition in alcohol abuse.*

tionship between consumption in a community and alcohol-associated problems, it is not surprising that there has been a corresponding increase in admissions for alcoholism, accidents associated with drinking, medical conditions associated with alcohol, and deaths from cirrhosis, as well as crime and industrial losses. In two hospital surveys in Glasgow approximately one quarter of all male emergency medical admissions were found to have some alcohol problem.

Alcohol exerts its influence on the gastrointestinal system at the points of ingestion, absorption, assimilation and utilisation (Fig. 2.5). Liver disease associated with alcohol is discussed on page 159. Alcohol has a direct toxic effect upon gastric and small bowel mucosa, pancreas and liver: malnutrition is no longer considered to be the sole factor. Secondary malnutrition is, however, common in alcohol abuse for a variety of reasons (Fig. 2.6) and can certainly lead to widespread complications. These include megaloblastic anaemia due to folate malabsorption and Wernicke – Korsakoff syndrome due to thiamine deficiency.

Other toxic substances

Food additives and contaminants are regularly ingested, usually in amounts too small to be noticed or important. In some instances these substances may be potentially carcinogenic, for example nitrites in relation to carcinoma of the stomach (see p. 94). A food contaminant, possibly of very great importance, is the fungal toxin Aflatoxin, which is found in grain 'spoiled' by the fungus *Aspergillus flavus*. It is a potential cause of liver damage and primary liver cancer (see p. 170) and has been incriminated in several large outbreaks of toxic hepatitis. No doubt other, as yet unidentified, mycotoxins could also be important. Ingestion of poisonous fungi such as *Amanita phalloides* leads to rapid and fatal liver failure. The outbreak of jaundice in Epping in 1953 is an example of poisoning with food contaminated by industrial solvents. Similarly, an outbreak of poisoning by contaminated cooking oil in Spain in 1981 resulted in a number of deaths.

Iatrogenic disease

Doctor-induced disease is common. Numerous drugs induce vomiting either as a direct result of their action (e.g. emetine), as a feature of overdosage (e.g. digitalis), or as an occasional side-effect (e.g. phenylbutazone). Many are similarly associated with diarrhoea, a notable example being antibiotics. These may act primarily by altering bacterial flora within the gut and allowing the emergence of superinfection, e.g. with the organism *Clostridium difficile* (see pp. 234 and 334). Aspirin has been shown to be associated with gastric ulcer (p. 77).

Food intolerance

This broad term covers a range of phenomena occurring within minutes or hours of ingestion. It includes:

i. True food allergy (see p. 17).
ii. Pseudo allergy – reactions due to release of histamine from ingested food (e.g. cheese, strawberries) with resulting urticaria.
iii. Toxic and pharmacologic reactions – due to traces of substances inducing vomiting or diarrhoea, often by imperfectly understood mechanisms.
iv. Idiosyncratic reactions – including lactase deficiency (see below), glucose-6-phosphate dehydrogenase deficiency (Favism, induced by eating beans, gooseberries, etc.), phenylketonuria and other inborn errors of metabolism.
v. Psychological intolerance – probably including many who regard themselves as 'allergic'.

Genetic Defects

Since the alimentary tract and liver are the major areas of assimilation and utilisation of nutrients and the site of much of the body's metabolic homeostatic processes it is not surprising that enzyme defects leading to disorder are numerous. Overall, however, they account for only a tiny proportion of gastrointestinal disease. In some instances, for example the extremely rare congenital chloridorrhoea, their importance lies in contributing to understanding the normal physiology or biochemistry.

An interesting exception to the great rarity of these enzyme defects is alactasia. This occurs in two forms. The infantile primary disease (which is uncommon) is found at or soon after birth on feeding with milk; there is complete absence of the beta-galactosidase enzyme lactase. In the normal subject, lactase activity falls in adult life as milk intake falls. In some cases the hypolactasia is severe, leading to symptoms of bloatedness, borborygmi and diarrhoea when milk is drunk. The prevalence is extremely high (50–90%) in certain ethnic groups, mainly non-caucasian. (This strange medical expression – 'caucasian' – has crept across the Atlantic and now pervades many medical texts; it refers to white-skinned people, very few of whom come from the Caucasus or have even heard of it.) The enzyme defect is independent of lactose intake and it is generally accepted that it is inherited as an autosomal recessive trait. Hypolactasia may also be due to transient or permanent structural disease of the small bowel (see p. 140).

Almost all enzyme defects are inherited as autosomal recessive traits. Structural defects tend to have autosomal dominant inheritance. An important example of this is familial colonic polyposis (see p. 204). Not only is polyposis relatively common but, most importantly, it is a premalignant condition. Indeed the risk is so great – approaching 90% in the fifth to sixth decades – that this inevitably determines management and demands total excision of large bowel mucosa. It also demands careful screening of relatives; excepting new mutations, first-degree relatives have a 50% chance of being affected. Penetrance is probably near complete in this condition.

In polygenic or multifactorial inheritance the simple Mendelian laws are inapplicable and the disease reflects variation at several gene loci. Here the genetic factor is less distinct and a background susceptibility requires one or more environmental triggers to produce disease. Most common disorders, including peptic ulcer and inflammatory bowel disease, will come within this category, and, in the majority of cases, the gene loci are completely unknown. Recently, however, a predisposing factor in some diseases has been shown to be associated with the Human Leucocyte Antigen (HLA) loci. For example coeliac disease, with a frequency of perhaps 1 in 1000 live births, has been shown to be associated with HLA DW3 (about 96% of patients compared with about 25% of the general population have this genotype). Clearly, however, only a tiny proportion of those with DW3 will develop the disease. A weaker association of coeliac disease with HLA B8 suggests linkage disequilibrium between this and DW3.

Hence most, if not all, disease has some genetic contribution with a varying degree of environmental component (Fig. 2.7).

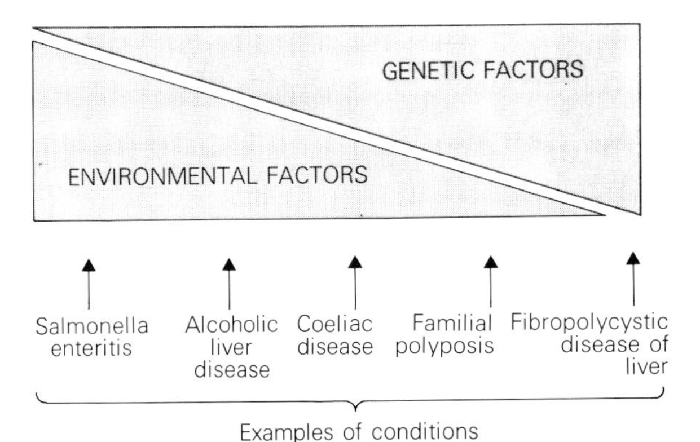

Fig. 2.7 *Relative interplay of genetic and environmental factors in disease.*

Immunological Factors in Disease

Normal immunological function and the gut

The alimentary tract plays a prime role in the body's immunological defences. This is not surprising when one considers the vast quantity of foreign protein antigen ingested during a lifetime; of all the body systems only the respiratory tract comes near to bearing the same antigenic load.

The neonate is immunologically immature, with a gut more permeable to antigens and a poor immunoglobulin response. It therefore depends to some extent upon its mother for immunological protection. Colostrum and human milk contain antibodies, of which bottle-fed infants are of course wholly deprived. The main intrinsic defences are constituted by lymphoid tissue (Gut Associated Lymphoid Tissue: GALT) which lines the gut from mouth to anus and constitutes no less than a quarter to a half of the mucosal mass. At birth, immature T-lymphocytes lie aggregated in follicles just beneath the mucosal surface (such as Peyer's patches). Specialised M-microfold cells, in a single-layered covering over the domes of the follicles, allow traces of antigen to enter and the lymphocytes are thereby stimulated. Some migrate to lymph nodes in the mesentery, thence to the thoracic duct and circulation and finally, by a remarkable homing-in mechanism, to the villous mucosa of the gut, coming to rest alongside the enterocytes (interepithelial lymphocytes or theliocytes, Fig. 2.8). In this process they become adapted to produce immunoglobulin, primarily IgA. IgA-producing cells constitute 80–90% of gut

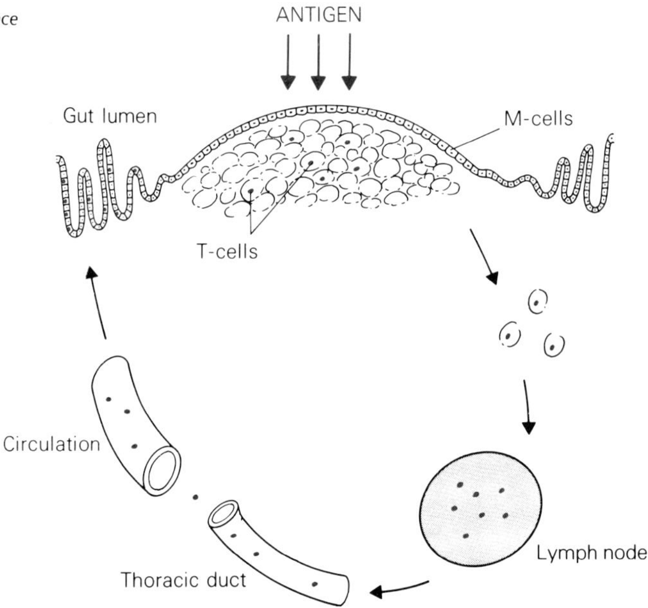

Fig. 2.8 *Stimulation of gut lymphocytes (T cells).*

immunocytes and are the primary antibody-producing cells (Fig. 2.9). Release of IgA occurs primarily into the gut lumen as a dimer attached to a glycoprotein called 'secretory component' or 'secretory piece' (Fig. 2.10). This component helps to protect against proteolysis. It may attach to IgM in patients with IgA deficiency. The function of liberated or secretory IgA is to reduce antigen absorption and to protect against bacteria (probably, in part, by reducing mucosal adherence: Fig. 2.11).

Some antigen is absorbed and can elicit a relatively weak systemic response – weak compared with local IgA response. It may be of considerable importance in protecting against tissue-damaging cell-mediated or Arthus type reactions to food and bacterial antigens in the wall of the gut. When local mechanisms are weakened and systemic response is increased, damaging reactions may occur.

The liver also plays an important part in the immunological defence system. The Kupffer cells are strategically placed to sequester antigens such as dietary proteins and bacteria, absorbed from the alimentary tract. Where the liver fails these antigenic substances effectively bypass the liver, as they also do with portasystemic shunting. In liver disease, non-specific rise in immunoglobulin (antibody) levels is common. The hepatocytes are not, however, responsible for immunoglobulin production. It is not yet clear what other immunological function the Kupffer cells have. Their

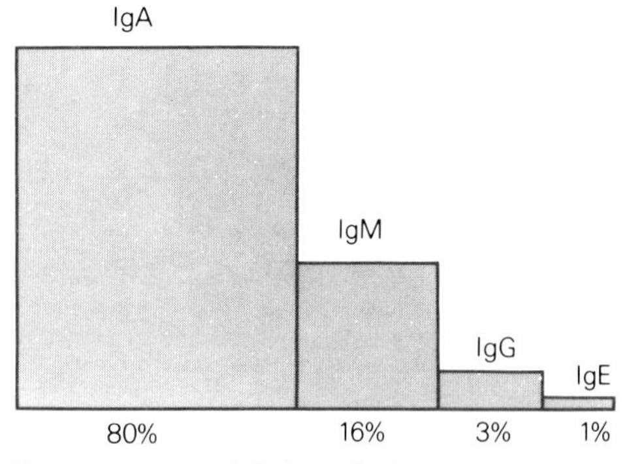

Fig. 2.9 *Immunoglobulin cell class in gut lymphocytes.*

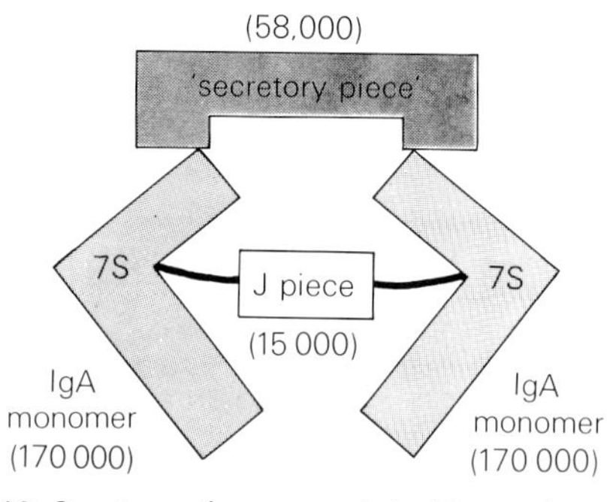

Fig. 2.10 *Structure of secretory IgA. (Figures in parentheses are molecular weights).*

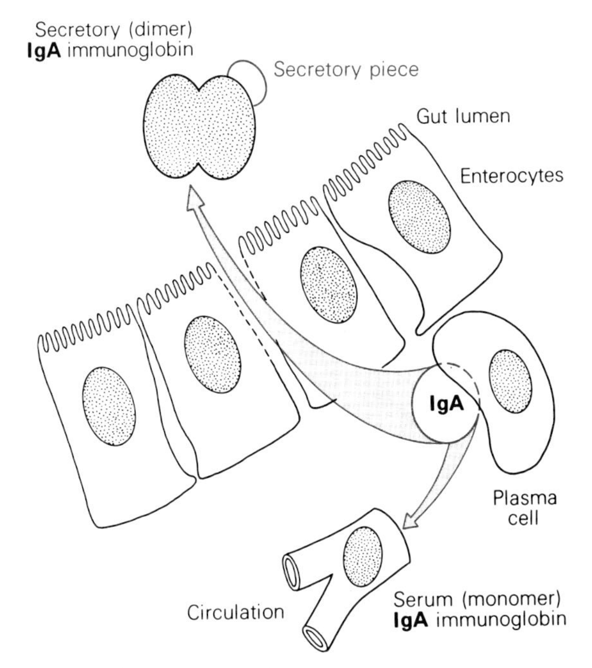

Fig. 2.11 *Release of IgA from plasma cells in wall of gut.*

phagocytic function is made use of in radionuclide imaging; the isotope (^{99}Tc) is tagged to a colloidal sulphur particle picked up by the Kupffer cells (p. 174).

Alimentary disorders associated with immunological abnormality

Numerous gut disorders have associated immunological features though in most cases it is not clear how much these are causally related or simply epiphenomena.

Food Allergy must be distinguished from food intolerance, and false allergies can arise by absorption of histamine. There are two true allergic reactions:

i. An *immediate* reaction arises from traces of antigen and is IgE-mediated (with high circulating IgE). There is usually severe vomiting and diarrhoea soon after ingestion of the food allergen and perhaps also asthma, angioneurotic oedema or even anaphylaxis. Foods such as strawberries, shellfish, egg-white, chocolate and food additives come into this category and are usually well recognised by the patient.
ii. A *delayed* reaction may occur, including abdominal pain, diarrhoea, eczema, headache, depression, arthralgia and, in children, failure to thrive. Large amounts of antigen may be involved – as in cows' milk intolerance. The diagnosis may be difficult and unsuspected. Carefully controlled food exclusion is the main test and the obvious treatment. Skin testing and the Radioallergosorbent Test (RAST) may be helpful in identifying IgE-mediated reacting subjects.

Sodium cromoglycate may help to reduce the allergic reaction to food where exclusion is impractible.

Chronic atrophic gastritis is a good example of an immunological disorder of the gut where infiltration of immunologically competent cells is associated with inflammation, functional loss and atrophy. Antibodies to gastric parietal cells may be detected in the blood. Atrophic gastritis is an invariable feature of Addisonian pernicious anaemia. In this disorder, in addition to non-specific parietal cell antibodies (in almost all cases) some cases show antibodies to intrinsic factor itself which is essential for vitamin B_{12} absorption. These intrinsic factor antibodies are in two forms:

i. blocking antibodies (preventing combination of vitamin B_{12} with intrinsic factor – IF).
ii. binding antibodies (reacting with vitamin B_{12}-IF complex and interfering with subsequent absorption).

There is a strong association (both in patients themselves and in their first-degree relatives) between pernicious anaemia and other so-called 'autoimmune' disorders such as juvenile (type I) diabetes, thyroid disease, idiopathic Addison's disease (hypoadrenalism) and arthritis.

Coeliac disease (see p. 130) is associated with immunological phenomena including reticulin antibodies, raised IgA and splenic atrophy, though the pathogenetic significance is unclear. There is a strong association with histocompatability antigens HLAB1, DW3 and B8. The possibly immunological link of coeliac disease with the later development of lymphoma is interesting.

Inflammatory bowel disease (IBD), both idiopathic proctocolitis, and Crohn's disease, shows some evidence of an immunological pathogenesis. Antibodies to colon cross-reacting with a common enterobacterial antigen (Kunin antigen) have been demonstrated, and there is growing evidence that both diseases represent differing immunological reactions to an insult, as yet unidentified. Lymphocytes in such patients can be shown to be cytotoxic to colonic epithelium. The extra-intestinal manifestations of IBD, such as uveitis, arthritis, erythema nodosum and possibly some liver disease, may be due to deposition of circulating immune complexes originating in damaged bowel.

Immunodeficiency diseases may be manifested in the gastrointestinal system. An example is hypogammaglobulinaemia which may be associated with small bowel dysfunction and malabsorption (p. 140).

Neoplasia

The gut is host to three of the world's most common malignant tumours – colo-rectal cancer, primary liver cell cancer, and cancer of the stomach. Comment has already been made about the possible role of ingested toxins in gastric carcinoma; the same may be true of hepatoma and mycotoxins, although in this case a clear association with hepatitis B infection has also been demonstrated (see p. 00). Indeed hepatoma is one of the best-established links between a virus and human cancer. This does not preclude an additive role for a dietary factor such as aflatoxin. Alcohol plays a role in oesophageal cancer, and balance of the diet may be important in colonic cancer. The gut also has the distinction of having tumours with the worst prognosis (e.g. pancreatic and gastric carcinoma) and also with quite good prognosis (e.g. carcinoma of colon), although these features may reflect the difficulty of recognition and diagnosis rather than virulence of the tumour. Considering the remarkable rate of turnover of small bowel mucosa it is surprising that small bowel malignancy is so infrequent.

Much interest in recent years has centred on oncofetal antigens in relation to cancer. Carcinoembryonic Antigen (CEA) was first described in colonic cancer; it is now known to be non-specific, and is found in association with other malignancies, and in some non-neoplastic conditions. Unfortunately these markers have not proved as helpful as originally expected in early diagnosis of cancer or in detecting a malignant change in a precancerous lesion (such as ulcerative colitis or familial polyposis). However, CEA is strongly positive in widespread metastatic colonic cancer and hence may have some usefulness, especially in long-term follow-up. Another oncofetal antigen, alpha fetoprotein (AFP), is positive in most cases of primary liver cancer but is again non-specific, being found in other tumours and non-neoplastic diseases.

Humoral Mechanisms

The gut as an endocrine organ

Although the discovery of secretin by Bayliss and Starling in 1902, and of gastrin by Edkins in 1905, marked the beginning of endocrinology as a separate discipline, it is only in recent years that the importance of the gut to the endocrine system has been appreciated. The advent of sensitive radioimmunoassay techniques has overcome some of the formidable difficulties of isolation and measurement and allowed the recent discovery of numerous peptides secreted by the gut which have the ability to act as hormones. Considerable difficulties of isolation and definition of action remain. Unlike other endocrine organs, the hormone-producing cells of the gut are diffusely scattered and not collected into recognisable glands. The situation is further complicated by the fact that several different endocrine cell types overlap in their distribution so that extracts from a piece of

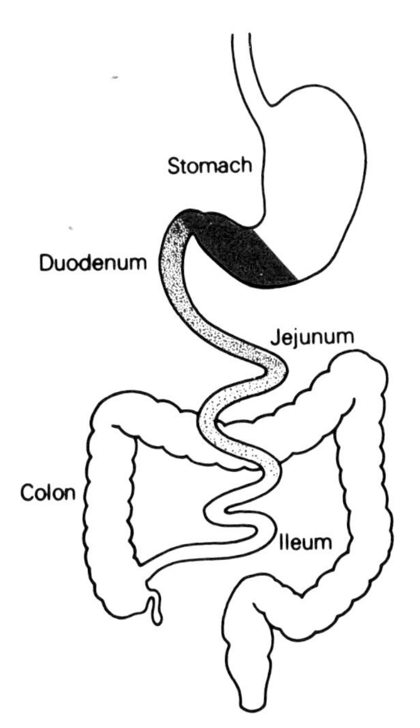

Fig. 2.12 *Human distribution of gastrin. Highest concentration in stomach.*

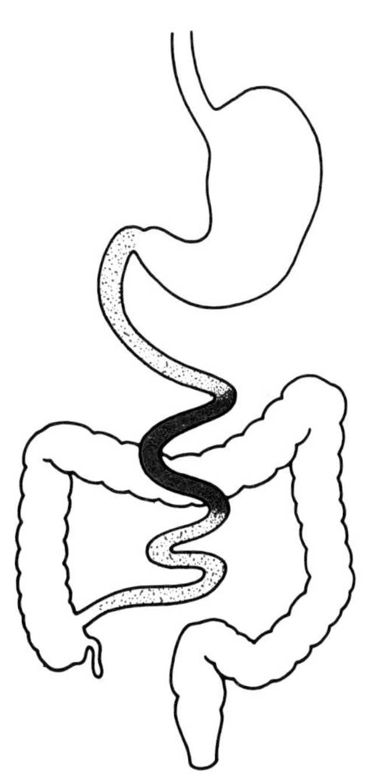

Fig. 2.13 *Human distribution of cholecystokinin. Highest concentration in jejunum.*

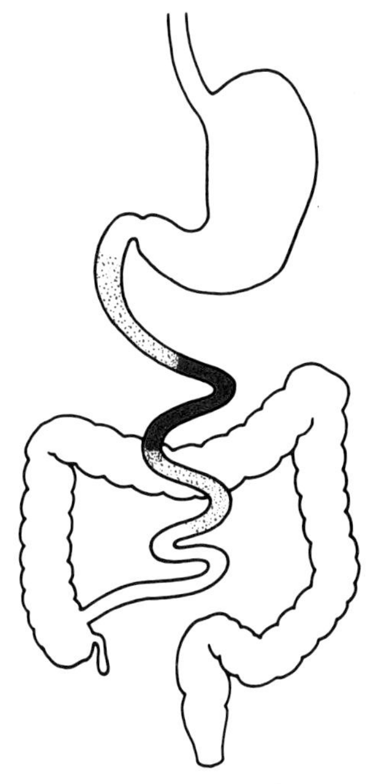

Fig. 2.14 *Human distribution of secretin. Highest concentration in duodenum and upper jejunum.*

gut mucosa may contain many different hormones (no doubt including those yet to be discovered) often with different actions. These problems have led to great difficulty in defining the action, interaction and distribution of hormones in the gut. The function of none of the known circulating gut. hormones is completely understood, and there remain several peptides secreted by the gut for which no physiological function can be found.

The importance of gastrin (p. 72), cholecystokinins (p. 103), and secretin (p. 103) is described elsewhere; their distribution is shown in Figs 2.12, 2.13 and 2.14. More recently-established hormones include pancreatic polypeptide (PP), gastric inhibitory peptide (GIP), vasoactive intestinal peptide (VIP), motilin, enteroglucagon, somatostatin, substance P, neurotensin, bombesin, and the endorphins.

Pancreatic polypeptide (PP). Discovered in 1972, the importance of this 36-amino-acid peptide remains unclear. In man, more than 90% of PP is found in the pancreas (Fig. 2.15), where it is present in both the exocrine glands and the islets of Langerhans. At peak levels in the blood (after a meal) there is reduction of the amount of bilirubin in the duodenum, associated, it is believed, with relaxation of the gall-bladder and contraction of the sphincter of Oddi. Enzyme and bicarbonate output from the pancreas is inhibited.

PP is not detectable in the blood after pancreatectomy and its secretion is grossly reduced in chronic pancreatitis; it is found in increased concentration in the blood of 50% of patients with pancreatic endocrine tumours (insulinoma, gastrinoma, glucagonomas and VIPomas) but as yet no clinical symptoms have been described which can be readily ascribed to high circulating concentrations of PP.

Gastric inhibitory peptide (GIP). GIP belongs to the secretin–glucagon family and is a peptide of 43 amino acids. It is found in high concentrations in the jejunum but is also present in the duodenum

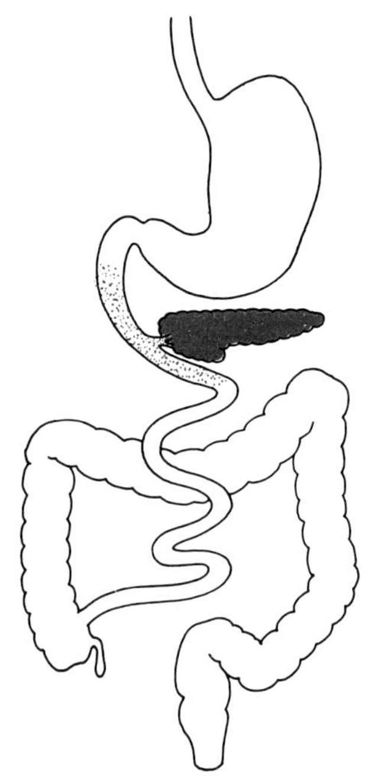

Fig. 2.15 *Human distribution of pancreatic polypeptide. Highest concentration in pancreas.*

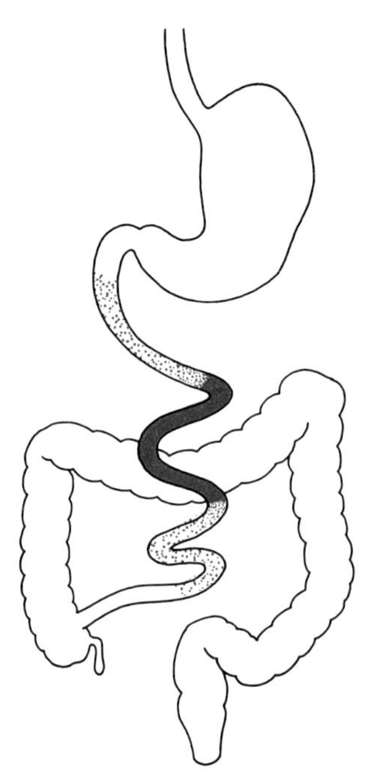

Fig. 2.16 *Human distribution of GIP. Highest concentration in jejunum.*

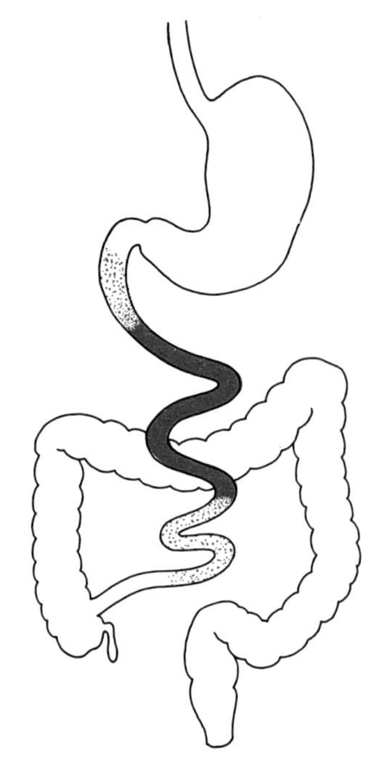

Fig. 2.17 *Human distribution of motilin. Highest concentration in duodenum and jejunum.*

and ileum (Fig. 2.16). It is released from the small bowel in response to carbohydrate and fat in a meal and its release is known to be inhibited by glucagon and somatostatin. Its secretion is diminished in coeliac disease and increased in obese diabetics. Its role is not yet clearly identified but it is believed that, in the presence of a high circulating blood glucose level, GIP is secreted from the gut and stimulates release of insulin from the pancreas (so-called entero-insular axis). Other postulated actions in man remain unproven.

Vasoactive intestinal peptide (VIP). This 28-amino-acid peptide also belongs to the secretin – glucagon family and can be found throughout the gastrointestinal tract. It is normally present in very large concentrations, and greatly exceeds the quantities of other gastrointestinal hormones. It is further unusual in that it is also found outside the gastrointestinal tract, notably in the brain where it probably acts as a neurotransmitter substance. Despite its wide distribution, plasma levels of VIP remain extremely low, largely because it is rapidly destroyed (by proteolytic enzymes in plasma) and has a half-life of less than one minute. This is fortunate; it is pharmacologically very potent, stimulating gastric acid secretion, releasing hepatic glycogen, stimulating small bowel and pancreatic secretion, and having very powerful vasodilatory effects on all arteries and arterioles. The only well-recognised pathological role of VIP is in the syndrome (described by Verner and Morrison in 1958) of severe, often fatal, watery diarrhoea associated with hypokalaemia and achlorhydria and islet cell adenoma of the pancreas – so-called 'WDHA syndrome', or 'VIPoma syndrome', in which high circulating levels of VIP are found as well as high concentrations within the adenoma. Occasionally, similar VIP-producing tumours may be found in the nervous system – ganglioneuromas, and ganglion neuroblastomas – presenting with identical symptoms.

Motilin. The sequence of the 22 amino acids of

motilin is quite unlike that of any other known gastrointestinal hormone. It is principally located in the duodenum and jejunum (Fig. 2.17) and is secreted by the enterochromaffin cells. Its main action in man seems to be to cause contraction of the pyloric sphincter (tending to cause gastric stasis) and stimulation of the lower oesophageal sphincter. Its actions in other species are often quite different and it has been shown that there is considerable species difference in its structure.

Enteroglucagon (EG). Glucagon (enteroglucagon) secreted by the gut exists in two forms, one of relatively high molecular weight (approx. 10 000) and the other with a molecular weight similar to pancreatic glucagon (approx. 3 500). Highest concentrations exist in the terminal ileum (Fig. 2.18) and there are also significant amounts in the colon. It is produced by a cell (the EG cell or L cell) which is found in the basal part of the mucosal glands, and it is believed that this cell produces both forms of EG. Its precise role remains speculative. Normally there is only a very small rise in circulating EG after a meal (as might be expected from its distribution) but in conditions associated with intestinal hurry or malabsorption there is increased release. There is a close correlation between the rise in circulating EG and the fall in plasma volume that occurs in the 'dumping syndrome' (see p. 91). Coincidental with the rise in circulating EG in dumping, the classical intestinal hurry of this syndrome gives way to gastrointestinal stasis. Whether this is due to EG release is not yet proven. Similar gastrointestinal stasis has been reported in EG-producing tumours.

A 'trophic' action of EG on gut mucosa in man remains unproven.

Somatostatin. Somatostatin, or growth hormone-release inhibiting hormone, is a 14-amino-acid polypeptide which, although initially found in the brain, was present in even greater quantities in the

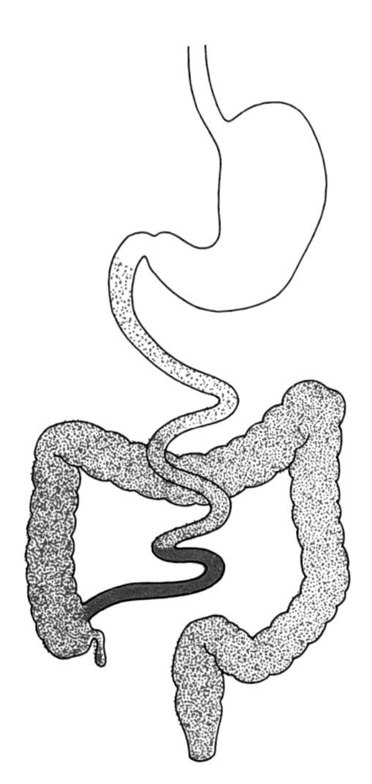

Fig. 2.18 *Human distribution of enteroglucagon. Highest concentration in terminal ileum.*

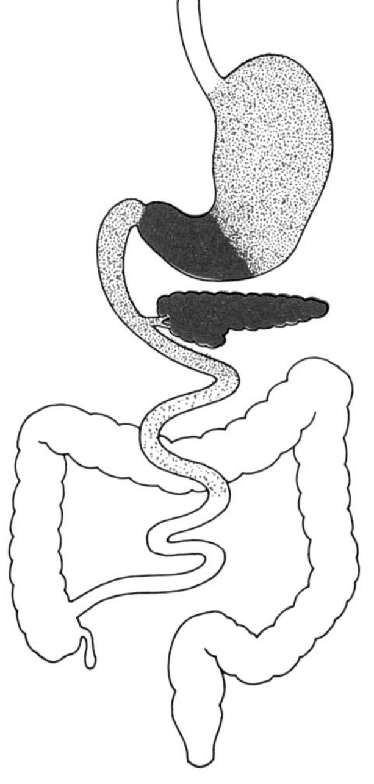

2.19 *Human distribution of somatostatin. Highest concentration in gastric antrum and pancreatic islets.*

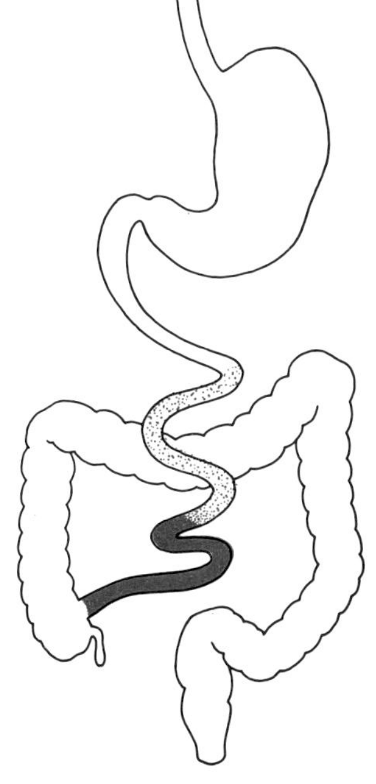

Fig. 2.20 *Human distribution of neurotensin. Highest concentration in lower ileum.*

gastric antrum and in the pancreatic islet cells (Fig. 2.19). Somatostatin strongly inhibits the release of growth hormone, TSH, insulin and glucagon, gastrin, motilin, GIP secretion, EG and PP. It is rapidly destroyed (has a half-life of less than one minute) and, like VIP, probably therefore does not normally act as a circulating hormone but rather as a locally-acting hormone or neurotransmitter.

Substance P. This is a small peptide consisting of 11 amino acids, widely distributed throughout the body but especially in the brain and spinal cord, salivary glands, pancreas, thyroid, kidney, smooth muscle, prostate and skin. In the gut greater quantities are found in the wall of the duodenum and colon. Despite its great potential importance, substance P remains only a possible hormone and probable neurotransmitter.

Neurotensin. Originally extracted from hypothalamic tissue, this 13-amino-acid peptide is found in largest quantities (over 80%) in the lower small bowel (Fig. 2.20). It has a wide spectrum of possible pharmacological actions but, like substance P, its role in the mechanism of gut symptoms or other disease states remains speculative.

Bombesin. This is a 14-amino-acid peptide (one of a family) which is found in the gut in small amounts, notably in the stomach and duodenum. It is also found in the brain, and probably constitutes yet another addition to the 'neurointestinal hormones'. Its role in physiology and pathology in man is not yet established, but in view of its wide distribution and the variety of its pharmacological activity it seems very likely that it will prove to be of considerable importance.

Endorphins and Enkephalins. This group of naturally-occurring peptides with opiate-like activity was discovered in the late 1970s. The first two discovered were the closely related pentapeptides, methionine and leucine enkephalin. The larger molecules of B and Y endorphins were discovered later. The endorphins are found only in the brain, whereas the enkephalins are found widely distributed in the gastrointestinal tract with greater concentrations in the gastric antrum. The enkephalins are rapidly broken down and therefore may have no in-vivo analgesic activity. Endorphins may induce analgesia for many minutes and their pharmacological action is quite distinct. In the gastrointestinal tract enkephalins may act physiologically in the same way as opiates but, like many of the other recently-discovered peptides, their precise role remains to be defined.

Conclusions

The full importance of the gut as an endocrine organ has yet to be appreciated. No doubt further hormones will be discovered, and the importance of those already isolated will become more firmly established. As well as leading to increased understanding of disease mechanisms, it seems certain that increasing knowledge will allow the development of new and accurate diagnostic tests. The financial and organisational implications for the health service are not yet clear.

Cellular Biochemical Mechanisms

Some diseases of the gut arise from fundamental changes in biochemical processes at an individual cellular level. This has already been alluded to when considering genetic and hormonal mechanisms of disease. A prime example of this kind of disease process is 'secretory diarrhoea'.

An understanding of the mechanisms of production of diarrhoea demands knowledge of the normal processes of fluid and electrolyte absorption (p. 117). Diarrhoea can arise in several ways, and these are described below.

Osmotic diarrhoea

The gut acts as a semipermeable membrane through which water can pass to equalise osmotic gradients. Nonabsorbed sugars; for example mannitol, may enter the colon and produce a considerable osmotic drive. Saline purgatives work similarly.

Defective permeability

This may arise in disease states, such as coeliac disease, where small solutes penetrate the jejunal mucosal barrier (normally very permeable) only poorly.

Impaired active transport

It seems likely that defective ion transport may occur as a result of lowered sodium/potassium ATPase activity caused, for example, by viral infection (e.g. Rotavirus in infantile diarrhoea).

Secretory diarrhoea

Much has been learned in recent years about this mechanism from detailed study of the highly lethal disease cholera, where the infection itself (by the bacterium *Vibrio cholerae*) is self-limiting but death is due to overwhelming losses of water and electrolyte. Similar 'choleraic' diarrhoea occasionally occurs in other infections, such as enteropathogenic *E. coli*, and is especially lethal in young small babies.

Cyclic AMP is formed on the basolateral membranes of intestinal villous epithelial cells from ATP and stimulates net secretion of sodium and water from cell to lumen (Fig. 2.21). The process of formation of cyclic AMP is catalysed by the enzyme adenylate cyclase which, in turn, is stimulated by several independent mechanisms. These include:

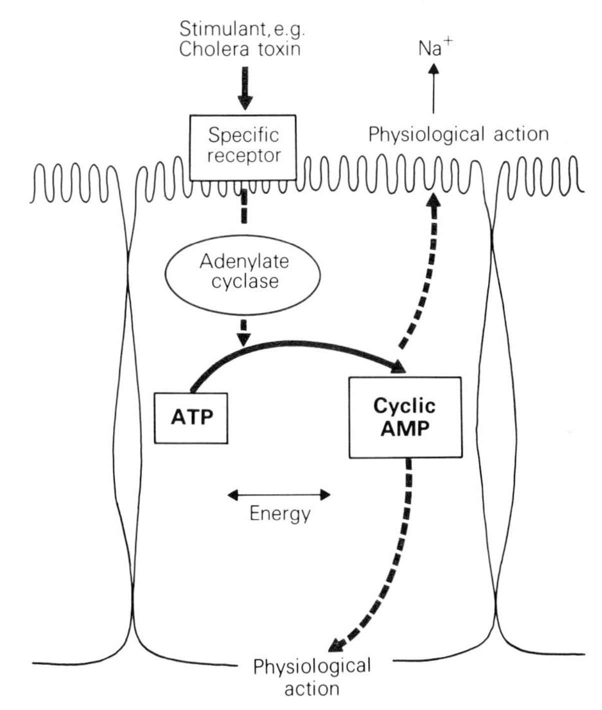

Fig. 2.21 *Action of adenylate cyclase and cyclic AMP.*

i. *Cholera toxin* (and some other bacterial toxins) which first bind to certain gangliosides on the villus cells; then a subunit of the toxin enters the cells and activates adenylate cyclase (Fig. 2.21).
ii. *Vasoactive intestinal peptide* (VIP) and possibly other hormones.
iii. *Prostaglandins* – notably F_2 and E_2 – produced endogenously. Increased synthesis of prostaglandins has been shown to occur in inflammatory bowel disease. This may explain, in part, the diarrhoea in those conditions and may also explain the response to drugs which have properties of inhibiting prostaglandin synthetase activity (such as the salicylate in sulphasalazine).
iv. *Deconjugated bile salts.* Deconjugation occurs when bile salts enter the colon, where they are broken down by bacterial action of the normal colonic flora. Abnormally large amounts of bile salts enter the colon in disease of the terminal ileum (e.g. Crohn's disease) and following surgical resection of this area, because bile salts are normally largely reabsorbed in the terminal ileum. The bile salt pool is depleted by such interruption of the enterohepatic circulation (see p. 147). Similarly, extensive bacterial colonisation of the small bowel (see p. 138), e.g. in tumours, strictures, diverticula and surgical bypass, can also lead to deconjugation. (Fig. 2.22).
v. *Long chain fatty acids.* The presence of poorly-digested or malabsorbed fats in stool (steatorrhoea) stimulates net secretion in the colon and leads to diarrhoea.

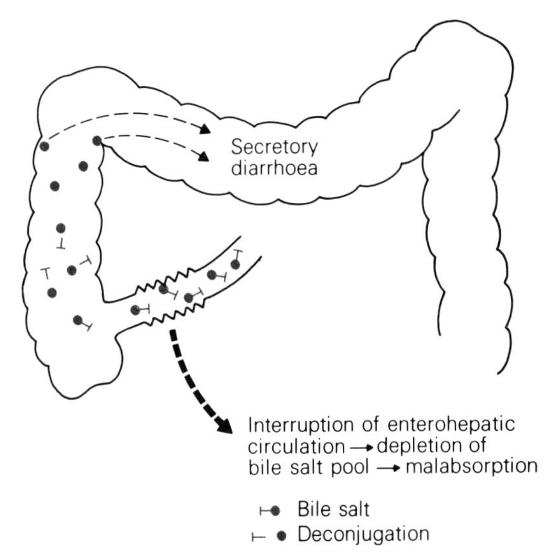

Fig. 2.22 *Diarrhoea in disease of the terminal ileum.*

Prostaglandins

In addition to the action on cyclic AMP mechanisms described above, the importance of this group of components in the alimentary tract is being increasingly recognised. The spasmogenic action on gastrointestinal motility of prostaglandins was recognised from the beginning by von Euler. More recently, their cytoprotective properties have been studied. Prostaglandins can protect gastric and intestinal mucosa from attack by bile acids, anti-inflammatory drugs, bacterial invasion, etc. This action is partly mediated through inhibition of acid secretion and stimulation of bicarbonate secretion, together with stimulation of mucus production. The role of endogenous prostaglandins, as distinct from the pharmacological action of exogenous prostaglandins, in this regard is not yet understood. There is evidence also that prostaglandins may protect the liver from damage.

Ageing and Degeneration

As the mean age of the population increases so diseases associated with degeneration become more prominent.

Vascular impairment

Acute ischaemia of the gut with rapid occlusion of a vessel is dramatic and associated with high morbidity and mortality (see p. 219). Chronic ischaemia is much less obvious and is difficult to diagnose. It may present as vague abdominal pain after eating, or malabsorption (where the small bowel is affected), or as ischaemic colitis (p. 219).

Loss of wall integrity

Frequency of diverticulosis, especially of the colon, increases with age and is present in at least 75% of those aged over 75 in Western countries. It is largely symptomless and fortunately only rarely leads to serious complications such as diverticulitis, pericolic abscess or bleeding (see p. 216).

Progressive loss of function

As yet very little is known of the effects of ageing on gut and liver function and it is remarkable how well gastrointestinal function is apparently maintained in the elderly compared with most bodily activities. Although malabsorption may occur, nutritional deficiency in the elderly is much more likely to be due to poor intake because of poverty, infirmity and loss of appetite.

'Small swallow' is one manifestation of the progressive loss of function in the pharynx and oesophagus in the elderly. Presbyoesophagus is also associated with considerable non-propulsive, non-peristaltic contractions – tertiary contractions.

EPIDEMIOLOGY

Alimentary tract disease is astonishingly common throughout the world. In the tropics, intestinal parasites are widespread; it has been calculated that about 1000 million people harbour roundworms and 500 million suffer from hookworm. Ten per cent of the world's population has amoebiasis: in Egypt, this infestation affects half the population. In Britain, gastroenterological disorders make up 11% of GPs' work, and their treatment costs equal those of the whole of the maternity services.

As well as producing a remarkable volume of ill-health, the diseases of the alimentary tract provide some striking examples of the varied incidence of disease in different countries, between the sexes, at various ages, and among families.

Colo-rectal cancer, diverticular disease and acute appendicitis are almost entirely found among the residents of Western-style civilisations, an association which has a very close relationship with the refined diet of these countries. Other diseases, such as peptic ulcer, have much more complicated origins, with gastric and duodenal ulcer behaving as two different diseases. Studies of the geographical distribution of cancer of the alimentary tract show remarkable examples of extremely high and very low incidence.

Somewhere in the varied pieces of epidemiological evidence, outlined below, will be the clues to the aetiology of gastrointestinal disease, of which at the moment we know so little.

Acute appendicitis

This is one of the conditions which has received special attention from epidemiologists because its incidence differs so much in different parts of the world. In Western Europe, North America, Australia and New Zealand, acute appendicitis is the commonest abdominal surgical emergency by far and yet it was hardly known until the later years of the nineteenth century, and was not properly described until 1886. Then Fitz, the Professor of Pathology at Harvard, made so clear a synthesis of post-mortem and clinical findings in 257 patients that surgeons had to recognise a new and dangerous disease entity. At that time the overall mortality was 26%; if the appendix had perforated, three out of four patients died.

It is very difficult to believe that a disease of such gravity could have been missed by generations of clinicians, so there must have been some change in the circumstances of North Americans and Europeans. It was during the 1880s that the mechanical roller-milling of flour was introduced into Western Europe and North America, and at the same time cheap beet sugar appeared on the market. As a consequence, the crude fibre content of the average diet must have fallen to 20–25% of what it had previously been (Fig. 2.23). The theory is that, with less bulk, the transit time of faeces through the bowel would be slower, allowing time for greater dehydration. The resulting more viscous faeces would be more likely to impact in the lumen of the appendix and form a faecolith, which would in turn produce the conditions for acute obstructive appendicitis.

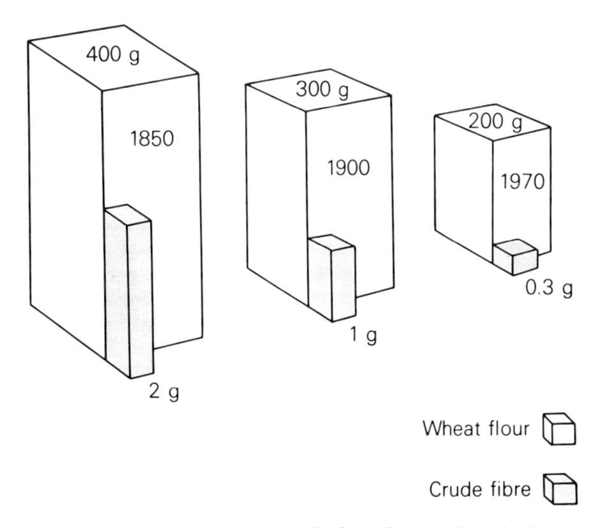

Fig. 2.23 *Daily consumption of wheat flour and crude fibre in Great Britain (1850–1970).*

This theory of deficient fibre in diet does seem to receive a great deal of support from epidemiological studies. Acute appendicitis is hardly seen in rural hospitals in Africa and India but it is relatively common among Africans who come to work in the cities and have to eat refined foods. When, during the Second World War, carbohydrate foods were less refined and more vegetables were eaten, some countries showed a decline in acute apendicitis. Fibre does not, however, seem to be the complete explanation: for instance, Eskimos taking their traditional carnivorous diet, with very little fibre, very rarely suffer acute appendicitis.

Alimentary Tract Cancer

These neoplasms are outstanding for the striking way in which they show areas of high and low geographical incidence. Much attention has naturally been paid to these differences in the hope that analyses of diet, environment or race would reveal important aetiological factors.

Carcinoma of the oesophagus

This provides a particularly striking example of areas of astonishingly high incidence. There is a belt stretching across Asia from North-Eastern China, through Soviet Central Asia, to the shores of the Caspian Sea, and there are also specific areas of Southern Africa, especially the Transkei, where incidence is 30–40 times as high as in Western Europe (Fig. 2.24). The other very striking feature of these areas is that, alongside an area of very high incidence, there will be, only a few miles away, a region showing only one-tenth of the frequency.

In spite of these contrasts, it has proved very difficult to identify the factors which produce the difference. The drinking of exceptionally hot beverages, the smoking of unusual tobaccos, with an underlying element of malnutrition have been postulated. Alcohol abuse is associated with a higher frequency.

Carcinoma of the stomach

Over the whole world, this is one of the commonest fatal cancers. Japan, Chile, Iceland and Finland have had, in that order, the unhappy distinction of the highest incidence. In Europe, nearly double the number of cases occur in the Eastern countries, such as Finland, with incidence diminishing westwards across Europe until France and England show the lowest figure. Across the Atlantic, the white citizens of North America show an even lower incidence (Fig. 2.25). Incidence throughout the Western World appears to be falling.

In spite of intensive study of diets there is very little definite information. It seems that dwellers in areas of high incidence tend to eat a lot of starchy food such as potatoes, rice and bread, and little fresh fruit or vegetables. There is a strong hint that eating a lot of smoked food may be harmful, and pickled vegetables and salted fish may also be significant. The role of nitrosamines is discussed on p. 94. High intake of alcohol and heavy smoking do not appear to be significant.

The other known aetiological factors are blood group A and pernicious anaemia (see p. 94).

There is much speculation and little hard fact in the search for the cause of gastric cancer but it does seem likely that differences in incidence are largely explicable in terms of variations in diet.

Table 2.2
Common Malignancies: Registrations in England and Wales, 1977

Men		*Women*	
Trachea, bronchus, lung	28 348	Breast	21 558
Colon and rectum	11 026	Colon and rectum	12 145
Other malignant disease of skin (not melanoma)	10 389	Other skin (not melanoma)	9 037
Prostate	7 694	Cervix and uterus	8 000
Stomach	7 346	Trachea, bronchus, lung	7 685
Bladder	5 962	Stomach	5 084
Pancreas	2 923	Ovary	4 406
Oesophagus	2 115	Pancreas	2 702
Testis	774	Bladder	2 276
Liver	498	Oesophagus	1 748
Gallbladder	483	Gallbladder	746
Small bowel	172	Liver	312
		Small bowel	169

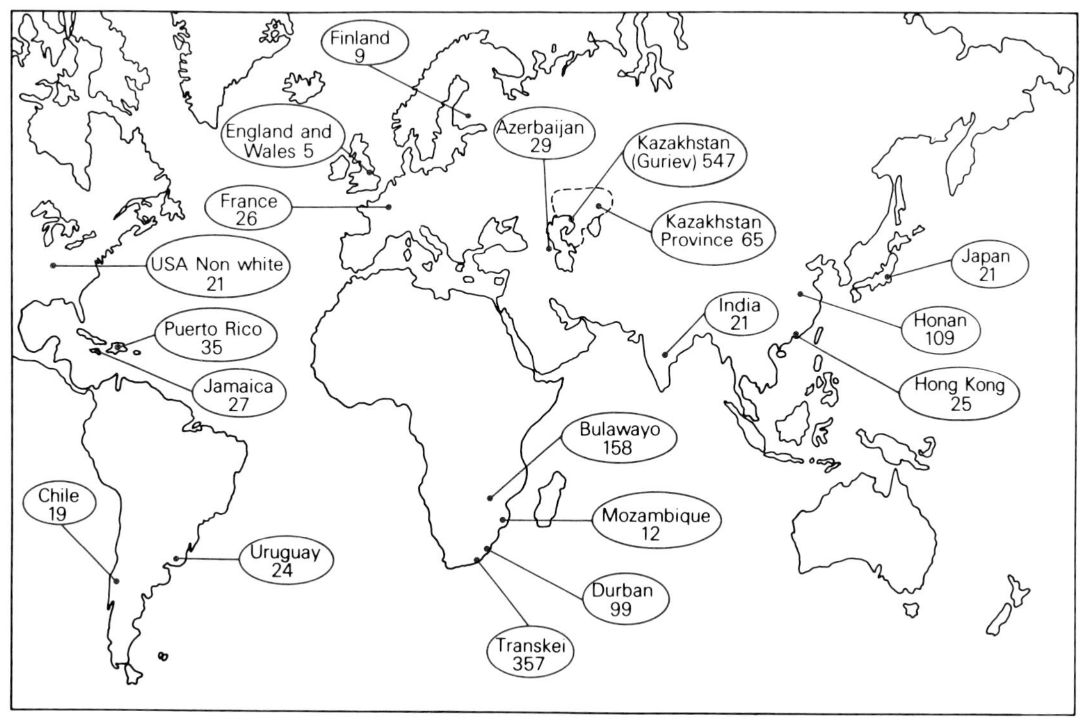

Fig. 2.24 *Carcinoma of oesophagus, annual incidence in males (per 100 000).*

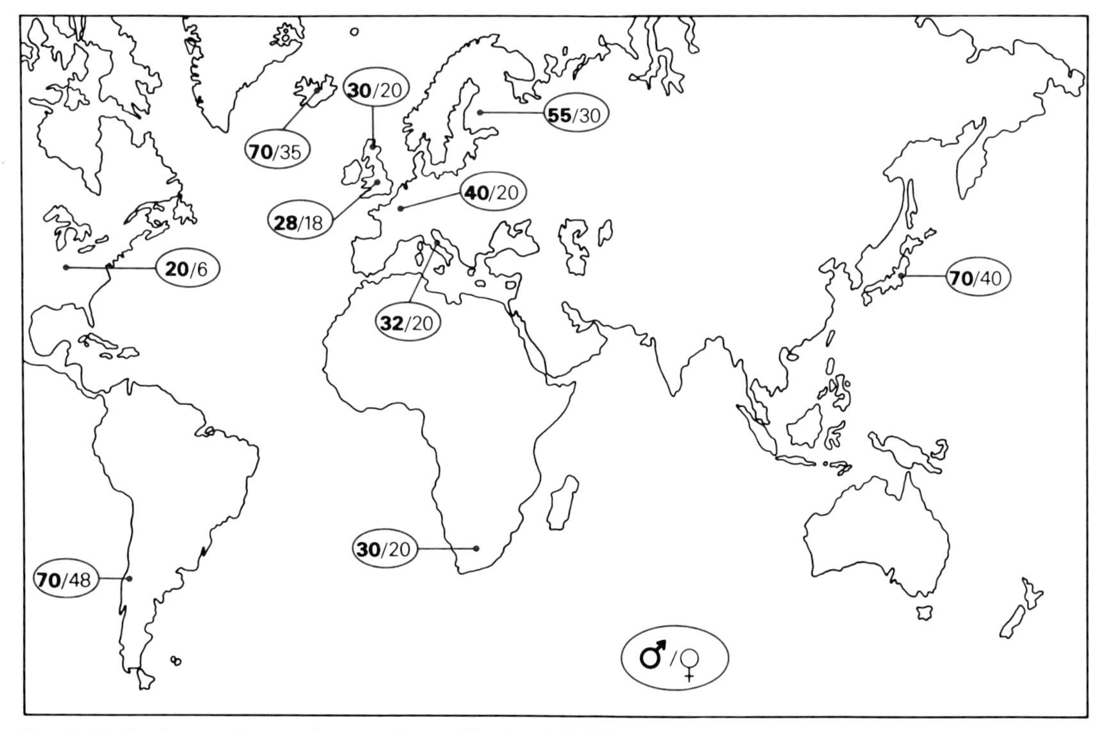

Fig. 2.25 *Carcinoma of stomach, annual mortality (per 100 000).*

Colo-rectal cancer

In Western communities, colo-rectal cancer is the second commonest malignancy, exceeded only by lung cancer among men and breast cancer in women (Table 2.2). This is true throughout North America, Northern Europe, Australia and New Zealand, with the highest incidence so far recorded being found in North Eastern Scotland and Connecticut, USA, where over 50 new cases occur per 100 000 population per year. In an Eastern European country, such as Romania, the incidence is only one-third that found in Scotland: among South African citizens the incidence is three-fifths of the Scottish figure among whites, one-fifth among Indians, and one-tenth among the Bantu. In Israel large bowel cancer is much commoner among immigrants from Europe than in those who come from Asia and Africa. Poles who migrate from their homeland to the USA or Australia show, within one generation, a rise in the incidence of colo-rectal cancer, from about 10, to 30 per 100 000 per year.

This pattern of incidence (Fig. 2.26), which closely resembles that of diverticular disease and appendicitis, strongly suggests that refined, low-bulk diets play an important part in aetiology. If this theory is true then it is not surprising that the incidence of colo-rectal cancer is roughly equal among men and women.

A great deal of work has been done on the bacterial content of the stools of people eating low and high fibre diets, on the action of bacteria on bile and animal fats, and on the possible consequent formation of carcinogens. If such agents were formed, they would tend to be diluted by the bulk of high-fibre diet stools, and the exposure of colonic mucosa to them would be reduced by the rapid transit through the colon. The converse would be true of low-fibre diets.

Carcinoma of the tongue

This is now one of the rare tumours of the Western World (less than 1% of all malignancies) but in South India it accounts for about 20%. This appears to be directly connected with the habit of chewing betel nut; the chronic malnutrition of the chewers may well contribute to epithelial instability and this is a good example of the way in which social circumstances and habits can contribute to disease.

The chance of developing a squamous cell carcinoma anywhere in the oropharynx is 15 times higher among those who regularly smoke tobacco and drink alcohol.

Primary carcinoma of the liver (hepatoma)

There are wide variations in world incidence of primary hepatoma; in some areas the rate is a staggering 98 per 100 000 per year (Fig. 2.27). It is commonly but by no means always associated with cirrhosis. This includes cirrhosis of various kinds including haemochromatosis, alcoholic disease and post-viral cirrhosis. There is now compelling evidence linking hepatitis B infection with development of the tumour (see p. 170), and integration of HBV-derived DNA into host DNA has been demonstrated. Interestingly this has recently also been found in hepatomas supervening upon alcoholic cirrhosis. The disease is commoner in males. The role of additional factors such as plant or fungal toxins as co-factors in hepatoma aetiology is as yet uncertain.

Diverticular Disease

The formation of diverticula in the colon, especially in the sigmoid, becomes increasingly common as age advances in the people of Western societies. Post-mortem studies show that 35% of British citizens over 60 years of age have diverticula but probably only 10% of these will have been patients who had symptoms of diverticulitis. In contrast, only five examples of colonic diverticula were found in a series of 3000 Bantu post mortems. It is perhaps significant that deaths from diverticular disease in Britain remained stationary during 1939–50, and then rose steadily again: it is suggested that this could be a consequence of the higher fibre content of wartime and early post-war food.

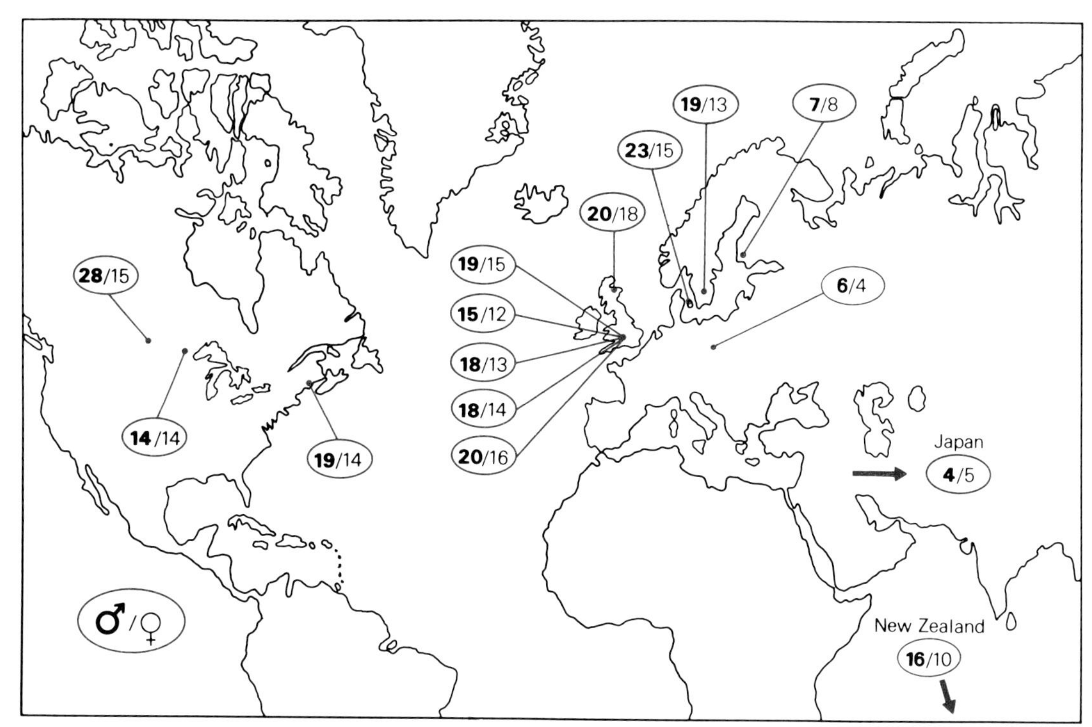

Fig. 2.26 *Carcinoma of rectum, annual incidence (per 100 000).*

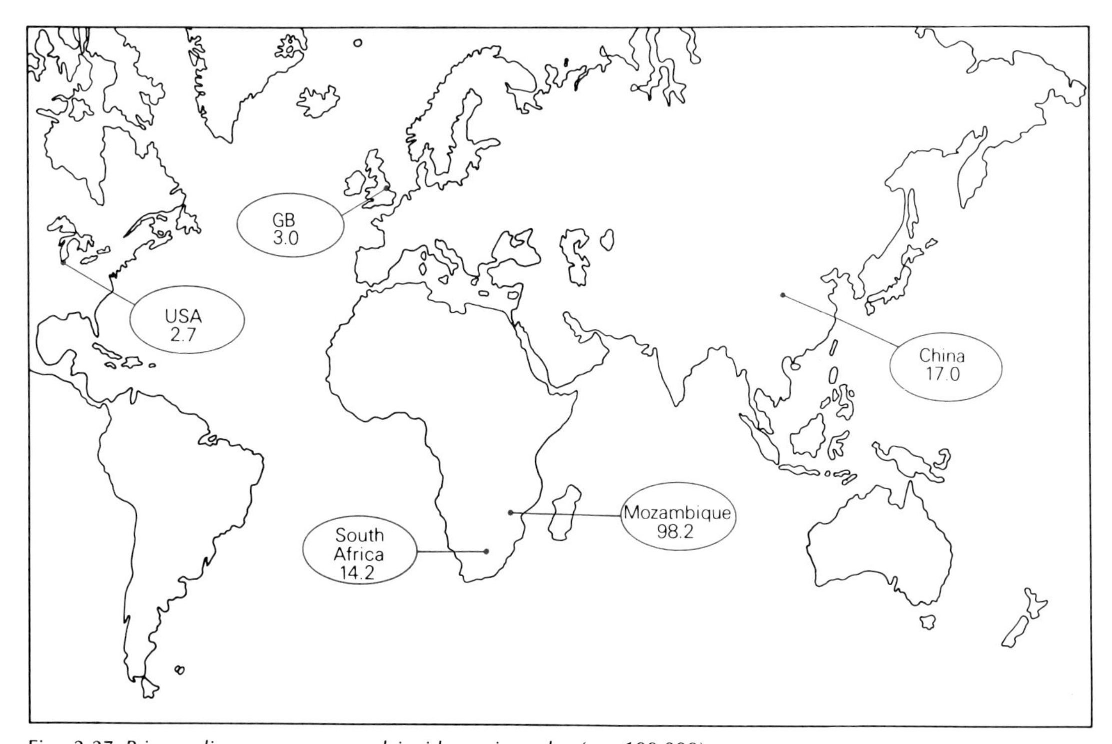

Fig. 2.27 *Primary liver cancer, annual incidence in males (per 100 000).*

Peptic Ulcer

In contrast to the distribution of large bowel disorders (which seems to bear such a close relationship to dietary habits) the occurrence of peptic ulcer is much more difficult to unravel and explain.

In the nineteenth century the predominant form in Great Britain was gastric ulceration among young women, who were almost always single, anaemic, and living away from home as housemaids or shop assistants. With the turn of the century this strange manifestation of ulceration seemed to melt away, to be replaced by a steadily-rising tide of duodenal ulceration, with men outnumbering women by about twelve to one. This was especially marked in Northern England and in Scotland where, by the 1940s, each district hospital was seeing one or two perforated duodenal ulcers each day.

Although duodenal ulceration has become progressively less prevalent over the past thirty years, peptic ulceration is still a very common condition and affects about 10% of the male population of Western countries. In one year during 1966–7 a total of 13 million working days were lost in England and Wales because of gastro-duodenal disorders.

Beyond Britain, peptic ulcer is common throughout Europe, North America and Australasia. A recent rise in gastric ulceration among women in Australia appears to be related to regular ingestion of aspirin.

However, tropical countries such as Africa and India also show some areas much affected by peptic, and especially duodenal, ulcer.

India has for long been known to have a high incidence of duodenal ulcer, but there are peculiar regional characteristics. It is common in the South, where it mostly affects poor young male labourers:

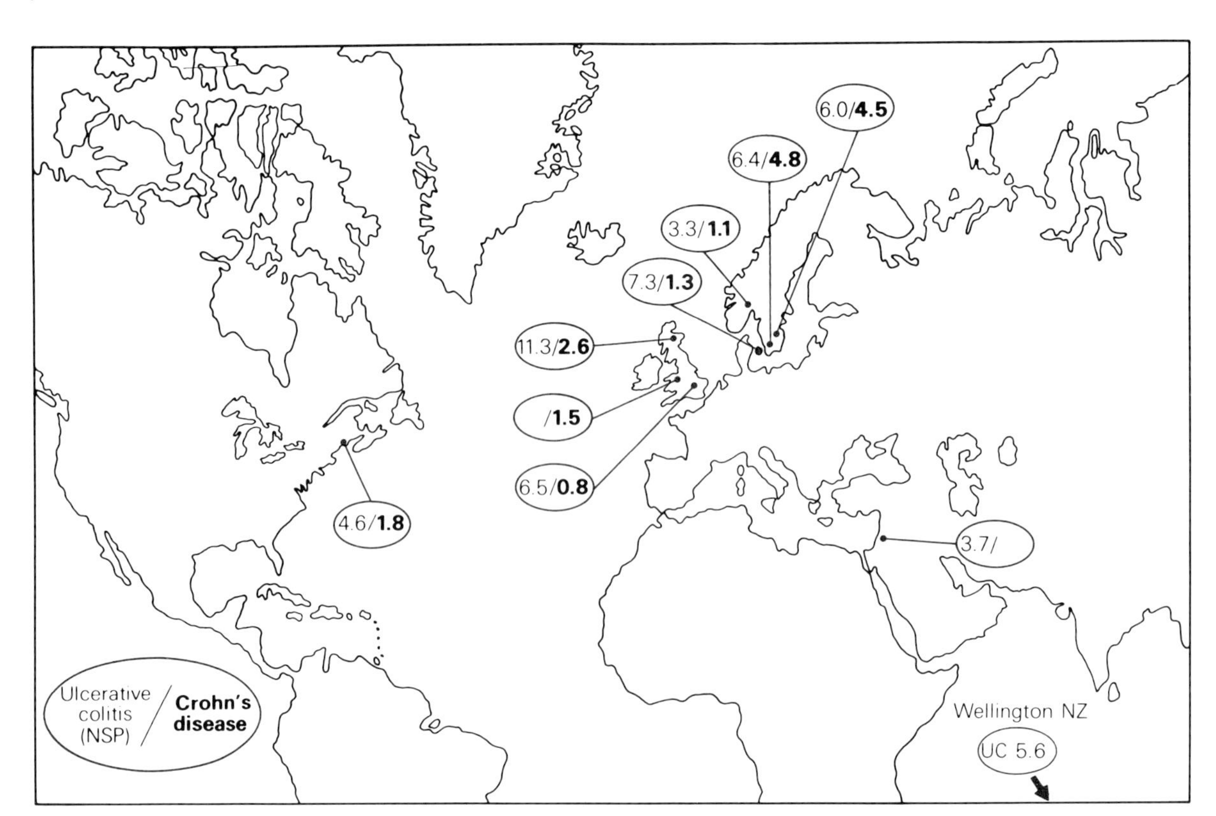

Fig. 2.28 *Inflammatory bowel disease, annual incidence (per 100 000).*

pyloric stenosis is a very frequent complication whereas perforation or haemorrhage are rare. The DU/GU ratio is 20:1 and male/female ratio 16:1. It is relatively uncommon in the North of India. Some workers relate this to diet, since people in the South eat polished rice and very hot curries whilst those in the North use unrefined wheat as their principal food source, made up into chapattis which require a lot of mastication.

The basic causative factors are hard to elucidate. There are marked differences in sex incidence, and for a few there is a strong familial incidence. Many surveys of dietary, drinking and smoking habits have been inconclusive. Young adults who avoid coffee and drink a lot of milk show a very low incidence of ulceration whilst smokers seem to show a slightly higher incidence than non-smokers. Drinking alcohol has little adverse effect, although taking alcohol and aspirin together certainly carries an increased risk of gastro-duodenal bleeding.

Inflammatory Bowel Disease (IBD)

Although Crohn's Disease (CD) is a general disease of the alimentary tract, and nonspecific proctocolitis (NSP), otherwise known as ulcerative colitis, is confined to the colon, they share many common characteristics.

In particular their geographical distribution is very similar to other large bowel diseases such as colo-rectal cancer and diverticular disease, (Fig. 2.28) and this suggests that a refined diet might be an important predisposing factor. It has, for instance, been shown that patients with CD eat more than twice as much sugar (150 g per day) as the general population (60 g). There are interesting, and as yet unexplained, differences in incidence within one country, e.g. Great Britain (Fig. 2.28).

There is certainly a familial factor in the incidence of inflammatory bowel disease: 1 in 10 patients with NSP have a relative with either NSP or CD. This is probably not due to an environmental factor because IBD is rare in the spouses of patients.

A large amount of work on possible viral or bacterial causes of IBD has been done, with inconclusive results.

Defective colonic metabolism may be important. Short-chain fatty acids, produced under anaerobic conditions in the caecum, are important for the health of the colonic mucous membrane, but in patients with NSP the utilisation of fatty acids is defective. This could make the colonic mucosa more susceptible to damage and would account for the localisation of UC to the large bowel only.

There is no evidence, in spite of many anecdotal reports, that psychological factors play any part in the *aetiology* of IBD.

3

Clinical Diagnosis and Investigative Techniques

Patients with alimentary tract disease are often embarrassed by having to talk about their diarrhoea or their piles, worried by recurrent bouts of pain or marked weight loss, anxious about the family at home and their job; by the time they come for help, a number are gravely ill. Many of these patients will need a number of investigations, which can be tedious or uncomfortable, and some will have to face the need for major surgery. Personal interest in, and sympathy for, the patient are personal attributes of the gastroenterologist which are as important as skill and experience. Shrewd reading of character is also needed because there are many patients whose psychological problems present with gastrointestinal complaints. Happily the need to take a full history from every patient combines very well with the need to make good personal contact during the first few interviews.

It is important to sit down and listen. Some patients are good at describing their symptoms whilst some describe what others think rather than what they feel, so the need for prompting varies greatly. It is most unwise to hurry over the taking of a history in the belief that the physical examination will yield the more important information. In gastroenterology this is rarely true. There are a number of essential GI symptoms and a clear account of each must be obtained.

Symptoms

Pain

Abdominal pain is the most important. It can be of two kinds: visceral and parietal. The abdominal viscera are insensitive to handling and cutting, but obstruction, causing distension, triggers stretch receptors; traction on mesenteries is painful; acid gastric juice stimulates pain receptors in the base of gastric and duodenal ulcers. Although the source of the pain in the viscus may be anywhere in the abdomen, the sensory fibres run back in the mesenteries of the alimentary tract to the spinal cord and the principal site at which the patient experiences pain is in the midline, where the primitive fore-, mid- and hind-gut originated. The level at which pain is felt depends on the site being stimulated. Thus oesophagitis causes substernal pain. The pain of an ulcer in stomach or duodenum, or of a stone in the biliary tree, is felt high in the epigastrium (Fig. 3.1). Obstructive appendicitis due to a faecolith impacted near the base causes quite severe pain around the umbilicus, whilst an obstructing carcinoma in the sigmoid colon will produce recurrent pain across the lower abdomen.

Visceral pain may be referred to other sites: it is characteristic of a stone impacted in the biliary tract for pain to be felt first below the xiphoid process and then for it to spread along the costal margin through to the back, around the angle of the right scapula.

When visceral pain arises from the paired renal tracts, the pain is felt on the affected side. A stone in the renal pelvis causes aching or colicky pain in the loin or, if the stone impacts lower in the ureter, the pain is felt low in the iliac fossa or in the testicle or labia. Acute retention of urine produces intense pain felt directly over the distended bladder.

Totally different from visceral pain is the pain which is experienced when the parietal peri-

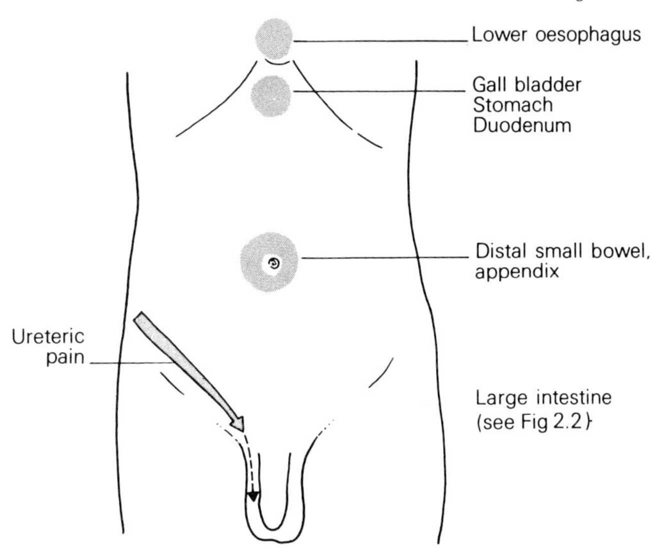

Fig. 3.1 *Areas of reference of visceral abdominal pain.*

toneum which lines the abdominal wall is subjected to irritation. This peritoneum (in contrast to the peritoneum covering viscera) is innervated by the appropriate thoracic spinal nerve which carries motor fibres to the abdominal wall musculature. When, for instance, acute appendicitis has developed sufficiently to cause inflammation in the abdominal wall peritoneum overlying it, this is felt as a steady aching pain well localised to the inflamed area: this accounts for the well-known shift of pain from around the umbilicus to the right iliac fossa. Movement or coughing conspicuously aggravates this type of pain so it is characteristic of such patients that they lie still and only move with caution. The irritation of the parietal peritoneum also sets up a reflex protective spasm in the overlying abdominal muscles which can be recognised, on palpation, as either a stiffening or even complete rigidity of the abdominal wall. This rigidity is classically seen when a duodenal ulcer perforates and the contents of the stomach flow out over the peritoneal cavity: there is immediate severe generalised abdominal pain from the chemical assault on the peritoneum lining the abdominal wall, and the whole abdominal musculature also immediately tightens up.

Blood can also irritate the parietal peritoneum; it is characteristic of a ruptured bleeding ectopic pregnancy in the fallopian tube that the blood shed into the abdominal cavity causes not only severe abdominal pain and muscle guarding but, when it reaches the under-surface of the diaphragm, it stimulates sensory fibres which run up the phrenic nerve and enter the cervical plexus. The pain is experienced in the distribution of the supraclavicular nerve branches of the cervical plexus, so shoulder-tip pain (Fig. 3.2) is characteristic of bleeding ectopic pregnancy (as it is of perforated peptic ulcer).

The *timing* of abdominal pain is very important. The patient who perforates a peptic ulcer or who suffers embolism of the superior mesenteric artery may be literally caught in the act of lighting a fire, washing up, crossing the road – the task being done at the moment of onset is precisely remembered and is highly characteristic of these emergencies. The pain of a duodenal ulcer is typically related to hunger, so it often wakens the patient at night and is relieved by a drink of milk or bicarbonate of soda: relapse tends to occur in spring and autumn.

The *character* of pain needs careful analysis.

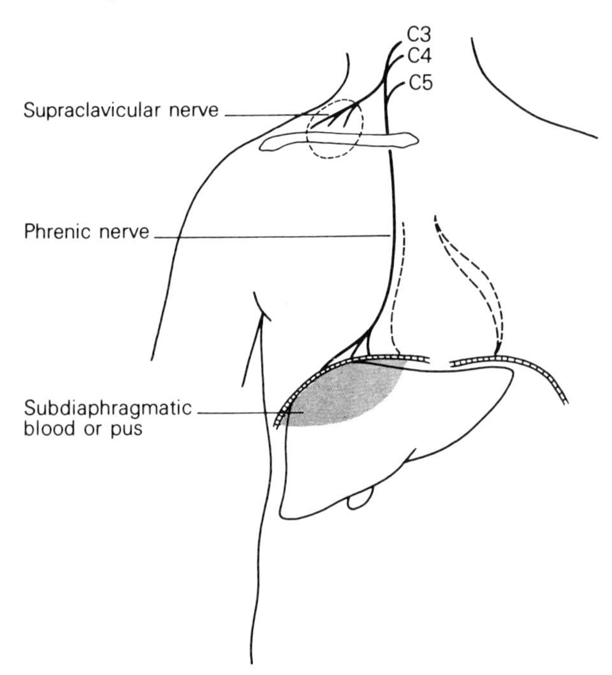

Fig. 3.2 *Shoulder tip pain and diaphragmatic irritation.*

The pain of acute small bowel obstruction is typically colicky, rising to a peak of severity and then fading away, to be followed in a few minutes by another spasm. However, so-called biliary and ureteric colic are usually steady pains, maintained over several hours, and often of great severity. The patient rolls about, seeking without success for an easier position. The pain of peptic ulcer is a duller, boring type of pain, but very persistent and repetitive.

Anorexia (see p. 7)

This is a common and important symptom. Almost everyone with an acute abdominal condition, such as acute appendicitis, loses any desire to eat. Some patients lose the urge to eat because eating brings on pain – this occurs in some patients with gastric ulcer and, an important group, with small bowel disease, such as Crohn's disease or chronic ischaemia. It is characteristic of patients with a gastric carcinoma that they lose their appetite early – often before there are any other symptoms or signs.

Nausea, retching and vomiting

Although a symptom experienced at some time by all, nausea is a psychic experience which is impossible to define. It may follow a bewildering variety of stimuli (e.g. labyrinthine stimulation, visceral pain, fear and unpleasant memories) and it is not known where the impulses arise. Nausea is commonly associated with excess salivation and often accompanied or preceded by yawning. Gastric peristalsis and tone are reduced, and there is frequently reflux of duodenal contents into the stomach which may account for the sour eructation which frequently precedes vomiting.

By contrast, much more is known about the mechanisms involved in retching and vomiting, the two very active symptoms which often follow nausea.

Retching is an uncomfortable and sometimes frightening symptom which usually precedes vomiting. There are short rapid respiratory movements against a closed glottis. The abdominal muscles contract powerfully and there is short violent downward contraction of the diaphragm. This leads to a rapid rise in intra-abdominal pressure. The pyloric end of the stomach contracts whilst the cardia relaxes and, as endoscopists can witness, the rapid rise in intra-abdominal pressure forcibly drives the cardia up into the lower end of the oesophagus, temporarily assuming the macroscopic appearances of a tumour. These dramatic movements are powerful, rapid and often repetitive and it is not difficult to see how they sometimes result in a Mallory–Weiss tear (see p. 320). It is believed that the upward movement of the cardia during retching is necessary to overcome the lower oesophageal sphincter pressure; otherwise the rise in intra-abdominal pressure (described above) on the short segment of intra-abdominal oesophagus (see p. 58) would ensure tight closure of the lower oesophageal sphincter and make vomiting difficult.

Vomiting occurs as the gastric contents are forced up to and out of the mouth, which opens a few seconds prior to stomach evacuation. The act of vomiting is controlled by a vomiting centre in the medulla. The afferent impulses arise in the alimentary tract and elsewhere. Receptors are well recognised in the pharynx, the pyloric region, and the entire bowel and biliary tract, and probably also exist in the mesenteric vessels and the heart. In the floor of the fourth ventricle there is also a chemoreceptor trigger sensitive to drugs such as digitalis, and to motion sickness and metabolic disturbances such as keto-acidosis and uraemia. The efferent control is via the vagi and sympathetic systems.

With such a variety of possible stimuli it is therefore not surprising that vomiting may be functional, or due to a great variety of organic and metabolic disturbances including: gastric, intestinal and biliary obstruction; drug intoxication, including alcohol; uraemia; ketoacidosis; food poisoning; infection; raised intracranial pressure; and physiological states such as pregnancy.

Vomiting is thus a non-specific symptom which may be due to many disorders outside the alimentary tract. However, when alimentary disease is suspected, the timing and the nature of the vomitus may provide clues to its cause. When vomitus is seen to contain food eaten many hours (or even days) before, this suggests gastric outlet obstruction (e.g. due to antral gastric ulcer or malignancy, or 'pyloric stenosis' due to chronic duodenal ulceration) or gastric stasis (e.g. post-vagotomy or diabetic neuropathy). By contrast, vomiting immediately after food is very suggestive of functional vomiting – but may occasionally be seen in pyloric channel ulceration. Early morning vomiting is characteristic of pregnancy, alcoholism (often induced as the alcoholic brushes his teeth in the morning), uraemia and so-called bilious vomiting (see p. 91). It is also of great clinical importance to note whether the vomitus contains blood or 'coffee grounds', indicating gastrointestinal bleeding (see Chapter 14), or is faeculent, indicating intestinal obstruction (see Chapter 13).

Hiccough

This is a troublesome symptom which can be of considerable significance, especially after abdominal surgery, when it should always suggest that there may be gastric distension or paralytic ileus. It also occurs in uraemia.

Heartburn

This is one of the commonest alimentary tract symptoms and originates in the lower oesophagus. Distension, acid, heat and cold applied to this area all produce the sensation of burning and distension beneath the lower sternum that everyone recognises as heartburn. It is especially associated with situations in which the competency of the gastro-oesophageal junction is impaired, e.g. sliding hiatus hernia, pregnancy, and obesity. It is also very common in cholelithiasis.

Diarrhoea and constipation

These terms require careful examination because they are very loosely used. Patients are inclined to say that they have 'diarrhoea' when they pass a stool several times a day, irrespective of whether it is fluid or solid. A useful arbitrary guide is to say that a normal person may defaecate as frequently as three times a day or as infrequently as once in three days. However, someone who moves the bowel more than three times a day does not have diarrhoea unless the faeces are fluid in consistency, whilst some very healthy people have been 'constipated' all their lives. The patient with a rectal carcinoma or proctitis who goes many times a day to the toilet to pass only blood and mucus must be watched for. The duration and precise character of the bowel disorder must therefore be determined by questioning. It is particularly important to detect a change in the individual's normal pattern of defaecation – whether it be towards diarrhoea or constipation, or alternation of both. Whenever possible, direct examination of a fresh stool should be made in every patient with diarrhoea: this is one of many useful findings at out-patient sigmoidoscopy (p. 44).

The causes of diarrhoea (see also p. 22) can be broadly grouped as:

1. Bacterial infection or parasitic infestation. This includes blind loop syndrome and gastro-colic fistula. (Chapter 15).
2. Inflammatory bowel disease (Chapter 10).
3. Neoplastic disease (Chapter 9).
4. Malabsorption (Chapter 7).

5. Drugs.
6. Disorders of motility.

This is a very broad group ranging from nervous tension before an examination to the effects of truncal vagotomy, and hormonal imbalance (thyrotoxicosis, Zollinger – Ellison syndrome). In many patients diarrhoea is a symptom of the irritable bowel syndrome. It should be remembered that the patient with faecal impaction complains of diarrhoea (see below).

Constipation (Table 2.1) is exceptionally difficult to define and many patients worry excessively about the sluggishness of their bowels when in fact they are perfectly healthy. In some of these, purgative abuse can be a problem. A careful history is of particular importance in assessing the true situation. The relatively sudden onset of constipation in a previously regular pattern of defaecation is always significant and suggests some mechanical narrowing of the bowel. This can be elucidated by thorough investigation. The hypothyroid patient is usually very constipated.

In the young and the elderly, faecal impaction can cause a confusing picture. Faeces accumulate in the rectum until a large semi-solid mass distends the whole rectum. The sensation of rectal fullness appears to be suppressed and all that these patients complain of is diarrhoea and soiling. Loose faeces often leak from the anus and the true diagnosis is immediately evident on rectal examination. Digital evacuation of the rectum (in children under anaesthesia) must be followed by an energetic and prolonged regime of diet, and regular laxatives to prevent recurrence.

Weight change

This can be highly significant: wherever possible, objective information should be obtained because patients' impressions can be very misleading.

Jaundice

Perhaps more a sign than a symptom, past episodes of jaundice may be of great significance. Jaundice due to gallstones is usually associated with pain, whereas pain is quite often unnoticed in neoplastic biliary tract obstruction. The jaundice of virus hepatitis is usually preceded by several days of malaise and anorexia, so the circumstances surrounding an attack of jaundice are very important. The pruritus of cholestatic jaundice is an important additional symptom. (See Chapter 8.)

Drug-induced symptoms

Many drugs induce gastrointestinal side-effects: e.g. nausea and vomiting (digoxin); constipation (opiates); diarrhoea (antibiotics); bleeding (aspirin); and jaundice (phenothiazines). It is therefore most important that a full drug history is taken.

Physical Signs

One of the advantages of taking a full history is that it gives the doctor an opportunity to observe the patient. Learning something of the patient's personality and outlook can be of great significance in management. Appearance and behaviour can provide a wealth of physical signs. Thus, the patient with peritonitis is anxious and tense and lies very still; the patient with intestinal colic has spells of restlessness and pain; the patient who has had a major alimentary tract haemorrhage will be pale and sweaty, and there may be the unmistakable odour of melaena around the bed.

Temperature, pulse and blood-pressure recordings are of great importance in abdominal emergencies, and recognition of the characteristic deep rapid acidotic respirations may give a warning that acute abdominal pain is connected with diabetic ketosis rather than a surgical emergency.

A full physical examination is not a matter of routine but an essential part of physical assessment. Cardiac, respiratory, neurological, urological and haematological diseases can all present with abdominal complaints and complications, so it would be a serious error to concentrate attention on the abdomen, important as that is.

Inspection of the abdomen (Fig. 3.3) is rewarding. The abdominal wall should rise and fall with respiration and any distension or visible mass is

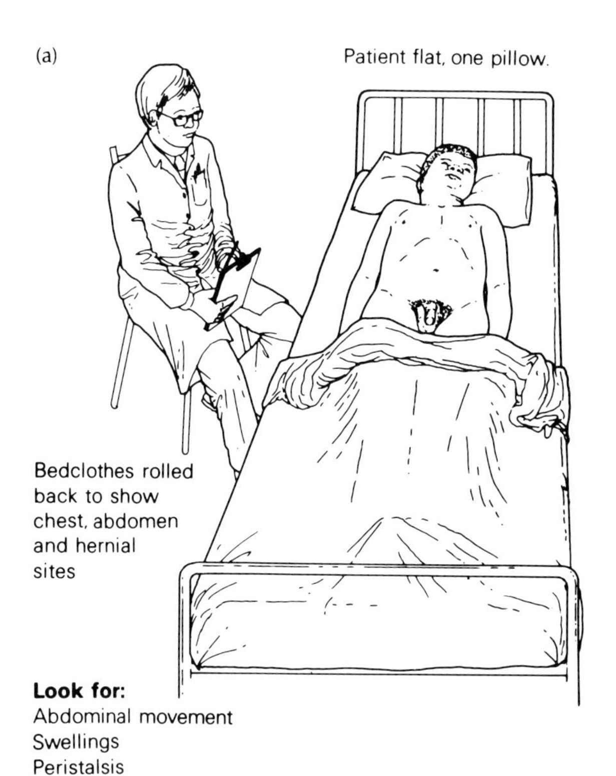

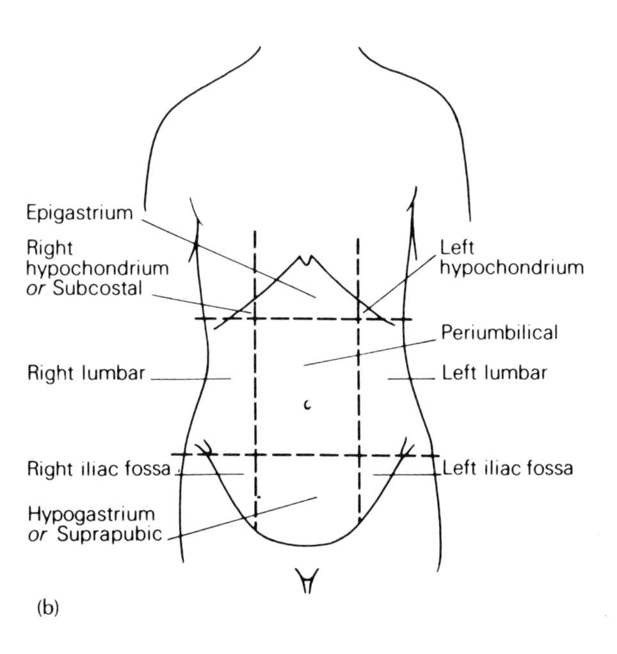

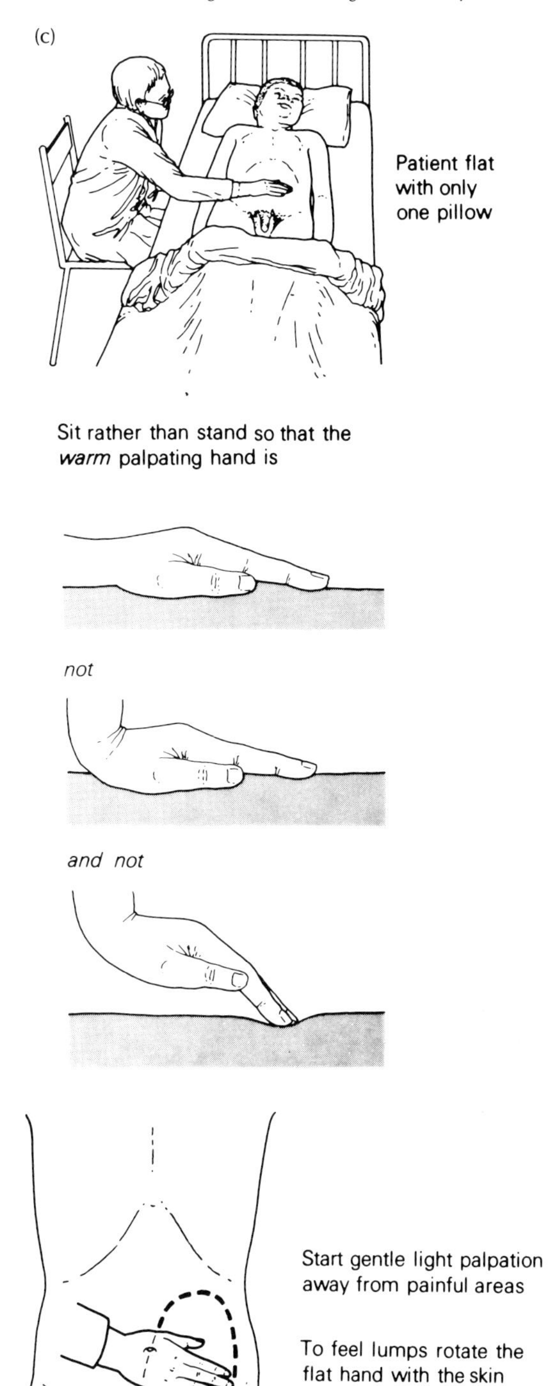

Palpation.

Fig. 3.3 *Examination of the abdomen. (a) Inspection. (b) Anatomical regions. (c) Palpation.*

(d)

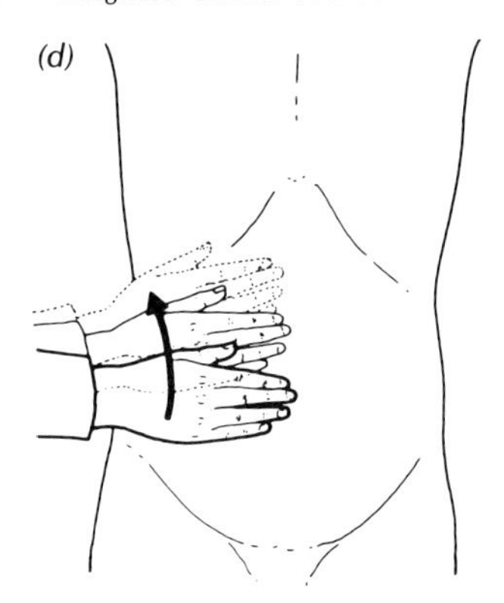

Start *low* over the right iliac fossa, and move upwards, hand parallel to costal margin

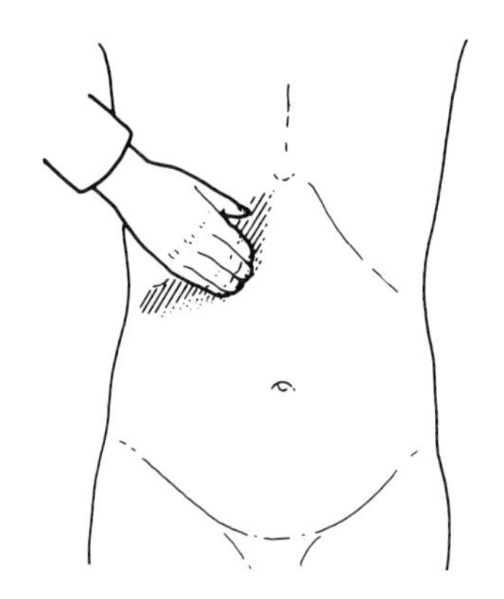

It is helpful to palpate across the costal margin and flex fingers around the liver edge, feeling it descend on inspiration

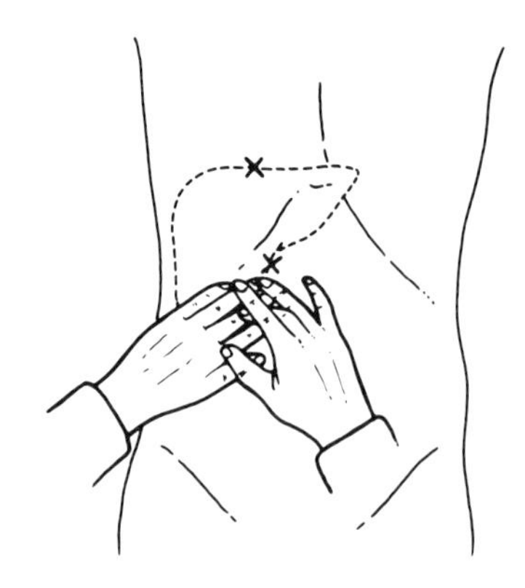

Always confirm liver size by percussing *upper* as well as lower edges of dullness

(e)

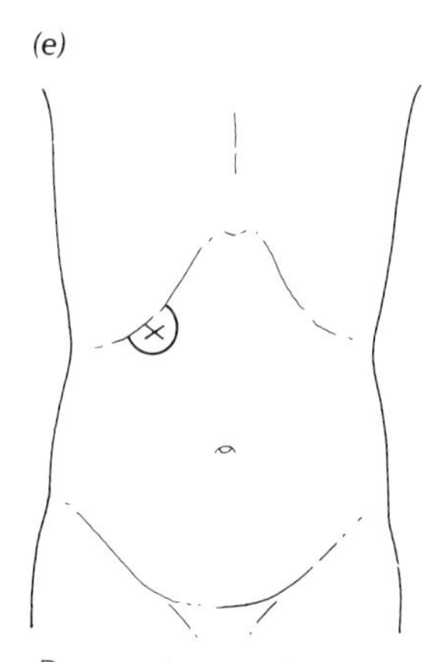

Deep under costal margin, on deep respiration, only felt if distended

(f)

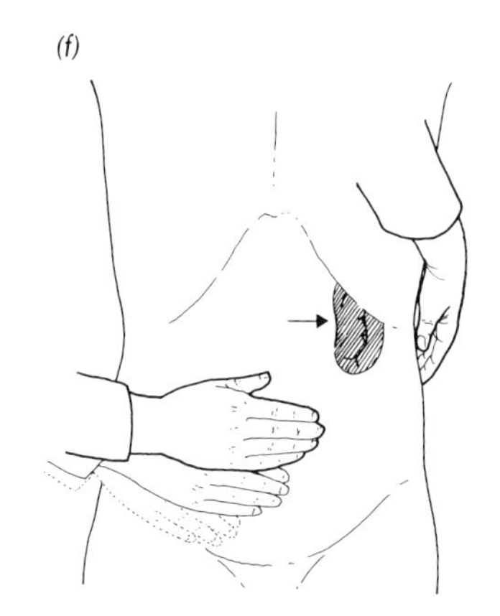

Start palpating at umbilical level, or lower
Most large spleens have a palpable notch
Moves on respiration
Left hand in loin may help

(g)

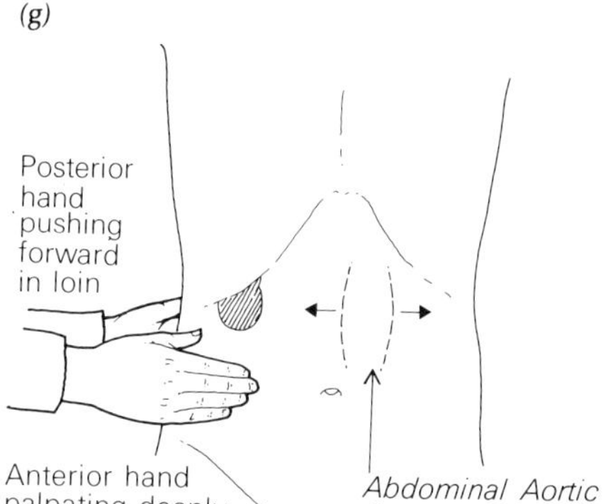

In most people the normal kidney is not palpable. It may be felt when — it lies low
— the patient is thin

Usually epigastric
Pulsatile and *expansile*

Fig. 3.3 contd.
(d) Examination of liver. (e) Examination of gall bladder. (f) Examination of spleen. (g) Examination of kidneys and aorta.

noted. If there is a history of copious vomiting, look for visible peristalsis. Occasionally loud peristaltic noises (borborygmi) are audible and always need further investigation. Careful *palpation* is essential (see p. 277). Palpation can discover or define masses, localise areas of tenderness, and demonstrate enlargements of liver, spleen or kidneys. *Auscultation* can pick up the vital signs of obstructive bowel sounds or an arterial bruit. *Percussion* is of great help in deciding whether abdominal distension is due to gas, fluid or enlargement of an organ. A fluid thrill or careful demonstration of the sign of shifting dullness will establish the presence of ascites (Fig. 3.4). A large central swelling of the lower abdomen will be dull if it is due to distension of the bladder or an ovarian cyst or a pregnancy, and resonance will then be found out in the flanks. (Fig. 3.5). Percussion can be of considerable help in determining the size of the liver and the spleen.

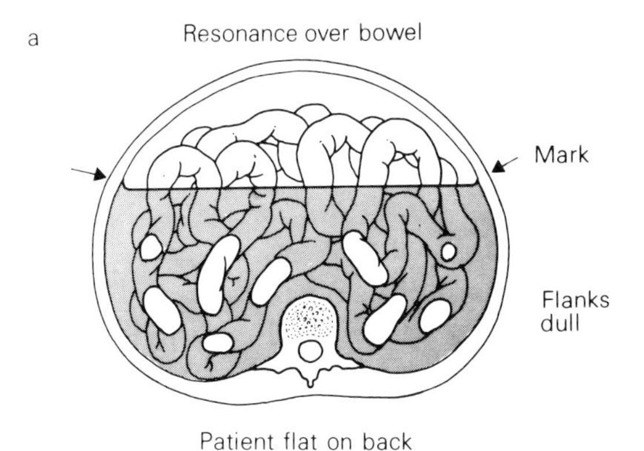

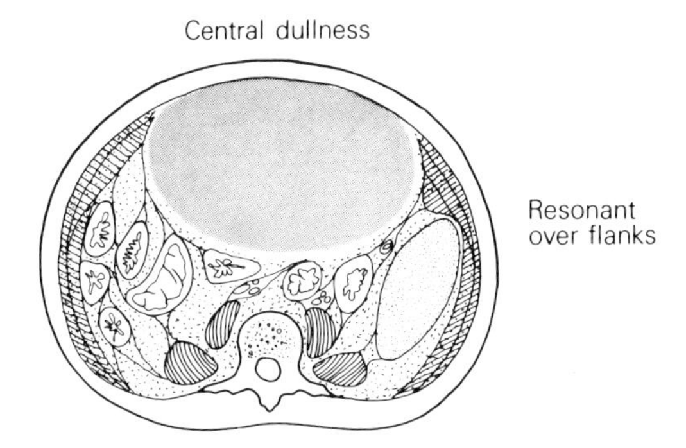

Fig. 3.5 *Signs of a full bladder or an ovarian cyst.*

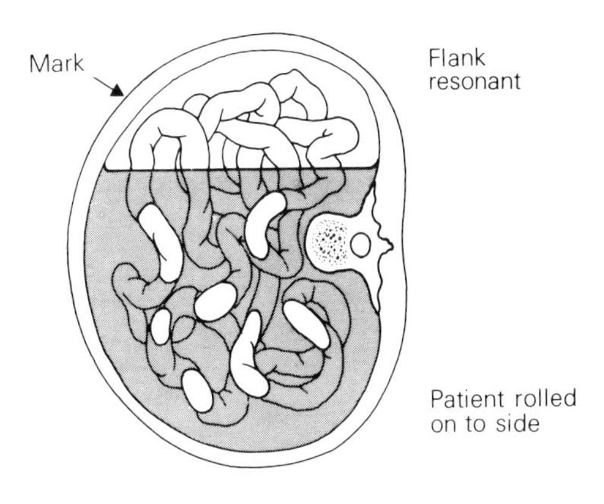

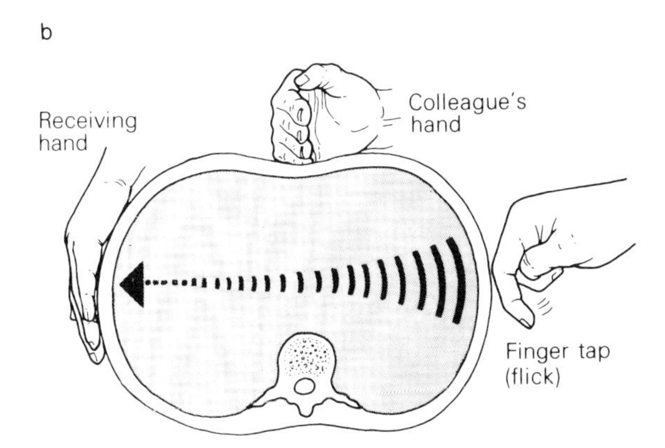

Fig. 3.4 *Signs of free fluid. (a) Shifting dullness. (b) Fluid thrill.*

No examination of the abdomen is complete without inspection and palpation of the inguinal and femoral hernial sites (Fig. 3.6).

Inguinal hernia

This can be seen at any age and in both sexes but, throughout life, it is much commoner in the male, whose inguinal canal has to transmit the spermatic cord. In babies, children and young adults, an inguinal hernia is due to persistent patency of the processus vaginalis (Fig. 3.7). If this has not closed by the time of birth it is not likely to close thereafter, and the appearance of an inguinal hernia in a baby is an indication for dissection of the sac from the spermatic cord and ligation of the neck of the sac – inguinal herniotomy. Inguinal herniae in babies under one year of age are especially likely to strangulate, so they should be operated on without delay. Later in life, inguinal herniae are more likely to be acquired. They may then be oblique (indirect), passing down the whole length of the inguinal canal, or direct, which means that the hernia has passed directly through a weakness in the posterior wall of the inguinal canal, medial to the inferior epigastric vessels, and pushed its way forward to emerge through the external abdominal ring (Fig. 3.8). Operative repair is usually advised, with only a few unfit patients being consigned to wearing a truss.

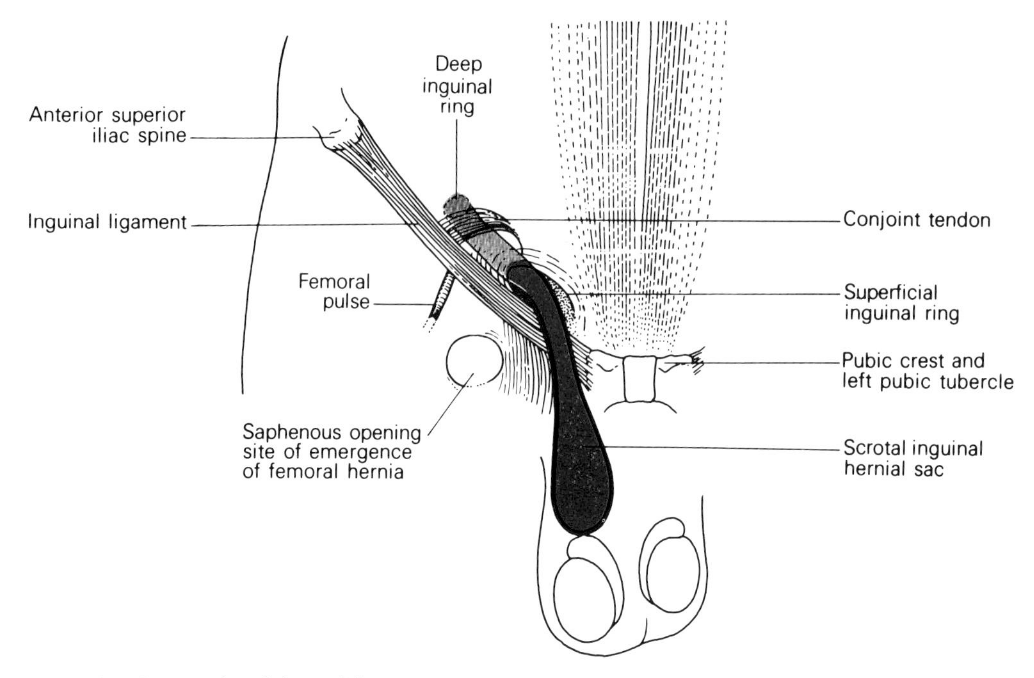

Fig. 3.6 *Landmarks of inguinal and femoral herniae.*

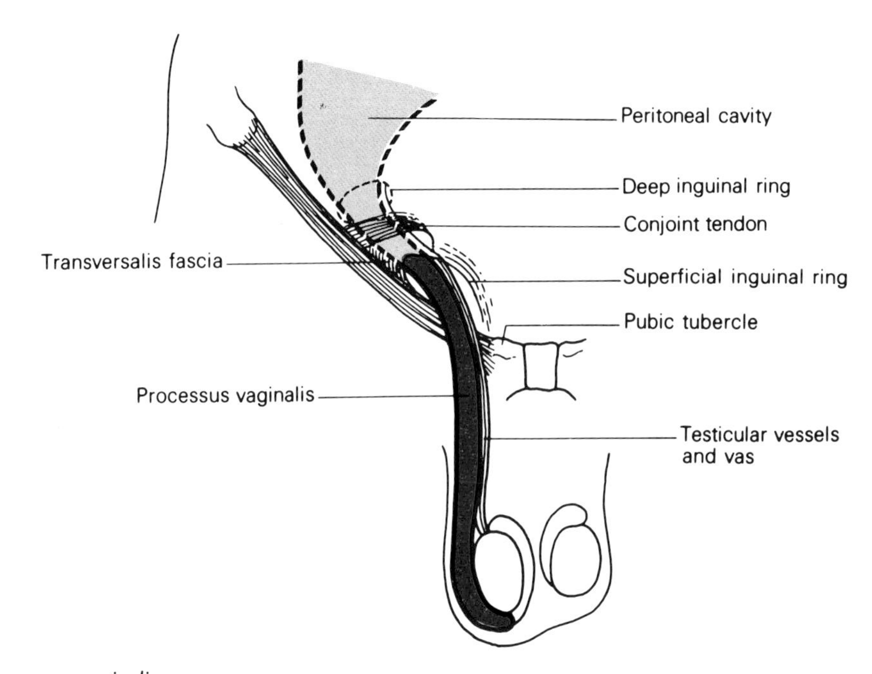

Fig. 3.7 *The processus vaginalis.*

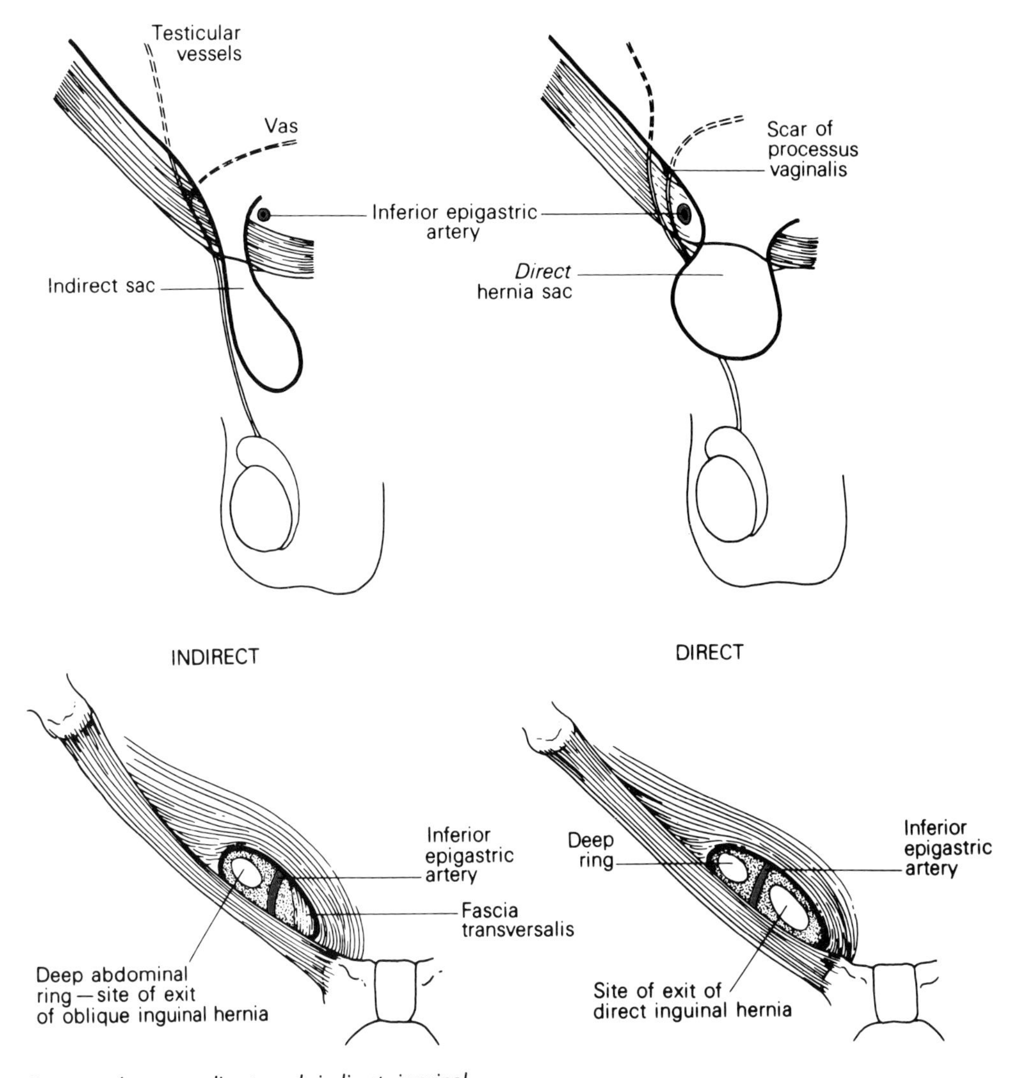

Fig. 3.8 *Differences between direct and indirect inguinal herniae.*

Femoral herniae

These are hardly ever seen in childhood, are rare in young adults and, after about the age of 40, are seen three times more often in women than in men. They cause few problems until strangulation occurs: one-third of femoral herniae present in this way, so all femoral herniae should be repaired as soon as possible unless the patient is quite unfit for operation.

In the early stages of development a femoral hernia will be impalpable, but as soon as the peritoneal sac has made its way down the femoral canal and turned forwards to emerge through the saphenous ring it will become palpable as a small bulge lying below the line of the inguinal ligament (Fig. 3.9).

It is important to be able to distinguish inguinal from femoral herniae; to do this, the line of the inguinal ligament must be established (Fig. 3.6). It is easy to find its lateral insertion, which is the anterior superior iliac spine, but some care is

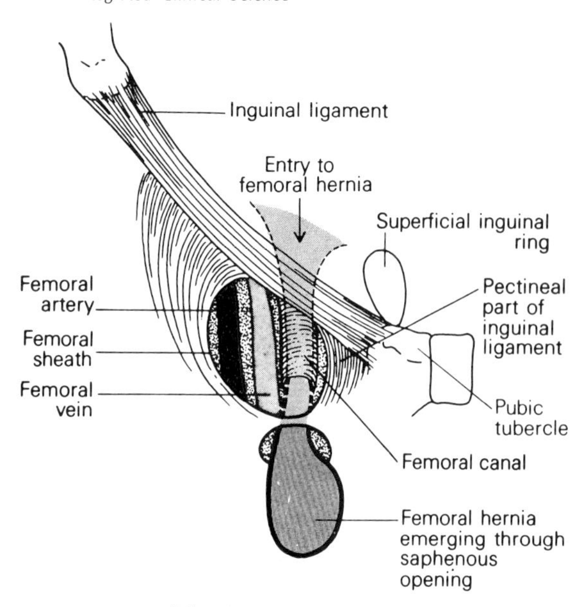

Fig. 3.9 *Femoral hernia.*

needed to find its medial point of attachment at the pubic tubercle. This is most easily done by palpating the pubic crest in the midline and then following its upper edge laterally until a bony prominence is felt at its lateral end. This is the pubic tubercle. The external abdominal ring lies immediately above and lateral to this point and in the male both tubercle and ring can be easily felt by gently invaginating the skin of the scrotum with the index finger: if a cough impulse is felt at the external abdominal ring then the patient has an inguinal hernia. If the lump and the cough impulse lie clearly below and slightly lateral to the pubic tubercle then the patient has a femoral hernia. If the position of the pubic tubercle is clearly established by palpation, it is generally not difficult to decide whether a patient has an inguinal or a femoral hernia: the patient usually needs to be examined both lying down and standing. When femoral hernia is diagnosed repair is fairly urgent because of the risk of strangulation.

Umbilical hernia

A true umbilical hernia is seen only in babies in whom the umbilical cicatrix has failed to close completely (Fig. 3.10). These herniae usually disappear by continued contraction of the ring of fibrous tissue at the umbilicus during the first 12–18 months of life; only a few need to be closed by operation.

Para-umbilical herniae

Usually seen in obese elderly people, these commence as a fatty hernia of the linea alba, close to the umbilical scar but not through it (Fig. 3.11). Coughing and straining pushes more fat through the defect and finally a protrusion of peritoneum occurs which, when large, often contains transverse colon as well as small bowel and omentum. The main danger of this hernia is strangulation, which is especially serious if it involves the colon because of the high risk of sepsis.

Diaphragmatic hernia

This very important form of concealed abdominal herniation is considered in Chapter 13.

Rectal and vaginal examination

These vital parts of physical examination of the

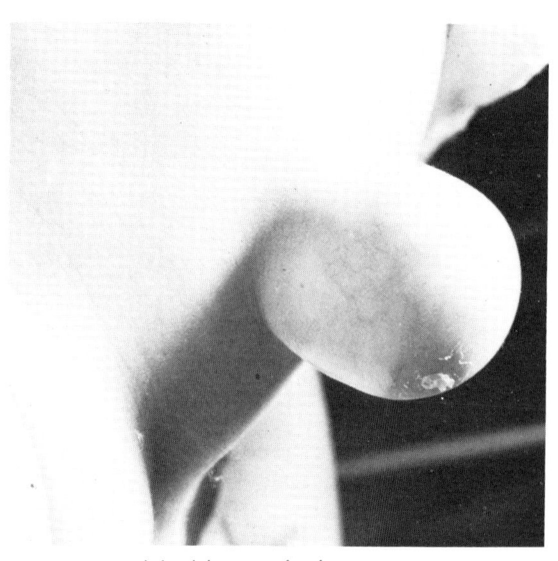

Fig. 3.10 *Umbilical hernia of infancy.*

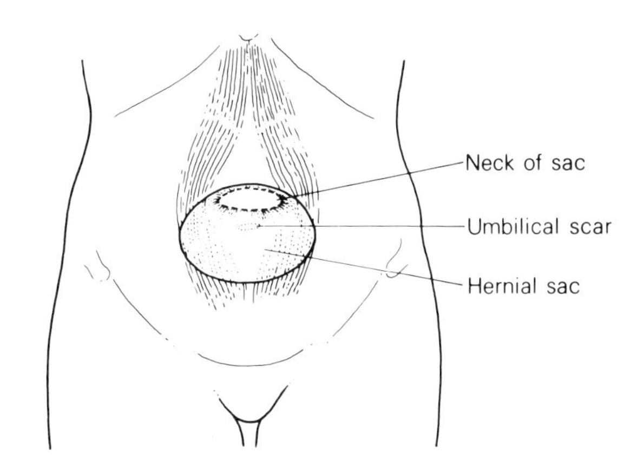

Fig. 3.11 *Para-umbilical hernia: note divaricated recti.*

abdomen not only allow detection of abnormalities of the vagina or rectum but provide access to the pelvis, which is beyond the reach of abdominal palpation. They are essential elements of a complete bedside assessment. Inspection of the anus may show prolapsed haemorrhoids, or an anal fissure or fistula (Chapter 11). The general appearance of the anus may give a vital clue to the diagnosis of Crohn's disease (Chapter 10).

Digital examination of the rectum can give information both about the rectum and the pelvic contents. This is always an uncomfortable examination and the comments of some patients are a warning to everyone to recognise how vividly some people remember previous experiences. At the same time, most patients recognise that this is a necessary examination, especially if a brief explanation is given. For right-handed examiners it is best to have the patient in the left lateral position with the buttocks at the edge of the couch or bed. This is not a dignified position for anybody and the patient is helped if the buttocks and thighs are covered with a blanket.

The modern disposable glove made of very thin plastic film is easily donned. Lubricate the right index finger well with KY jelly, separate the buttocks with the left hand, and make a careful inspection of the anal region. Then draw the extended index finger gently over the anus several times before placing the pulp of the distal phalanx over the anus and exerting gradual increasing pressure, while flexing the distal interphalangeal joint. The anus will tend to relax (unless pathologically tight due to fissure or stricture) and the whole length of the flexed index finger can be introduced without much discomfort. Gently rotate the finger so that all the rectal wall within reach of the finger is palpated – in this way benign or malignant neoplasms of the lower rectum can be identified. Then turn attention to the extrarectal structures which can be felt through the rectal wall. Anteriorly, in the male is the prostate and in the female the cervix. Above these structures lies the recto-vesical or recto-vaginal peritoneal pouch (Fig. 3.12). This is an important extension of the peritoneal cavity because an inflamed pelvic appendix can lie within it – far from the anterior abdominal wall and only accessible to rectal examination. Sometimes a carcinoma in the sigmoid colon, or an ovarian neoplasm, can be felt lying in the pouch. In general peritonitis or intraperitoneal haemorrhage, pus or blood will lie in the pouch, and pressure upon it with the rectal finger will produce pain. In ectopic pregnancy, palpation over the cervix is characteristically exceptionally painful.

For vaginal examination the patient is usually

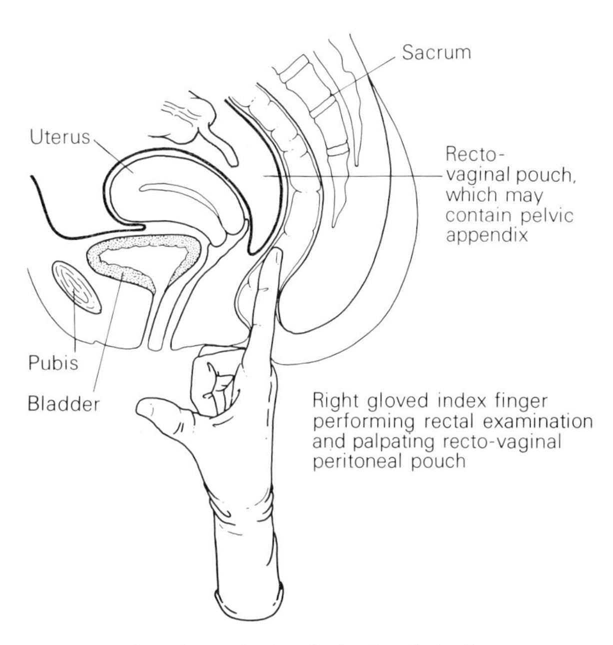

Fig. 3.12 *Rectal examination in the female (peritoneum outlined in red).*

examined in the left lateral position. The important results of this examination for the gastroenterologist are that some uterine and overian swellings present with abdominal complaints, and pelvic abscesses in the female are particularly easily detected on vaginal examination.

Proctoscopy

This is the only way in which most haemorrhoids can be visualised. It is carried out with a short internally-illuminated tube which, with its obturator in place, is passed through the anal canal so that the tip lies in the lower rectum. The obturator is withdrawn and the light cable attached. The whole length of the anal canal can be inspected as the instrument is slowly withdrawn (Fig. 3.13). If the patient is asked to strain, internal haemorrhoids will bulge into view and fibrous polyps of the anal canal will be seen; in the case of third-degree haemorrhoids, they will be seen to prolapse outside the anus as the proctoscope is withdrawn.

Injection of haemorrhoids (p. 249) is carried out through a proctoscope.

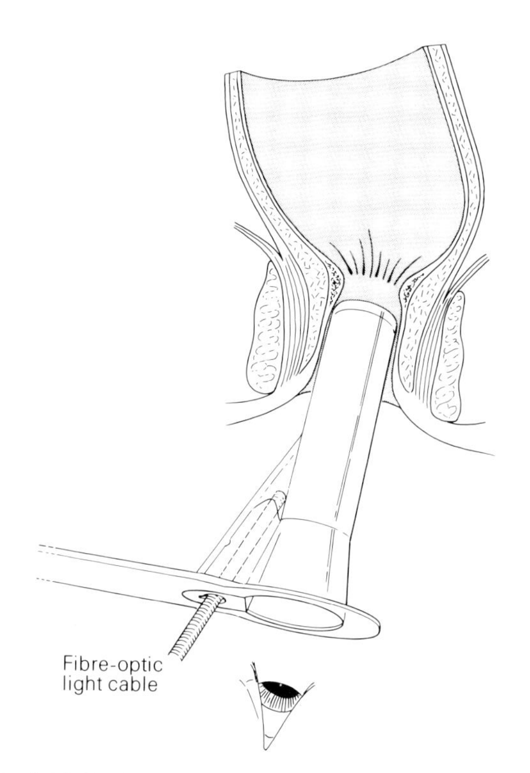

Fig. 3.13 *Proctoscopy.*

Sigmoidoscopy

This is a vital part of out-patient examination of the patient with rectal symptoms. It is a mistake to think that the rectum should be prepared for sigmoidoscopy. It is much more valuable to pass a small (1.5 cm diameter) sigmoidoscope on the first attendance of the patient in the clinic, because this allows a view of the unprepared rectum – traces of blood and stool may be seen which are valuable clues that would otherwise be washed away.

Gently performed, this should not be an unduly uncomfortable examination. The patient lies in the left lateral position with the buttocks over the side of the couch. After introducing the sigmoidoscope through the anal canal, the obturator is removed and the telescope attached. The rest of the examination is performed under visual control, the sigmoidoscope barrel being moved to follow the

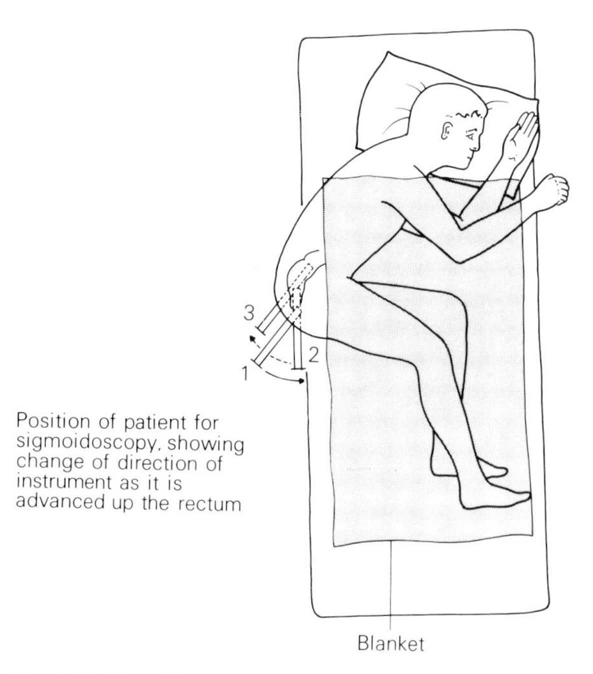

Fig. 3.14 *Sigmoidoscopy.*

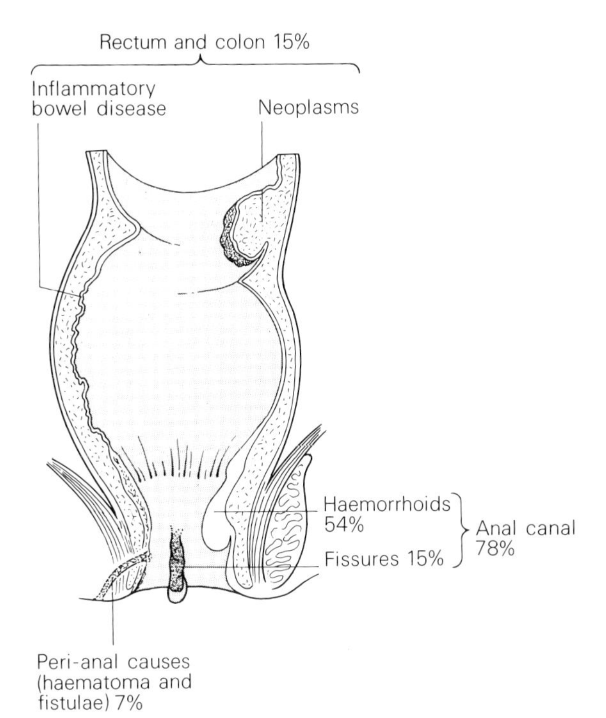

Fig. 3.15 *Relative frequency of common causes of anorectal bleeding. The remaining 9% with bleeding from anal canal were thought to be constipated.*

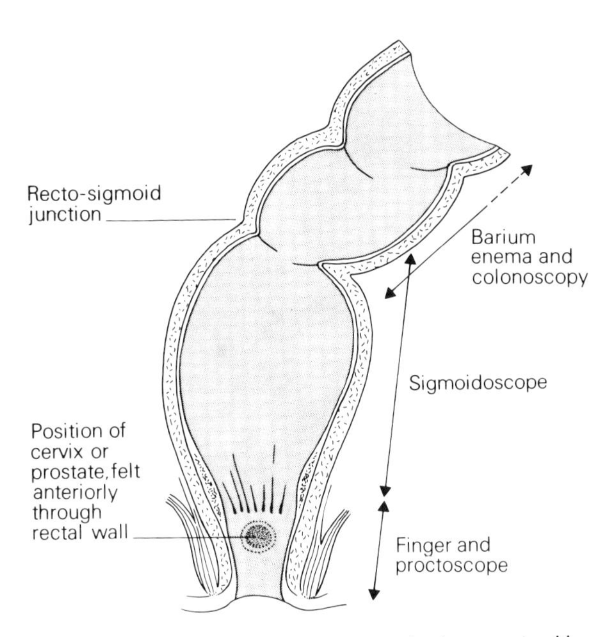

Fig. 3.16 *Areas of anal canal, rectum and colon examined by finger and by endoscopy.*

curves of the rectum and sigmoid. Being a rigid tube, the sigmoidoscope cannot always pass the rectosigmoid bend, when this is an acute angle, but often much of the sigmoid can be inspected (Fig. 3.14).

In at least four out of every five patients complaining of rectal bleeding, the origin can be established during the first out-patient visit by careful inspection of the perianal area, with digital, proctoscopic and sigmoidoscopic examinations (Fig. 3.15). In about 10% of patients, further investigation by barium enema (and sometimes by colonoscopy) will be needed to establish the source of bleeding, because it lies further up the colon, beyond the range of the sigmoidoscope (Fig. 3.16).

INVESTIGATIVE TECHNIQUES

While important clinical decisions can be made solely on the basis of history and bedside signs – in some instances they may, indeed, have to be, e.g. in the acute abdomen – gastroenterology depends as much as other specialties upon supplementary tests. These fall into four groups:

i. Tests of structure.
ii. Tests of function.
iii. Tests of inflammation or injury.
iv. Specific disease indicators.

Some tests of structure and function are more discriminant than others, and by and large the more discriminant are also the more uncomfortable or invasive. X-rays have played, and continue to play, a central role in alimentary disease, but two major advances in 1960s and 70s have revolutionised gastroenterology. The first, an extension of radiology, is the emergence of scanning techniques, ultrasonic, radionuclide and computer-assisted tomographic. The second is the development of fibre-optic systems, allowing direct visualisation of the gut virtually throughout its extent. A lateral development, or spin-off, from these advances is 'interventional radiology' and 'interventional endoscopy', i.e. the adaptation of the techniques for therapeutic purposes.

Tests of Structure

Radiology

X-rays are important in both acute and chronic disease, in all parts of the gut, from pharynx to anus, and the biliary tract (less so in liver and pancreatic disease), and in all severities of disease.

Plain abdominal x-rays. These are often underrated. They are an essential for all hospital admissions with abdominal pain, vomiting or diarrhoea. In episodic acute abdominal pain, the importance of erect and supine films taken during an attack of pain cannot be overemphasised.

In general, plain x-rays give three types of information, both radio-opaque and radiolucent:

i. *Calcification* may be seen in stones, both biliary (about 10–20% of gallstones are radio-opaque) and renal (about 80–90% of renal calculi are radio-opaque). Calcium is sometimes seen in chronic pancreatitis and in hydatid cysts in the liver. It also occurs in the lower abdomen and pelvis in some ovarian cysts, calcified fibroids, and (harmless) phleboliths and calcified lymph nodes.

ii. *Soft-tissue shadows* may be useful in showing hepatomegaly, splenomegaly and tumour masses. Fluid (ascites) shows as a 'ground-glass' haziness throughout the abdomen. Foreign bodies are occasionally seen.

iii. *Radiolucent gas shadows* may give crucial information. Gastric dilatation shows as a mixed radiolucent/radio-opaque picture. Absence of the normal gas bubble in the fundus of the stomach suggests achalasia. Some small-bowel gas is normal. When excessive, as in obstructed bowel, dilated loops may be seen (see p. 280). In such cases it is essential for the radiographer to obtain erect as well as supine films, when fluid levels may be visible. Similar fluid levels may also occur in gastro enteritis. A characteristic 'sentinel' loop of small bowel may be visible in pancreatitis. Similarly, inflammatory lesions such as appendicitis and abscess may be revealed by small tell-tale loops or one or two fluid levels. Dilatation of large bowel occurs in severe inflammatory bowel disease (see p. 221) and in obstruction, as by carcinoma (see p. 295) or intussusception. A characteristic loop occurs in sigmoid volvulus (see p. 297) Gross dilatation occurs in megacolon and Hirschprung's disease (see p. 265). Faecal stasis is visible in severe constipation.

Free gas in the peritoneum (see p. 280) follows perforation of a viscus, such as duodenum or stomach in peptic ulcer, or colon in inflammatory bowel disease. This is seen best in an erect film, beneath the diaphragm on one or other side. Gas may, alternatively, track upwards in retroperitoneal spaces and even into the mediastinum.

Contrast radiology. Contrast materials can be used to outline the alimentary lumen, biliary and pancreatic ducts, fistulae, and arteriovenous systems.

Luminal Contrast Radiology. Two contrast media are used:

Barium sulphate is a radio-dense material which can be refined to be of low viscosity and low flocculation.

Diatrozoate methylglucamine (Gastrografin) is an iodinated liquid giving poor contrast pictures, but is safe to use where perforation of a viscus or intestinal obstruction are suspected. Its high osmotic effect can cause dehydration, especially in tiny infants, and it is highly irritant to the lungs, causing pulmonary oedema, so it should not be used in patients with dysphagia.

Barium swallow and meal. A barium swallow (using thick barium) is useful for outlining the oesophagus, identifying strictures, tumours, or external compression, and for assessing motility. Since oesophageal problems often arise or are associated with gastroduodenal disease, a 'barium swallow' is rarely, if ever, indicated without an accompanying 'barium meal'. As with all contrast radiology, skilled screening is essential. Where neuromuscular disorders are suspected, especially at pharyngeal level, a cine film or videotape is very helpful to allow slowed-down replay and analysis of motility. Deep inspiration or a valsalva manoeuvre are required to demonstrate varices (see p. 321). Tipping may be used to demonstrate hiatal incompetence (e.g. a hiatus hernia). In pharyngeal lesions, aspiration of barium is a risk.

The barium meal x-ray can be improved by adding a gas-forming tablet or liquid to the thin barium. This leads to distension of the stomach (and duodenum) and light coating of the wall with barium, which produces a 'double contrast' picture (Fig. 5.2). Irregularities of the mucosa and rugae, small polyps, larger tumours and ulcer craters should all be visualised. Producing atony or 'paralysis' by an injection of hyoscine butylbromide (Buscopan) or glucagon may help, especially in the duodenum. In addition to intrinsic defects, external displacement or compression, e.g. by an enlarged liver or pancreas, should be readily seen.

Barium meal and endoscopy. There is no doubt that endoscopic examination in upper alimentary disease is diagnostically superior to x-ray in virtually all respects, especially since it allows direct vision and biopsy. However, a barium meal is more convenient, is less invasive (and has virtually no risks), involves no time-consuming sedation, and is available almost everywhere. It also has the added advantage over endoscopy of demonstrating motility disorders and extrinsic displacement. The cost of the two procedures is closely comparable.

Barium 'follow-through' examination. Either during a standard barium meal or, preferably, as a separate exercise (using a smaller quantity of barium), the contrast may be followed in its transit through the small bowel. A non-specific malabsorption pattern (clumping and flocculation) may be seen, or tumours and ulcers in the wall be shown up. It is of value in patients with suspected malabsorption and in recurrent (but not acute) small bowel obstruction (Fig. 7.20). The quality of the picture may be improved by a double contrast technique, injecting barium followed by air through a tube passed (under screening) into the duodenum – the so-called 'small bowel enema' (see Fig. 7.21). Neither of these techniques is of any value for assessing the colon.

Barium enema. In this technique the colon and terminal ileum are demonstrated by barium run in through a catheter placed in the rectum (usually with a retaining balloon). There are two important caveats:

a. Since the barium enema x-ray is *not* an adequate demonstration of the rectum, procto-sigmoidoscopy should *precede* x-ray in all but exceptional circumstances.
b. Perforation of the bowel is a risk especially in fulminant colitis, toxic dilatation and diverticulitis.

Hence, most x-ray departments wisely restrict barium enema requisition to hospital consultants and not general practitioners (barium meal is available to practitioners in most British regions).

Again, a double contrast or air contrast technique greatly enhances the value of a barium enema examination.

Adequate preparation to produce a clean colon is essential and, except in inflammatory disease, involves laxatives and cleansing enemas. The whole procedure is usually uncomfortable and, for frail or elderly patients, quite exhausting.

Polyps, tumours, diverticula and the changes of inflammatory bowel disease are the principal abnormalities detectable.

Biliary contrast radiology. All the biliary contrast materials are iodine-containing compounds excreted, like bilirubin, almost exclusively in bile (a little renal excretion may also be seen). Oral compounds include sodium ipodate (Biloptin), ipanoic acid (Telepaque), and iocetamic acid (Cholebrin). Ingestion is preceded by plain abdominal films in case calcified stones are present. Side-effects are commonly mild. Intravenous agents (e.g. meglumine ioglycamate) are essential if visualisation of the bile ducts is required, but side effects can be severe and occasionally fatal (anaphylaxis) and they have to a considerable extent been replaced by newer techniques (see p. 173).

The indications and use of biliary contrast radiology, including the direct technique of percutaneous cholangiography and endoscopic retrograde cholangiography, are described below and in Chapter 8. Ultrasonography has had a significant impact on biliary radiology; it should be considered in cases where there is doubtful cholecystography or when normal x-rays are obtained in a patient with a very typical history; it is the first investigation of choice in obstructive jaundice.

Arteriography. Arterial contrast x-rays are occasionally used to outline the hepatic, pancreatic or mesenteric vessels. Indications include hepatic space-occupying lesions of uncertain nature, suspected vascular anomalies (e.g. angiodysplasia), ischaemic disease of the gut and, occasionally, pancreatic tumours.

An important use is the detection of obscure bleeding in the colon or small bowel. If blood-loss is continuing faster than 1–2 ml/minute, the area of bleeding may be identifiable, but this means that a time-consuming x-ray must be performed in an ill patient and requires special apparatus and considerable skill; it is therefore most commonly effective in enthusiastic centres. The approach is retrograde via the femoral artery, using a Seldinger type catheter (threaded through a direct stab cannula), and may be carried out under local or general anaesthetic (see p. 319).

Imaging techniques

A variety of techniques have been developed during the 60s and 70s which have complemented x-rays and greatly improved the diagnostic capacity of the clinician.

Computer-assisted tomography (CT). This is an extension of x-rays where paired x-ray tubes and photomultipliers are placed opposite each other and rotated, allowing multiple 'cuts' to be made of organs under vision. The subject must remain still. Contrast materials may be used to assist anatomical display. A computer builds up an image from the multiple recordings and selected areas can be shown by sequential display of individual tomographic slices.

CT scanning has considerably assisted in diagnosis of pancreatic disease, since the pancreas is singularly inaccessible to most diagnostic techniques; tumours, cysts and abscesses are commonly well seen. Tumours and lymph-node enlargement elsewhere in the abdomen are visible, and CT scanning has a useful place in the staging of lymphomas. The use of this technique in liver disease is discussed on p. 172. A major disadvantage of CT scanning is its high capital and running costs.

Radionuclide scanning. Imaging with isotopes is used especially in liver disease (p. 174) but also in pancreatic and alimentary disorders. Its use in diagnosis of pancreatic disease, where radioactive seleniomethionine is employed, has largely been abandoned because of difficulties in interpretation.

Imaging using technetium-labelled sulphur colloid has been used to demonstrate oesophageal function and gastric emptying. It can also be used to demonstrate a Meckel's diverticulum, where it is taken up by ectopic gastric mucosa in the diverticulum.

Use of radioactive Gallium citrate (^{67}Ga) can show up intra-abdominal lymph-node enlargement as well as abscesses.

Tagging of red cells with radioactive chromium can be used to detect sources of alimentary blood loss (p. 319).

Ultrasonic scanning. Ultrasound is a simple, safe, and relatively cheap technique that is now very widely used in the diagnosis of liver, pancreatic, biliary and alimentary tract disorders. It can be safely used repeatedly, even in pregnancy, and involves little or no discomfort to the patient. Its main disadvantage is the fairly high operator and observer dependency and much depends upon the skill and experience of those involved.

The technique is shown in Fig. 3.17. Ultrasound is the first line of investigation in the jaundiced patient (see p. 174) and is reasonably good at detecting intrahepatic parenchymal dis-

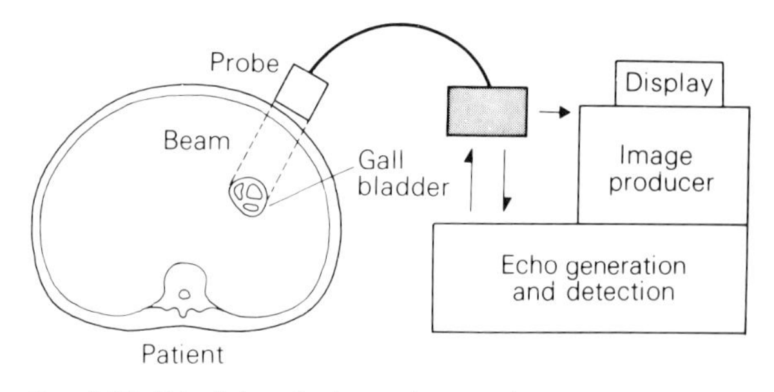

Fig. 3.17 *Principles of ultrasonic scanning.*

ease. The pancreas can often be demonstrated, as long as there is not too much intestinal gas, and its outline detected. Ultrasound is particularly useful in detecting and delineating intra-abdominal abscesses, e.g. in the pelvis and under the diaphragm, and is therefore particularly valuable in investigation of PUO and postoperative sepsis.

Fibre-optic endoscopy of the gastrointestinal tract

The rapid development in the past decade of flexible fibre-optic instruments for examination of the alimentary tract has greatly increased diagnostic accuracy. Moreover, the introduction of the fibre-optic gastroscope and colonoscope has undoubtedly been a powerful stimulus for radiologists to improve their techniques and in particular to use air-contrast in the radiological examination of the gut. Barium studies and fibre-optic examination of the gut are complementary. The information obtained by barium studies depends on several variables, including the skill and experience of the radiologist. Expertise and experience are just as necessary for accurate and reliable endoscopic examination. Usually barium studies precede endoscopic examination.

Glass fibres have the ability to allow total internal reflection of light, and therefore also of images (Fig. 3.18). This was a British discovery, and the instruments, which are produced in Japan and the USA, consist basically of two bundles of thousands of fine glass fibres. One flexible bundle transmits light from a special light source into the gut, and the other carries the image back to the observer's eye. Each instrument carries an air channel, to allow air distension of the gut and to allow the passage of a clearing jet of water (Fig. 3.19). In addition, a biopsy channel allows the passage of flexible forceps for biopsy under direct vision and, if required, cytological brushings may be taken through the same channel. Suction may be applied through these instruments to remove gut secretions or blood. More recently, further adaptations have allowed diathermy to be used (via the biopsy channel) under direct vision. A photographic attachment allows visual records to be kept for each patient. Because of anatomical considerations, it was initially necessary to have both end-viewing and side-viewing instruments to ensure complete visualisation of the oesophagus, stomach and duodenum. More recent modifications have, however, increased the fields of vision (Fig. 3.20) so that side-viewing instruments are only needed for specialised examinations such as ERCP (See below). In days of financial stringency this is an important consideration as these instruments are expensive to buy and repairs are costly. They must be carefully handled and meticulously cleaned after use.

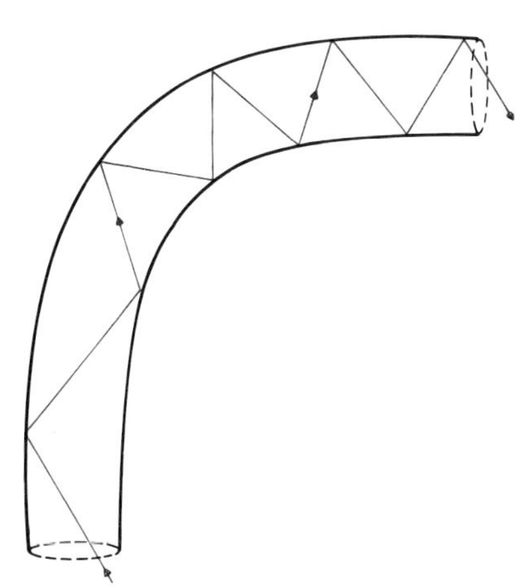

Fig. 3.18 *Principle of fibre-optics. Light entering each fibre is transmitted by repeated internal reflection. Each fibre is coated with glass of a lower optical density to prevent leakage of light.*

Endoscopy should be carried out by a trained doctor in purpose-built or adapted accommodation with the help of suitably trained nursing staff. The patient should be examined on a table which can be quickly tilted if required, and all the usual resuscitation equipment should be readily available.

Apart from the frail or very elderly, patients with advanced cardiorespiratory diseases, and people travelling from a distance, oesophago-gastro-duodenoscopy is usually performed on an out-patient basis. Before examination of the upper alimentary tract each patient is asked to fast from the previous evening. Next morning the patient reports to the endoscopist, who will usually have seen and examined the patient previously. The

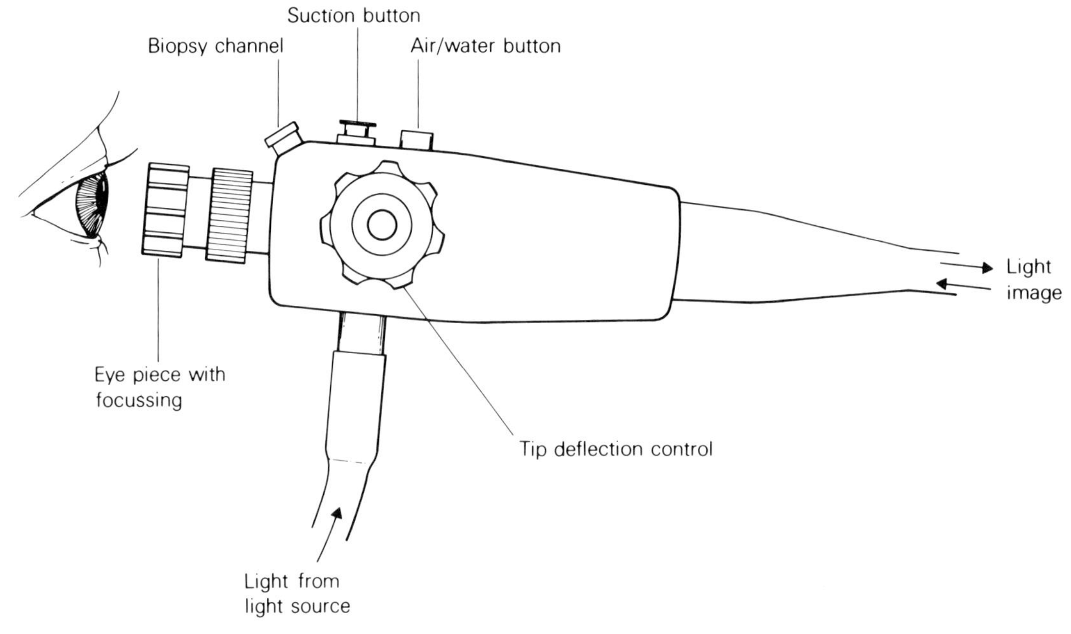

Fig. 3.19 *Controls of fibre-optic endoscope.*

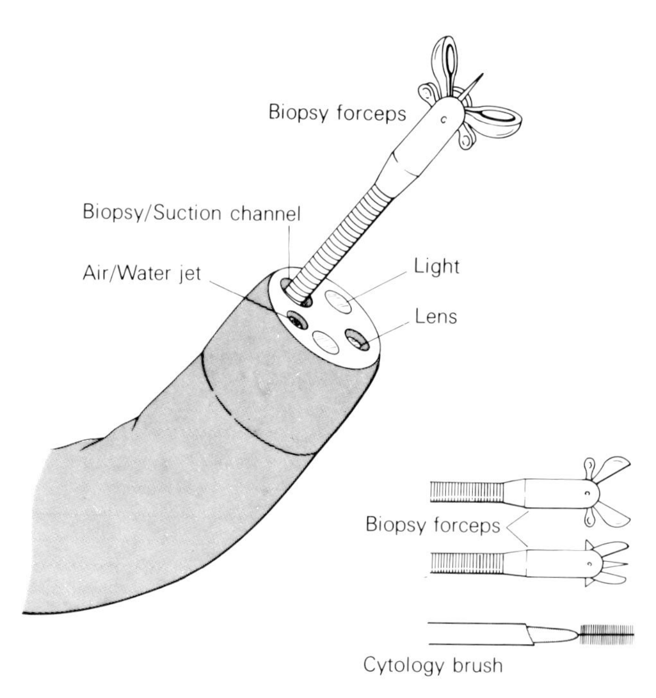

Fig. 3.20 *Distal end of a forward-viewing endoscope, with instruments which can be passed down the biopsy channel.*

nature of the examination is explained and the patient is reassured if necessary. Local anaesthetic is applied to the patient's oropharynx by spray and the patient is sedated using intravenous diazepam. The latter, if properly used, induces amnesia without hypnosis, allowing full patient cooperation throughout the examination. After the examination the patient is observed in a recovery area and is usually able to return home (accompanied) approximately 2 or 3 hours later.

For 2 days before *colonoscopy* the patient goes on a low residue/fluid diet. A laxative is taken on the evening before the examination, and on the day of the examination the bowel is thoroughly emptied by the administration of an enema (repeated if necessary). For a satisfactory examination the bowel preparation must be thorough. As well as sedation it may sometimes be necessary to use an analgesic (e.g. pethidine) to alleviate the discomfort produced by colonic distension. It is, however, usually possible to perform colonoscopy on an out-patient basis.

Although fibre-optic endoscopes have been adapted for therapeutic use, their principal value lies in diagnosis.

All patients who present with true dysphagia should proceed to endoscopy (usually preceded by barium swallow and meal examination). Most causes of dysphagia (see p. 59–68) are readily diagnosed by endoscopy and, most important, histological or cytological confirmation is obtained. Disorders of the pharynx may be more readily diagnosed by radiology or by direct pharyngoscopy. Because of the poor correlation between macroscopic appearances at endoscopy, histology of oesophageal biopsies, and the severity of a patient's symptoms, the fibre-optic endoscope has proved disappointing in the elucidation of oesophageal pain (see p. 58). Nevertheless all patients suspected of having oesophageal pain should proceed to endoscopy; the findings should be correlated with those of the barium meal, the acid perfusion test, and manometry (p. 59).

The value and limitations of fibre-optic endoscopy in gastrointestinal haemorrhage including laser- and electro-coagulation are considered in detail elsewhere (p. 326).

It is very rarely necessary to confirm the radiological diagnosis of a duodenal ulcer by endoscopy, but this examination is valuable in monitoring the healing of gastric ulcers and in the early diagnosis of gastric cancer (see p. 95). Fibre-optic endoscopy often correctly diagnoses patients whose symptoms suggest peptic ulcer disease but whose radiological studies are negative ('X-ray-negative dyspepsia': see Chapter 5).

Endoscopic retrograde cholangio-pancreatography (ERCP) is a technique carried out in specialist centres which is of value in the diagnosis of jaundice (see p. 173) and some pancreatic pathologies (see p. 107). The patient is prepared in the standard fashion for upper gastrointestinal endoscopy, and the examination is carried out on an x-ray table with screening facilities. The ampulla of Vater is identified and cannulated with a special

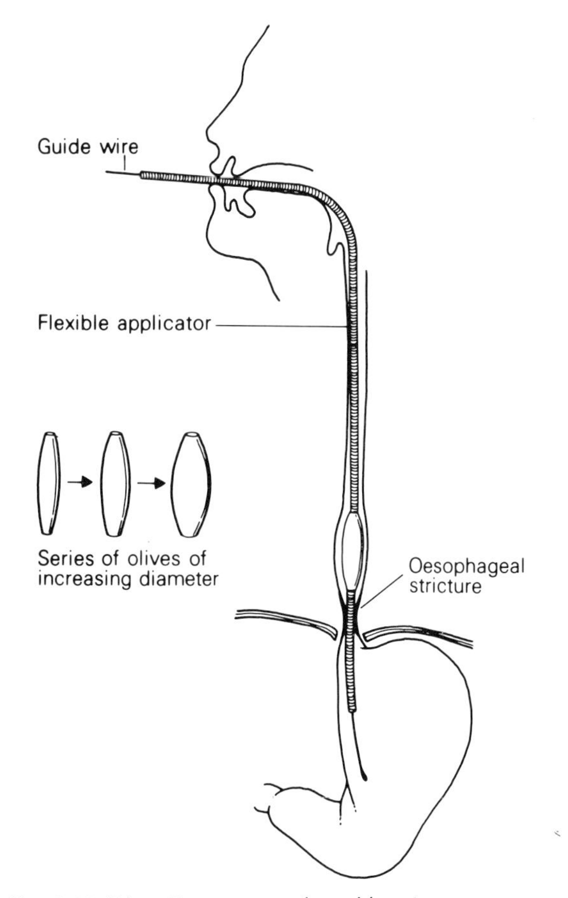

Fig. 3.21 *Eder – Puestow oesophageal bougies.*

tube passed down the biopsy channel, and the biliary system and the pancreatic ducts are visualised by the injection of contrast medium down the cannula.

The fibre-optic endoscope finds the following therapeutic applications in the upper alimentary tract:

1. *Sclerotherapy* for oesophageal varices (see p. 65).

2. *Bouginage of benign oesophageal stricture.* The endoscope is passed and the stricture identified. A fine wire is then passed down the biopsy channel and through the stricture. The endoscope is carefully withdrawn over the wire, leaving the wire *in situ*. A flexible applicator, onto whose end a series of 'olives' of increasing diameter may be screwed, is then threaded over the guide-wire and through the stricture (Fig. 3.21). Repeated gentle dilatation is then possible by gradually increasing the diameter of the olive passed. This procedure may be safely carried out under diazepam sedation, but in patients with very tight or high strictures it is best done under general anaesthetic.

3. *Sphincterotomy* (of the ampulla of Vater). Some patients with obstructive jaundice due to impaction of stones in the common bile duct are not fit for standard surgical treatment (p. 182). In some specialised centres it is now possible to widen the ampullary opening (sphincterotomy) using a special diathermy knife passed down the biopsy channel of the endoscope. It is then possible to introduce a collapsible basket device into the bile duct and extract the stone via the sphincterotomy. This procedure requires considerable skill and, as the patients in whom this procedure is carried out are usually frail, carries a definite mortality risk. Using the endoscope it is also possible to pass small prostheses through strictures in the common bile duct and relieve the distressing itch in obstructive jaundice (see p. 184).

The *colonoscope* is both a diagnostic and therapeutic instrument. It finds great value in providing histological confirmation of colonic lesions suspected of malignancy on barium enema examination. It provides a valuable method of both

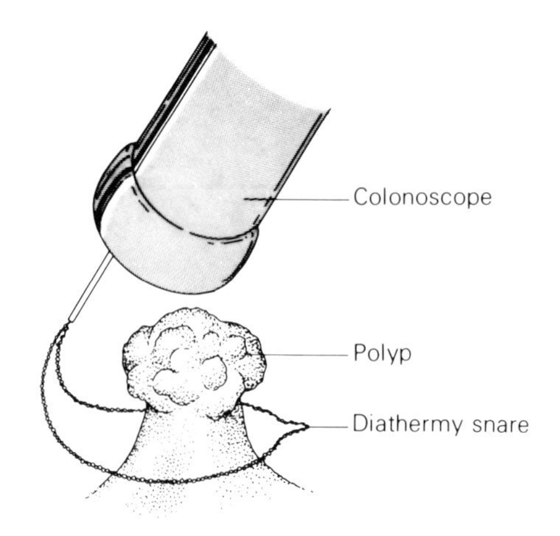

Fig. 3.22 *Diathermy removal of colonic polyp.*

establishing the extent of colonic involvement, and monitoring the progress, of patients with inflammatory bowel disease (p. 233). Its value in the diagnosis of the patient suspected of having colonic bleeding is described in Chapter 14. Colonoscopy is dangerous in patients with severe inflammatory bowel disease, because there is a real risk of perforating the badly diseased colon. Extensive diverticular disease of the colon (especially sigmoid) increases the risk of accidental perforation.

Colonoscopy finds its main therapeutic application in the removal of colonic polyps. The patient is prepared in the usual way, the whole of the colon is examined, and the situation of all polyps carefully identified. A diathermy loop ('snare') is then passed down the biopsy channel (Fig. 3.22), the polyps are snared and are then removed by diathermy after inflation with carbon dioxide.

Other investigative techniques, which vary very widely according to the system involved, include:

Tests of function
Tests of inflammation or injury
Specific disease indicators

These are more appropriately dealt with in the relevant chapters.

4

The Mouth, Pharynx, Tongue and Oesophagus

INTRODUCTION

The mouth, tongue, pharynx and oesophagus are concerned with mastication, initiation of digestion (with salivary amylase) and the transport of food to the stomach. Disorders of these organs often cause distressing symptoms which, because they interfere with swallowing, may lead to serious malnourishment. The neoplasms of this area are of a high degree of malignancy: their early diagnosis is of the greatest importance and treatment is still a major challenge to surgeons and radiotherapists.

MOUTH AND PHARYNX

Diseases of the mouth and pharynx are multitudinous and are often manifestations of either skin or systemic disorders. Only those conditions which have a bearing on gastrointestinal disease are described here.

Stomatitis

Simple catarrhal stomatitis

Poor oral hygiene in febrile illnesses, dehydration, dental sepsis, smoking and alcoholism are the main causes. The mucous membrane is reddened and sore and the tongue is covered with a dry brown fur. Halitosis is present. Treatment consists of preventive hygiene and mouthwashes with hydrogen peroxide.

Nutritional deficiences

Vitamin C deficiency results in hyperaemic, purplish, oedematous and friable gums. However, it is important to realise that in edentulous patients the first sign is perifollicular purpura on the legs, the oral features being absent.

In riboflavin deficiency, a magenta rough tongue with cheilosis and angular stomatitis is seen.

A 'raw beef' tongue, characteristic of vitamin B_{12} deficiency, is seen mainly in patients with pernicious anaemia.

Pellagra, owing to a deficiency of nicotinic acid, results in a sore, bright red buccal mucosa and glossitis in conjunction with dermatitis of exposed skin resembling severe sunburn, with diarrhoea and dementia. A pale atrophic smooth tongue with or without aphthous ulceration may indicate iron or folate deficiency. Nutritional deficiencies in Great Britain are seen in the impoverished elderly, alcoholics, the immigrant population, food faddists, and in patients who have had a gastrectomy or who suffer from malabsorption.

Aphthous stomatitis

Aphthous ulceration is a common affliction which is found in otherwise healthy children and adults, but patients with coeliac and inflammatory bowel disease are particularly at risk. The lesion is extremely painful and commences as a small vesicle on the buccal mucosa or tongue, which breaks down to leave a yellowish ulcer with an erythematous halo: healing can take up to two weeks. In one form, quite large ulcers, of more than 1 cm diameter, appear and may persist, acquiring secondary infection, so that biopsy may be needed to distinguish them from carcinoma.

Treatment starts with attention to dental hygiene, and removal of any rough corners on teeth or dentures. Local application of a corticosteroid as hydrocortisone or betamethasone is usually sufficient, but occasionally a course of systemic corticosteroid is required to achieve healing. There is a strong tendency to recurrence, which may continue over several years.

Viral stomatitis

Herpes simplex type I virus, herpes zoster, Coxsackie group A viruses, measles and other viruses often cause a stomatitis. Herpes simplex usually affects children, who develop numerous vesicles which ulcerate and coalesce causing severe pain. A liquid diet and early local treatment with iodoxuridine may be efficacious. Systemic vidabarine is reserved for severe cases or those with complications such as encephalitis. Glandular fever, probably the commonest cause of viral stomatitis, causes palatal petechiae and an acute pharyngitis and tonsillitis with an overlying creamy adherent membrane.

Bacterial stomatitis

This occurs with a streptococcal sore throat, diphtheria and syphilis. The most striking example is Vincent's stomatitis (which can sometimes become epidemic as in 'Trench mouth'), which produces ragged yellow sloughing ulceration with marked hyperaemia, oedema and friability of the gums, 'Vincent's organisms' (*Borrelia vincenti*) and fusiform bacilli of the genus Bacteroides, which are anaerobic commensals of the healthy mouth, are found in large numbers in the acute phase and the disease responds to penicillin.

Fungal stomatitis (Thrush)

Thrush is due to an infection with *Candida albicans* and is often found in infants, in patients with debilitating illness such as cancer and diabetes, in the immunologically incompetent, and following antibiotic and steroid therapy. White sloughs of superficial ulceration occurring on the gums, palate and buccal mucosa coalesce to form a white membrane which, if detached, leaves an erythematous surface. Effective treatment is available using nystatin suspension, amphotericin B lozenges or miconazole oral gel.

Allergic stomatitis

Allergy to denture plastic is rare. Eosin in lipstick is a common cause of allergic cheilitis.

Granulomatous stomatitis and cheilosis

This is a rare but painful and disfiguring complication of Crohn's disease.

Blood dyscrasias

Stomatitis is a distressing feature of acute leukaemias.

Heavy metals and drugs

Blue discolouration of the gums is produced by lead poisoning. Drug therapy can also produce oral effects, e.g. Candidiasis in antibiotic therapy.

TONGUE

In many patients with stomatitis there is also involvement of the tongue.

Ulceration

Simple ulceration

This is caused by repeated trauma, such as damaged teeth or badly fitting dentures.

Syphilitic ulceration

The mouth and tongue are the most usual extragenital sites for a primary chancre, which develops into a painless ulcer associated with regional lymphadenopathy. The diagnosis is made by the demonstration of the spirochaetes of *Treponema pallidum* by dark-ground illumination in a scraping taken from the base of an ulcer, and by serological investigation.

Tubercular ulceration

This is now very rare. It consists of a very painful shallow ulcer with undermined edges located on the dorsum of the tongue, usually near its tip.

CANCER OF THE ORAL CAVITY

Almost all the neoplasms in the mouth are squamous cell carcinomas. Incidence has fallen remarkably over the past 30 years and now about 2500 new cases are seen annually in England and Wales (about 1% of all malignant tumours). There is strong association with heavy smoking and chronic alcohol abuse, and betel nut chewers are also very much at risk (p. 28). Syphilis used to be an important factor.

The sites involved are the tongue (50%), the cheeks, the gums and the floor of the mouth. These lesions usually start as small hard lumps which ulcerate, become painful, and do not heal: some are papillary in character. Carcinoma of the anterior two-thirds of the tongue presents with local pain or a lump or ulcer, but in the posterior third it generally presents with dysphagia or, unhappily, with a lump in the submandibular region or neck from metastases in lymph nodes.

Neoplasms of the oropharynx and hypopharynx are, like tumours of the posterior one-third of the tongue, out of sight; they nearly always present with local pain and dysphagia, and sometimes with metastases in cervical nodes. Diagnosis requires very careful inspection and palpation of the area, often under general anaesthesia, with biopsy of any suspicious area. Lymphomas of the tonsil are sometimes seen. Carcinoma close to the larynx (postcricoid carcinoma) may cause hoarseness as well as dysphagia.

All these tumours are difficult to treat successfully so it is vital to obtain a biopsy of any questionable lesion in the mouth. Close collaboration between surgeon and radiotherapist is essential from the start of treatment. Very radical resection, including block dissection of the cervical lymph nodes, plays an important part in management.

Leukoplakia

This is a chronic condition characterised by smooth white patches, often fissured, which occurs commonly on the dorsum of the tongue but also affects the buccal mucosa. Its importance lies in that in some cases it is a precancerous state. Surgical biopsy is therefore essential. If hyperkeratosis or dysplasia are seen, then wide excision and/or radiotherapy are recommended.

SALIVARY GLAND DISEASE

There are three pairs of glands – parotid, submandibular and sublingual – that secrete saliva, which is a mixture of water, salts, mucus and ptyalin. Saliva moistens the mouth, making speech comfortable, assisting mastication and swallowing by liquefying the food taken into the mouth, and also plays a minor part in starch digestion through the action of ptyalin.

The parotid is purely a mucus-secreting gland. The stimulus to secretion comes through the postganglionic parasympathetic fibres running in the auriculotemporal nerve. The submandibular gland contains both musuc-secreting cells and serous cells which produce ptyalin. Parasympathetic fibres to the submandibular and sublingual glands come from the submandibular ganglion, which is suspended from the lingual nerve.

Saliva has a pH of about 7.0, and ptyalin (which is an amylase) slowly digests starch to maltose, but this process is quickly arrested when food mixes with gastric acid. The secretion of saliva is stimulated both by the sight of food and by taste, especially of acid substances.

Infection

Mumps

This is an infectious viral disease, with an incubation period of 17–21 days, which usually causes bilateral parotid swelling. Occasionally orchitis, meningitis, and pancreatitis are complications.

Acute suppurative parotitis

This is now a rare condition, seen occasionally in the course of a fever, of alimentary disease, or following an abdominal operation. Dehydration and poor oral hygiene are contributory factors. An ascending infection with *Staph. aureus* or *Strep. pyogenes* results in an acutely painful swollen gland. Rehydration and antiobiotics usually result in a cure and only rarely is surgical drainage required.

Recurrent parotitis

This usually affects children and causes recurrent pain and swelling in one gland. Dilatation of the duct (sialectasia), strictures, or calculi may be present. Massage of the gland, sialogogues, and antibiotic therapy are of assistance. Strictures and calculi must be dealt with surgically and, rarely, removal of the gland may be needed.

Sjögren's syndrome

This condition, which is uncommon, is more-or-less confined to women over 40 years of age. Salivation and lacrimation are scanty, which leads to recurrent dryness of the mouth (xerostomia), conjunctivitis sicca (xerophthalmia) and swelling of the salivary glands. Some have associated rheumatoid arthritis, sarcoidosis, or primary biliary cirrhosis.

The blood shows anaemia and hypergammaglobulinaemia, and autoantibodies are present. Biopsy of a salivary gland shows a dense lymphocytic infiltration.

The most important aspect of treatment is to provide 'artificial tears', as eyedrops, to compensate for the diminished secretion from the lacrimal glands.

Heerfordt's uveo-parotid fever

The combination of parotid swelling, acute iridocyclitis, and fever occasionally occurs in patients with sarcoidosis.

Salivary Calculi

Stone formation occurs principally in the submandibular gland because this gland has a long duct and secretes a mucoid saliva. On eating, the patient experiences a painful swelling of the gland, of variable severity. On examination the gland may be enlarged and tender and a stone is often palpable under the tongue. An x-ray may confirm the presence of a stone. Removal of a stone close to the orifice of the duct is feasible. If one or more stones are impacted in the gland then glandular removal is necessary: care must be taken not to injure the lingual or hypoglossal nerves.

Salivary Tumours

Pleomorphic adenomas ('mixed' tumours)

These are the most common tumours affecting salivary tissue; 90% occur in the parotid. Most present in the fifth decade, equally in the two sexes.

Histologically, these tumours are adenomas but, because they have no true capsule and a lobulated surface, they are liable to recur if treated by enucleation only.

The patient presents with a painless lump, often in the lower pole of the gland, which is well-defined and firm. Superficial parotidectomy with wide excision of the tumour, but with exposure and preservation of the facial nerve, usually results in an excellent prognosis. Inadequate surgery, however, is followed by recurrence.

Occasionally an adenoma arises in the submandibular salivary gland and is treated by complete removal of the gland.

Adenolymphoma

This benign, soft and cystic tumour accounts for

10% of parotid tumours; it occurs usually in men over the age of 50. Prognosis is good following local removal.

Carcinoma

This occurs equally in both sexes over the age of 50 and usually involves the parotid gland. Clinically the patient presents with a rapidly-growing, hard and painful tumour, with early involvement of the facial nerve. Radical removal with block dissection of the regional lymph nodes is carried out, though the prognosis is generally poor. Postoperative radiotherapy must be considered.

THE OESOPHAGUS

Anatomy and Physiology (Fig. 4.1)

It is helpful to regard the oesophagus as a muscular tube lined by very sensitive stratified squamous epithelium. It is about 25 cm long and runs from the upper oesophageal sphincter (formed from the inferior constrictor fibres of the cricopharyngeus muscle) to the lower oesophageal sphincter lying at the gastro-oesophageal junction. In the cervical region, the oesophagus lies adjacent to the thyroid gland, trachea, and carotid arteries. In the thorax, the aortic arch often indents the oesophagus, making a useful endoscopic landmark. It then passes close to the left main bronchus and the left atrium. Finally, leaving the posterior mediastinum, it turns to the left and anteriorly to enter the abdomen through the oesophageal hiatus to join the cardiac end of the stomach. Its close proximity to all these vital structures means that neoplasms quickly become irremovable.

The blood supply of the oesophagus comes from the aorta, left gastric artery, bronchial, and inferior thyroid arteries. The azygos vein drains the upper two-thirds while the remainder is served by the gastric veins, thus forming a connection between the systemic and portal systems. In portal hypertension the flow may be reversed, leading to the development of oesophageal varices.

The oesophagus is lined with squamous epithelium which has a shell-pink colour and shows a

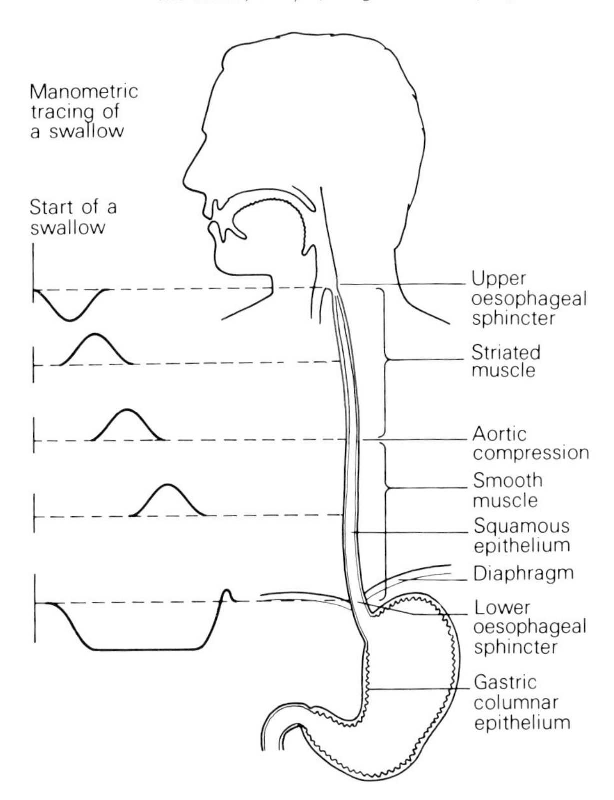

Fig. 4.1 *Anatomy and physiology of the oesophagus.*

delicate vascular pattern when viewed endoscopically. This contrasts with the reddish-brown columnar epithelium seen below the junction with the gastric mucosa.

The upper one-third of the oesophagus, including the cricopharyngeal sphincter, consists of striated muscle activated by a barrage of vagal nerve impulses which, when interrupted, causes the sphincter to relax during the initiation of a swallow. At this point the lips, palate, posterior fauces and glottis are closed and the musculature of the tongue, pharynx and mouth act in unison to propel a bolus of masticated food through a relaxed upper oesophageal sphincter. Manometric studies have shown that the latter generates pressures from 40–60 mmHg preventing regurgitation of oesophageal contents into the larynx. The lower one-third of the oesophagus consist of smooth muscle and the terminal 3–4 cm constitutes the anatomically inconspicuous but physiologically distinct lower oesophageal sphincter.

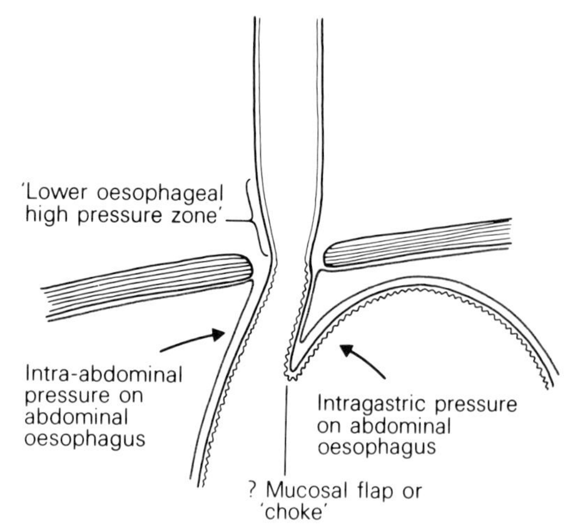

Fig. 4.2 *Factors preventing oesophageal reflux.*

Primary peristalsis, initiated by a swallow, is a coordinated pressure wave sweeping down the oesophagus at a rate of 2–4 cm/sec, obliterating the lumen and then propelling the bolus of food into the stomach. Secondary peristalsis commences at a local level, often due to local stimulation by food residues or reflux of acid into the oesophagus.

The factors which have been suggested as preventing gastro-oesophageal reflux (Fig. 4.2) include the lower oesophageal sphincter, diaphragmatic squeeze, an intra-abdominal segment of the oesophagus, and a mucosal 'choke' effect of the loose fundal folds lying just below the oesophago-gastric junction. However, it is now generally accepted that the most important factor is the resting tone of the lower oesophageal sphincter and its responses to stress, i.e. a rise in intra-abdominal pressure. The basal pressure is 15–20 mmHg and this relaxes on swallowing. Lower oesophageal pressure is decreased, and the risk of reflux therefore accentuated, by fatty foods, chocolate, alochol and smoking. Drugs with an anticholinergic action have the same effect.

Symptoms of Oesophageal Disease

Reaching an early diagnosis in diseases of the oesophagus is greatly facilitated by taking an accurate history and realising the significance of commonly used (or abused) terms.

There are three kinds of pain which originate in the oesophagus: heartburn, oesophageal spasm, and impact pain.

Heartburn

This, the best known and very common symptom, refers to a retrosternal burning pain which radiates towards the throat. Its occurrence is usually related to the ingestion of a heavy meal and to posture, being aggravated by bending, stooping and recumbency. Obesity and the wearing of constrictive clothing around the abdomen are also aggravating factors. Accompanying symptoms are: the regurgitation of bitter gastric contents into the mouth; waterbrash (the sudden filling of the mouth with a clear slightly salty fluid excreted by the salivary glands); and odynophagia (impact pain), particularly when taking alcohol or hot liquids. Acid and bile regurgitation should not be confused with oesophageal regurgitation of undigested food from the obstructed oesophagus which can occur in achalasia, strictures and tumour.

Oesophageal spasm

Pain in the chest may arise from diseases of the musculoskeletal system, pleura, aorta, mediastinum, diaphragm and occasionally from the biliary system, stomach, duodenum and pancreas. However, from a clinical point of view the differentiation of oesophageal from that of ischaemic heart pain is the most important (Table 4.1). A good history is invaluable, but may not ensure differentiation between the two.

Pain originating from both the myocardium or the oesophagus is often central; it may be severe, tight, or crushing in quality and may have the same radiation to the jaw, arms and back. The pain of oesophageal spasm, however, often has a burning quality and is more likely to affect the lower chest and radiate to the back. Myocardial pain is usually related to effort but may occur at night (angina decubitus), after heavy meals, and on emotion. The pain of oesophageal spasm often

Table 4.1
Comparison of Cardiac and Oesophageal Pain

Cardiac pain	*Oesophageal pain*
Wide radiation from mid-line	Wide radiation – including to back
Commonly radiates to arms – especially left arm	May radiate to arms
Commonly effort-related	Not usually effort-related
May follow eating	Commonly follows eating
Relieved by nitrites	Relieved by nitrites
Bernstein test negative	Bernstein test positive
Manometry normal	Manometry abnormal

occurs spontaneously, though it is more likely to occur during meals and is sometimes associated with dysphagia, heartburn, and symptoms of the irritable bowel syndrome. It also occurs commonly on recumbency, presumably owing to increased gastro-oesophageal reflux.

Impact pain (odynophagia)

This means pain which is felt when a bolus of food impinges on a raw area of mucosal injury, such as may occur in reflux oesophagitis, candidiasis, after ingestion of corrosive chemicals, after irradiation, and at the site of a neoplasm. Impact pain is aggravated by irritants, e.g. alcohol, or by taking very hot or very cold foods.

Dysphagia

When true dysphagia is present, the patient experiences difficulty with swallowing – either in the form of pain or a feeling of obstruction – within 10 seconds of the pharyngeal phase of swallowing. Few patients can indicate the level of obstruction quite accurately. This symptom usually implies oesophageal (or pharyngeal) pathology and has to be distinguished from *pseudodysphagia*. The latter is experienced after (rather than during) a meal. The patient then does not experience 'bolus' obstruction but instead is aware of epigastric 'fullness', and 'lump' in the throat which does not interfere with swallowing and may disappear with swallowing, or a sensation of food 'sitting' in his neck or chest. Some of these patients may be shown to have a hiatus hernia, other disorders of the stomach or upper alimentary tract, or sometimes no obvious pathology. Very few patients with pseudodysphagia have disorders of the oesophagus.

Small swallow is a term sometimes applied to a particular form of difficulty with swallowing. The old, the anorexic, or the depressed may be able to swallow their saliva and can drink but (presumably by cortical inhibition) cannot bring themselves to swallow food. The so-called small swallow of the elderly may have no obvious cause or may reflect pharyngo-oesophageal obstruction from intrinsic or extrinsic causes. Further investigation is therefore indicated. Small swallow may also result from soreness or dryness of the mouth or pharynx (see p. 53 and 55).

Flatulence

Excessive belching is usually consequent on aerophagy, in anxious individuals or in those who bolt their food. Belching is occasionally due to putrefaction of food in those with gastric outlet obstruction and in these cases patients will usually proffer the information that it is foul-smelling.

Globus hystericus (see p. 8)

Motility Disorders of the Pharynx and Oesphagus

Pharyngeal pouch

Aetiology. Although the upper oesophageal sphincter relaxes promptly on commencement of a swallow, premature closure of this sphincter be-

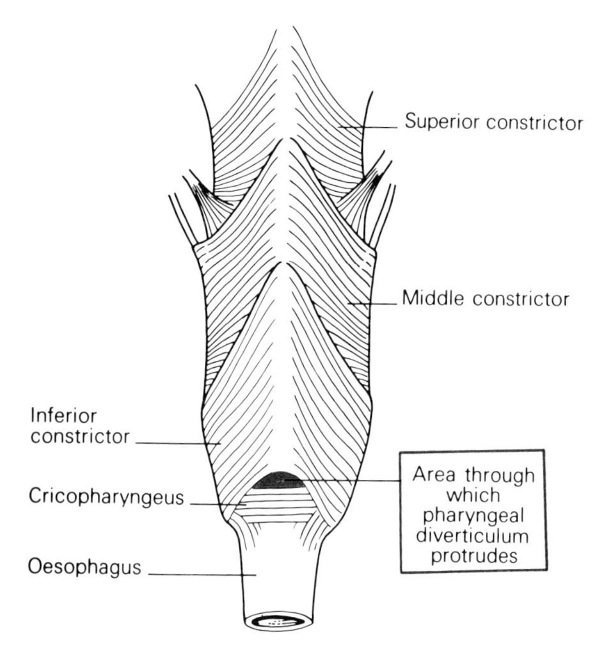

Fig. 4.3 *Posterior view of the pharynx.*

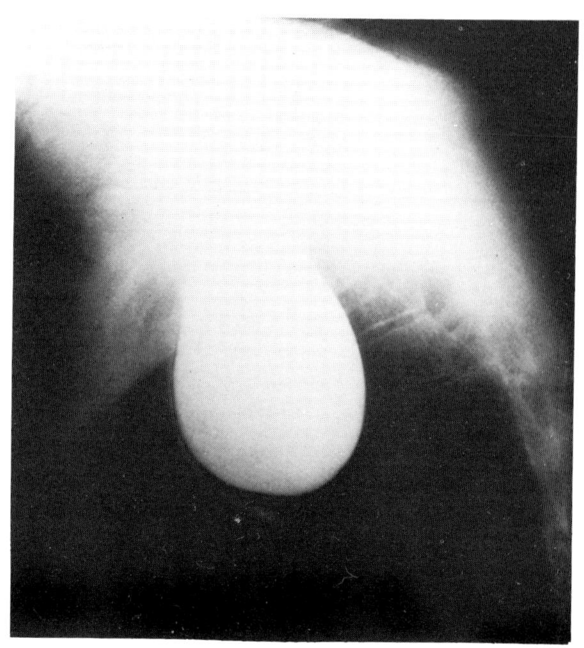

Fig. 4.4 *Barium swallow: pharyngeal pouch.*

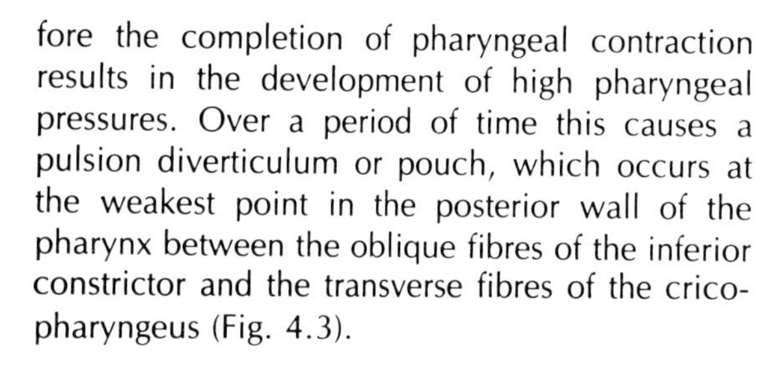

fore the completion of pharyngeal contraction results in the development of high pharyngeal pressures. Over a period of time this causes a pulsion diverticulum or pouch, which occurs at the weakest point in the posterior wall of the pharynx between the oblique fibres of the inferior constrictor and the transverse fibres of the crico-pharyngeus (Fig. 4.3).

Clinical features. A pharyngeal pouch occurs more commonly in men. Initially a sensation of food sticking in the throat is followed by gurgling noises, regurgitation of food, and halitosis caused by decomposition of food in the pouch. A swelling may occur postprandially at the left side of the neck.

Investigation. The pouch is confirmed by a barium swallow performed in the recumbent position (Fig. 4.4).

Management. Surgical excision of the pouch and primary closure result in a cure. Cricopharyngeal myotomy in addition has been recommended.

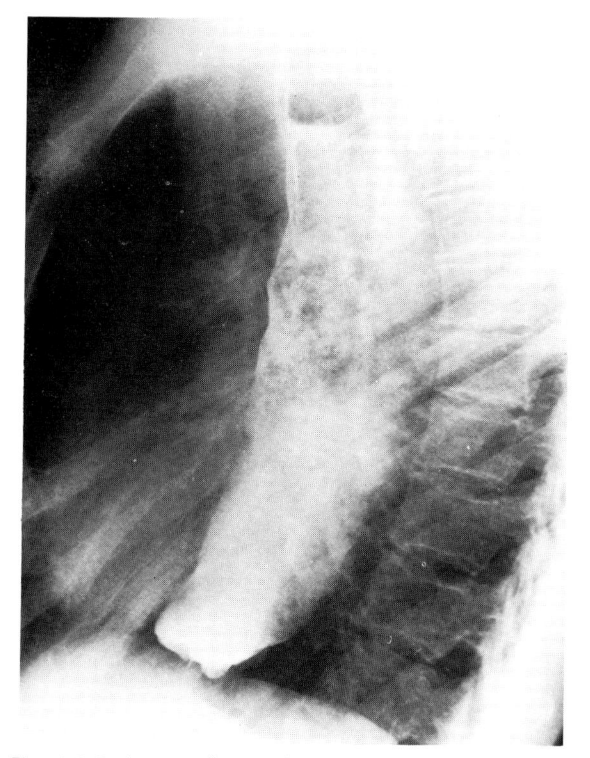

Fig. 4.5 *Barium swallow: achalasia.*

Neuromuscular pharyngeal disorders

The symptoms of pharyngeal dysphagia have already been described. Diseases affecting the central nervous system, peripheral nerve, motor end plate, and muscle can all cause dysphagia by impairment of pharyngeal muscle contraction and coordination, and also by interfering with upper oesophageal sphincter relaxation during a swallow.

Brain stem lesions such as pseudobulbar palsy, motor neurone disease, and poliomyelitis cause inhibition of upper oesophageal sphincter relaxation and hence dysphagia.

Myasthenia gravis and myotonia dystrophica cause reduction of upper oesophageal sphincter tone, allowing spill-over of oesophageal contents into the larynx and consequent symptoms.

The strength of striated muscular contraction is impaired in dermatomyositis and also in lower motor neurone disease.

In scleroderma, the lower oesophageal muscle atrophies, and so peristalsis is impaired.

Management is difficult. Specific treatment is available for myasthenia gravis. In selected patients with distressing symptoms, pulmonary aspiration, and weight-loss, consideration may be given for upper oesophageal sphincter bouginage. In scleroderma, hiatal incompetence is common, and oesophagitis may be severe enough to require fundoplication.

Achalasia

This is a fairly unusual but potentially serious cause of dysphagia. Incidence is believed to be about 1 per 100 000 per year. The basic lesion is failure of relaxation of the lower oesophageal sphincter. Post-mortem studies show degeneration of ganglion cells in the myenteric plexus of the oesophageal wall: this results in the complete loss of coordinated peristaltic activity in the lower two-thirds of the oesophagus, and failure of the sphincter to relax on swallowing. Non-propulsive tertiary contractions occur, causing pain.

Clinical features. Characteristically a history of intermittent dysphagia, especially for fluids, extending over several years is obtained in a middle-aged patient of either sex. The dysphagia gradually worsens and becomes persistent; often, patients develop the trick of standing up, drinking a glass of water and performing the valsalva manoeuvre to force food into the stomach. Weight loss and malnutrition are rare until the later stages. Episodes of severe spontaneous chest pain occur, and may lead to confusion with ischaemic heart disease, especially in the earlier stages before oesophageal dilatation has taken place. Regurgitation of undigested food is common, but lacks the sour taste of gastro-oesophageal reflux. Overspill of oesophageal contents at night leads to coughing, wheezing, and repeated episodes of chest infection and aspiration pneumonia.

Investigation. A chest x-ray may show a widened mediastinum due to the dilated oesophagus. A fluid level may be seen in the oesophagus, but is characteristically absent from the stomach. Rarely, pulmonary fibrosis and bronchiectasis are seen. A barium swallow reveals a sigmoid (or cucumber) oesophagus, absent or disorganised peristalsis, retained food residues in the oesophagus, and a smooth tapering at the lower oesophageal sphincter (Fig. 4.5). Endoscopy is essential to allow close inspection and biopsy of the narrowed area: the major concern is to make sure that the narrowing is not due to a carcinoma at the oesophago-gastric junction. In achalasia, despite the retention of food debris the endoscope passes into the stomach with surprising ease. Manometry, in which pressures at different levels in the oesophagus can be measured synchronously, shows failure of peristalsis, non-peristaltic tertiary contractions, an exaggerated response to cholinergic drugs, and failure of the lower oesophageal sphincter to relax during a swallow. This test is especially useful in the early stages of the disease, when confusion with ischaemic heart disease is most likely.

Treatment. In healthy patients, approximately 80% obtain satisfactory relief of symptoms following an adequate Heller's cardiomyotomy in which a longitudinal incision is made through all the muscle coats down to the mucosa. In some patients, rupture of the circular fibres in the lower oesophageal sphincter can be achieved using a pneumatic bag: the length of benefit obtained is extremely variable, but this procedure can easily be repeated.

Chagas disease

A flagellate protozoan, *Trypanosoma cruzi,* is responsible for this disease, which is spread by bug bites and is endemic in South America. The initial stages are characterised by fever, lymphadenopathy and hepatosplenomegaly but later features develop which are identical to those of primary achalasia. These are due to destruction of the ganglion cells in the myenteric plexus, caused by liberation of a neurotoxin by the parasite. The heart and colon are also affected. Cardiomyotomy may be required for relief of symptoms.

Diffuse spasm of the oesophagus

Aetiology and pathophysiology. Patients complain of severe substernal pain which is often quite suggestive of angina. Non-propulsive contractions of the lower two-thirds of the oesophagus are the hallmark of this disorder, and positive diagnosis requires the performance of oesophageal manometry. Muscle hypertrophy often ensues; the ganglion cells of the myenteric plexus remain intact. Lower oesophageal sphincter function is usually normal. Stimulation of the afferent nerve endings in the oesophageal mucosa, usually by acid reflux, and rarely by carcinomatous infiltration, may be responsible in part for the spasm. Patients with the irritable bowel syndrome are particularly prone to diffuse oesophageal spasm and this may be a manifestation of a total gut dysmotility disorder.

Clinical features. Oesophageal pain is the presenting feature, though two-thirds of patients will have experienced episodic and variable dysphagia for fluids and solids, often over many years.

Investigations. A barium swallow is often normal, but it may show non-propulsive contractions which, if prominent, give an appearance of a 'corkscrew' or 'beaded' oesophagus. Manometry confirms the abnormality of peristalsis in the lower two-thirds of the oesophagus, the tertiary contractions often being provoked by a swallow. Oesophagitis and carcinoma can be sought for by endoscopy.

Management. Patient reassurance and trust are of paramount importance, since medical and surgical treatment has little to offer. If reflux is present this should be treated energetically. Glycerine trinitrate sublingually may alleviate pain and dysphagia and can be used prophylactically before meals if the discomfort is largely confined to the prandial period. Anticholinergic drugs are even more disappointing. In severe cases, balloon dilatation should be tried: cardiomyotomy is performed occasionally, though it is not without risk.

Sideropenic web (Paterson – Brown – Kelly or Plummer–Vinson syndrome)

This unusual condition occurs predominantly in females of middle age with an iron-deficiency anaemia. The classical features are koilonychia, glossitis and dysphagia due to a thin web of oesophageal mucosa at the postcricoid level (Fig. 4.6). Oesophagoscopy is essential for diagnosis and, if the rigid oesophagoscope is used, the web can be broken by manipulation of the tip of the instrument. The anaemia must continue to be treated.

This condition will not necessarily recur, but continued supervision is important because there is an increased risk of occurrence of postcricoid carcinoma.

Lower oesophageal (Schatzki) rings

These are a rare cause of intermittent dysphagia. A mucosal ring lies at the junction of squamous and columnar epithelium and causes occasional difficulty in swallowing meat – 'steak house syndrome'. The rings are seen in a barium swallow but are difficult to identify on endoscopy (Fig. 4.7).

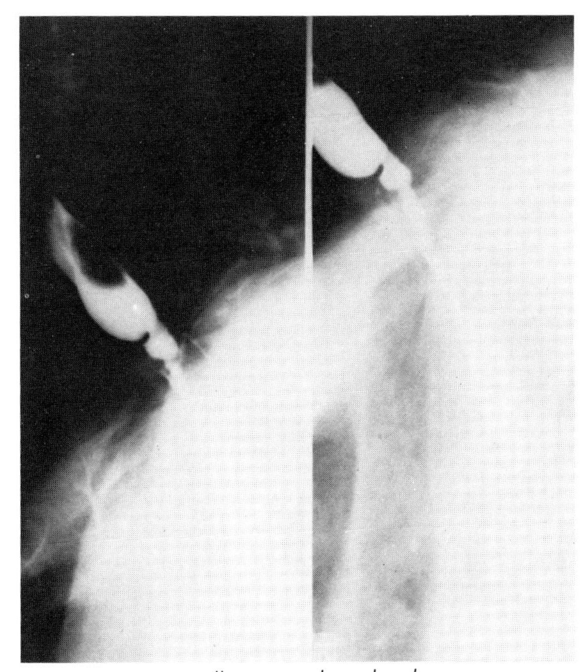

Fig. 4.6 *Barium swallow: oesophageal web.*

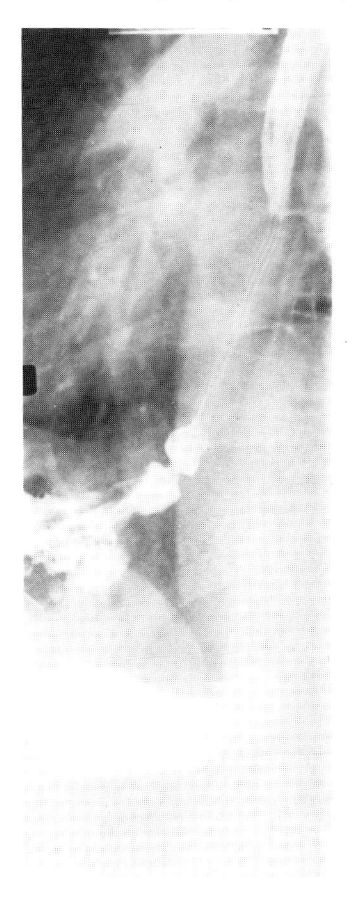

Fig. 4.7 *Barium swallow: Schatzki ring.*

Gastro-oesophageal Reflux

Everyone is familiar with the experience of discomfort after a heavy meal which is usually termed heartburn; this is due to the acid contents of the stomach refluxing across the gastro-oesophageal junction and stimulating the pain receptors in the lower oesophagus. In most people this is a temporary phenomenon but, in a substantial minority, symptoms of heartburn and regurgitation are frequent and severe enough to make them seek relief.

The major factors which prevent reflux (Fig. 4.2) are the resting tone in the lower oesophageal pressure zone and the compressive effect of intra-abdominal pressure on the abdominal oesophagus. In the past, the presence of a sliding or axial hiatal hernia (Fig. 4.8) was thought to be the major cause of gastro-oesophageal reflux (and it is still a very important association (Fig. 4.9): but major reflux can occur without a demonstrable hernia and this appears to be due to loss of tone in the lower oesophageal sphincter or pressure zone (irrespective of whether it lies above or below the diaphragm).

Secondary peristalsis, which sweeps refluxed gastric contents back into the stomach, helps to reduce the effects of reflux.

Because the oesophago-gastric junction is more or less intact, reflux is not a feature of para-oesophageal hernia (Fig. 4.10). These herniae may be silent, but they can cause acute symptoms if the greater curvature rotates up into the peritoneal-lined sac as a gastric volvulus: this can cause gastric obstruction and, occasionally, strangulation.

The effects of gastro-oesophageal reflux

Acid and pepsin are the major irritants. However, if duodenogastric reflux also occurs, e.g. after

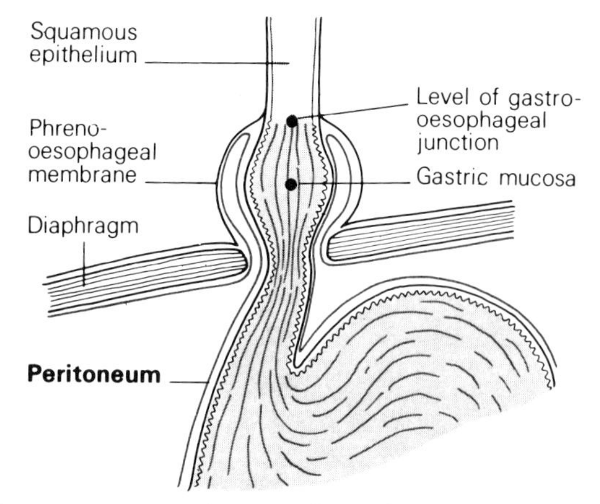

Fig. 4.8 *Type I axial (sliding) hiatus hernia.*

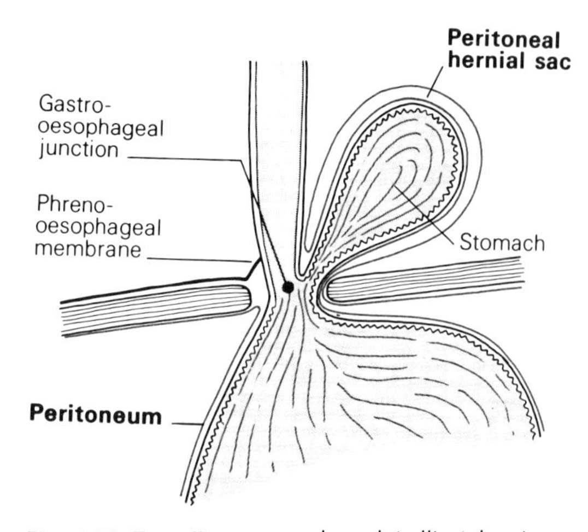

Fig. 4.10 *Type II para-oesophageal (rolling) hernia.*

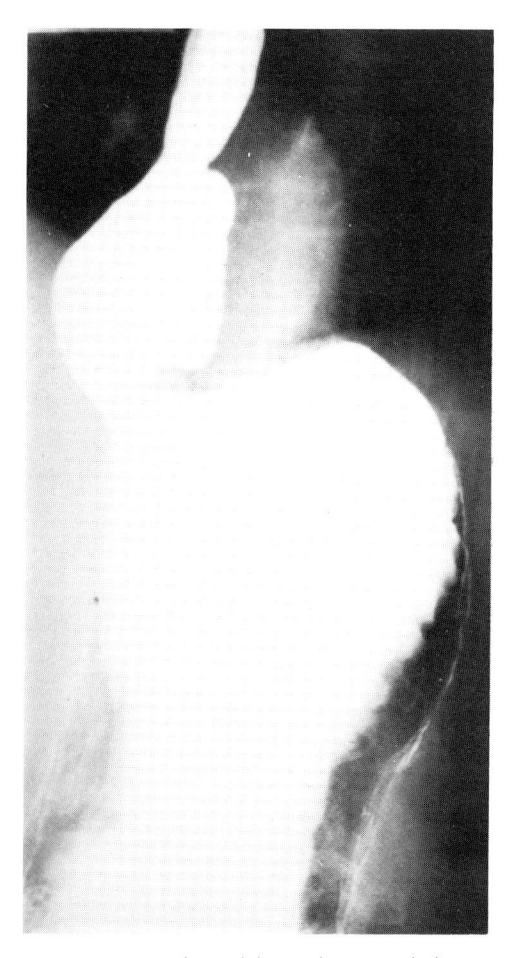

Fig. 4.9 *Barium meal: axial hiatus hernia with free gastro-oesophageal reflux.*

partial gastrectomy, then bile, bile salts, pancreatic enzymes and lysolecithin (a product of fat digestion) may all have a similar irritant effect.

Gastro-oesophageal reflux has three main effects:

i. Heartburn or pyrosis. This symptom, with acid regurgitation into the mouth, is diagnostic of reflux. The intensity of the symptoms may not correlate with the appearance of the oesophagus on endoscopy or microscopy, e.g. marked heartburn may occur with a surprisingly normal-looking oesophagus, but the converse is also true.

ii. Oesophagitis. Normal oesophageal mucosa consists of three layers. The squamous epithelium consists of a basal layer (occupying 10% of the total thickness) and a stratified zone. The lamina propria has papillae which extend less than two-thirds of the way towards the surface epithelium. The muscularis mucosae underlies the lamina propria (Fig. 4.11). Reflux, owing to its irritant nature, causes increased shedding of epithelial cells, compensatory hyperplasia, and finally inflammation. On biopsy there is at first an increase in the basal cell layer from 15% up to about 30% of epithelial thickness and lengthening of the papillae of the lamina propria. Inflammatory cells are later found in the lamina propria and, finally, ulceration and fibrosis may occur.

Recurrent ulceration and fibrosis lead to the development of a peptic stricture, usually at the

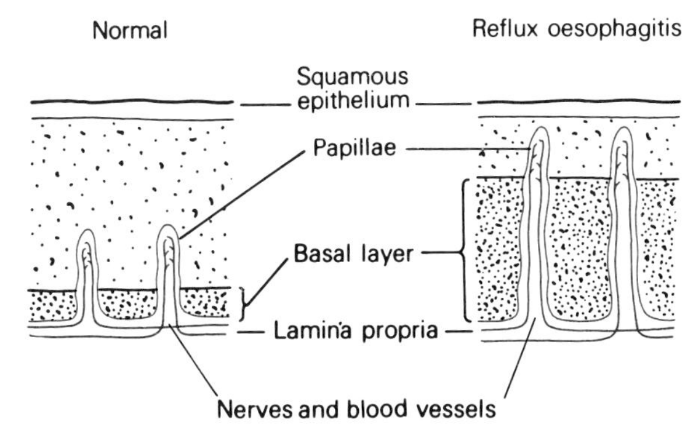

Fig. 4.11 *Histology of: normal oesophagus; reflux oesophagitis.*

squamo-columnar junction, causing a slowly progressive dysphagia for solids.

Barrett's oesophagus, in which columnar epithelium lines the lower oesophagus (Fig. 4.12), may occur as the result of replacement of the squamous epithelium during healing as a consequence of repeated episodes of oesophagitis, or may be due to a congenital abnormality. This condition may predispose to:

high peptic stricture
chronic gastric ulcer lying within the oesophagus
development of adenocarcinoma.

iii. Disordered oesophageal motility. Non-peristaltic contractions interfere with the clearance of refluxed acid into the oesophagus, and a vicious cycle ensues. Oesophageal spasm may aggravate the pain.

Diagnosis and investigations

The diagnosis of reflux is usually made on a detailed history. Anaemia and obesity may be present on physical examination.

Routine investigations. When there is oesophagitis the haemoglobin, red cell indices and film may confirm an iron deficiency anaemia due to chronic blood loss. Hiatus hernia without oesophagitis is not an explanation for anaemia. A chest x-ray and electrocardiogram may help in the diagnosis of chest pain.

Radiology. In the head-down position a barium contrast examination may be able to demonstrate reflux (Fig. 4.9), though the failure to show reflux radiologically does not exclude it because reflux can be intermittent. Radiology can also show severe oesophagitis and a peptic stricture.

Endoscopy and biopsy/cytology. Endoscopy is the only way to diagnose oesophagitis positively. Severity is assessed by the presence or absence of friability and bleeding, ulceration, and stricture formation. Endoscopy and biopsy is essential to exclude oesophageal carcinoma. Moreover, inflammatory changes may be seen with the microscope, although the oesophagus looks normal to the naked eye.

Bernstein acid perfusion test. Following a strict protocol, 0.1N sodium chloride or 0.1N hydrochloric acid is perfused into the oesophagus, the patient having no knowledge of the perfusate at a particular time. The reproduction of the patient's

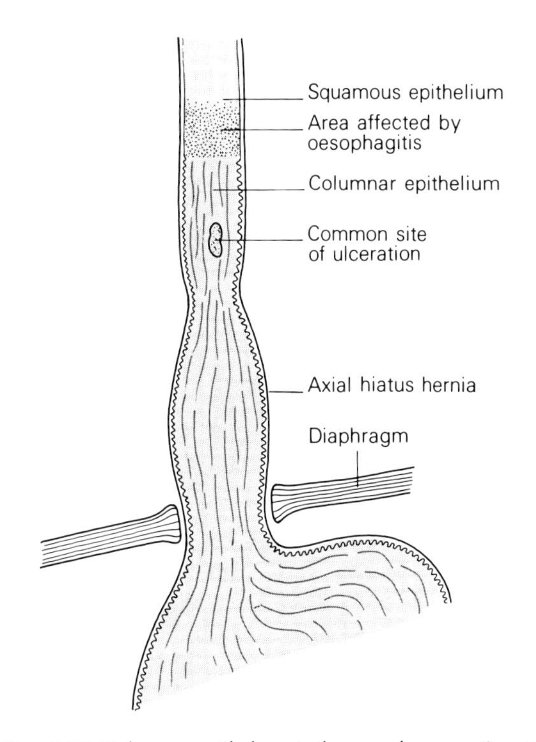

Fig. 4.12 *Columnar epithelium in the oesophagus, or Barrett's oesophagus.*

symptoms on infusion with hydrochloric acid is highly suggestive that gastro-oesophageal reflux is the problem. However, normal controls often experience pain with acid perfusion.

Oesophageal pH recording. By using a swallowed glass electrode, the number and duration of reflux episodes can be recorded, especially those occurring at night. The method is cumbersome and needs admission to hospital: its use is mainly restricted to intensive investigation and research.

Medical management of gastro-oesophageal reflux

Most people will suffer from transient heartburn from time to time, usually following dietary indiscretion. In these cases simple advice and the use of an antacid is all that is required. In more persistent heartburn cases, the advice given falls into two broad categories: that based on physiology and the use of specific pharmacological agents (Fig. 4.13).

Advice based on physiology. The basic aim is to reduce factors which raise intra-abdominal pressure. Of these, much the most important is obesity. The majority of patients troubled by reflux are overweight, and there is almost always a striking improvement in symptoms if they return to their proper weight. Measures to reduce passive reflux at night include raising the head of the bed on blocks 20–30 cm high, and avoidance of late meals. Squatting, rather than bending, to pick up objects and avoidance of tight clothing around the abdomen are helpful. It is doubtful whether the avoidance of fats and alcohol is of value except insofar as this helps weight reduction.

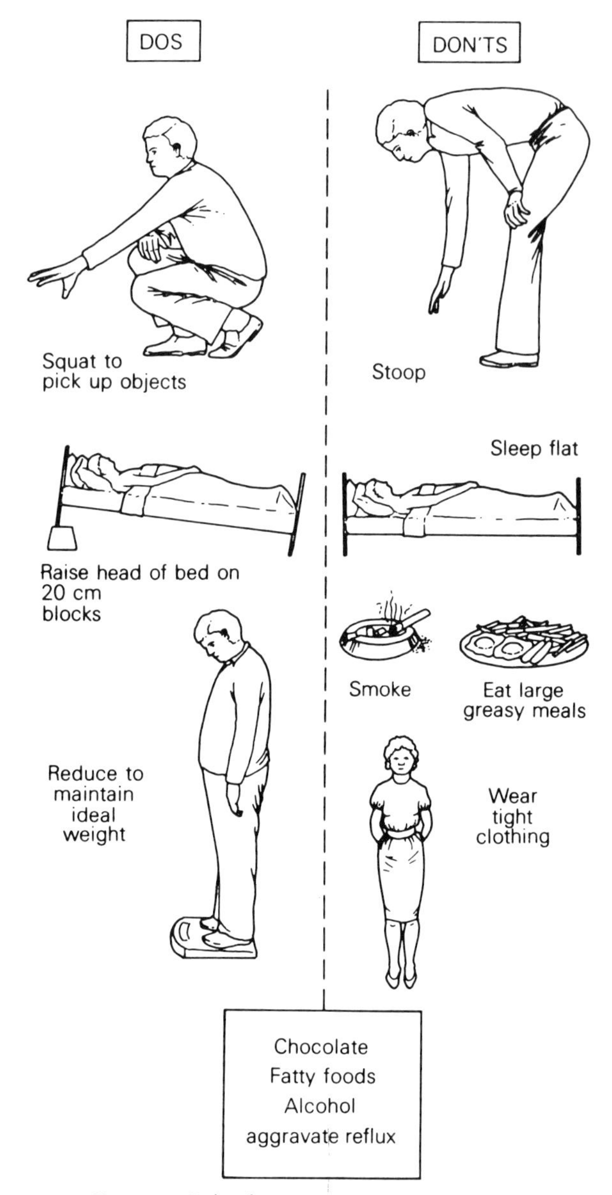

Fig. 4.13 *Rules for preventing reflux.*

Specific pharmacological agents. These have three main mechanisms of action: to reduce acid, to prevent reflux and to increase mucosal resistance.

Neutralisation of acid can be achieved by using fairly large doses of antacids, which should be given one and three hours after meals and on retiring to bed. Antacids work by coating the oesophagus, a property enhanced by a defoaming agent (e.g. dimethicone), neutralising the acid within the oesophagus and, to some extent, in the stomach, and also by increasing lower oesophageal sphincter pressure. Antacids with hydrotalcite, a bile acid-binding preparation, may be used in those who have biliary reflux.

The use of H_2-receptor blockers (e.g. cimetidine and ranitidine), potent inhibitors of acid and pepsin secretion, has been somewhat disappointing. Although most trials indicate some symptomatic relief from heartburn, the effect on oesophagitis seems to be minimal.

Metoclopramide promotes normal peristaltic activity in the oesophagus, stimulates gastric emptying, and may increase lower oesophageal sphincter tone. A combination of an antacid with alginic acid forms a floating viscous raft which acts as a barrier to reflux.

An increase in mucosal resistance is claimed with carbenoxolone, a derivative of liquorice, especially when combined with an antacid and alginate. Unfortunately, carbonoxolone has a mineralo-corticoid effect and, in the elderly, urea and electrolytes, blood pressure and weight must be regularly measured.

Surgery

Peptic strictures can be dilated under diazepam sedation by passing olive dilators over a guidewire introduced through the stricture under direct vision at endoscopy (Fig. 3.21). The size of the Eder–Puestow dilators is gradually increased and, if necessary, the procedure can be repeated at intervals.

Patients in whom symptoms are severe and unresponsive to medical treatment, and especially those with oesophagitis, should be considered for surgery. Only a minority of children with hiatus hernia have oesophagitis; when it occurs, however, it can quickly lead to a severe stricture so it is important to be ready to operate on this group.

The operation may be performed in one of two ways:

1. Through an abdominal incision, the upper end of the stomach is fully mobilised and the oesophago-gastric junction reduced into the abdomen. The widened oesophageal hiatus in the diaphragm is then restored to its normal size by suturing the right and left arms of the crura together. Finally a cuff of stomach is wrapped around the lower oesophagus – Nissen's fundoplication (Fig. 4.14).

2. Through a left intercostal incision, the lower end of the oesophagus and the upper stomach is freed, working through the wide oesophageal hiatus. A fundoplication is then done and sutured to the margins of the hiatus (Belsey Mark IV operation).

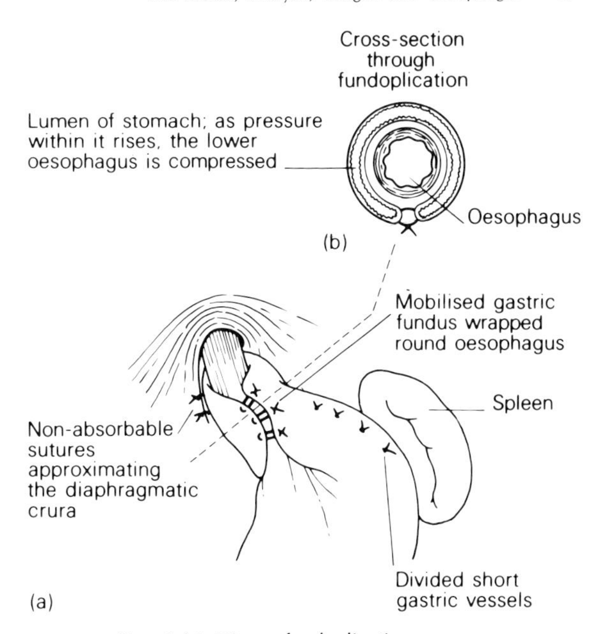

Fig. 4.14 *Nissen fundoplication.*

Oesophageal Neoplasms

Benign tumours are very uncommon, and most are submucous leiomyomas.

Malignant neoplasms of the oesophagus account for some 3% of malignant tumours in Britain. There are wide geographic variations in incidence (see p. 26).

Roughly twice as many men as women are affected. About 80% of neoplasms are squamous cell carcinomas of varying malignancy, and about 85% occur at or below the level of the aortic arch. In the lower one-third, many of the neoplasms are adenocarcinomas, usually carcinomas of the oesophago-gastric junction which have spread proximally: however, in some patients the lower oesophagus is lined by columnar epithelium and they seem to be particularly prone to development of a carcinoma. All carcinomas of the oesophagus tend to spread longitudinally in the submucous plane and so resection needs to be particularly radical. Direct spread to the adjacent pleura and diaphragm is rather likely to occur, and metastasis to lymph nodes around the left gastric pedicle and the hilum of the lung all make radical resection difficult.

There is a particular association of postcricoid and upper oesophageal carcinoma with iron-deficiency anaemia (Plummer–Vinson). Risk factors include the imbibing of alcohol by smokers, achalasia, Barrett's oesophagus, hereditary tylosis and chronic oesophagitis.

Clinical features and diagnosis (Fig. 4.15)

It is characteristic of these patients that they have had no heartburn or trouble with swallowing until the acute onset (often over 2–3 days) of dysphagia. This is initially for solids and then for liquids, often with marked weight loss and impact pain. A barium swallow may show an irregular narrowing, often with a shouldered edge: however, an early carcinoma may be missed and endoscopy in every patient is essential. The diagnosis is confirmed at endoscopy by the macroscopic appearance, and by histology obtained on biopsy and brush cytology.

Peptic Stricture	**Carcinoma**
Usually a long history of heartburn	Usually no dyspeptic history
Dysphagia	
Gradual onset	Usually sudden onset, e.g. one day a piece of meat sticks and has to be regurgitated
Variable in degree	Steadily progressive
Barium swallow	
Smooth narrowing Fig. 4.15a	Irregular, asymmetrical narrowing Fig. 4.15b Can be *negative* in early carcinoma
Oesophagoscopy (Never to be omitted in any patient with dysphagia)	
Oesophagitis above a sudden smooth-sided narrowing	Normal oesophagus above the stricture, the surface of which may be pale, friable, nodular. But may need repeated biopsy or brush cytology before diagnosis confirmed

a

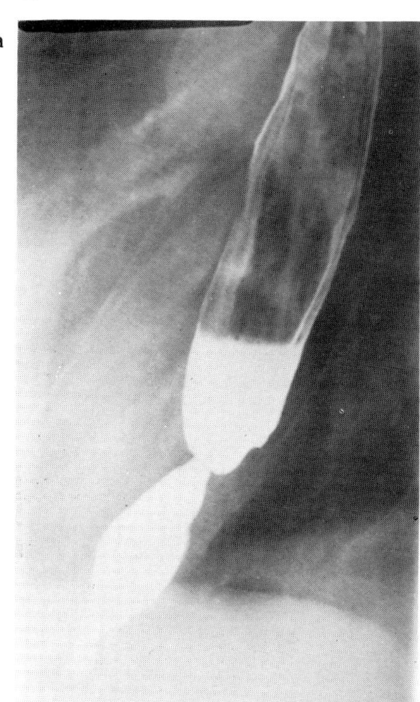

b

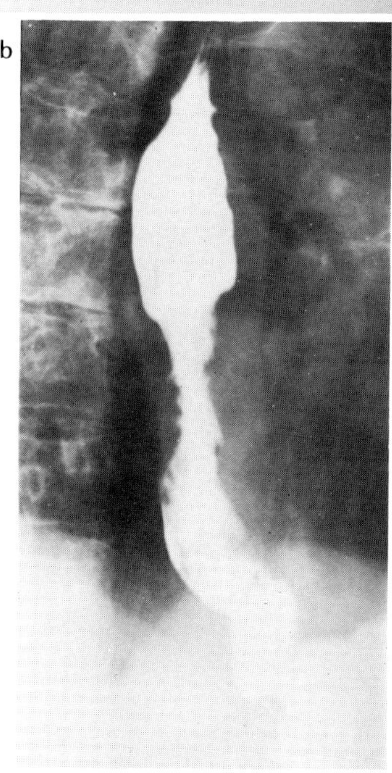

Fig. 4.15 *Comparison of benign and malignant strictures. Radiographs: (a) Peptic stricture. (b) Carcinoma of oesophagus.*

Treatment

Oesophageal carcinoma is not often curable, but a great deal can be done, both by surgery and radiotherapy, to relieve the progressive dysphagia which is the most distressing symptom.

Surgical resection is used for carcinomas of the middle and lower third, whenever that is feasible. The most usual procedure is to perform a wide resection of the oesophagus along with a cuff of stomach, and to bring the mobilised stomach up into the chest for the oesophago-gastric anastomosis (Fig. 4.16). Total oesophagectomy is now favoured for high carcinomas lying around the level of the aortic arch; the whole oesophagus is mobilised and removed through thoracic and cervical incisions, and the stomach is then brought up and anastomosed to the upper oesophagus in the neck, at the level of the thyroid gland.

Carcinomas of the upper one-third, which are almost always squamous cell neoplasms, generally respond well to radiotherapy, and this is preferred to resection.

Unhappily, a number of patients are no longer resectable when they present, and in these cases relief can usually be given by insertion of a plastic cuffed tube through the carcinoma: this is done either endoscopically or by operation. Intubation can give considerable relief of dysphagia.

In spite of modern advances in nutritional support and intensive care, the operative mortality remains around 10%, and the 5-year survival rate is also about 1 in 10.

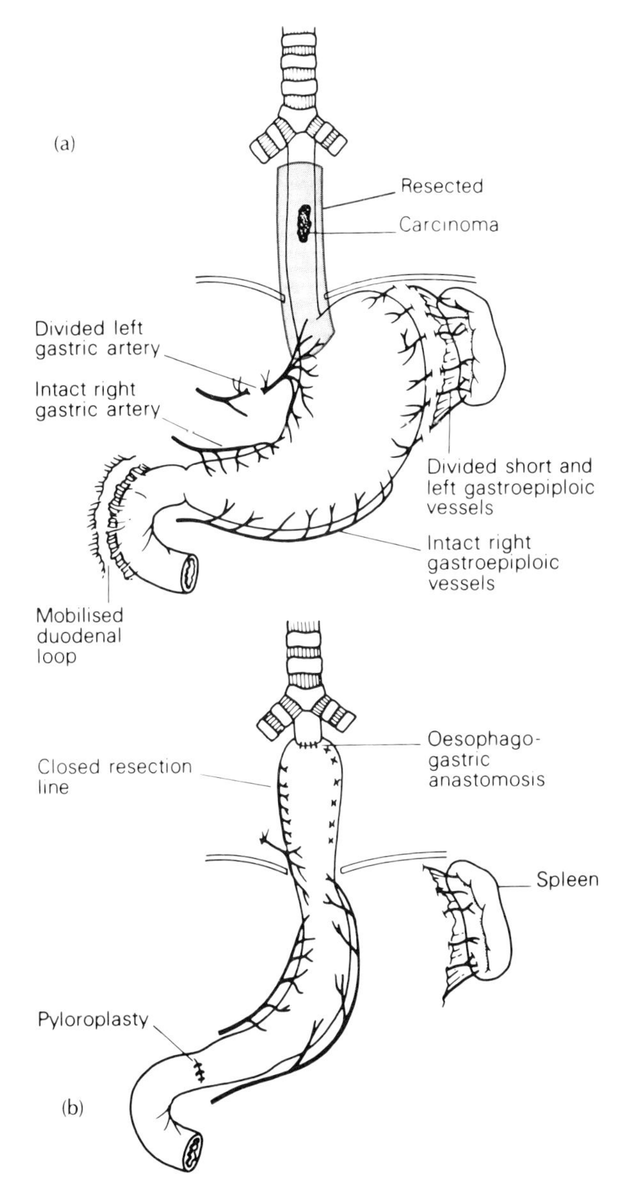

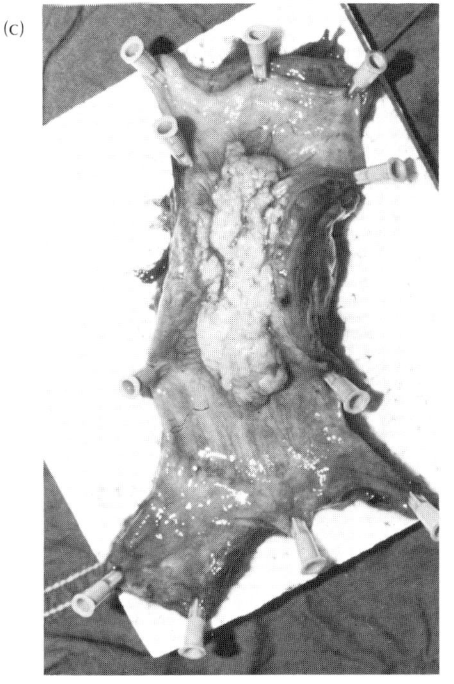

Fig. 4.16 *Surgery for carcinoma of oesophagus. (a) Diagram of tissue resected in Lewis oesophagectomy. (b) Reconstruction in Lewis oesophagectomy. (c) Photograph of specimen.*

5

Stomach and Duodenum

Although the stomach and duodenum lie in continuity and are often considered together they are in many ways dissimilar. Their functions are very different: peptic ulcer is much commoner in the duodenum; primary malignant disease is almost unheard of in the duodenum but all too often seen in the stomach.

ANATOMY

Half of the normal stomach is hidden under the costal margin (Fig. 5.1) but when the stomach is obstructed the greater curvature may lie well below the umbilicus and the important physical sign of visible gastric peristalsis may be seen.

It is customary to divide the stomach arbitrarily into three parts: the fundus, the body, and the antrum (Fig. 5.2). The *fundus* is the uppermost part of the stomach; the *body* extends from the gastro-oesophageal junction to the region of the incisura; and the *antrum* stretches onwards down to the pylorus (see microscopy, p. 72).

The important structures in the neighbourhood of the stomach are shown in Figs 5.1 and 5.3. These explain how a carcinoma of the greater curvature can produce a gastro-colic fistula, how a posterior penetrating gastric ulcer can erode the pancreas or the splenic artery, and why a posterior duodenal ulcer not infrequently penetrates to and erodes the wall of the gastro-duodenal artery; both events cause very grave gastric haemorrhage.

The stomach has three main layers: there is an outer serosal coat, absent only along both curvatures and at the gastro-oesophageal junction; a muscular coat whose fibres run in three definite layers – outer longitudinal, middle circular fibres (most prominent at the pylorus where it forms the pyloric sphincter), and inner oblique coat (most prominent in the body); the inner lining is the mucous membrane. Especially in the body and

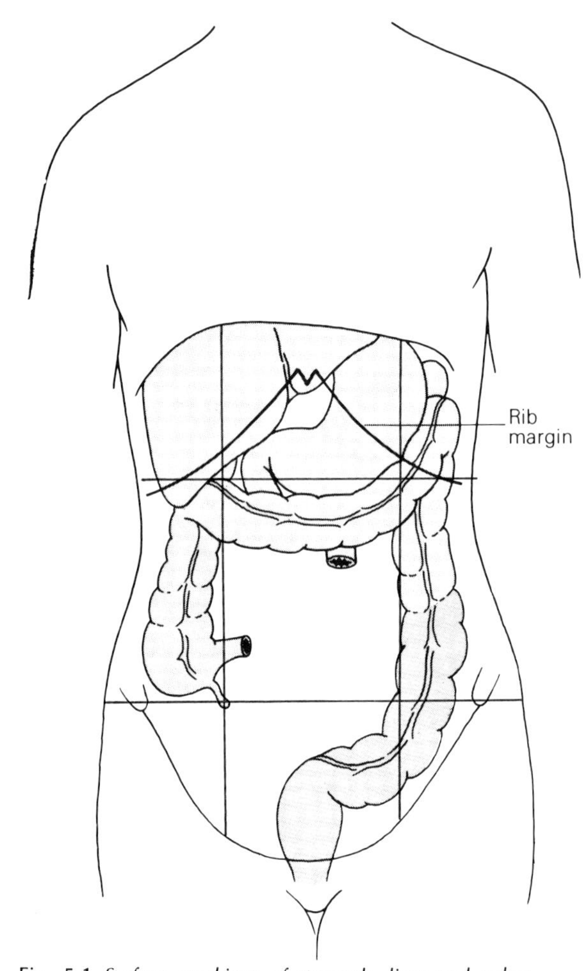

Fig. 5.1 *Surface markings of stomach, liver and colon.*

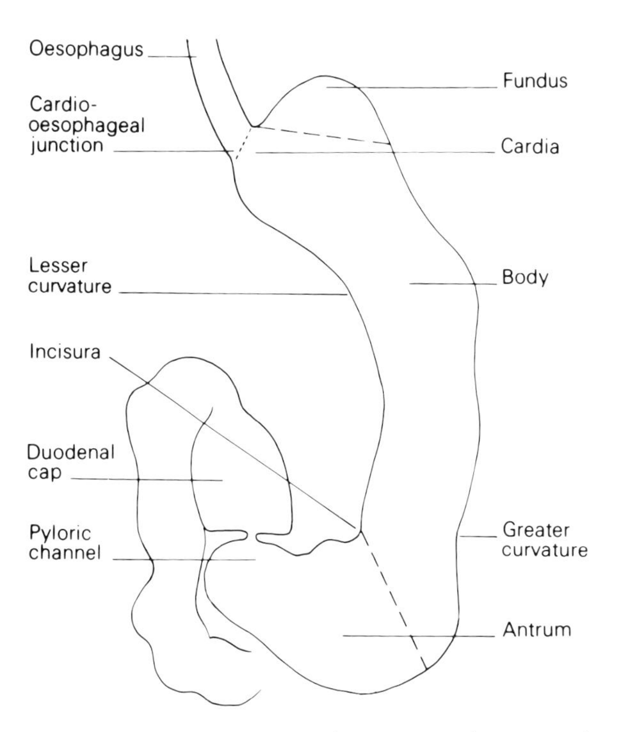

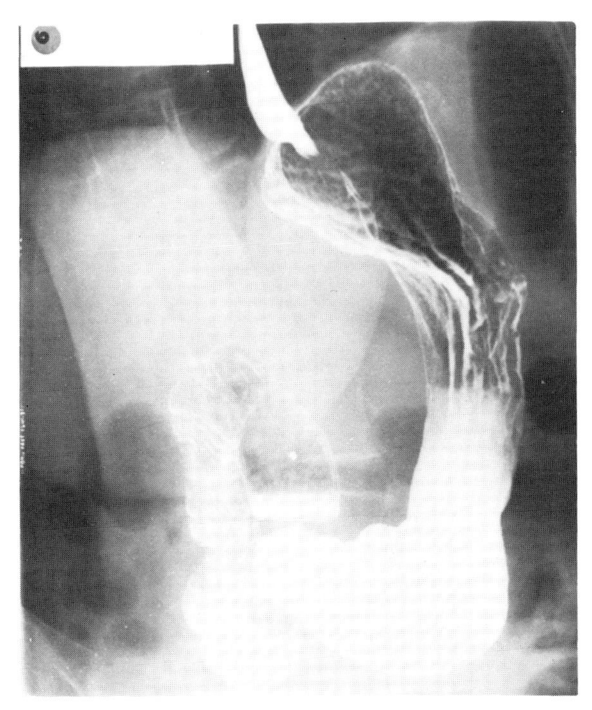

Fig. 5.2 *Anatomy of the stomach. Air-contrast barium meal showing normal stomach and normal duodenal cap.*

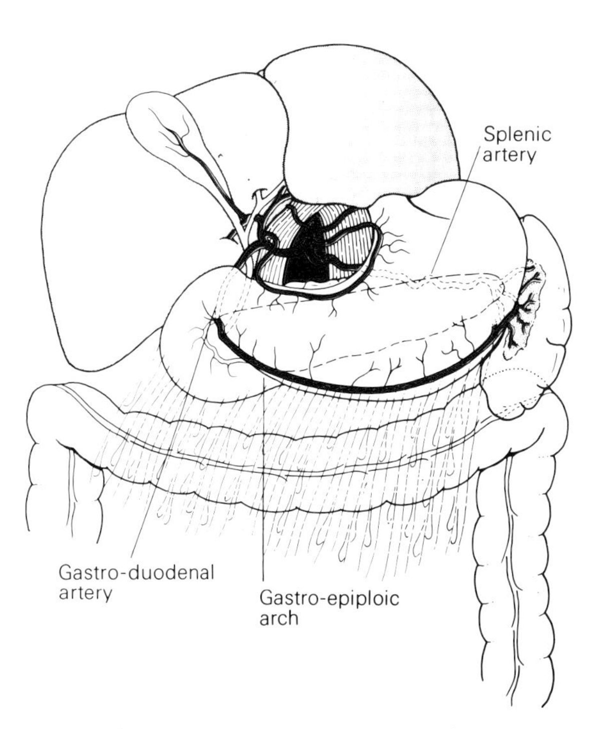

Fig. 5.3 *Blood supply and relations of stomach.*

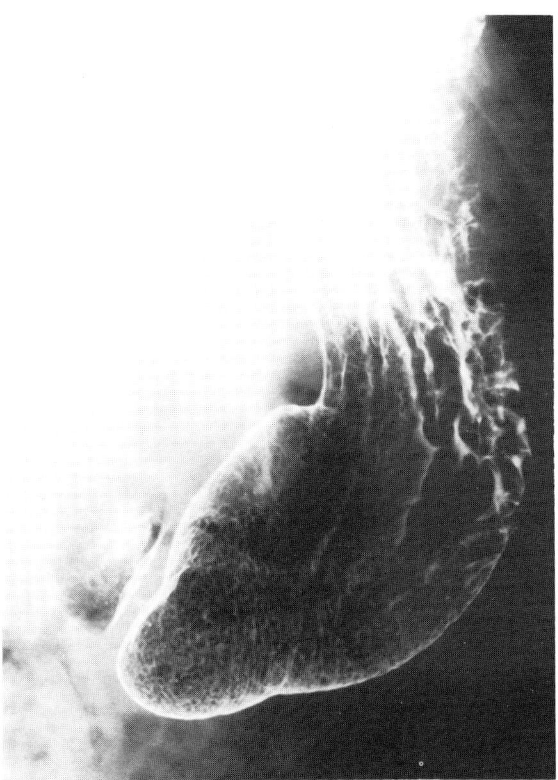

Fig. 5.4 *Air contrast barium meal showing gastric rugae.*

along the greater curvature, the mucosa is thrown up into folds called rugae (Fig. 5.4), so that the surface area of the mucosa is very much greater than that of the muscular wall of the stomach.

When the rugae are flattened by gastric distension, the mouths of innumerable gastric pits can be seen.

Microscopy (Fig. 5.5)

Between three and seven glands open into each gastric pit.

The neck cells are responsible for the replacement of surface epithelium, which has a turnover of 2–3 days. The mucous neck cells (goblet cells) are found most commonly around the cardia and in the antrum. The chief (or peptic) cells are situated mainly in the deeper parts of the glands and are readily identified by their prominent zymogen granules, which contain pepsinogen. The parietal (oxyntic) cells, which are mainly sited in the more superficial parts of the glands, contain intracellular canaliculi and secrete hydrochloric acid.

In the antrum, there are large numbers of pyloric glands, (secreting mucus) and G cells (Fig 5.6). G cells secrete gastrin, of which the two major forms are little gastrin G 17 and big gastrin G 34 (the

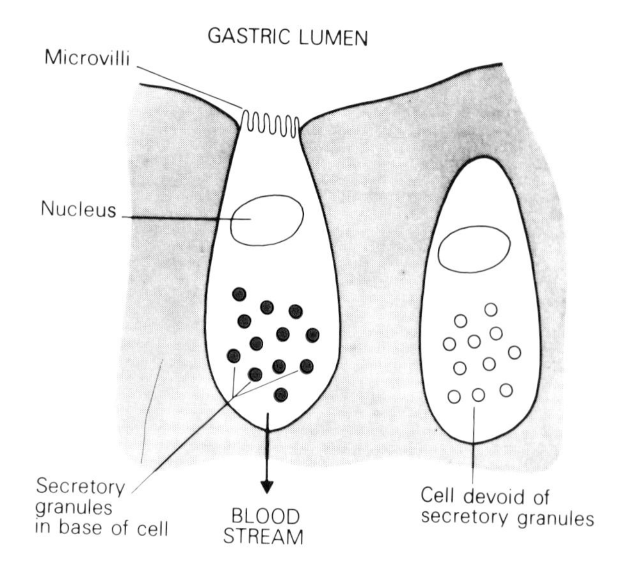

Fig. 5.6 *Sketch of a G cell.*

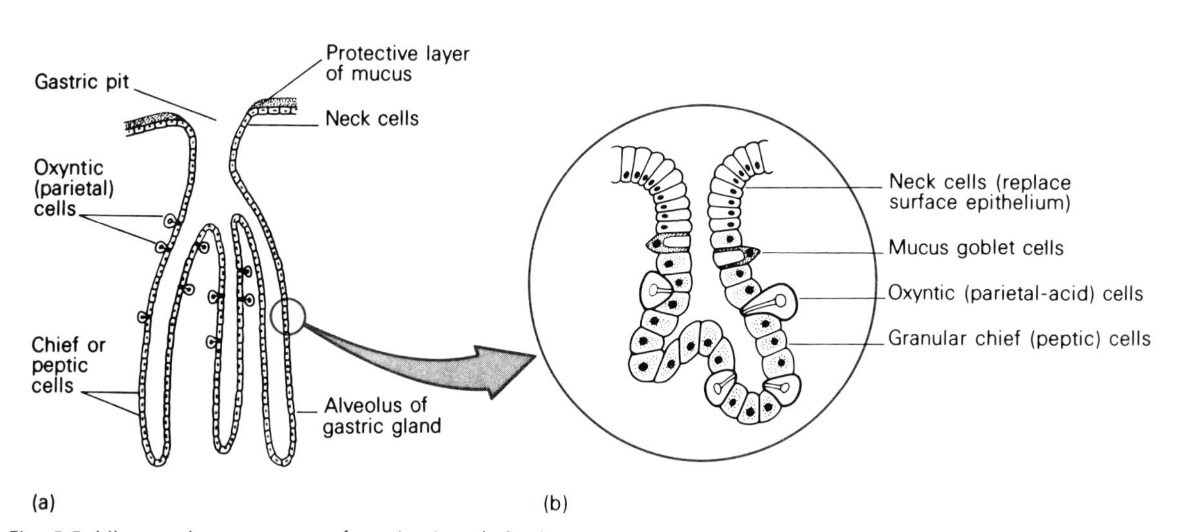

Fig. 5.5 *Microscopic appearances of gastric pit and glands.*

numbers indicate the number of amino-acid residues in the peptide chain). G cells are also present in the proximal duodenum, mainly producing G 34 (see p. 75). The junction between antral and body mucosa may be visible but is more precisely drawn by measuring surface pH. Gastric ulcers mostly occur on or below this mucosal junction. It is interesting that this junction migrates proximally with age: ageing is also associated with gradual atrophic changes in the gastric mucosa (see p. 81).

Blood Supply

The stomach is well supplied with blood. The left gastric, the right gastric, the gastroepiploic arcade, and the short gastric vessels from the splenic artery provide a rich arterial anastomosis. The venous drainage follows the arterial system and drains into the portal venous system. Lymphatic channels follow the arteries.

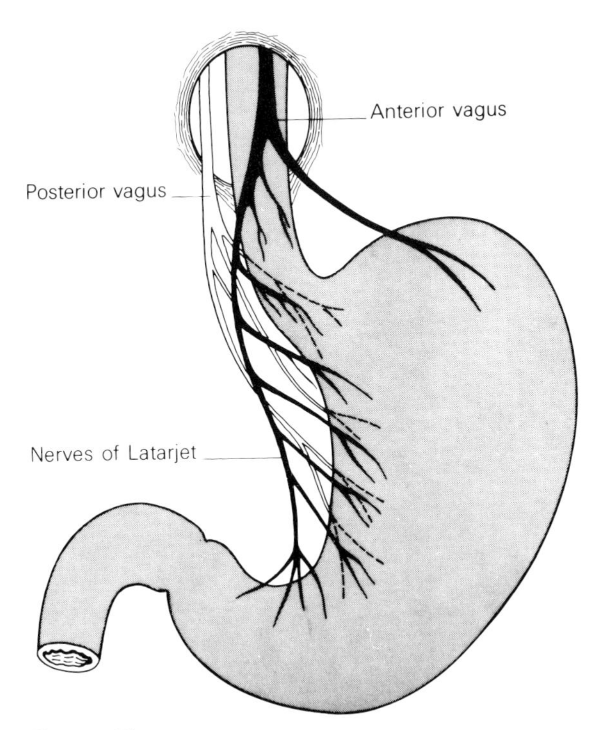

Fig. 5.7 *The vagus nerves.*

Nerve Supply

Sympathetic nerves from the coeliac axis follow the arterial supply. The important supply comes from the parasympathetic nervous system via the vagus nerves, which have both motor and secretory functions. Both branches enter the abdomen through the oesophageal hiatus, the anterior nerve closely applied to the front of the abdominal oesophagus and the posterior vagus lying behind and to the right (Fig. 5.7). The two nerves run distally within the lesser omentum (where they are called the nerves of Latarjet) and supply the stomach, pylorus and intestines.

PHYSIOLOGY

Functions of the Stomach

As a reservoir

During eating, contractions of the stomach are inhibited and 'receptive relaxation' occurs.

Gastric emptying depends on the contractions of the antrum, and is completed in 1–4 hours. The rate of emptying depends on:

1. The amount of food present. About 3% of the gastric contents is released per minute.
2. The osmotic relationship of the contents. Gastric secretion renders food isotonic and maximal emptying only occurs when this is achieved, usually after about 2 hours. Fatty meals delay emptying.

It is important to remember that the pyloric closing mechanism not only regulates gastric emptying but prevents reflux of duodenal contents into the stomach. The study of patients after pyloroplasty shows that bile can be highly irritating to gastric mucosa and can cause a troublesome gastritis. One of the particular virtues of highly selective vagotomy (see p. 90) is that it leaves untouched the complex of antrum, pyloric sphincter and proximal duodenum, with its nerve and blood supply completely intact, so the regulation of gastric emptying can proceed normally.

Commencing digestion

The food taken into the stomach is wetted by gastric secretion and then churned by gastric contractions against a closed pylorus.

The secretion of hydrochloric acid has two functions: the hydrolysis of food and the activation of pepsinogen (produced in the zymogen granules of the parietal cells) (Fig. 5.8). Pepsin splits protein into polypeptides and peptones (see Chapter 7).

Antibacterial action

Gastric juice undiluted by food has a pH of about 2.0, and this is sufficient to render gastric juice sterile. If gastric acid secretion is reduced by disease, drugs or surgery, there is an increased likelihood of bacterial growth.

Commencing absorption of some elements of food

The stomach has the capacity to absorb some water, alcohol, certain drugs, and glucose from hypertonic glucose solutions, but this is only of minor importance in supporting life. The presence of an acid pH may be important in permitting the normal absorption of iron from the duodenum, perhaps by aiding the reduction of ferrous to ferric iron. This mechanism may be impaired when surgery alters gastric pH.

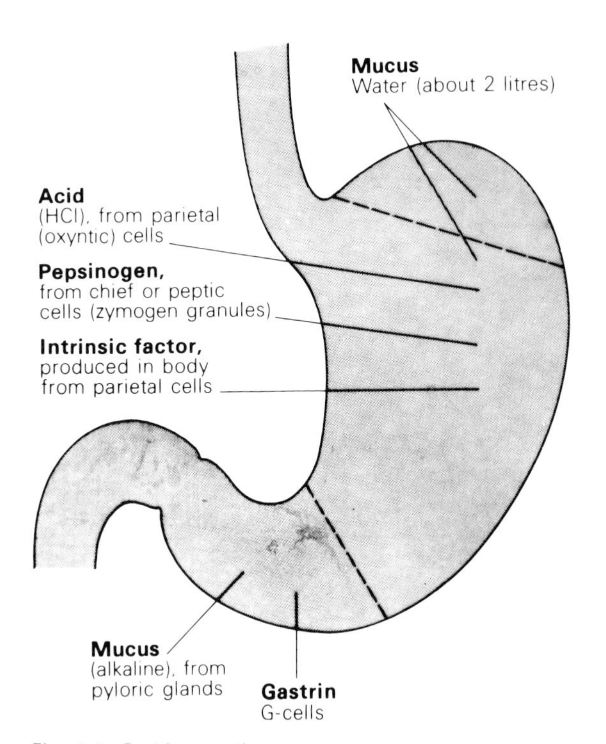

Fig. 5.8 *Gastric secretions.*

Haemopoiesis

The secretion of intrinsic factor in the body of the stomach is necessary for the normal absorption of vitamin B_{12} in the ileum (see p. 121).

The 'gastric mucosal barrier'

An organ which contains both acid and pepsin must have some mechanism to save it from autodigestion. This barrier is not normally easily penetrated by hydrogen ions, but a drug such as aspirin, or bile refluxing through the pylorus, seriously increases the permeability of this barrier.

Gastric Secretion

It is possible to divide gastric secretion into basal secretion – that which occurs after a meal has been digested – and postprandial secretion.

Basal secretion

This is generally higher in the morning than in the evening, and at a minimum during sleep. Basal acid secretion tends to be above normal in duodenal ulcer patients, and is probably largely under vagal control.

Postprandial secretion

Three phases are distinguished, although they greatly overlap (Fig. 5.9).

Cephalic or neural (Fig. 5.10). This is stimulated by the sight, smell or even the anticipation of food, and is mediated by the vagus nerve.

Gastric (Fig. 5.11). This phase is stimulated by food or other distension of the stomach. It is mainly humoral but is also in part vagally mediated. The main humoral agent is gastrin, but many other chemical messengers have been identified (see p. 19).

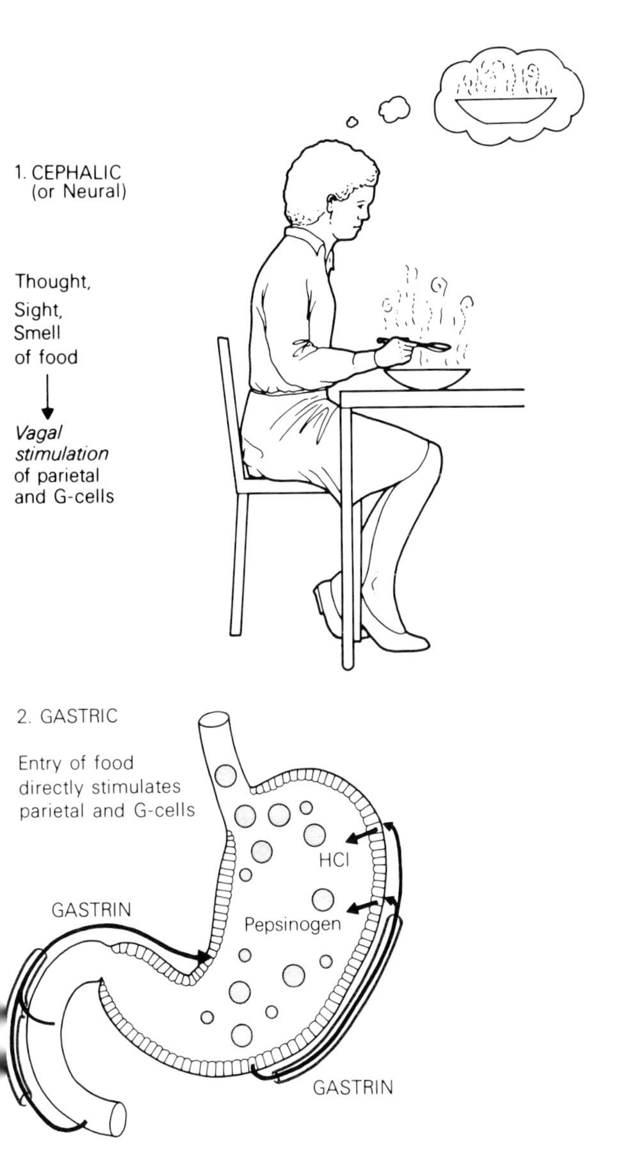

Fig. 5.9 *The phases of gastric secretion.*

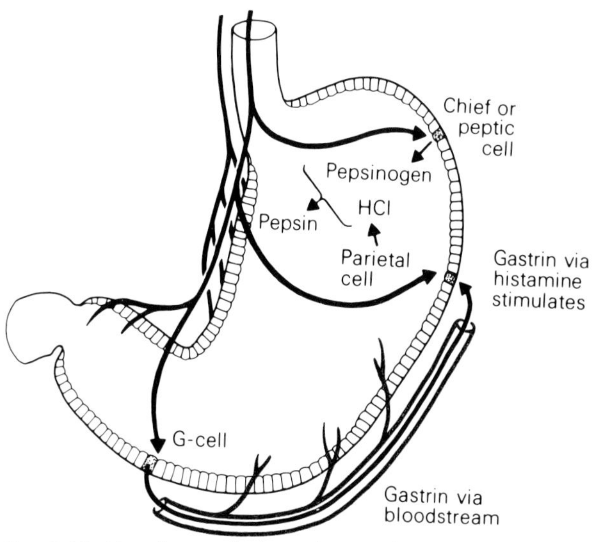

Fig. 5.10 *Neural control of gastric secretion.*

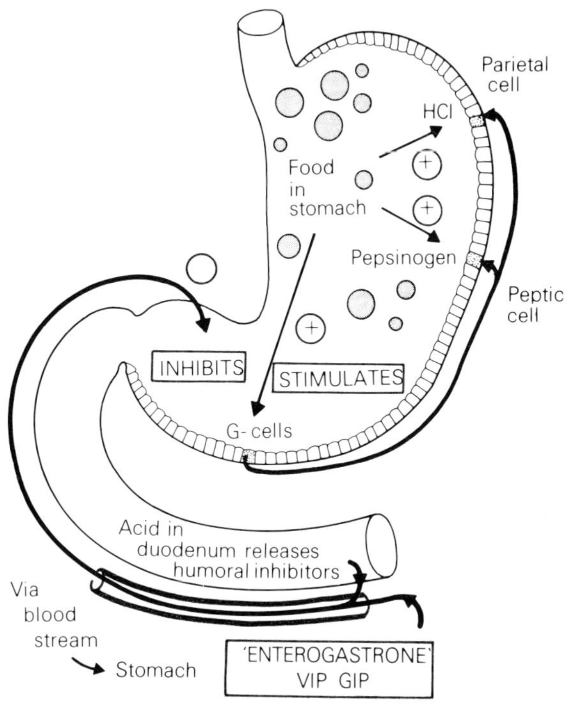

Fig. 5.11 *Humoral control of gastric secretion.*

Intestinal. This phase is initiated by the passage of food into the duodenum and upper jejunum. It is entirely humoral, and contains both stimulatory and inhibitory elements. The mechanism of intestinal stimulation of gastric secretion is not yet clear, although gastrin can be released from the upper duodenum.

There is now clear evidence that the presence of fat in the duodenum inhibits gastric secretion in man. This appears to be due to the release of an enterogastrone, which may or may not be distinct from secretin and cholecystokinin. The upper small intestine also secretes gastric inhibitory polypeptide (GIP) and vasoactive intestinal peptide (VIP), which both inhibit gastric secretion (see p. 18).

The three phases – cephalic, gastric and intestinal – are coordinated and concurrent. In man, as opposed to experimental animals, vagal release of gastrin seems to be of minor importance.

Gastric Function Tests

In the past, these were much used in diagnosis and in the planning of surgical treatment, but indications for their use are now strictly limited to the following situations:

1. In the rare event of the suspicion that a patient has Zollinger–Ellison syndrome (see p. 78).
2. To confirm the diagnosis of Addisonian pernicious anaemia. Pentagastrin (a synthetic pentapeptide, simulating gastrin) is injected and acid output measured by analysis of samples of gastric juice: in PA there is total achlorhydria due to atrophic gastritis.
3. To test the completeness of a previous operation to denervate the stomach (Hollander's test). Insulin is injected to produce hypoglycaemia. This stress stimulates the vagus via the hypothalamus: if some vagal fibres to the stomach are still intact, then acid output will rise.

ANATOMY AND PHYSIOLOGY OF THE DUODENUM

The duodenum is to a considerable extent retroperitoneal, which is an important point to remember because rupture of the duodenum can be silent until retroperitoneal cellulitis is well established. The wall is like the rest of the small intestine in having outer longitudinal and inner circular layers of muscle, with a villiform mucosa arranged in circular folds.

Brunner's glands are very similar in appearance to the pyloric glands of the gastric antrum but produce an alkaline secretion which, with bile and pancreatic juice, probably provides important protection against the digestive effects of gastric juice.

Within the loop of the duodenum lies the pancreas, thus pancreatic tumours may invade and obstruct the duodenum.

Fibre-optic endoscopy now allows direct inspection of the whole of the duodenum and, via the ampulla of Vater, retrograde catheterisation allows the biliary and pancreatic ducts to be visualised (ERCP, p. 51).

PEPTIC ULCER

Aetiology

A peptic ulcer is a breach in mucous membrane which is within or close to mucosa producing hydrochloric acid and pepsin. The common sites are therefore stomach and duodenum, less commonly lower oesophagus, and rarely jejunum or (in the case of Meckel's diverticulum, see p. 272) the ileum.

The cause of peptic ulceration remains unknown (see p. 30), but there are some clues to the reason for its occurrence in certain individuals. Gastric acid plays an important part, insofar as benign peptic ulcers are exceedingly rare in patients with achlorhydria (e.g. in pernicious anaemia), and they nearly always occur – and are exceedingly troublesome – in severe hypersecretion, as in the Zollinger–Ellison syndrome (p. 78). Some duodenal ulcer patients secrete more gastric acid than do normal people, both at a basal level and in response to pentagastrin. In about 50% of duodenal ulcer subjects, however, the acid secretion lies within the normal range, whilst the majority of gastric ulcer patients are hypochlorhydric. It is therefore clear that excess acid production cannot be the sole mechanism and others must operate to reduce the resistance of the mucosa to ulceration.

Factors which certainly contribute are:

Sex

Men are more prone to peptic ulceration than women, and this is particularly true for duodenal ulceration. In Western Europe the male: female ratio for duodenal ulcer (DU) is about 4:1, and for gastric ulcer (GU) it is about 2:1. (However, there are considerable geographical differences in these ratios – see p. 30).

Family history

When a teenager presents with a duodenal ulcer there is almost invariably a close relative who also has the condition.

The relatives of patients with a gastric or duodenal ulcer are three times more likely to have a similar ulcer. However, DU families do not suffer more gastric ulceration than the general population nor do GU families particularly suffer from DU.

Blood group O is particularly associated with the occurrence of duodenal, but not gastric, ulceration. Non-secretion of ABO substances is associated with the development of a duodenal ulcer.

Diet

The striking difference in the incidence of duodenal ulceration between the North and the South of India has been explained on the basis of a marked difference in diet (p. 30). In Western countries there is no evidence to incriminate any particular food, with the possible exception of coffee.

Smoking

There is no clear evidence that heavy smoking induces peptic ulceration (though there is a strong suspicion of this among many clinicians). However, healing of an ulcer is certainly delayed by continuation of smoking.

Alcohol

There is no proof that excess alcohol ingestion is an important aetiological factor. Modest drinking seems to be associated with a lower incidence of ulceration.

Drugs

The drug which is most clearly associated with gastric ulceration is aspirin. Habitual use of aspirin-containing analgesic powders has been clearly related to the recent rise in gastric ulceration among Australian women.

Other non-steroidal anti-inflammatory drugs, such as indomethacin and phenylbutazone, are also liable to cause gastric ulceration. Both appear to have a direct toxic effect on the gastric mucosal barrier.

There is no proven association between drug ingestion and duodenal ulceration. For a long time there has been a clinical suspicion that corticosteroids induce peptic ulceration but this is not proven. Simultaneous ingestion of alcohol and aspirin together carries a particular risk of bleeding from acute gastric erosions.

There is now strong evidence that prostaglandins are crucially important in mucosal protection. Some drugs – including aspirin, indomethacin, and other non-steroidal anti-inflammatory agents – inhibit prostaglandin synthesis.

Stress

For a long time it has been believed that the busy young executive, constantly under pressure from above and below, is especially liable to duodenal ulceration. This is not proven, and there is evidence that DU occurs more often among the self-employed and the unemployed. Gastric ulcer is commoner among poorer sections of the community.

There is an important connection between

trauma and peptic ulceration. It has long been recognised that severe burns (Curling's ulcer) and head injuries (Cushing's ulcer) can occasionally be associated with acute, deeply-penetrating ulcers of duodenum or stomach, which are particularly likely to bleed or perforate. Gravely ill septic patients, especially those with severe abdominal injuries, are particularly likely to suffer stress peptic ulceration: there is now good evidence that these can largely be prevented by effective prophylactic antacid administration.

Zollinger–Ellison syndrome

For a long time it has been recognised that there are a few patients whose tendency to produce a peptic ulcer is so strong that recurrent ulceration rapidly follows standard gastric surgery and only ceases after total gastrectomy. In 1955, Zollinger and Ellison described two patients whose gastric hypersecretion and recurrent ulceration was associated with a non-β cell tumour of the pancreas. Subsequently Gregory showed that these were gastrin-secreting neoplasms (gastrinomas), of which about 60% are malignant and many are multicentric.

Patients, usually of middle age, tend to have a history of dyspepsia over several years and then, following gastric surgery, rapidly form a recurrent ulcer and complain of diarrhoea. The ulcer is either in the duodenum (quite often post-bulbar) or the jejunum, and both haemorrhage and perforation are likely to occur. If a further gastric operation is performed, recurrence rapidly follows again.

The diagnosis is confirmed by estimating the serum gastrin level, which is many times above the normal range of 30–120 pg/ml.

If possible a tumour in the pancreas is localised and removed, but this can only be done in a few patients. Cimetidine and ranitidine are valuable for relieving the most severe symptoms in patients with multiple or metastatic lesions. Total gastrectomy is still sometimes a useful, if severe, treatment.

Figures 5.12 and 5.13 show the aetiological factors believed to be important in the origin of gastric and duodenal ulceration.

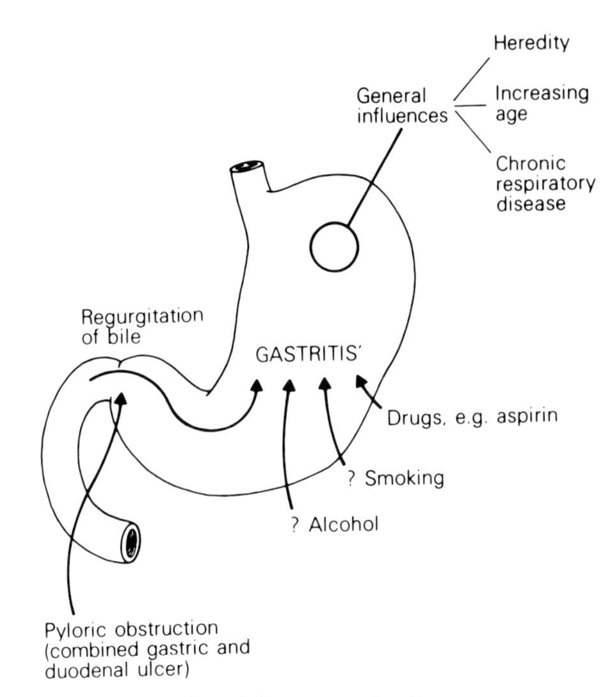

Fig. 5.12 *Aetiological factors: gastric ulcer.*

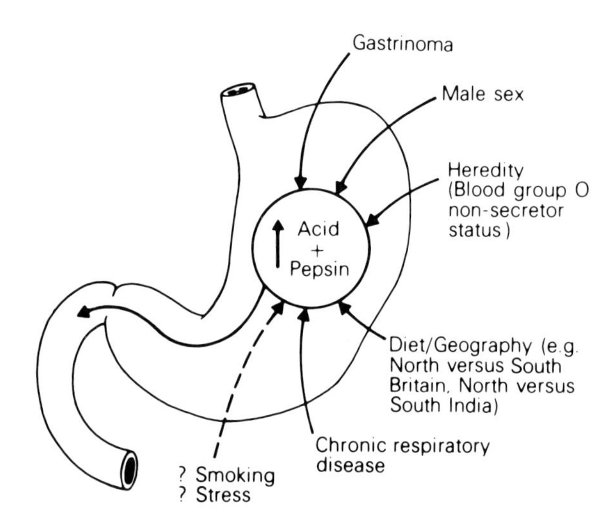

Fig. 5.13 *Aetiological factors: duodenal ulcer.*

Pathology

Gastric Ulcer

Acute gastric erosions (small shallow ulcers which appear rapidly and heal without scarring) can occur as a result of acute insults to the stomach.

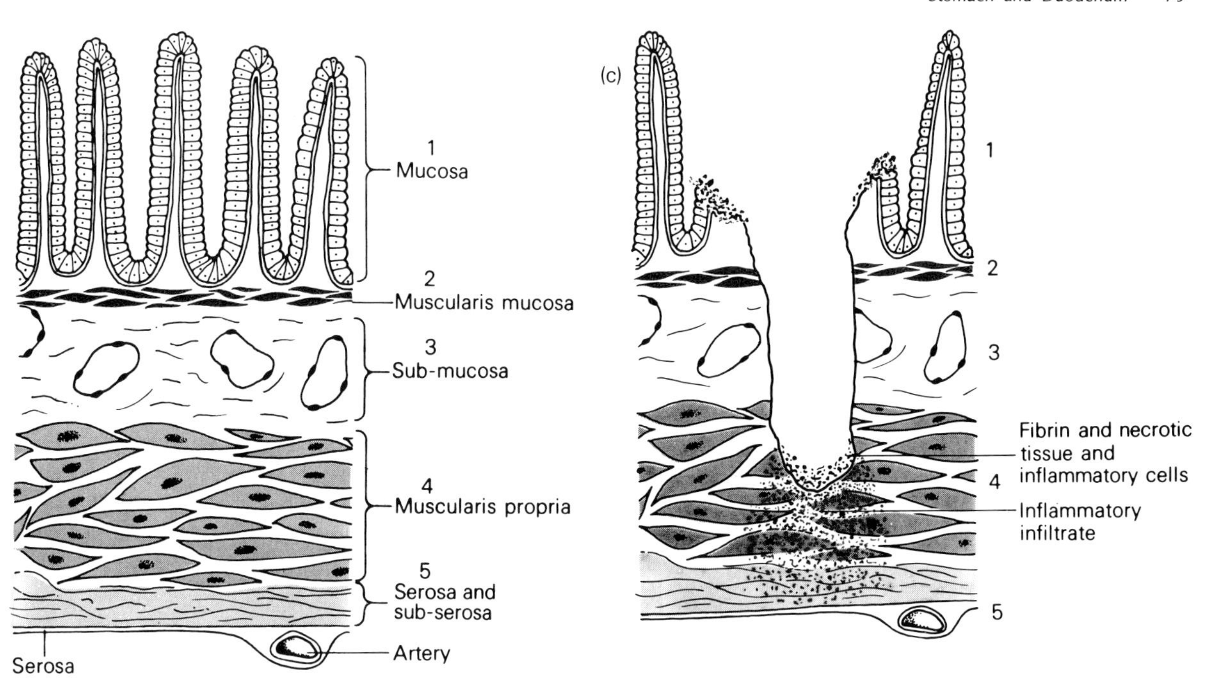

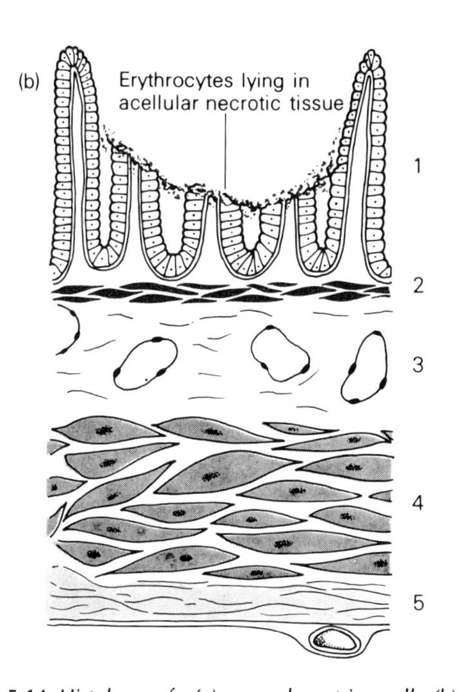

Fig. 5.14 *Histology of: (a) normal gastric wall, (b) acute haemorrhagic erosion, (c) acute gastric ulcer. (The numbers in each diagram refer to the layers labelled in (a). See also Figs 5.16, 5.31 and 5.32).*

These include an alcoholic binge, aspirin ingestion, and acute severe illnesses. These ulcers often penetrate to the submucosal vascular plexus and can cause a major haematemesis (Fig. 5.14b), and may progress to an acute ulcer (Fig. 5.14c).

Chronic gastric ulcers tend to occur close to the line of junction of antral mucosa with body mucosa (Figs 5.15, 5.16, 5.17). They are usually single and 2 cm or less in diameter, although there is a strong tendency for posterior ulcers to enlarge and penetrate into the body of the pancreas: occasionally the splenic artery is eroded, causing very severe haemorrhage (Fig. 5.18). Free perforation of a gastric ulcer into the peritoneal cavity is considerably less common than perforation of a duodenal ulcer, but carries a worse prognosis. This is because gastric perforations are often large and therefore more difficult to close securely: they also cause a severe degree of peritoneal contamination, so the postoperative recovery in these patients can be complicated. Furthermore, some gastric carcinomas present with perforation, and it can be very difficult to identify these at the time of emergency operation. It is therefore a rule that a biopsy of a perforated gastric ulcer should be

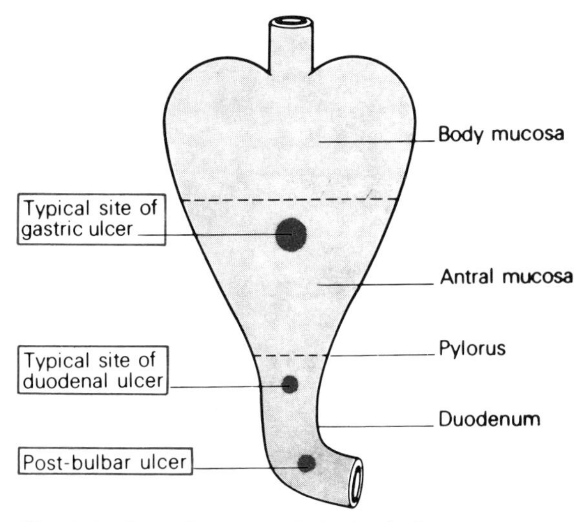

Fig. 5.15 *Sites of gastric and duodenal ulcers.*

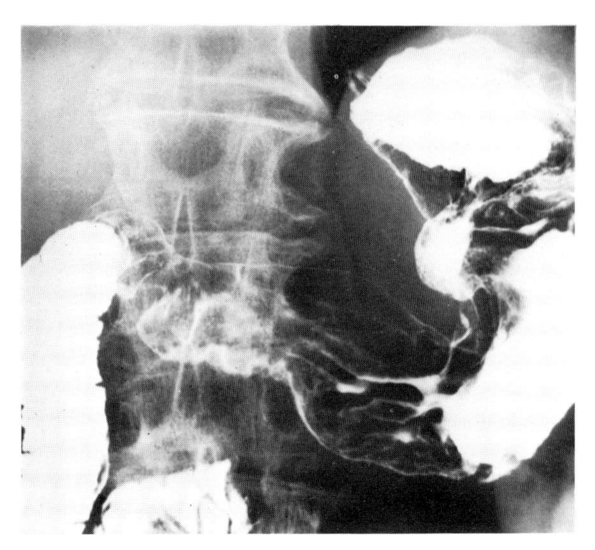

Fig. 5.17 *Barium meal showing penetrating ulcer of lesser curvature.*

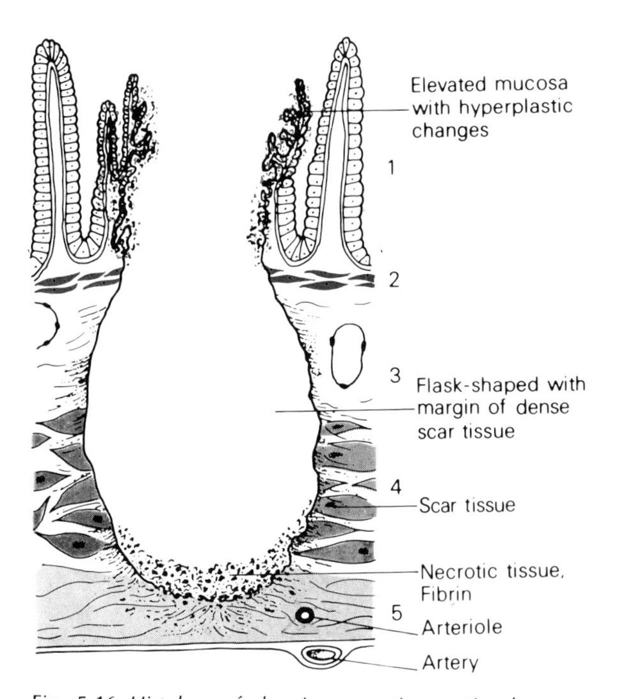

Fig. 5.16 *Histology of chronic penetrating peptic ulcer.*

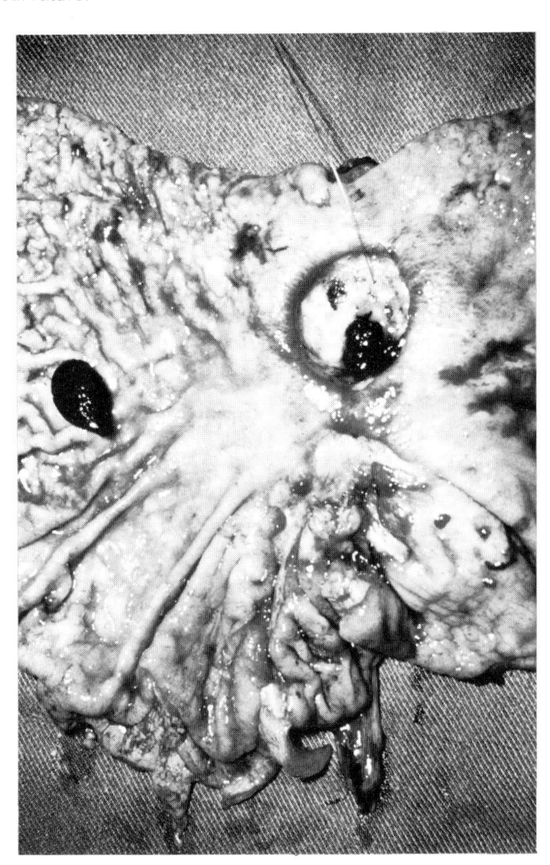

Fig. 5.18 *Penetrating gastric ulcer which has eroded an artery (cannulated) causing severe haemorrhage.*

obtained: in many cases the best way to achieve this is to perform an immediate partial gastrectomy. This gives a complete removal of the ulcer and circumvents the problem of achieving sound closure of a large perforation.

The difficulty of distinguishing between a

benign gastric ulcer and an early gastric cancer is very real. Even the advent of endoscopy has not always made this distinction easier, because both can look alike. The ability to take biopsies from the edge of the ulcer can be of crucial importance, but malignant change is not necessarily present in all parts of the ulcer and so negative histology does not exclude a carcinoma. It is now believed to be very rare for carcinomatous transformation (ulcer cancer) to occur in a chronic gastric ulcer.

Chronic atrophic gastritis, and its possible relation to peptic and neoplastic ulceration of the stomach, is the subject of much controversy and speculation. This condition is a slowly progressive atrophy of the gastric mucosa, with a reduction of the number of peptic and parietal cells in the mucosa of the body, and of the glands in the antrum, causing a reduction in output of acid and pepsin and of intrinsic factor. There is an important tendency to metaplasia of gastric to intestinal-type mucosa, which is accompanied by increased nuclear activity and high mitosis counts.

In duodenal ulcer, the gastritis is localised to the antrum and may be a response of the gastric mucosa to hyperacidity. In chronic gastric ulcers and carcinomas, the changes of gastritis are much more general but the antrum is always affected. It is thought that the chronic gastritis is probably present first and a peptic ulcer follows because the atrophic mucosa is less able to resist the factors which cause the peptic ulcer.

The relationship of chronic gastritis and carcinoma of the stomach is considered on page 94.

Gradual change of gastric mucosa towards atrophy is a natural occurrence as the individual grows older and is particularly noticeable over 70. Other factors which are associated with chronic gastritis are the long-term ingestion of salicylates, constant drinking of very hot fluids, low socio-economic class, and possession of blood group A. Consistent heavy alcohol drinking is not established as a factor.

Duodenal ulcer

The major aetiological factors are summarised in Fig. 5.13.

Acute ulcers may appear in the duodenum in conditions of stress; Curling's ulcer is a unique form of this (see p. 78).

Chronic ulcers mostly occur in the bulb of the first part, just distal to the pylorus, and 50% are situated on the anterior wall. A few ulcers occur more distally, at the junction of the first and second parts, and are known as post bulbar ulcers (Fig. 5.15).

The fluctuating activity that is so characteristic of duodenal ulcer is reflected in periods of active ulceration, when symptoms are severe, followed by remission, when healing with fibrosis occurs (Fig. 5.19). This fibrosis causes the scarring and pouching of the duodenal cap typically seen in barium meals (Fig. 5.20). Repeated episodes of fibrosis over the years may eventually lead to such marked contraction of the duodenum that it presents an obstruction, which is generally known as 'pyloric stenosis' (Fig. 5.21).

Active anterior ulcers may perforate: active posterior ulcers may penetrate the pancreas, and cause severe back pain. If the gastroduodenal

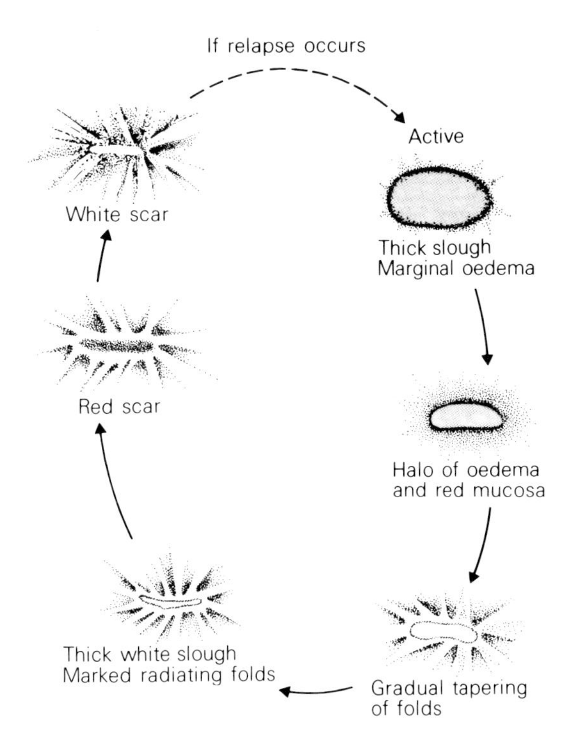

Fig. 5.19 *Life cycle of benign peptic ulcer.*

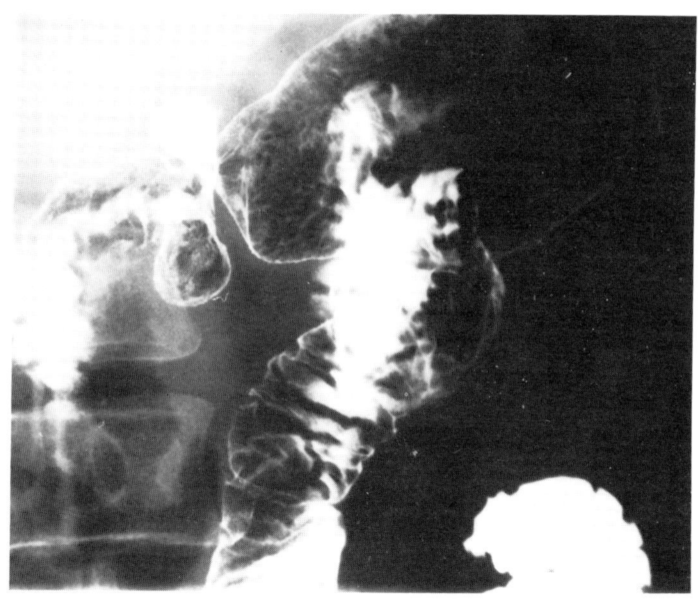

Fig. 5.20 *Barium meal of typical 'clover-leaf' deformity of chronic duodenal ulcer.*

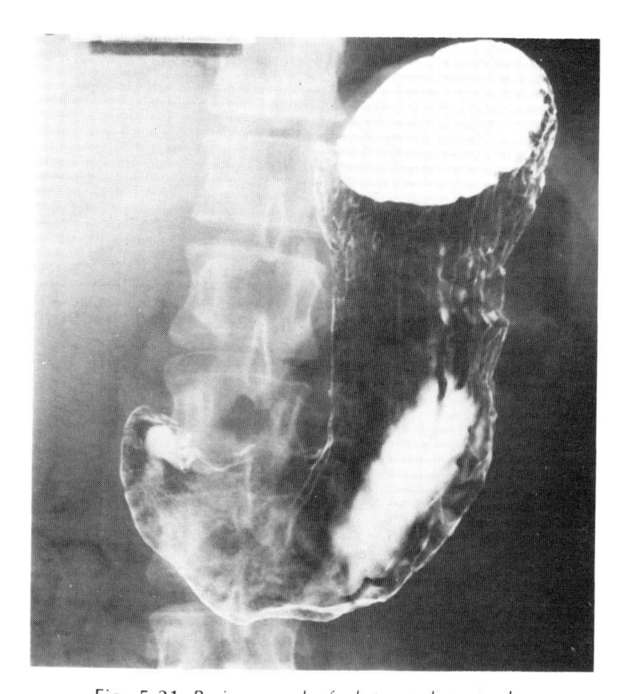

Fig. 5.21 *Barium meal of obstructed stomach.*

artery (see Fig. 5.3) is eroded, this causes particularly severe haemorrhage which requires very urgent surgical arrest.

Combined gastric and duodenal ulcers

In about 20% of all peptic ulcers, a gastric and a duodenal ulcer coexist. Generally, the duodenal ulcer appears first and, in about two-thirds of cases, causes some degree of pyloric hold-up: the gastric ulcer seems to follow a period of gastric stasis. Haemorrhage complicates combined ulceration unduly often.

Clinical Features of Peptic Ulcer

The symptoms and signs of both gastric and duodenal ulcers are considered together since, despite many claims to the contrary in the past, the clinical distinction is difficult and the overlap considerable.

Pain

The predominant symptom of peptic ulcer is pain or discomfort. This is commonly epigastric, but may also be felt in the right upper quadrant, around the umbilicus, and even in the lower abdomen. Radiation to the back may occur with posterior ulcers. Pain is commonly related to meals, coming on up to two hours after food. In some duodenal ulcer patients, hunger pain is relieved by eating. Nocturnal pain, commonly around 2–3 am, is also a feature, especially of duodenal ulcer. Pain is usually short-lived and is commonly relieved by antacids. This suggests that pain may arise from acid 'bathing' the ulcer, and there is some experimental evidence to support this.

Heartburn

Burning discomfort substernally, radiating upwards in the midline, suggests incompetence of the cardia and may occur in peptic ulcer as well as hiatal hernia.

Vomiting

This is sometimes a feature and, because it may relieve pain, may be self-induced. When persistent, it suggests gastric outflow obstruction, and the patient may notice food from a previous day's meals. Stenosis of the gastric outlet leads to copious projectile vomiting, often late in the day. At the bedside, a gastric succussion splash may be detectable. This valuable sign, indicating gastric outlet obstruction, is elicited by gently rocking the pelvis and abdomen from side to side while listening for a characteristic loud splashing sound. (NB: this can be heard in healthy people within two hours of drinking.) Both patient and doctor may be surprised bv the volume of the vomitus, which reflects the fact that gastric secretions may amount to two litres per day.

Anorexia

This rare symptom should raise the suspicion of malignancy.

Tenderness

This is a consistent sign of peptic ulcer, and point tenderness is a strong indicator of organic disease. Some ulcers, however, notably those on the posterior wall of the stomach and duodenum, may be quite free of tenderness. The patient with DU often indicates with one finger the site of pain.

Periodicity (Fig. 5.22)

This is a striking feature of the symptoms and signs of peptic ulcer. Furthermore, activity of the ulcer cannot be judged on symptoms and physical signs alone; some ulcers may remain 'silent' for long periods. Some otherwise silent ulcers may present with anaemia from blood-loss. Both haematemesis

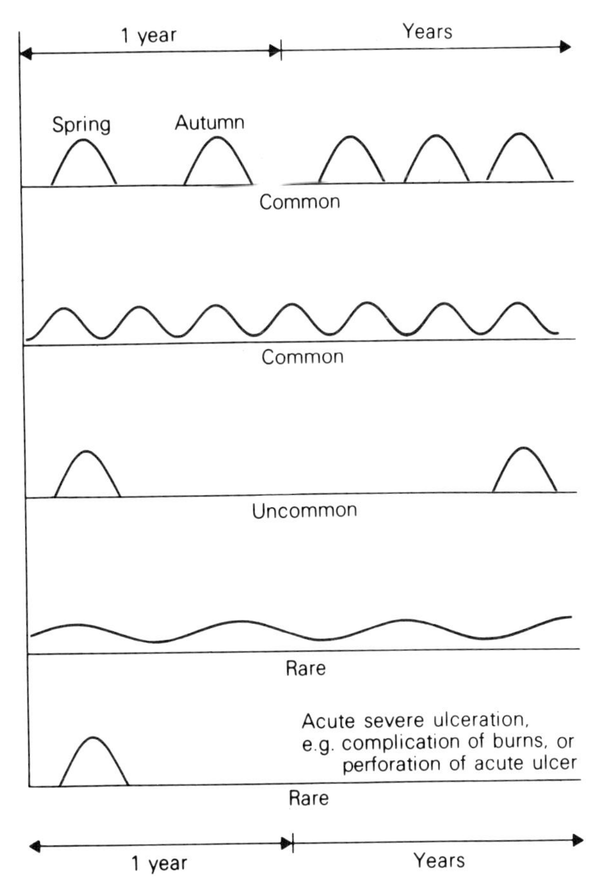

Fig. 5.22 *Patterns of symptomatic behaviour of duodenal ulcers.*

and melaena, and perforation, may occur without any prior warning.

Atypical clinical presentation is not uncommon in three particular situations:

Recurrent ulcer after operation
Young children
The elderly.

In all these, the site of pain may be variable and the relation to eating less obvious.

Diagnosis

Barium meal

This remains the standard method. Gastric ulcers show as a niche of barium – commonly on the lesser curve, rarely on the greater curve. When on the posterior wall of the stomach they are difficult to detect. Double contrast barium radiology greatly improves the pick-up rate. Benign gastric ulcers usually show regular radiating rugal folds (Figs 5.17 and 5.18). Duodenal ulcers are usually diagnosed from deformity of the cap and only occasionally is a frank crater diagnosed with any certainty (Fig. 5.20). Hence a barium meal is a poor indicator of progress or activity since fibrous scarring may be permanent. Therefore 'follow-up' x-rays are not normally indicated in DU.

Endoscopy

This provides a definitive answer in most cases; in experienced hands it will detect 95% or more of both gastric and duodenal ulcers (see Chapter 3). It is the first investigation of choice if there has been previous gastric surgery and in acute gastrointestinal bleeding. Where suspicion of an ulcer is reasonably strong, a 'normal' barium meal should be followed by endoscopy, because a proportion of peptic ulcers cannot be demonstrated even by the best radiology.

Positive identification of a DU on x-ray does not normally require confirmation by endoscopy; findings of a GU on x-ray are, by contrast, an indication for endoscopy, since direct vision and biopsy can greatly increase diagnostic precision in excluding cancer (see p. 81).

As already mentioned (p. 76), acid studies no longer hold an important place in the diagnosis or management of peptic ulcer.

Differential Diagnosis

A careful history is an important part of reaching a diagnosis but it is surprisingly difficult, in many patients, to differentiate peptic ulceration from gall-bladder dyspepsia, and both possibilities may have to be investigated. Hiatus hernia, reflux oesophagitis, and carcinoma of the stomach can all cause dyspeptic symptoms, and chronic pancreatitis causes recurrent epigastric pain. Pain after meals is characteristic of any obstructing lesion in the small bowel, which may be due to neoplasm, Crohn's disease or chronic intestinal ischaemia.

Medical Management of Peptic Ulcer

The aims of management (Table 5.1) are threefold:

To relieve symptoms
To secure healing of the ulcer
To prevent relapse.

Gastric and duodenal ulcers share some common characteristics, but they also show some important differences which influence management. The most important of these differences is the fact that any gastric ulcer may be malignant. For this reason the management of gastric ulcer must include:

a. An initial evaluation, with direct visualisation (endoscopy) and biopsy. Even with this, some malignant ulcers will be missed.
b. Early referral for surgery in the event of non-healing. This generally means referral to the surgeon if, after approximately two months of effective treatment, endoscopic follow-up shows that the ulcer is still unhealed.

Both GU and DU can be acute and transient (as, for example, following stress) or chronic and

Table 5.1
Suggested Plan for Management of Peptic Ulcer

General Measures

Regular relaxed meals
No tobacco
Avoidance of gastric irritants: Alcohol
Drugs, e.g. salicylates, other non-steroidal anti-inflammatory drugs
Reduction of stresses as far as possible
– in occasional cases: sedation
In severe cases: bed rest for 1–2 weeks

Symptomatic Relief

For pain, heartburn, discomfort
Antacids Balanced magnesium/aluminium salts preparation
In patients with costive stools –
Magnesium salts (e.g. Mist. Magnesium Trisil. BPC)
10 ml three times daily 1 hour after food and at night
In patients with loose stools –
Aluminium salts (e.g. aluminium hydroxide gel, BPC)
10 ml three times daily 1 hours after food and at night

For nausea and vomiting
Metoclopramide or domperidone 10 mg three times daily orally or intramuscularly

Specific Healing

Gastric ulcer

Colloidal bismuth (De-Nol) 5 ml in 15 ml water half-an-hour before meals and at night 4–6 weeks. No significant side effects

Carbenoxolone (Biogastrone) 100 mg three times daily one week, then 50 mg three times daily 5 weeks. Watch for oedema, blood pressure, hypokalaemia

Cimetidine (Tagamet) 200 mg three times daily 400 mg nightly or ranitidine (Zantac) 150 mg twice daily 4–6 weeks (as yet the role of H_2-receptor blockers is not conclusively proved)

Duodenal ulcer

Cimetidine (Tagamet) 200 mg three times daily 400 mg nightly or 400 mg twice daily 6–8 weeks or ranitidine (Zantac) 150 mg twice daily 6–8 weeks

Colloidal bismuth (De-Nol) 5 ml in 15 ml water or one tablet three times daily and at night 6–8 weeks

'High dose' antacid regimes, e.g. Maalox 10 ml two-hourly and at night

Maintenance Therapy (prevention of recurrence)

No satisfactory regime available or advised.
No available evidence of any drug altering the long-term natural history.
In selected cases – Cimetidine (Tagamet) 400 mg twice daily or 400 mg at night (side effects – enzyme rises, muscle pains, diarrhoea, impotence, gynaecomastia, interference with drugs such as warfarin or phenytoin)
Ranitidine (Zantac) 150 mg daily

relapsing over many years. Medical treatment can therefore be tailored to the natural history, and in DU this means that relapses can be treated symptomatically and empirically. Prolonged remission of both GU and DU may occur even after many years of relapses (Fig. 5.22).

There is no convincing evidence that diet in any way alters the natural history of peptic ulcer, and 'bland' or 'gastric' diets have a place only during symptomatic treatment of relapse. Milk is a traditional treatment which gives considerable relief of symptoms. However, if acid is important in aetiology, milk is not logical therapy because initial buffering is followed by vigorous rebound stimulation of acid output.

Trials of any treatment in peptic ulcer must take into account the high healing rate with placebo. In fact, placebo effect is very important when it is remembered that the presence of an ulcer crater, proven on endoscopy, is not necessarily related to the presence or absence of symptoms.

Gastric ulcer (Table 5.1)

The strong association with salicylates, and possibly other anti-inflammatory drugs, means that these should be avoided.

Symptomatic relief is achieved with antacids, as in DU, although the mechanism is unclear.

Healing of GU may be facilitated by bed rest, and the value of cessation of smoking is stronger than it is for DU. As in DU, H_2-receptor blocking drugs (cimetidine and ranitidine) have been widely used and advocated, although the unequivocal evidence of their efficacy is still lacking and long-term safety is not assured. Bismuth colloid (De-Nol) promotes healing and deserves wider usage. Carbenoxolone has been shown to be effective but has significant side-effects, especially in the elderly, in whom GU is so common. It must therefore be used with caution, with regular checks for fluid retention, rise in blood pressure, and hypokalaemia. A thiazide diuretic with extra potassium supplements may be used.

Unfortunately there is as yet no convincing evidence that medical treatment prevents relapse.

Duodenal ulcer

With a duodenal ulcer there is, for practical purposes, no risk of malignancy and since complications such as bleeding, perforation and stenosis are relatively rare (in comparison to the frequency of duodenal ulcer itself) the management, be it medical or surgical, is based upon the severity of the patient's symptoms.

The natural history of ulcers in asymptomatic remission is unknown. In patients with proven DU, prophylactic surgery with the aim of avoiding bleeding or perforation is only indicated in rare situations, e.g. deep sea mariners and, perhaps, those on long-term ulcerogenic drugs.

Symptomatic relief of duodenal ulcers can usually be achieved with the sensible use of antacids, bearing in mind that aluminium salts (e.g. aluminium hydroxide) are constipating, and that magnesium salts (e.g. magnesium carbonate) are laxative. Balanced combinations (e.g. Maalox) are logical and widely used. Sodium bicarbonate gives rapid relief but, as with other alkalis, can if used excessively (especially in combination with milk) lead to alkalosis, calcium deposition, and renal failure (milk-alkali syndrome).

Certain bland foods, notably milk, are widely favoured by patients for rapid relief. They have the theoretical risk of rebound stimulation of acid secretion and are probably best avoided in the traditional night-cap advice.

Symptomatic relief can also be obtained with anticholinergics such as propantheline, but the effective dose almost always produces unpleasant side-effects. Inhibitors of acid output such as cimetidine or ranitidine are effective but should *not* be used on a demand basis. Nausea and vomiting may be controlled with specific anti-emetics such as metoclopramide (10 mg given half an hour before meals).

Healing of DU may be achieved in a high proportion of patients (70–80%) by a number of agents. However, the natural history of ulcers is one of relapse and remission and all controlled trials of such drugs show a considerable placebo response. Furthermore, general measures which may play some part in facilitating ulcer healing include:

physical rest
sedation to control anxiety and stress
stopping smoking
regular regimen of food and curtailment of excess alcohol.

Drugs shown to facilitate healing of DU include the following:

i. Antacids – but only in very large doses.

ii. Bismuth compounds: Dipotassium tricitrato-bismuthate (Denol) is said to operate by coating the ulcer base with a protein coagulum and may have antipeptic but not antacid activity. The tongue and stool are temporarily blackened during the 4–8 weeks of the course. Relapse occurs but probably less quickly than with the H_2-receptor blockers.

iii. H_2-receptor blockers (see Figs. 5.23, 5.24). These drugs, cimetidine and ranitidine, are a major advance in ulcer management but show the disadvantage of all similar therapsy, i.e. relapse. Side-effects of cimetidine include a rise in transminases and gynaecomastia. The long-term toxicity is unknown and on present knowledge these drugs should be used with caution on a long-term basis. Many patients can be adequately treated by repeated courses during relapses but frequent relapses suggest the need for surgery. H_2-receptor blockers are the drugs of choice for ulcers due to Zollinger–Ellison syndrome where the primary tumour cannot be extirpated, and may obviate the need for total gastrectomy.

iv. Sucralfate – a compound of sucrose octasulfate and aluminium hydroxide – probably acts similarly to bismuth but, although promising, its efficacy is as yet undecided.

v. Liquorice derivatives are of uncertain value. Deglycyrrhizinated liquorice (Caved-S) has been widely used, but its place is unproven. Position-released carbenoxolone (Duogastrone) has been shown to facilitate healing in a few trials but carries the risks of steroid-like effects, e.g. hypertension, water retention and hypokalaemia.

Prevention of relapse in DU is difficult or impossible to achieve medically. Low doses of cimetidine (200–400 mg at night) or ranitidine

$CH_2CH_2NH_2$ — HN, N (imidazole ring)

HISTAMINE

$CH_2SCH_2CH_2NHCNHCH_3$ (C=S); CH_3; HN, N (imidazole ring)

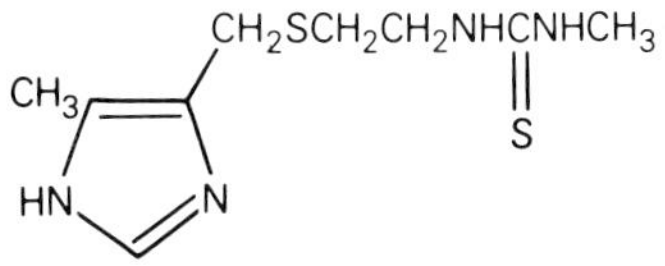

METIAMIDE
(no longer used because of side-effects)

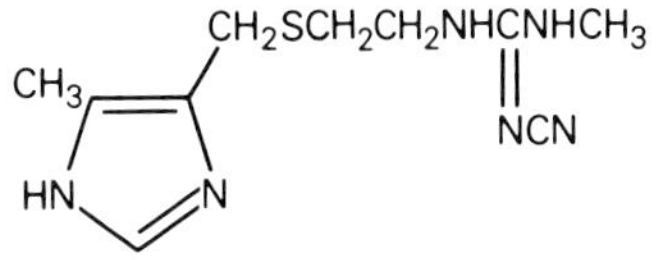

$CH_2SCH_2CH_2NHCNHCH_3$ (C=NCN); CH_3; HN, N (imidazole ring)

CIMETIDINE
Dose: 200 mg three times daily and 400 mg at night — or 400 mg twice daily.
Maintenance therapy after 1–2 months: 400 mg at night.

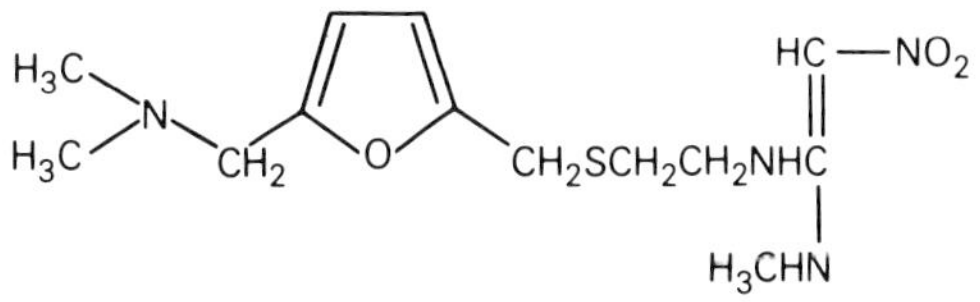

$(H_3C)_2N$–CH_2–(furan, O)–$CH_2SCH_2CH_2NHC(=HC—NO_2)$–$H_3CHN$

RANITIDINE
Dose: 150 mg twice daily.
Maintenance therapy. 150 mg at night.

Fig. 5.24 *The H_2-receptor blocking drugs.*

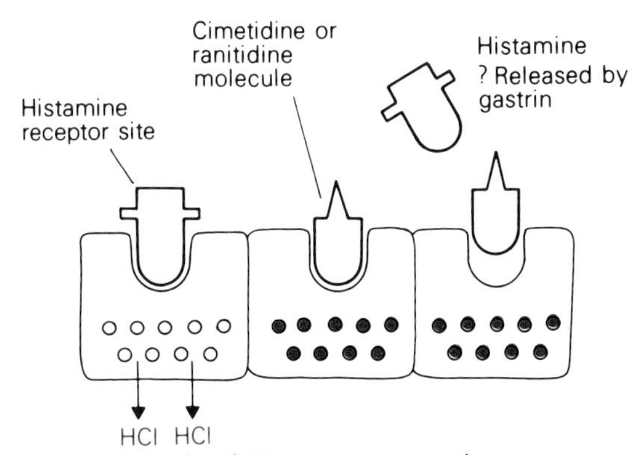

Fig. 5.23 *Principle of H_2-receptor antagonism.*

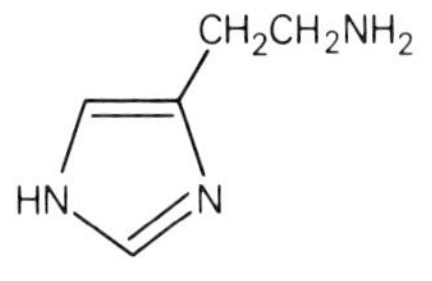

(150 mg at night) may prove of value but are expensive and of unknown long-term toxicity or value. There is no evidence that any dietary manipulation is of value in long-term management.

Surgical Treatment

There are three main reasons for undertaking surgical treatment of a peptic ulcer:

1. Failure of medical treatment. With development of more effective antacids over the past 15 years, there are now fewer patients coming into this category. However, patients who have genuinely sought to achieve healing by adjustments to their mode of living, stopping smoking, regulation of drinking and diet, and adherence to drug treatment, and who continue to relapse should generally be offered surgical treatment.
2. Gastric ulceration in which malignant change is possible.
3. The occurrence of serious complications, e.g. haemorrhage (Chapter 14), perforation (Chapter 13), and pyloric stenosis.

Chronic duodenal ulcer

The original operation, which had great popularity between 1920 and 1940, was gastrojejunostomy (GJ: Fig. 5.25). This seemed to have a magical effect on the symptoms of chronic duodenal ulcer and was indeed a highly successful operation for many patients. However, it became clear with further experience that the complete failure of this operation to control hypersecretion led, in many cases (nearly 50% over the years), to recurrent peptic ulceration, usually on or near the stoma. This ulceration was open to all the complications of the orignal duodenal ulcer and was sufficiently common and serious to invalidate GJ. The operation is now occasionally used for very elderly or infirm patients with pyloric stenosis.

All other operations aim, in one way or another, to reduce the level of acid secretion. Partial gastrectomy (PG) was for many years the standard treatment for chronic duodenal ulcer and produced a high level of satisfactory results. In view of the severity of the ulceration in the duodenum, the Polya type of gastrectomy was nearly always

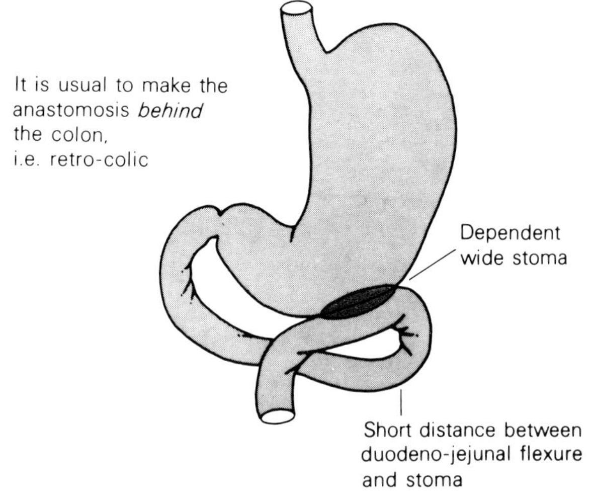

Fig. 5.25 *Gastrojejunostomy.*

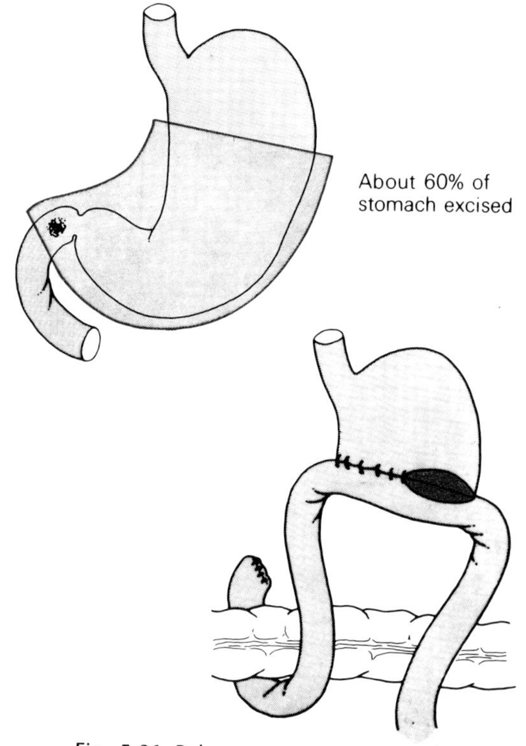

Fig. 5.26 *Polya gastrectomy.*

chosen (Fig. 5.26). By removing the first part of the duodenum and the gastric antrum, all G cells producing gastrin are excised. By removing a substantial part of the body, the level of gastric secretion of acid is reduced by about 70%. Recurrence of peptic ulceration is fairly unusual (about 3%). In spite of the radical nature of the surgery, at least 80% of patients obtained an excellent result, but the main drawbacks to this operation were:

1. Closure of the scarred duodenum could be very difficult and the result of a leak from the duodenal suture line was very serious. The mortality of Polya gastrectomy was consequently about 5%, which was too high to be acceptable.
2. The reduction in gastric capacity was a problem in some patients (especially women) who ate such small meals as to produce a serious loss of weight.
3. Various functional sequelae such as dumping and bilious vomiting (see p. 91). Late anaemia is a problem, especially in women under 50 years, and can be due to deficiency of iron and intrinsic factor. There is some evidence of an increased risk of carcinoma in the gastric remnant.

These defects led, in the 1940s, to a search for other operations for chronic duodenal ulcer, which was still a very common disease. Dragstedt introduced truncal vagotomy in 1943. Because the whole stomach and duodenum were denervated, many patients showed delayed gastric emptying and so a drainage procedure had to added–either pyloroplasty or gastrojejunostomy.

A procedure widely known as 'vagotomy and drainage' (V & D: Fig. 5.27) has become very popular for duodenal ulcer because it is technically simple and very safe, with a mortality below 1% and 75% of patients obtaining a very good result. However, the denervation of the whole of the upper alimentary tract means that many patients have some looseness of the stools and, for a few, diarrhoea is a great nuisance. The drainage procedure means that sphincteric control over gastric emptying is lost so 'dumping' (p. 91) and bilious vomiting occur in about 10% of patients. Recurrence of ulceration, either in the duodenum or at the stoma, is a complication in about 8%, although

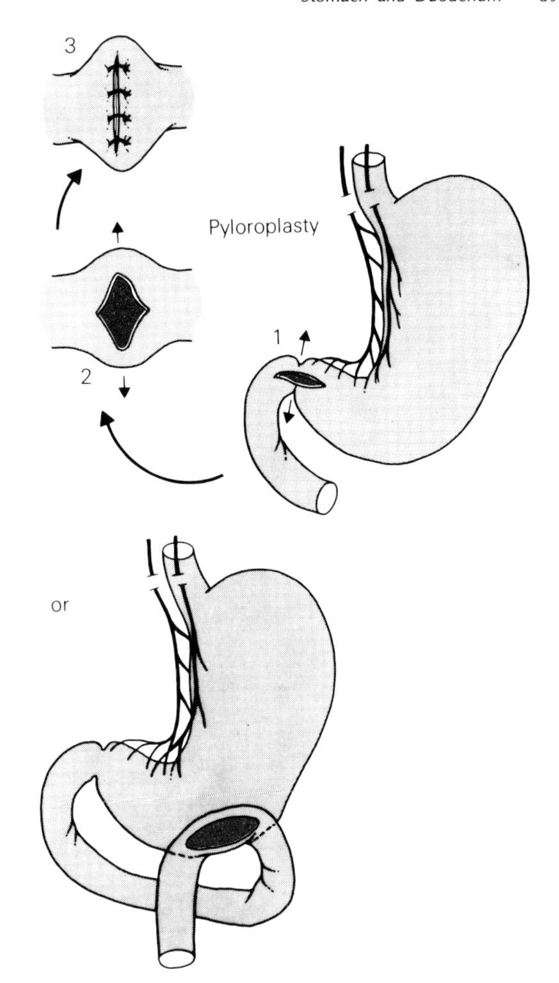

Fig. 5.27 *Vagotomy and drainage.*

it is lower if the vagotomy is very carefully and thoroughly done.

Recurrent ulceration in about one in ten patients prompted the search for a more effective operation and one suggestion which became very popular around 1955–65 was vagotomy and antrectomy (V & A: Fig. 5.28). This procedure not only denervated the stomach but removed the area of mucosa responsible for gastrin production, thus lowering acid output by about 90%. Recurrent ulcer is, as a result, very rare and occurs at most in 1 in 100 patients.

On the other hand, V & A means that patients suffer from the disadvantages of both truncal vagotomy and of gastrectomy. Nowadays V & A

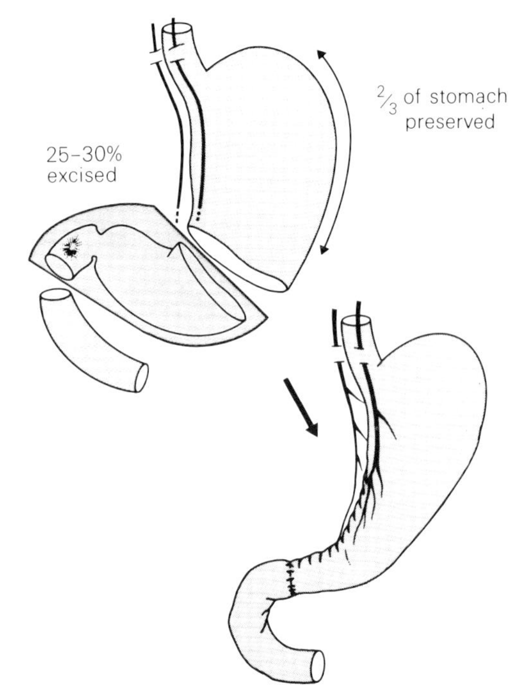

Fig. 5.28 *Vagotomy and antrectomy.*

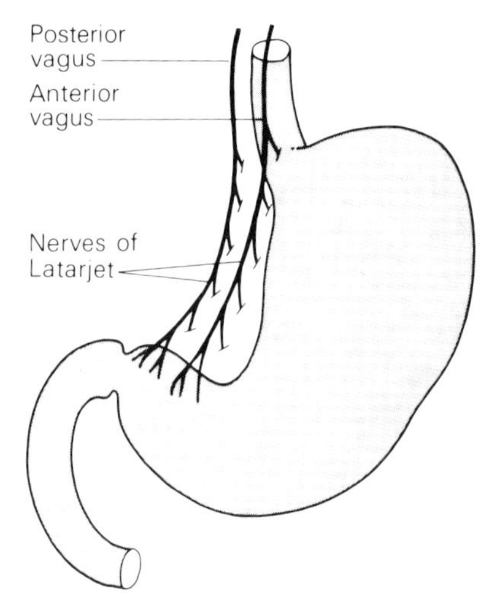

Fig. 5.29 *Highly selective vagotomy.*

would probably be reserved for a well-built young man with a strong family history of duodenal ulceration, and would certainly be avoided in thin patients.

The most recent operation to be developed is 'highly selective vagotomy' (HSV), which is by far the most physiological of all operations on the stomach. The aim is to totally denervate the stomach, with the exception of the pyloric sphincter and the adjacent area of antrum normally innervated by the nerves of Latarjet (Figs. 5.7 and 5.29). As a consequence, the antrum and pylorus can still act as a normal emptying mechanism for the stomach, whilst denervation of the mucosa of the body leads to a major drop in the secretion of pepsin and acid.

Comparing HSV with V&D, diarrhoea should be less troublesome because vagal branches to the liver, gall bladder, pancreas and intestine are preserved. Dumping and biliary reflex into the stomach should not occur through an intact pylorus. Clinical trials have confirmed the truth of these claims.

HSV and V&D both have a very low mortality (less than 1%) and they share a similar ulcer recurrence rate of about 8%: this figure is lower in the hands of surgeons with much experience of the operation, who can secure a total parietal cell denervation.

HSV alone is not a suitable operation for patients with servere duodenal fibrosis and pyloric stenosis: in these patients, dilatation of the duodenum or a drainage procedure must be added.

Chronic gastric ulcer

Whereas most chronic duodenal ulcers can be managed by careful medical treatment, the chronic gastric ulcer often requires surgical treatment. This is because medical treatment fails to heal a substantial number of gastric ulcers, there is always a doubt whether the ulcer is in fact a carcinoma, and the complications – haemorrhage and perforation – carry an unduly high mortality. Thus, when the physician finds that a gastric ulcer has failed to heal after one reasonable course of medical treatment, there is a strong indication to advise surgical intervention.

The surgical treatment of chronic gastric ulcer is dominated by the need to establish whether there is carcinomatous change within it. The most reliable way to do this is to remove the ulcer

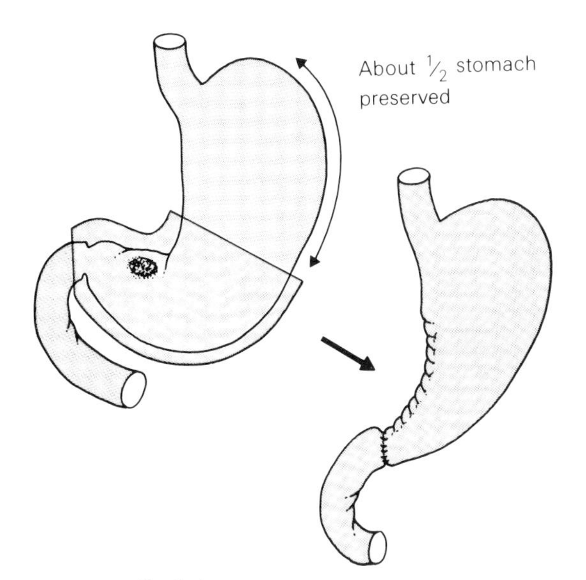

Fig. 5.30 *Billroth I gastrectomy.*

completely by partial gastrectomy; a Billroth I gastrectomy (Fig. 5.30) is the preferred method. This allows complete removal of the ulcer and joins the stomach to the duodenal stump by end-to-end anastomosis. This promotes good mixing of the gastric contents with the bile and pancreatic secretions. The great majority of patients secure a good result with this operation.

Some surgeons have suggested local excision of the ulcer, with vagotomy and drainage.

After-effects of gastric surgery

Most gastric operations provide a satisfactory result for a majority of patients. This depends partly on wise selection of patients for surgery and on the nature and quality of the surgery provided. However, even with the greatest care, there are a minority of patients who do not secure a satisfactory result. Reasons for this include:

1. Recurrent ulcer. This may be due to failure to perform a complete vagotomy or, in partial gastrectomy, to remove enough of the body of the stomach where acid and pepsin is produced.

If medical treatment does not provide enough relief, a failed vagotomy is usually treated by performing a partial gastrectomy, whereas a vagotomy is performed if recurrent ulceration follows partial gastrectomy.

Recurrent ulceration after gastrectomy for gastric ulcer is most unusual.

2. Post-vagotomy diarrhoea. Many patients who have a truncal vagotomy remark that their bowel moves more freely and many welcome this. In a small minority (3–4%) diarrhoea occurs, which can be quite troublesome. There is little specific treatment but generally the diarrhoea improves with time.

3. Bilious vomiting can occur after any operation which destroys the pylorus. It can occur after a Billroth gastrectomy so it is not necessarily due, as used to be thought, to the afferent loop of a gastro-jejunal anastomosis being suddenly emptied. These patients vomit pure bile and rarely lose their meals so they remain well nourished. However, the unpleasantness of repeated bilious vomiting may make it necessary to abolish it by reconstructing the anastomosis.

4. Dumping is an unpleasant feeling of faintness, sweating, dizziness and sleepiness which comes on after a meal and requires the patient to rest (and preferably lie down) until it passes off. There may be a feeling of epigastric discomfort which can be followed by vomiting of bile.

These effects are due to the rapid emptying of food from stomach into jejunum. The bowel is presented with a hyperosmolar meal which is promptly diluted by hypersecretion: this results in a fall in plasma volume of as much as 700 ml, which is why the patient feels faint. (Similar effects can be produced in normal people by the intrajejunal instillation of hypertonic glucose solution.)

Generally, dumping tends to improve with time. Small meals taken more often, avoidance of very sweet puddings, and separating the ingestion of food and of drink can all help. Some patients have to accept that they must sit down, with their feet up, for half an hour after the main meal.

Avoidance of dumping is one of the particular advantages of HSV.

5. Anaemia is an important complication of partial gastrectomy. Hypochlorhydria reduces the amount of iron absorbed in the jejunum and some

years after gastrectomy as many as half the patients may have an iron-deficiency anaemia. Less vitamin B_{12} is absorbed because of deficient production of gastric intrinsic factor, and this may, over a space of time, produce a megaloblastic anaemia.

6. *Osteomalacia* is occasionally seen after partial gastrectomy. This appears to be due to a deficiency of vitamin D and is partly due to poor intake and partly to a degree of malabsorption.

7. *Weight loss* can be a serious complication of radical gastric surgery: insufficient stomach is left to allow a normal meal to be eaten. This can usually be overcome by taking small nourishing meals frequently but it is an important reason for being wary of performing a gastrectomy on thin young people. The occurrence of some steatorrhoea in some patients after gastrectomy will also contribute to a failure to regain weight.

8. Rebound hypoglycaemia occurs in a few.

The present restricted use of partial gastrectomy means that most of these complications are now unusual.

GASTRIC NEOPLASMS

Gastric Cancer

Gastric cancer is currently the third most common malignancy, but its incidence in the Western World is falling. As a consequence the mortality from this cancer is falling steadily (30% in the past 10 years in the USA). This is fortunate, since there has been no improvement in surgical results for gastric carcinoma in the past 30 years (less than 10% of patients survive at 5 years). In Japan the incidence of gastric carcinoma is higher (Fig 2.25) and much finance and medical effort are directed to its early detection. This has stimulated a complete reappraisal of the classification of both early and advanced gastric cancer (Fig 5.31 and 5.32). Japanese work has also led to reports of 5-year survival rates as high as 90% among patients diagnosed before the tumour has spread beyond the lamina propria. There are a few small reports from the Western World of similar results, suggesting that claims that the Japanese may be

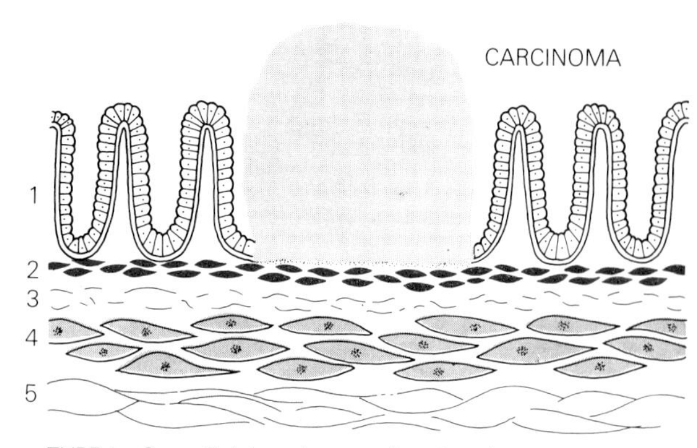

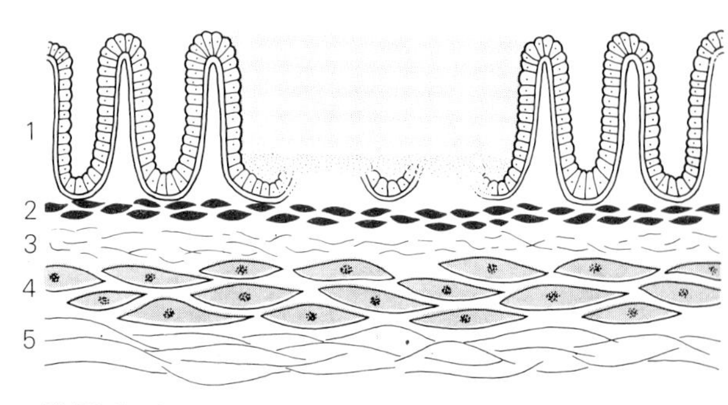

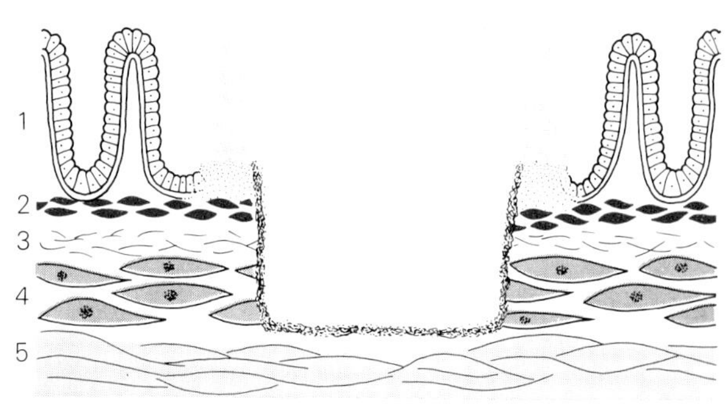

Fig. 5.31 *Japanese classification of early gastric cancer. (Numbers explained in Fig. 5.14a.)*

dealing with a less active malignancy may not be entirely true.

Pathology

The great majority of malignant tumours of the

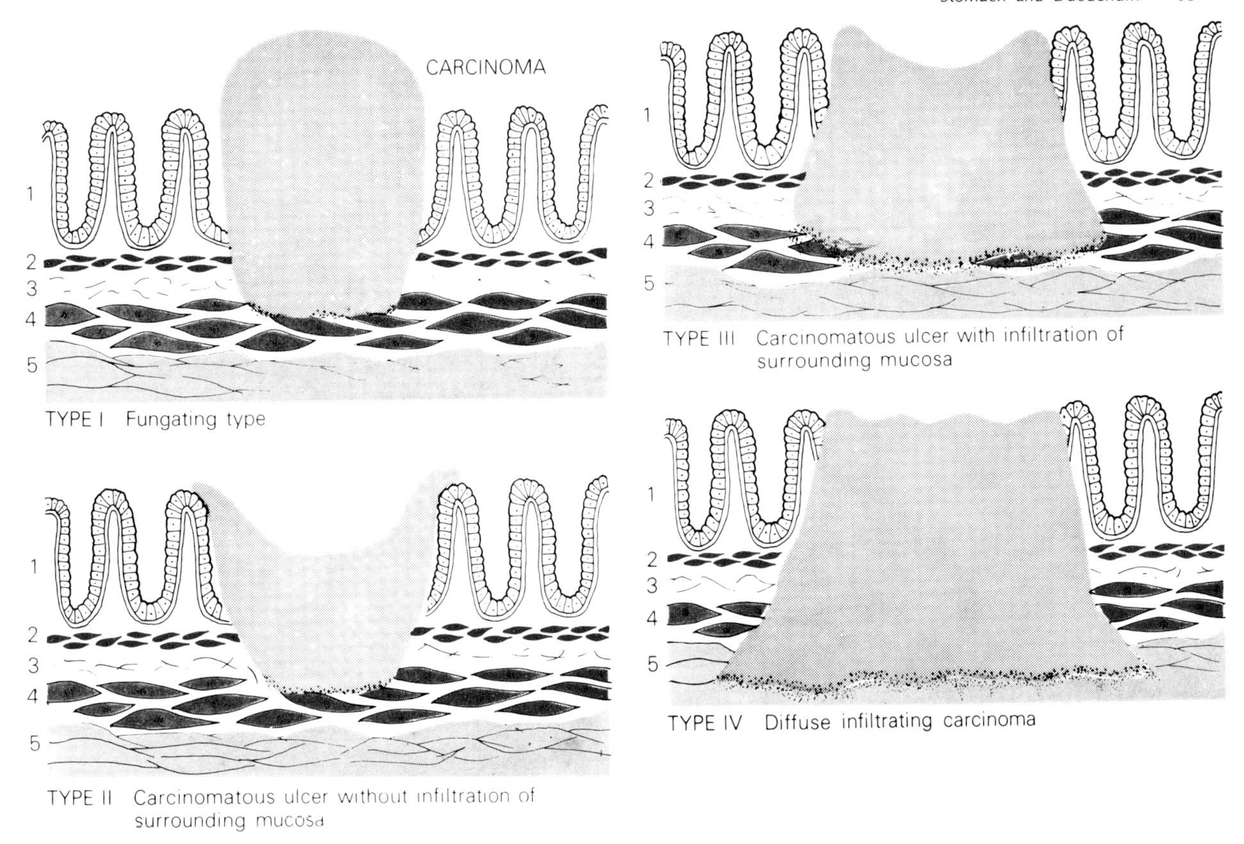

Fig. 5.32 *Borrmann classification of advanced gastric cancer.*

stomach are adenocarcinomata; sarcomata and lymphomata are much less common.

The tumour may take the form of a fungating polypoid structure (Fig. 5.33) which, when present in the fundus of the stomach, may infiltrate the lower end of the oesophagus causing obstruction and true dysphagia. In other patients the tumours may take the form of an ulcerating lesion, with 'heaped up' or 'rolled' edges (Fig. 5.34), in the antral region, sometimes causing gastric outlet obstruction. In the elderly especially, the tumour may take the form of a diffusely infiltrating scirrhous carcinoma producing the so-called 'leather bottle' stomach or 'linitis plastica' (Fig. 5.35), recognisable by its rather constricted appearance (on barium studies) and inability to distend or to transmit peristalsis normally. In general, gastric cancers arise most frequently on the greater curve of the stomach.

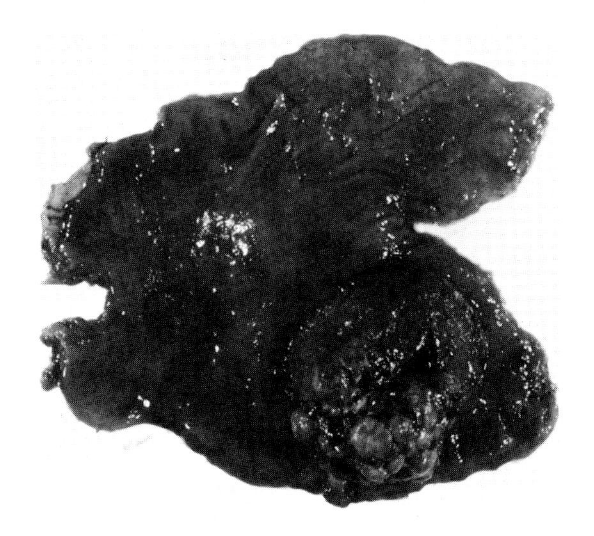

Fig. 5.33 *Polypoid carcinoma of stomach.*

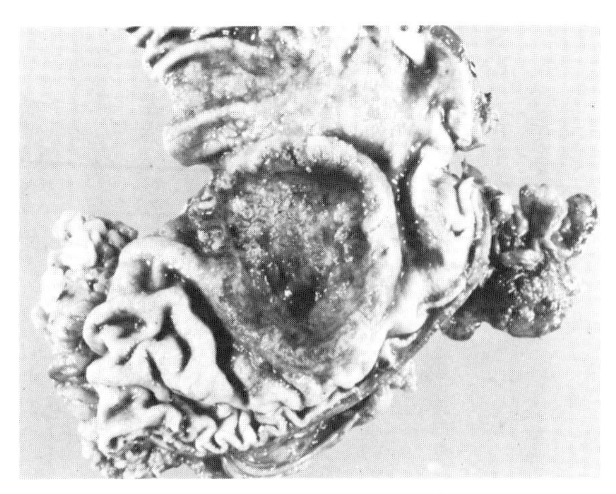

Fig. 5.34 *Ulcerating carcinoma of stomach.*

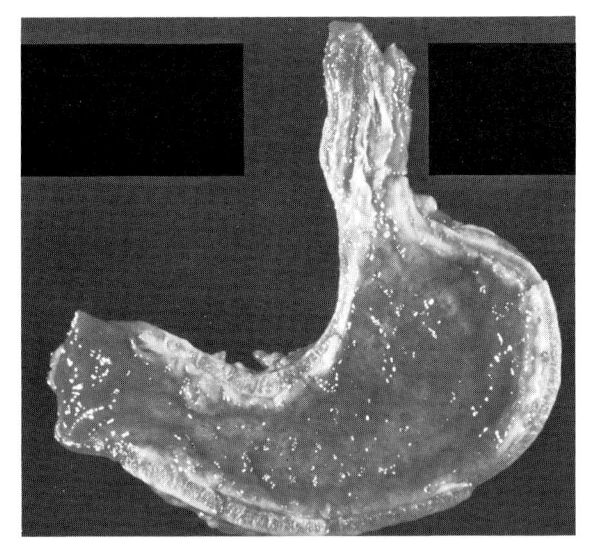

Fig. 5.35 *'Leather bottle stomach' (linitis plastica).*

As well as local spread to pancreas, spleen or transverse colon, local and distant lymphatic spread is common. It is important to realise that the often described spread to the left supraclavicular note (Virchow's node) is a late sign (Troisier's sign) which usually signifies advanced disease. Metastases to liver and peritoneum are common. Transperitoneal spread to the ovaries (Kruckenberg's tumour) is less common. Blood-borne metastases to brain and bone are infrequent and late.

Benign tumours of the stomach are relatively infrequent. Leiomyomata (locally infiltrative) are usually asymptomatic (see p. 97). Adenomatous polyps are more frequent and are often associated with atrophic gastritis and achlorhydria. They are considered by some to be premalignant, but the evidence is conflicting.

Aetiology (see also p. 26).

Gastric carcinoma occurs in the fundus in males twice as often as it does in females. In the antrum the sex frequency is equal. This tumour occurs with increasing frequency from middle age onwards but can occasionally manifest earlier. Carcinoma of the stomach is said to be three times more common in unskilled workers, and there is a possible association with mining, working in the rubber industry, and working with asbestos. Nevertheless, the cause of gastric cancer remains unknown, though predisposing factors are recognised.

Conditions associated with hypochlorhydria or achlorhydria carry an increased risk. Patients with pernicious anaemia have a three- to four-fold increased chance of developing gastric carcinoma (and this is independent of the known association between blood group A and liability to pernicious anaemia or gastric carcinoma). Chronic atrophic gastritis (not superficial gastritis) is associated with an increased risk of the same order. With the passage of years there appears to be an increasing risk of carcinoma developing in the gastric remnant of patients who have had partial gastrectomy. The nitrites in gastric juice are found in greater concentrations after gastrectomy, suggesting that nitrosamine formation may be important.

There is little convincing evidence that benign gastric ulcers become malignant. Any apparent increase in the risk of malignancy is probably attributable to initial misdiagnoisis of a gastric carcinoma as a 'benign' gastric ulcer.

There is some evidence for genetic predisposition. Gastric carcinoma occurs with slightly higher frequency in the families of patients with gastric carcinoma or pernicious anaemia. There is good evidence that it is 20% more common in patients with blood group A. The reported differences in incidence between Eastern and Western populations almost certainly reflect environmental rather than genetic influences.

Although there has been much research into possible carcinogens in food, there is no clear-cut evidence for this. Neither cigarette smoking nor alcohol consumption increase the risk. There is no convincing evidence that either benzpyrene in smoked fish, or aflatoxin in spoiled grain, increase the risk. There is circumstantial evidence incriminating nitrosamines, either ingested, or produced by the interaction of nitrites and secondary amines in the stomach. Nitrites are commonly used in food preservatives, and secondary amines may be present when food is imperfectly preserved. Thiocyanates present in saliva, gastric juice and bacteria can, in theory, catalyse the above reaction but evidence for this actually happening is inconclusive. There is, however, some evidence to suggest that gastric carcinoma occurs more frequently where nitrate (from which nitrites can be formed) concentrations in water are high. It is also known that vitamin C inhibits the reaction of nitrosation. This may explain the negative correlation between gastric carcinoma and eating green vegetables. Imbalance in trace metals in soil may be transferred to plants, and this has been suggested as a possible explanation for the high incidence of gastric carcinoma reported in North Wales, where it has been shown that there is a relative disproportion of zinc to copper in the soil. Brackens grow well in such soils and they do contain substances shown to be carcinogenic to cattle. The importance of these observations for man remains unclear.

Clinical features

The symptoms associated with gastric carcinoma are extremely variable, often insidious, and usually appear too late to allow early diagnosis and cure. Anorexia, weight loss, nausea, vomiting and dysphagia are common late symptoms but haematemesis or melaena are rare. Abdominal pain is very variable in site, frequency and severity; when present, it is often aggravated by food. Sometimes the pain is constant and sometimes it is related to movement or posture. Despite the variable and late symptomatology, the following conditions should arouse suspicion of carcinoma of the stomach, and at present offer the best hope for early diagnosis.

1. Recent onset of 'heartburn', or flatulence in the middle-aged or elderly patient.
2. Unexplained hypochromic microcytic, or 'mixed' anaemia.
3. The presence of the associated conditions such as pernicious anaemia described above.

By the time clinical signs are present there can be little hope of a surgical cure. The presence of hepatomegaly, an epigastric mass, Troisier's sign, ascites and breathlessness (due to anaemia and effects of lymphatic spread to the lungs) signify advanced malignancy.

Once suspected, the clinical diagnosis may be most easily confirmed by barium meal (Fig. 5.36).

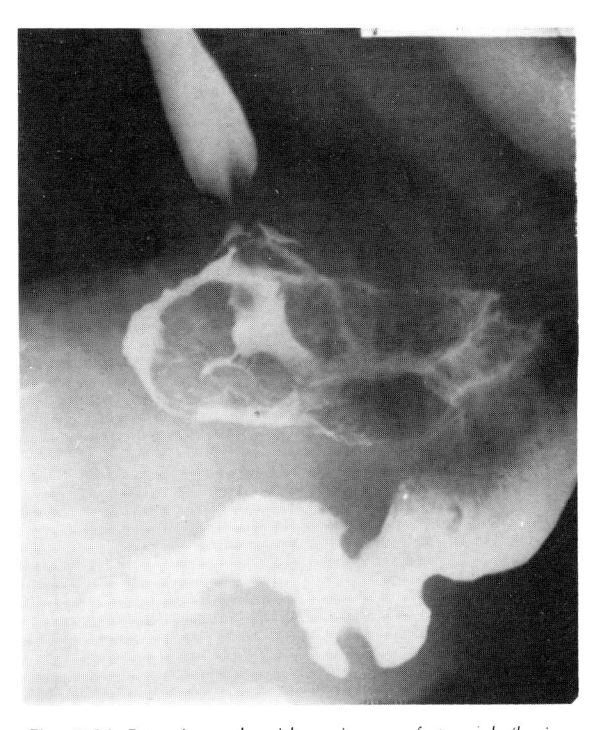

Fig. 5.36 *Extensive polypoid carcinoma of stomach (barium meal).*

Supportive evidence may be obtained in the form of a positive test for occult faecal blood, the presence of an iron deficiency anaemia, or abnormal liver function tests. A positive tissue diagnosis is only possible, however, by gastroscopy and biopsy and/or cytologic brushings.

It is an important principle that any patient with a 'benign' gastric ulcer on barium meal examination, or any other unusual radiographic abnormality, should undergo endoscopy combined with multiple biopsy and, if available, brush cytology. This will allow the early detection of a malignant ulcer with at least a chance of cure, and will minimise the risk of the incorrect classification of an early malignancy as a 'benign' gastric ulcer. There can be no place for a trial of medical treatment as a means of differentiating between a peptic ulcer and carcinoma because apparent 'healing' of ulcerating malignancies is well documented.

Treatment of carcinoma of the stomach

Treatment is surgical, and laparotomy should generally be undertaken because removal of apparently advanced tumours is occasionally followed by unexpectedly good results.

Subtotal gastrectomy (Fig. 5.37). Most carcinomas can be removed by excising two-thirds to three-quarters of the stomach, and anastomosing jejunum to the gastric remnant. In the course of such an operation, it is not uncommon to remove the body of the pancreas and the spleen along with the specimen, when a carcinoma has involved the pancreas. The great omentum is removed because it is often the site of transcoelomic spread of the carcinoma.

Total gastrectomy (Fig 5.38). When the carcinoma lies close to the oesophagogastric junction, then the abdominal oesophagus must be included in the resection to secure clearance of invaded tissue. Reconstruction is usually effected by bringing up a loop of upper jejunum through the transverse mesocolon and joining the end of the oesophagus to the top of the loop. It is wise to carry out long

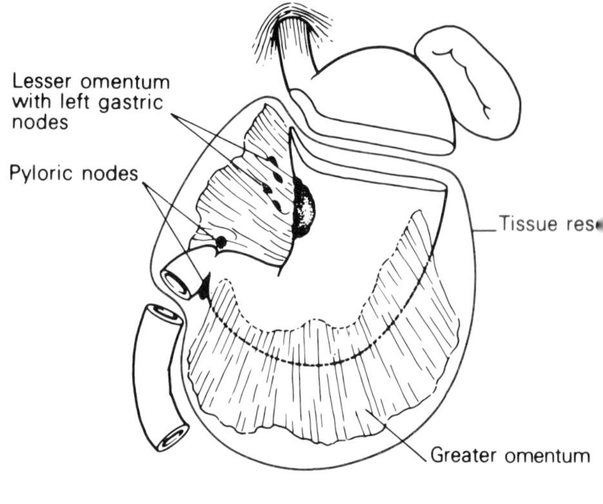

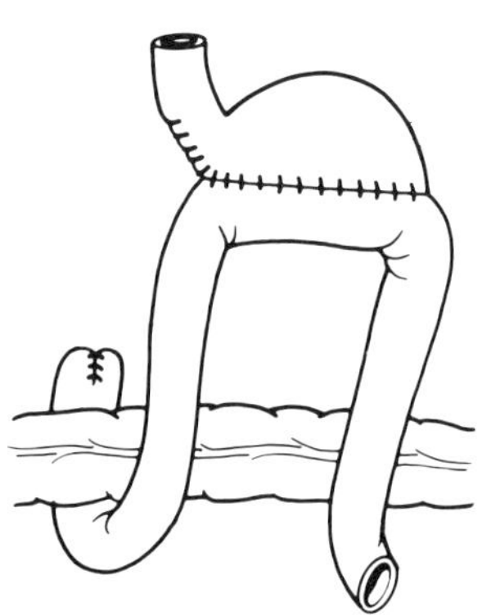

Fig. 5.37 *Radical subtotal gastrectomy.*

entero-anastomosis between the ascending and descending jejunal loops.

Oesophago-gastrectomy (Fig. 5.39). When the carcinoma invades the gastro-oesophageal junction then more oesophagus must be removed and the anastomosis can only be made by extending the abdominal incision into the left chest. This allows the diaphragm to be split down to the oesophageal hiatus and reveals the whole of the stomach as well as the lower oesophagus lying in the posterior mediastinum.

A very radical operation can then be performed, with removal of the upper half of the stomach, together with the spleen, and the whole of the left

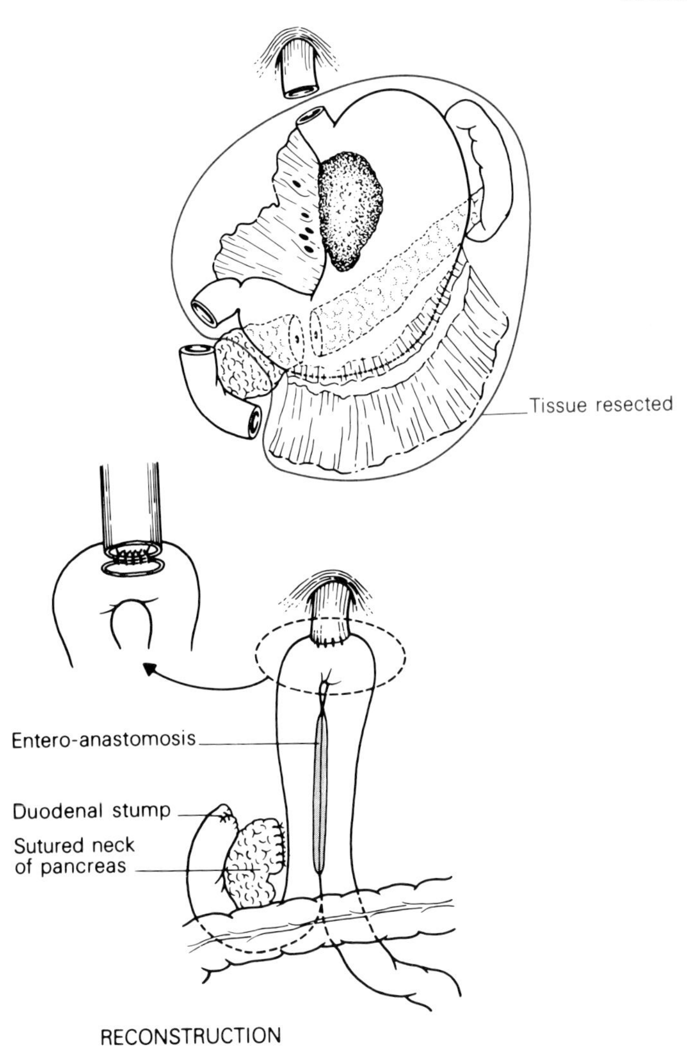

Fig. 5.38 *Radical total gastrectomy, including splenectomy and distal pancreatectomy.*

gastric artery and the coeliac lymph nodes.

Reconstruction is often effected by closing the distal half of the stomach, bringing it up as a tube, and joining the open end of the oesophagus to an incision into the front of the gastric pouch.

The diaphragm is carefully closed around the stomach, and the chest wall and abdominal incision sutured with an underwater drain to evacuate the left pneumothorax.

About 60% of carcinomas of the stomach can be resected by one or other of these rather major procedures. The mortality of the abdominal gastrectomies is about 5%, and for the thoraco-abdominal operations it is about 10%.

Most recurrences after gastric surgery occur around the stomach bed, and so the prospects for improving the prognosis for patients with gastric cancer may lie in performing more radical surgery. Adjuvant chemotherapy with drugs at present available has not produced useful results.

Leiomyoma

This unusual gastric tumour arises from the muscu-

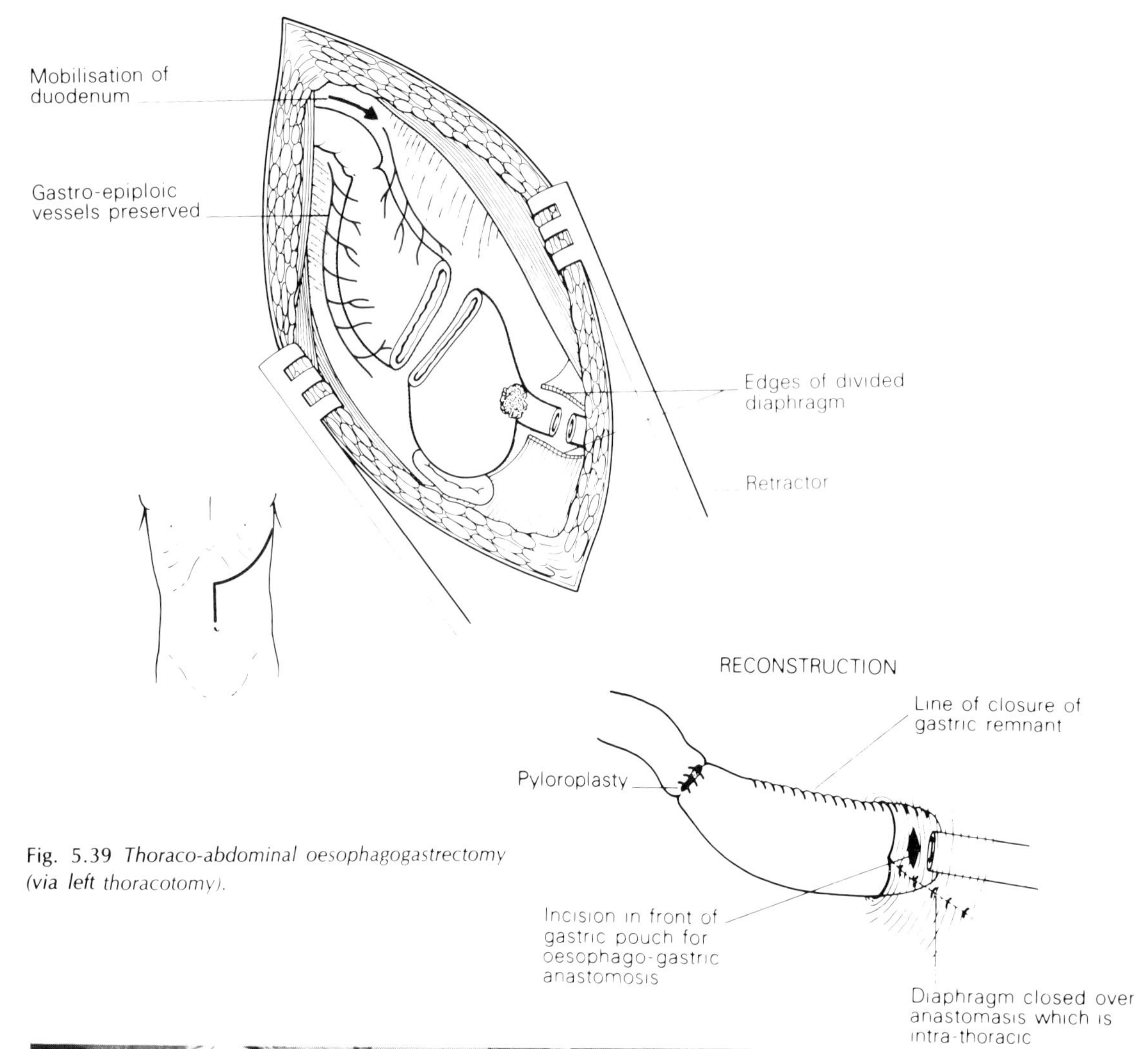

Fig. 5.39 *Thoraco-abdominal oesophagogastrectomy (via left thoracotomy).*

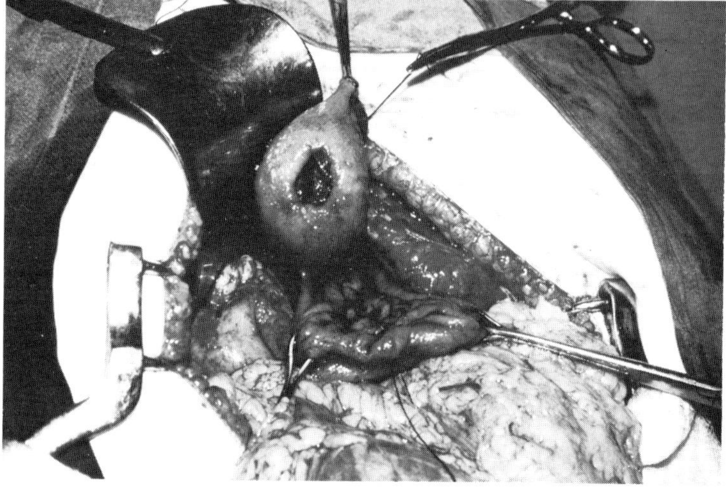

Fig. 5.40 *Leiomyoma of stomach: typical ulceration of fundus of tumour, causing haemorrhage. The leiomyoma has been delivered through a gastrotomy.*

lar wall. It may be benign, or have a sarcomatous element and be locally infiltrative. Symptoms are few and, by the time of diagnosis, the tumour is often pedunculated. It is characteristic for an ulcer to form on the apex and this may bleed and cause a haematemesis (Fig. 5.40). Wide local removal is usually the correct treatment.

Lymphomas of the Stomach and Intestines

Lymphomas of the gastrointestinal tract are uncommon. About one-half arise in the stomach, but they represent only 1–2% of all gastric neoplasms: in the small bowel, many present as an emergency, either as a perforation with peritonitis, or with intestinal obstruction. There is an association with coeliac disease (p. 13).

In all parts of the alimentary tract, lymphomas are likely to be mistaken for carcinomas, and the true diagnosis is only made at histopathological investigation. Fortunately radical surgical resection is the best treatment, although in a number of patients it can be usefully supplemented with radiotherapy and chemotherapy.

6

The Pancreas

The pancreas, partly due to its anatomical position, was one of the last organs in the body to receive the critical attention of anatomists, physiologists and clinicians. Despite much study over the past 20 years, the pathophysiology of the pancreas remains poorly understood, and diseases of the exocrine pancreas remain among the most difficult both to diagnose and treat.

EMBRYOLOGY

The pancreas is derived from two endodermal outgrowths from the foregut, which appear around the fourth week of gestation (Fig. 6.1). The ventral outgrowth develops into the inferior aspect of the head and the main pancreatic duct of Wirsung. The dorsal outgrowth forms the remainder of the gland and the accessory duct of Santorini (which remains patent in 70% of adults). Normally, complete fusion of both the ducts and parenchyma of these two parts of the pancreas occurs (Fig. 6.2): failure of complete migration of the two parts occurs rarely, resulting in the formation of an annular pancreas, which can cause duodenal obstruction. The outlet of both the bile duct and the duct of Wirsung on the ampulla of Vater is the result of the common origin of the bile duct and ventral pancreas. The ampulla lies at the point of separation of fore- and mid-gut and therefore the blood supply of the pancreas is derived from both the coeliac axis and the superior mesenteric artery (Fig. 6.3). The pancreatic acini develop about the third month and are connected to the main pancreatic ducts via small secretory ductules.

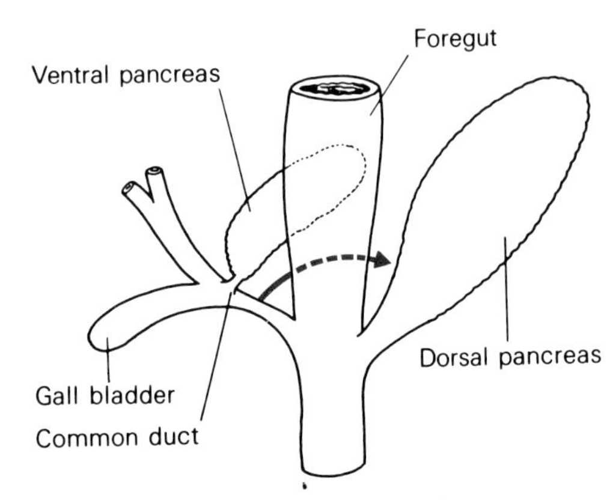

Fig. 6.1 *Pancreas at 5–6 weeks fetal life.*

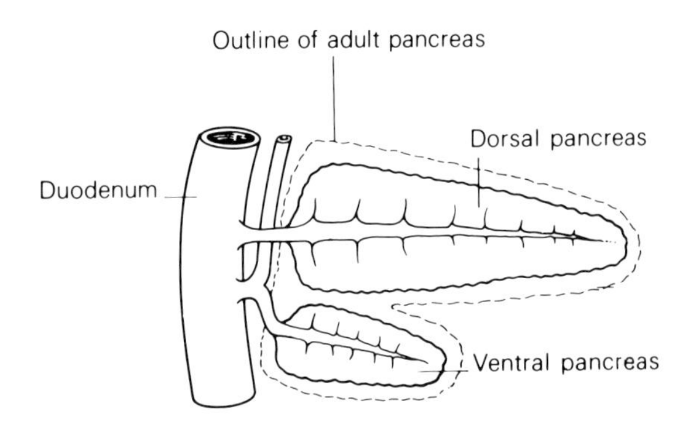

Fig. 6.2 *Pancreas at approximately 7 weeks fetal life.*

ANATOMY

The pancreas lies retroperitoneally on the posterior abdominal wall, within the duodenal loop and

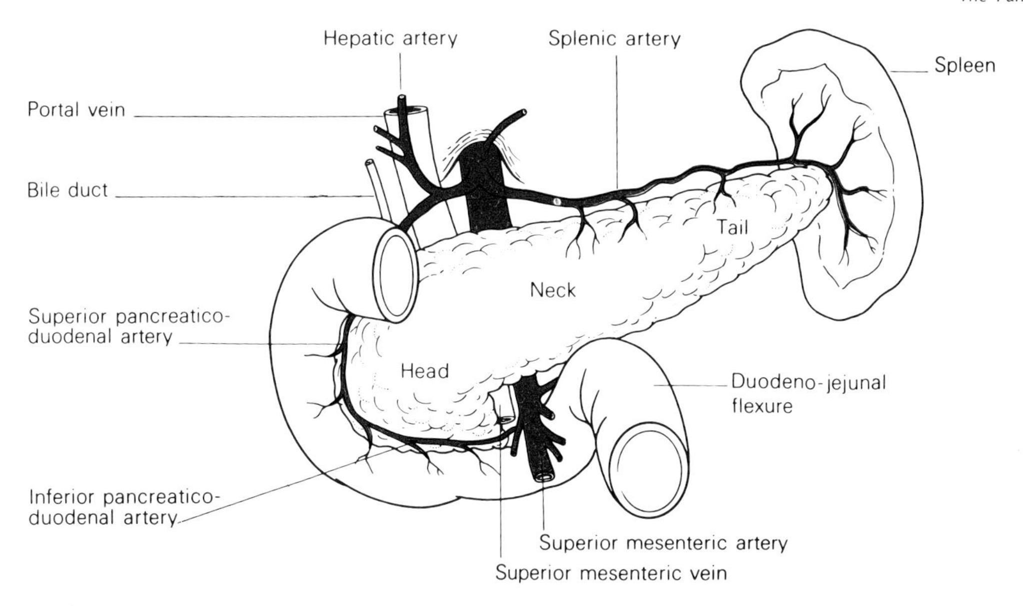

Fig. 6.3 *Relationships and blood supply of pancreas.*

behind the stomach. Immediate relationships are depicted in Fig. 6.3. The splenic vein lies behind the pancreas and runs medially to join with the superior mesenteric vein to form the portal vein. The normal texture of the gland is soft and fleshy (Greek, *pan* all; *kreas* flesh). Histologically, the pancreas consists of clusters of acini (Fig. 6.4) which form lobules separated from each other by areolar tissue. Each acinus is a sphere of pyramidal cells, their apices ending in the central lumen. Each acinus is drained by a pancreatic ductule, the ductular epithelium extending into the central lumen to form the centro-acinar cell. The ductule drains into an intralobular duct which then drains into an interlobular duct: these unite to form the main pancreatic duct.

The nerve supply of the pancreas comes from both the sympathetic system (via the coeliac plexus) and the parasympathetic (via branches of the vagus nerve).

Both histologically and physiologically, there has been a tendency to think of the pancreas in two distinct entities, namely the exocrine and endocrine elements. Many have been slow to appreciate the delicate and important portal cir-

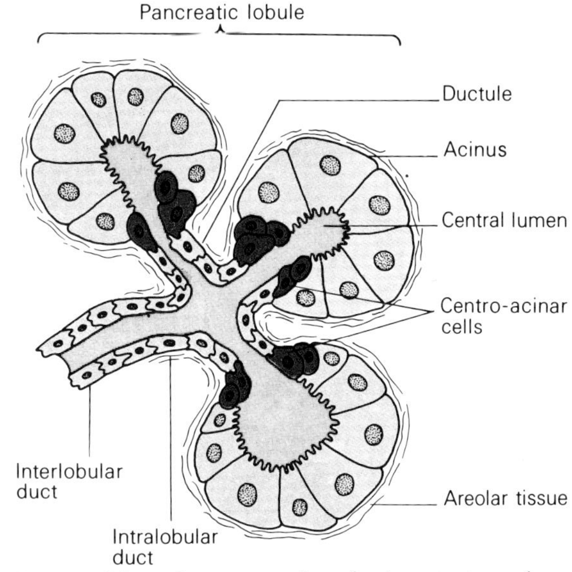

Fig. 6.4 *Schematic representation of acinar structure of exocrine pancreas.*

culation within the pancreas whereby blood in the arterioles goes initially to the capillaries of the islets of Langerhans and then to supply the adjacent acinar cells. This vascular arrangement indicates that products of the islet cells probably have an influence on acinar tissue secretion. While in many animals the alpha (glucagon) and beta (insulin) cells are arranged peripherally and centrally respectively within the islet tissue, with the D (somatostatin) cells in an intermediate position, this is not so in man. The cells are more irregularly disposed and several other cell types within the islets have been identified. The overall volume of endocrine tissue within the pancreas is approximately 1%, with the number of individual islets varying from several hundred thousand to two million in man. They are evenly distributed throughout the pancreas.

PANCREATIC SECRETIONS

Under basal conditions the pancreas produces 1.5–2.0 litres of juice in 24 hours; this is rich in bicarbonate (and is therefore alkaline), enzymes (which are proteins), and electrolytes. In response to various stimuli the volume of secretion can rise to 4 litres.

Principal Enzymes

Amylase

This hydrolyses glycogen and starch.

Lipase

Together with the essential protein cofactor co-lipase, this hydrolyses neutral fat to fatty acids and glycerides in the presence of bile salts (provided the latter are present in the correct concentrations).

Trypsinogen, chymotrypsinogen and procarboxy-peptidase

These protein-splitting enzymes are secreted in an inactive form from the zymogen granules within the acinar cells and are activated mainly by enterokinase secreted in the small intestine (notably duodenum). Enterokinase splits a small peptide fraction off the trypsinogen molecule, converting it to the active trypsin. Once formed, the trypsin activates the other pancreatic proteases.

Trypsin and chymotrypsin break up proteins within food into oligopeptides comprising 2–4 amino acids, which are hydrolysed further into individual amino acids during transport through the small intestinal cells.

Although efficient pancreatic exocrine secretion is essential to health, it is well documented that up to 40% of ingested fat and protein may be absorbed when there is little or no remaining pancreatic function (either due to disease or surgical resection). This is because amylases, lipases and peptidases are secreted in small quantities into the gut from sources other than pancreas. These alternative pathways of digestion sometimes allow survival in a clinical situation that initially looked hopeless.

The Anatomical Basis of Pancreatic Enzyme Secretion

All the pancreatic enzymes are secreted from the acinar cells at a very rapid rate. It is thought that the enzymes are formed at the ribosomes on the outer surface of the cisternae of the rough endoplasmic reticulum (Fig. 6.5). The enzyme protein then moves through the cell for further elaboration in the golgi apparatus, and onward to the condensing vacuoles. Energy in the form of ATP is needed for this movement. Once in the vacuoles, the enzyme proteins are concentrated and the vacuoles become visible, on electron microscopy, as zymogen granules. The final step is exocytosis: the zymogen granule fuses with the apical cell membrane, which then ruptures to allow rapid release of the zymogen contents into the acinar lumen.

Control of Pancreatic Secretion

Pancreatic secretion is under hormonal and nervous control, the precise mechanisms being un-

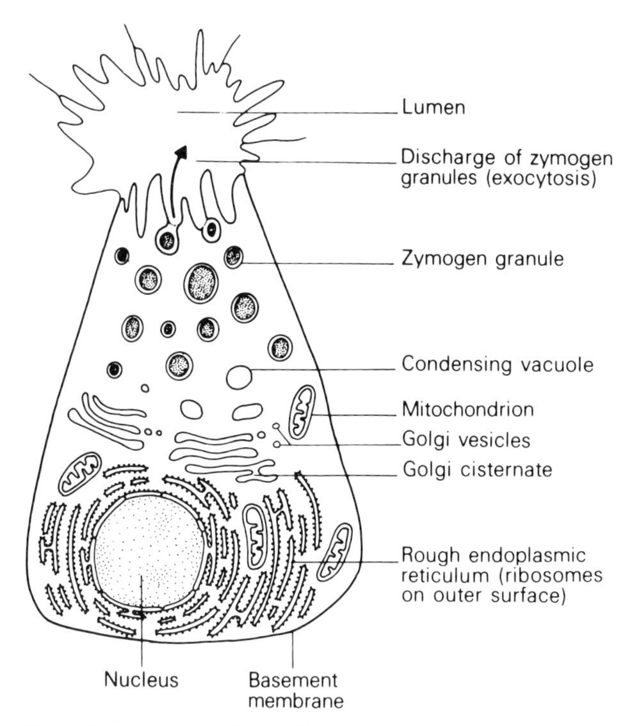

Fig. 6.5 *Pancreatic acinar cell.*

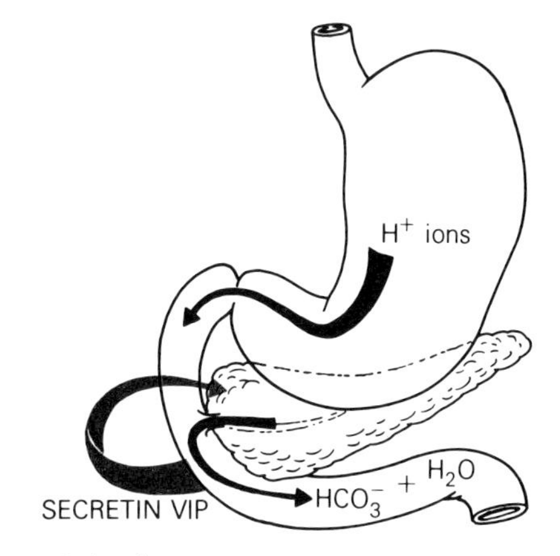

Fig. 6.6 *Role of secretin/VIP in pancreatic secretion.*

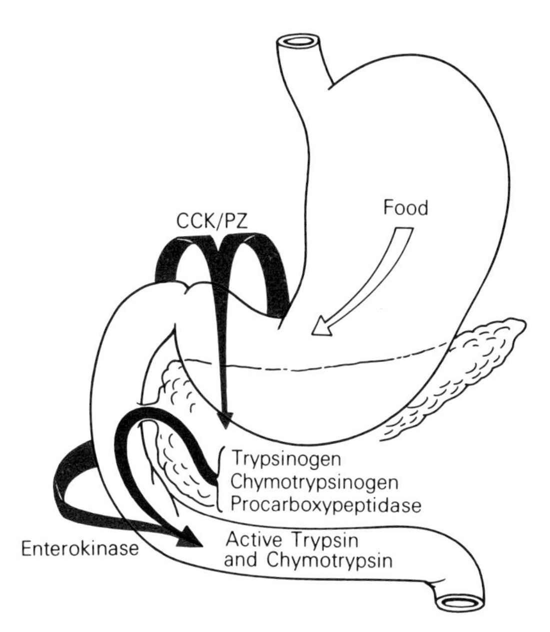

Fig. 6.7 *Role of cholecystokinin/pancreozymin in pancreatic secretion and of enterokinase activation.*

certain: the following summary reflects current evidence.

Hormonal control

The principal hormones controlling pancreatic secretion are:

secretin
vasoactive intestinal peptide (VIP)
cholecystokinin / pancreozymin (CCK / PZ).

Secretin and VIP (Fig. 6.6) are both secreted in the duodenum in response to hydrogen ions entering the duodenum from the stomach, particularly after a meal. Reaching the pancreas through the blood stream, they stimulate the pancreas to release fluid rich in bicarbonate and water, with a low enzyme content. The main result is to neutralise acid entering the duodenum.

CCK/PZ (Fig. 6.7) is released into the blood from the gastric antrum and duodenum by the presence of food and stimulates the acinar cells to secrete a juice rich in enzymes (amylase, lipase and trypsinogen) but low in volume and bicarbonate content. In the duodenum, trypsin is liberated from trypsinogen by the action of enterokinase, which is secreted in the duodenal mucosa.

The effects of gastrin, glucagon, somatostatin,

calcitonin, bombesin, motilin and other peptides on pancreatic secretion are complex and as yet unclear.

Nervous control

This remains uncertain, although it is known that stimulation of the vagus increases pancreatic secretion. There is a cephalic phase of secretion on sight and smell of food. Gastric and intestinal phases of secretion are also described. Neurohormonal interactions are important, and the rate of gastric emptying has a measurable effect on pancreatic secretion.

DISEASES OF THE PANCREAS

Whilst acute pancreatitis is quite frequently seen, and carcinoma is one of the commoner neoplasms, the other chronic diseases of the exocrine pancreas are relatively uncommon: they are however almost always serious, with high morbidity and mortality.

Pancreatitis

A useful classification, suggested at the Marseilles symposium of 1965, is as follows:

1. Acute pancreatitis: returns to complete normality.
2. Recurrent acute pancreatitis: repeated attacks, with return to normality between attacks.
3. Chronic pancreatitis: permanent impairment of function.
4. Relapsing chronic pancreatitis: relative freedom between attacks.

In practice, the differences between categories 3 and 4 may be difficult to establish with certainty.

Aetiology

In the recent past, gallstones were considered to be the usual cause of acute pancreatitis, but in a number of countries, e.g. Sweden and the USA, alcohol abuse is now the principal aetiological factor. Alcohol abuse remains the principal cause of chronic pancreatitis. Other causes include:

local obstructing mechanisms such as carcinoma, fluke infestations of the biliary tree
trauma: postoperative or accidental
viral infection (mumps, coxsackie B, hepatitis)
hyperlipoproteinaemia
hyperparathyroidism
drugs, e.g. azothiaprine, corticosteroids
familial pancreatitis

Acute Pancreatitis

Acute pancreatitis is an important and frequent cause of acute abdominal pain which, until the last few years, has been relatively neglected. This is partly because it is fairly difficult to diagnose positively at the bedside and, in the most severe cases, difficult to treat successfully. Recently it has received some well-merited attention with the result that most patients are now quickly recognised, and methods and standards of treatment have been considerably improved.

Clinically, this is a diagnosis which it is easy to miss. In the typical patient there is acute onset of severe upper abdominal pain, sometimes after a rich meal. Repeated vomiting is characteristic. The pain tends to be constant and of the severity of a perforated peptic ulcer: in strong contrast to this, the early abdominal signs may be surprisingly slight – the patient is clearly in severe pain but there may be only modest upper abdominal tenderness and guarding. This disparity between symptoms and signs should always suggest acute pancreatitis because, even though inflammation is severe, the pancreas is a retroperitoneal organ and does not at first produce signs on palpation of the anterior abdominal wall.

In a severe attack, the primary phenomenon is an excretory duct inflammatory change with subsequent inflammation of the pancreatic lobule, leading on to necrosis of adjacent pancreatic parenchyma. Between 30–60% of patients have associated gallstones and 10–50% (depending on locality) will recently have drunk an excess of alcohol. More rarely, acute pancreatitis follows an abdominal operation or blunt abdominal trauma, and it occasionally complicates hypotension due to septicaemia or myocardial infarction. Fat necrosis, manifested as multiple small white plaques on the peritoneal surface of organs near the pancreas, is a characteristic feature. In the most severe cases of acute pancreatitis the necrosis of the pancreatic parenchyma is likely to lead to considerable haemorrhage into and around the pancreas: occasionally this can be seen as bruising in the subcutaneous tissue of the left flank (Grey Turner's sign). Secondary infection of such a haematoma is a real risk and late pancreatic abscess is a most serious complication. If there is no secondary infection, erosion of pancreatic tissue may lead to extravasation of secretions into the lesser sac, producing a pancreatic pseudocyst: this occurs in 5–10% of all patients, in half of whom spontaneous regression will take place, whilst the remainder will require drainage.

The diagnosis of acute pancreatitis should be suspected in all patients admitted with acute upper abdominal pain (Fig. 6.8), and it is now customary to estimate the serum amylase in all such patients. The normal level is 70–300 international units/l, and values above 1200 units strongly support the diagnosis. However, it must be remembered that the serum amylase can be markedly elevated in a few patients with conditions requiring surgical treatment, e.g. a perforated peptic ulcer or infarcted bowel, so all patients need very careful assessment and continued observation. A urinary amylase level in excess of 3000 units/l (normal 300–1500) is a valuable confirmation of the diagnosis.

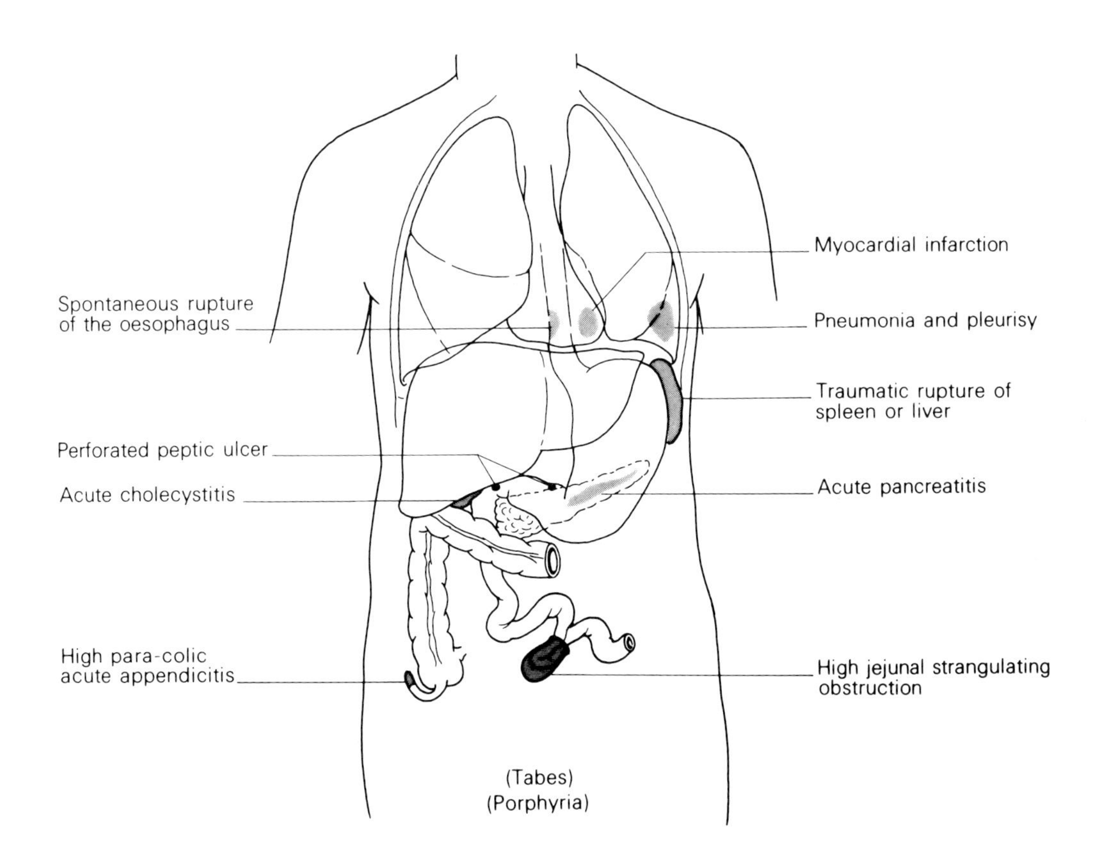

Fig. 6.8 *Differential diagnosis of sudden severe epigastric pain.*

Management

The management of 70% of patients with acute pancreatitis is simple, because the disease runs a benign course and these patients can be discharged after a few days of treatment with intravenous fluids, nasogastric suction and analgesics. Gradual restoration of diet to normal, the avoidance of alcohol, and early surgical removal of gallstones (if shown to be present), result in survival of 99% of these patients.

The most important aspect of management is to identify patients who have a severe attack, which carries a mortality rate of 20%. The grading scheme (Table 6.1) helps in this assessment. These patients are prone to failure of several organs; respiratory failure is the major hazard and the cause of 65% of deaths.

Central venous pressure measurements, hourly urine volumes, and half-hourly pulse and blood-pressure measurements are essential. Renal insufficiency may be a big problem and it is best prevented by provision of a sufficient volume of intravenous fluid – as much as 6 litres may be required in the first 24 hours. Up to half of these fluids may need to be colloidal solutions, including blood and plasma. Humidified oxygen should be administered by face mask and serial blood gas analysis performed: if hypoxaemia does not improve, mechanical ventilation will be needed for a few patients.

Some clinicians advocate the use of peritoneal lavage, but the value of this is at present undecided. Hypocalcaemia is often seen: it is usually secondary to loss of albumin in the inflammatory exudate and is corrected with albumin and calcium. The initial problem in these severe cases is one of anticipating and avoiding system failures.

Table 6.1
Indicators of Severe Acute Pancreatitis†

WBC > 15 000/mm^3
Glucose > 10 mmol/l (no diabetic history)
Urea > 16 mmol/l (no improvement on i.v. fluids)
Pa_{O_2} < 60 mmHg (8 kPa)
Calcium < 2.0 mmol/l
Albumin < 32 g/l
Lactic dehydrogenase > 600 units/l
Aspartate transaminase > 200 units/l

†Severe pancreatitis is present if any three of these measurements are positive. The greater the number of factors positive, the worse the prognosis.

A few patients remain gravely ill and toxic, and then a pancreatic abscess must be suspected. Ultrasonic scanning can be of great help in diagnosis. These patients are likely to be bacteraemic and they always require surgical drainage, when large pieces of sloughing pancreas require removal. A sustained catabolic phase may occur in severe acute pancreatitis, which will require a period of parenteral feeding: this can also be an integral therapeutic step in closure of a pancreatic fistula. Pseudocysts of the pancreas, which usually cause much less disturbance, will generally require internal drainage into the stomach or a loop of small bowel, but may be amenable to needle aspiration under ultrasound control.

A frankly diabetic state may occur in severe pancreatitis and insulin may be required temporarily, although islet cell function usually recovers satisfactorily.

Chronic Pancreatitis

The frequency of chronic pancreatitis in a community is proportional to alcohol consumption. With the exception of some tropical countries, other non-alcoholic causes are numerically insignificant.

Alcohol increases the protein content of pancreatic juice, with precipitation of protein plugs, leading to obstruction and focal distal dilatation of the smaller draining ducts. There may be calcification and sometimes stone formation within the ducts. Ultimately, severe destruction, fibrosis and atrophy leads to gross distortion of the gland, with pain and loss of function (Fig. 6.9).

Clinical features

Presentation is commonly in the third or fourth decades. Most patients present with pain, usually in the epigastrium or upper quadrants, radiating to

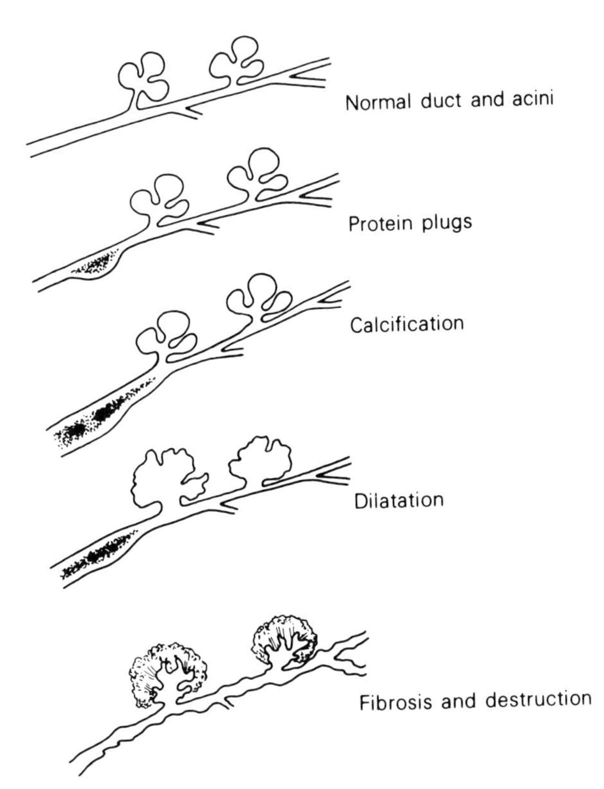

Fig. 6.9 .*Stages in development of chronic pancreatitis.*

the back. Acute severe attacks may supervene upon more chronic pain, often associated with eating. The combined effects of fear of eating, alcohol abuse and malabsorption lead to weight loss in 90% of patients. Steatorrhoea occurs in at least 50%, and diabetes in 75% of patients.

In addition, chronic pancreatitis may present with biliary obstruction and cholangitis. It can also cause duodenal obstruction. Rarely, obstruction of the splenic vein is followed by splenomegaly, formation of oesophageal varices, and bleeding, or the development of ascites. The distinction from carcinoma of the pancreas, especially where weight-loss is pronounced, may be very difficult.

Investigation

Many attempts have been directed at developing functional tests. If a tube is passed into the duodenum, direct sampling of pancreatic juice in response to injected secretin/pancreozymin, or a Lundh test meal, can be attempted. Steatorrhoea can be assessed by collection of faeces and estimation of fat content. Impaired glucose tolerance indicates severe damage to the gland. More recently, either a fasting level of pancreatic polypeptide, or serum levels in response to a standard stimulus, represents a new and potentially important move in the assessment of pancreatic function (Table 6.2).

Radiology may help by showing calcification within the pancreas in a plain abdominal x-ray, indentation of the stomach and duodenum by the enlarged pancreas in a barium meal, and obstruction of the bile ducts in a cholangiogram. A pancreatogram, obtained by direct injection of the duct of Wirsung at endoscopy (ERCP), may show multiple stenoses and dilatation of the duct system: cytology of pancreatic juice can also be obtained at the same time. Ultrasonography and computerised tomography are both able to provide excellent images of the state of the pancreas (Fig. 6.10).

Treatment

Correction of malabsorption is easy. This is managed directly by oral administration of pancreatic

Table 6.2
Tests to Assess Pancreatic Function

With tube in duodenum	*Tubeless* (urine collections)
Secretin – pancreozymin	Benzoyl – tyrosyl – aminobenzoic acid (BTP) test: measures recovery of urinary para-amino benzoic acid (PABA)
Lundh test meal*	
Faecal collections	Fluorescein dilaurate (FDL) test
Faecal fat	*Others*
Dual isotope fat absorption	Isotope breath test
	Pancreatic polypeptide

*Lundh test meal: a radio-opaque weighted tube is passed through the nose and, under x-ray screen control, the tip is sited in the second part of the duodenum. After collecting a fasting specimen of juice, a balanced meal of fat (corn oil), protein and glucose is given, which stimulates pancreatic secretion. Samples are analysed for amylase and trypsin content, both of which are reduced in chronic pancreatitis.

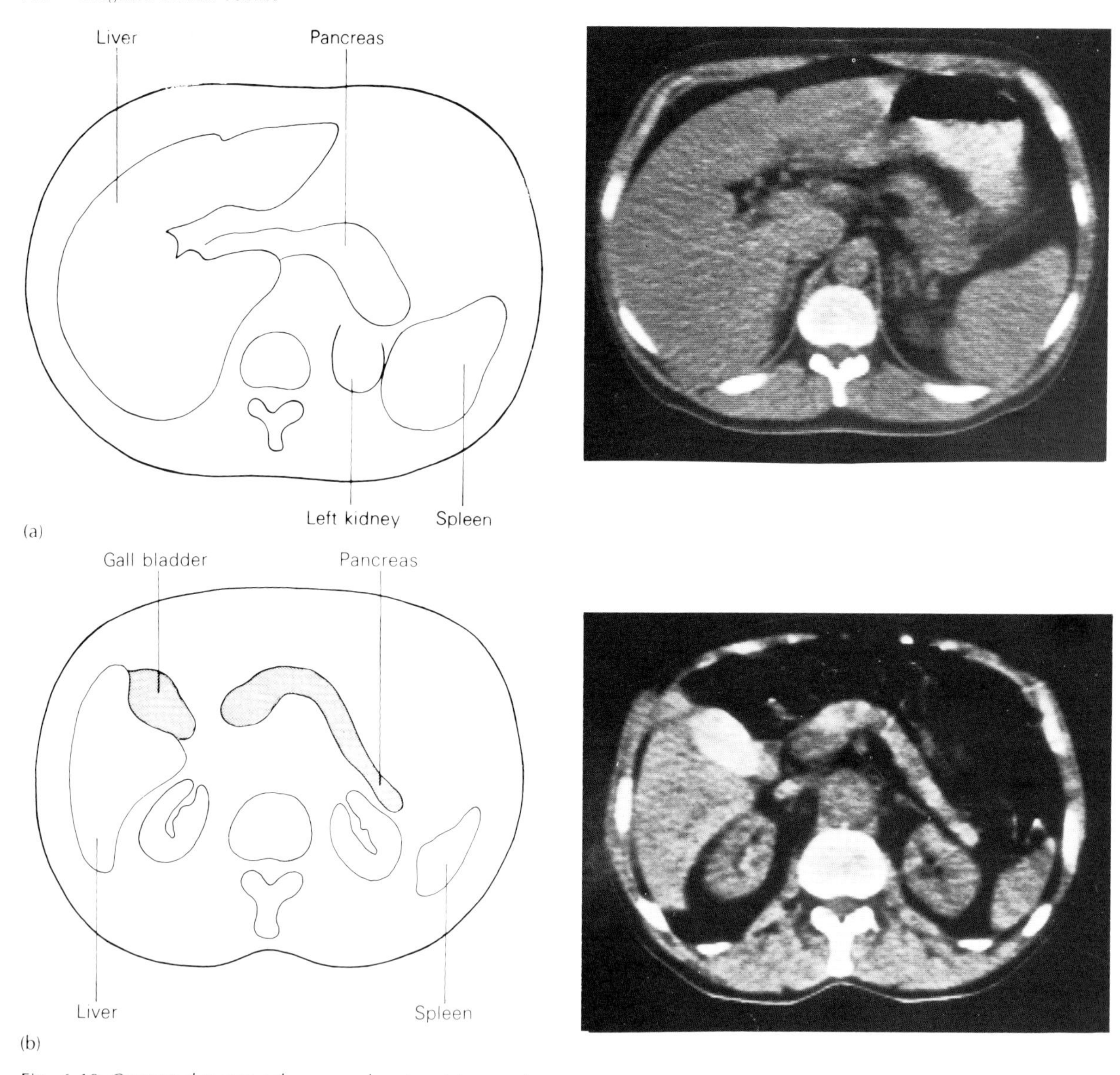

Fig. 6.10 *Computed tomography scans showing: (a) normal abdomen, pancreas; (b) calcified gall bladder and pancreas.*

extract with antacids, and indirectly by the addition of fat-soluble vitamin supplements and medium-chain triglyceride oil preparations.

Control of pain is, by contrast, difficult. Analgesics may be required in increasing dosage and frequency, and addiction is all too likely to occur. The surgical treatment of the pain of chronic pancreatitis rests on two approaches. the first is internal drainage of an obstructed main pancreatic duct, often into a loop of jejunum; or a sphincteroplasty on the ampulla of Vater may allow removal of stones from the pancreatic duct. The second approach is resection of the most diseased area of pancreas, ranging from distal pancreatectomy to pancreatico-duodenectomy (Whipple's operation) and, rarely, to subtotal or total pancreatectomy.

Another approach is to block the sensory nerves around the coeliac axis with carefully placed injections of 50% alcohol or phenol, but the beneficial effects rarely last more than a few months. Recently total main duct occlusion has been tried, with a blocking substance, Ethibloc, injected via an endoscope: this hardens and leads to death of the exocrine pancreatic tissue, but results are variable.

Complications

A pseudocyst may arise, and the patient usually experiences discomfort, pain or vomiting. While it may show on barium meal, ultrasonography and CT scanning are the most useful tests. Usually the cyst is drained into the stomach.

Pancreatic ascites probably arises from leakage from a cyst or pseudocyst or ductual rupture. It is rare. Pleural effusions may also occur.

Cystic Fibrosis

Cystic fibrosis (mucoviscidosis; fibrocystic disease of pancreas) is by far the commonest cause of pancreatic disease in childhood and is possibly the commonest lethal single-gene disease. It is transmitted as an autosomal recessive trait and the incidence is of the order of 1 in 1500–1800 live births in the Western World. Its cause is not yet fully understood, treatment is wholly supportive, and death usually supervenes from the respiratory complications during adolescence or early adulthood.

It is important not to regard this as purely a disease of the pancreas. The essential feature is alteration of all exocrine secretions:

- thick 'sticky' mucus in the gut, respiratory and genital tracts
- scanty concentrated secretions of pancreas (and salivary glands), with low bicarbonate but normal enzyme levels.
- increased ion concentrations (sodium, potassium, chloride and others) in sweat (chloride content in excess of 60 mmol/l).

The pancreas is from birth hard and knobbly with fibrosis and cystic dilatation of the ducts. Cirrhosis of the liver is a later feature. The lungs are normal at birth but repeated infection (notably with *Staph. aureus, Haemophilus influenzae* and *E. coli*) produces bronchitis, bronchiectasis, fibrosis, emphysema and cor pulmonale. Almost all patients eventually develop almost ineradicable pulmonary infection with *Pseudomonas aeruginosa*.

Presentation

In the newborn. Owing to the scanty pancreatic and intestinal secretions the meconium in the small bowel is exceptionally viscid and this can cause intestinal obstruction (meconium ileus) when the terminal ileum is plugged with sticky solid meconium. A diatrizoate enema (Gastrografin), administered under x-ray control, may succeed in dislodging the sticky solid meconium from the ileum so that it can then pass through the wider colon, but surgical relief is often necessary, which may involve resection of a length of the plugged-up ileum (see p. 264).

Infancy. From birth onwards there is a constant threat of recurrent respiratory infections. As these progress, the child may become cyanotic, barrel-chested and stunted, with a productive cough and finger-clubbing.

Older babies may have episodes of abdominal pain due to obstruction (meconium ileus equivalent), and occasionally present with rectal prolapse. Failure to thrive is due either to pancreatic insufficiency (with malabsorption and pale bulky offensive stools) or to recurrent respiratory infection.

Jaundice is a rare early sign. Cirrhosis is a late feature. Diabetes mellitus may occur (Fig. 6.11).

Diagnosis

Diagnosis is confirmed by:

1. Sweat test – high electrolyte content, especially sodium and chloride. This test requires some skill to effect collection and analysis of the inevitably small quantities of sweat.
2. Demonstration of malabsorption.

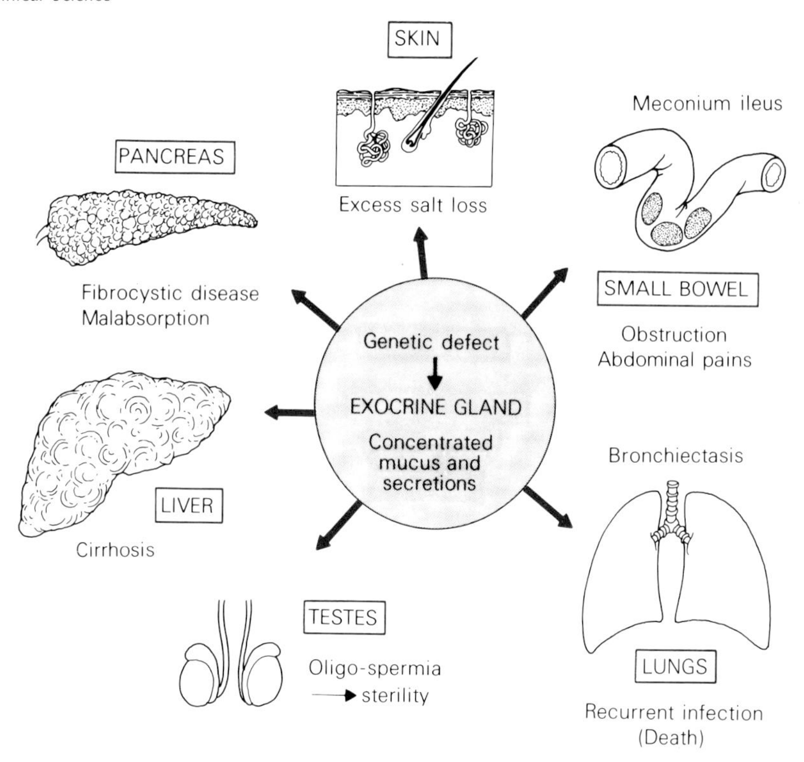

Fig. 6.11 *Widespread effects of cystic fibrosis.*

3. Pancreatic function tests. These tests have not often been done, since they generally require the passage of a duodenal tube, and the performance of the more complex pancreozymin and secretin tests (Table 6.2). Any infant with failure to thrive or recurrent respiratory infections should be suspected of having cystic fibrosis.

Treatment

The ideal treatment for cystic fibrosis would be a pharmacological treatment which restored secretions to normal, but this is not available. The treatment of meconium ileus is considered on page 265.

Malabsorption requires a high-protein-calorie diet with limited fat intake. Energy intake can be supplemented by medium-chain triglyceride oil. Pancreatic supplements are given *with* each meal, preferably sprinkled on to food. Relatively large doses are needed because pancreatic enzymes are inactivated by gastric acid, so antacids are also prescribed. Extra vitamins are wise, as well as salt supplements in very hot climates. Regular supervision by a qualified dietician is important.

Respiratory infections are the major problems, requiring repeated and sometimes continuous antibiotics according to the organism sensitivities, together with mucolytic inhalations and physiotherapy with postural drainage.

These patients require devoted and committed care from physician and parents, and many now survive to adult life, though with a limited expectation.

Genetic counselling may be required: as the inheritance is autosomal recessive, there is a 1 in 4 chance of each offspring of (heterozygote) parents being affected.

Other Rare Causes of Pancreatic Insufficiency

In addition to cystic fibrosis, and distinct from it, other very rare causes of pancreatic insufficiency have been described. The most important of these is Schwachman's syndrome, where congenital pancreatic atrophy and enzyme deficiency is associated with intermittent neutropenia. There may be an associated chondrodystrophy.

Carcinoma of the Pancreas

This is a tumour of considerable importance. Its incidence is steadily increasing in Western countries and it is particularly unresponsive to available treatments. This is largely due to the position of the pancreas, which means that, by the time the diagnosis is made, fewer than 5% of all pancreatic carcinomas are suitable for radical excision. In the USA, where it is the third commonest cause of cancer death, some 22000 die each year from this neoplasm. Incidence is claimed to be twice as high in smokers as in non-smokers, and in diabetics compared with non-diabetics, but this has not been explained.

Histologically, carcinoma of the pancreas is usually a well-differentiated adenocarcinoma arising from duct epithelium, and 60–70% arise in the head of the gland. As a consequence, the lower end of the bile duct is usually involved, causing obstruction and jaundice. Spread to adjacent organs, lymph nodes, and the liver is common.

Broadly, carcinoma of the pancreas presents in one of two ways. Carcinomas in the head are generally silent until the patient becomes jaundiced, although on questioning patients often remember noticing some epigastric discomfort: this may go through to the back, and in a minority of patients is troublesome. Weight-loss, anorexia and diarrhoea are fairly common.

When the carcinoma arises in the body or tail, the patient generally presents with persistent deep epigastric pain, often going through to the back: flexion of the spine may ease the pain and is a helpful diagnostic symptom. Jaundice is rare. An abnormal glucose tolerance test or frank diabetes occurs in more than one-third of cases.

The deep situation of the pancreas means that, apart from jaundice, signs are few. Malignant obstruction of the lower end of the bile duct is often, though by no means always, reflected in the distended gall bladder being palpable (Courvoisier's sign), which is a rare finding in calculous jaundice (p. 180).

Many investigations are unhelpful but ultrasonography, and particularly CT scanning, may provide accurate visualisation of pancreatic tumours. Percutaneous transhepatic cholangiogra-

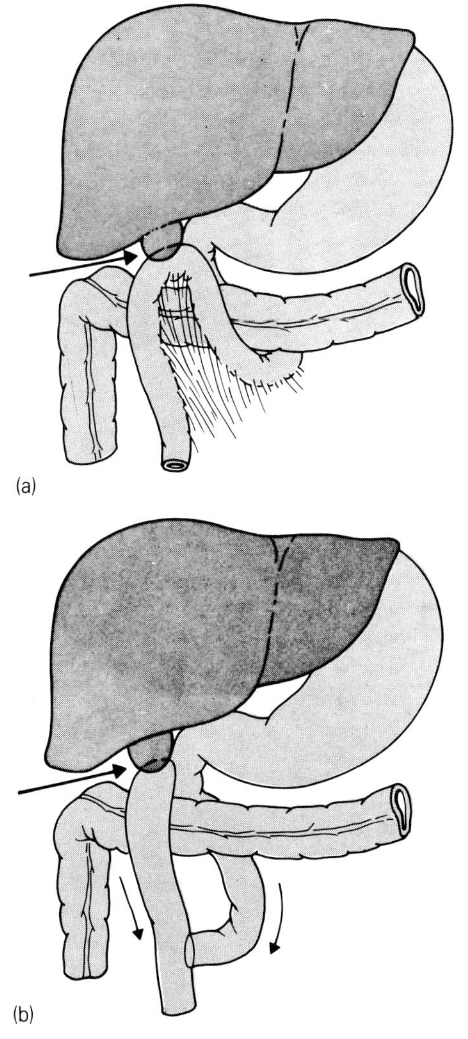

Fig. 6.12 *Cholecystjejunostomy. (a) In continuity. (b) Via a Roux-loop.*

phy may be very helpful in localising the site of obstruction in jaundiced patients, and duodenal endoscopy should identify the rarer resectable tumours of the ampulla of Vater, whilst ERCP (with or without cytology) may demonstrate a carcinoma of the lower end of the bile duct (and occasionally a carcinoma of the pancreas). In the elucidation of persistent pancreatic pain, ERCP may help to distinguish chronic pancreatitis from a carcinoma of the body of the gland.

Very few carcinomas of the head of the pancreas are removable but jaundice can nearly always be relieved by cholecyst-jejunostomy, which allows the distended biliary tree to be decompressed via the cystic duct and gall bladder. Two methods of anastomosis are used (Fig. 6.12). Some carcinomas are already invading the duodenal loop at the time of the laparotomy, and then a gastrojejunostomy must also be done to forestall the development of complete duodenal obstruction.

Rarely, an early localised carcinoma of the pancreas can be treated like a carcinoma of the ampulla or lower end of bile duct by radical pancreato-duodenectomy (Whipple's operation; see p. 183).

The prognosis, even with a drainage operation, is very limited: 6–9 months is the usual period of survival. Neither chemotherapy nor radiotherapy have proved helpful.

Carcinomas of the body and tail are never suitable for radical resection although palliative excision occasionally eases back pain.

7

Absorption and Malabsorption

The central function of the gut is the ingestion, digestion, absorption and assimilation of food. These processes must be seen as a closely integrated and interdependent system whose efficiency depends upon the macroscopic and microscopic structure of the gut and upon the neurohumoral control of secretion and motility.

Digestion is initiated by cooking, chewing and denaturation by gastric acid. It continues chemically within the intestinal lumen by the action of enzymes largely bound to the surface or in the cytoplasm of intestinal mucosal cells. (enterocytes). The enzymes are most densely situated in the mid-jejunum.

STRUCTURE OF SMALL BOWEL

The small bowel is an astonishing organ. It has the fastest turnover of any body tissue. Its lining cells (enterocytes) acquire their highly specialised functions, mature, perform a vital role in completing digestion and effecting absorption, die and are shed into the gut lumen all in the space of a few days. A large surface area is required for absorption and this is achieved by a remarkable series of anatomical devices: mucosal folds of Kerkring, villi and microvilli on the enterocyte surfaces (Fig. 7.1). These morphological features convert a simple tube into a surface which if opened out

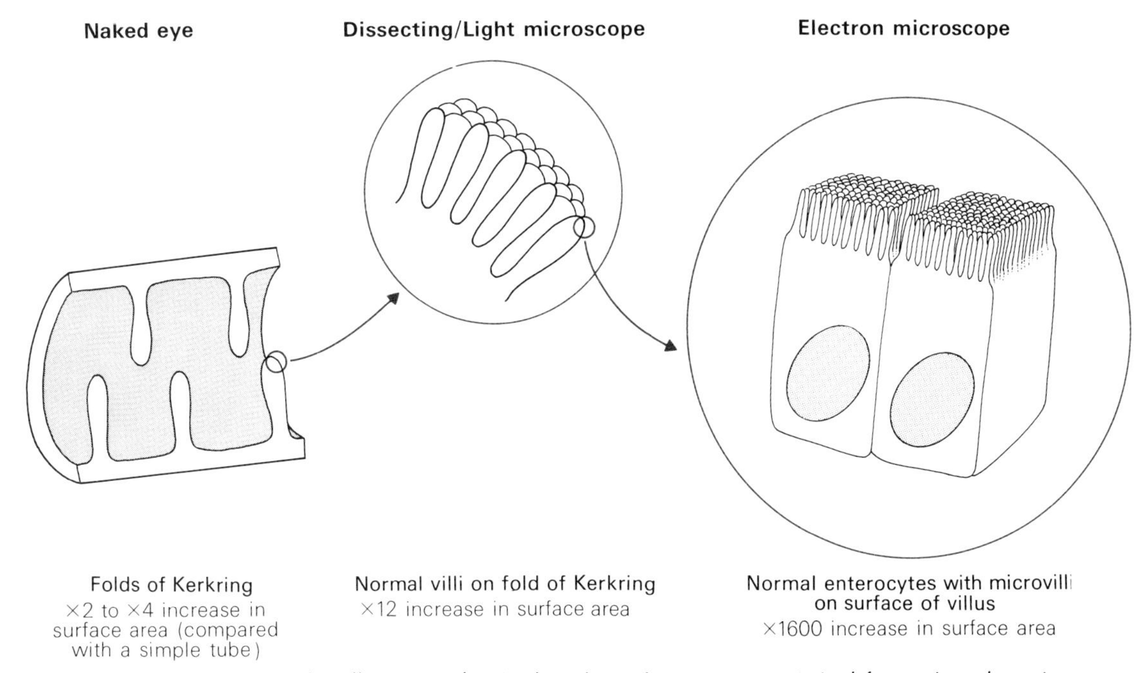

Fig. 7.1 *Normal structure of small intestine, showing how the surface area is maximised for nutrient absorption.*

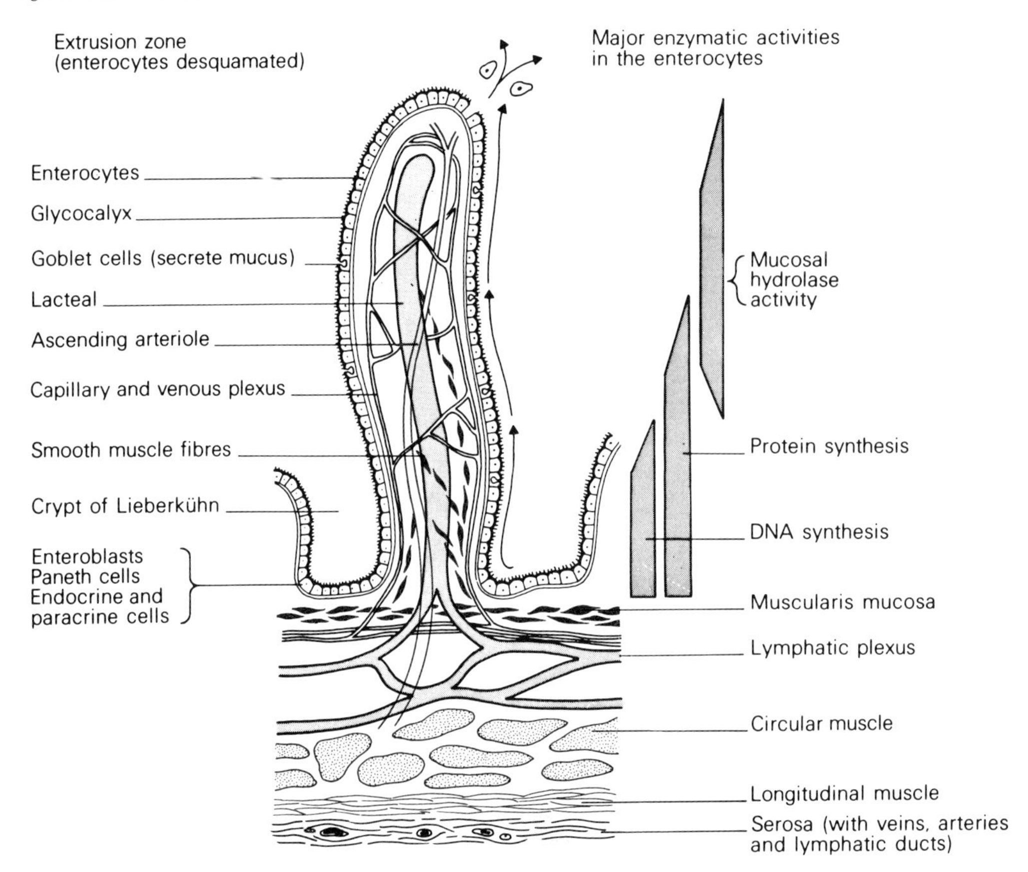

Fig. 7.2 *Anatomical and biochemical aspects of villus.*

would cover a doubles tennis court. The small bowel has striking powers of adaptation. Survival is possible with as little as 25 cm of surviving bowel following resection (e.g. because of ischaemic necrosis). This adaptation is achieved in part by hypertrophy and elongation of the existing villi (see p. 137). The small bowel has a central role in the immunoprotective system of the body (see p. 15).

The whole of the small bowel is a vast endocrine organ harbouring numerous humoral cells (p. 18).

In the villus (Fig. 7.2), muscle fibres running from the muscularis mucosae to the lacteals contract during absorption and pump lymph from the lacteals into the lymphatic vessels whence it passes into the mesenteric lymphatics. The villous capillary network is supplied by a central arteriole and drained by venules discharging into the portal vein radicles. Since the capillaries are fenestrated, cross-diffusion can occur, leading to a 'counter-current multiplier' system and concentration of nutrients at the villus tip. This hyperosmolarity facilitates intestinal water absorption (Fig. 7.3). Diffusion of oxygen from the arteriole low down in the villus means that the tip is more liable to hypoxia (probably thereby contributing to death and shedding of cells from the tip).

Enterocytes are highly organised cells (Figs 7.4 and 7.5). They are formed in the bases of the crypts of Lieberkuhn from precursor cells (enteroblasts) whence they migrate out of the crypts and along the villus like an escalator to the tip where they are shed – a process occupying only some 4–6 days in all. Maturation and elaboration of function occurs during this short life-span and can be related to specific micro-anatomical structures (Fig. 7.5).

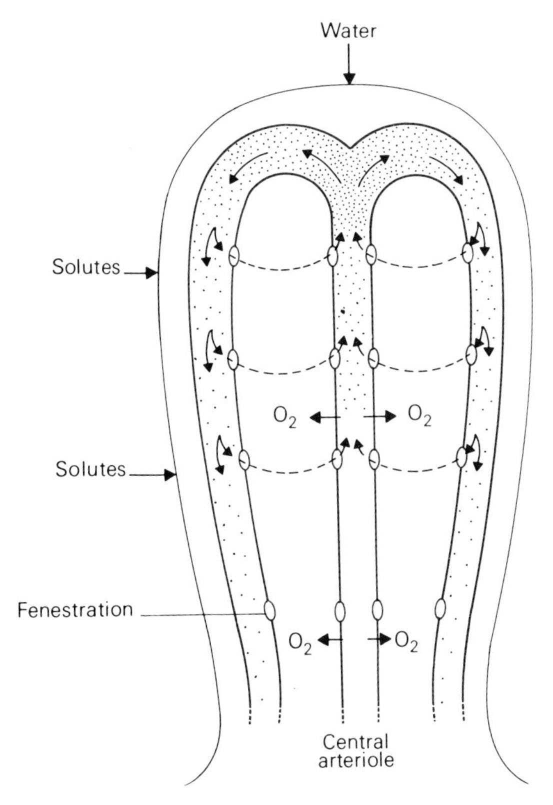

Fig. 7.3 *Villus 'counter-current multiplier system'.*

Glycocalyx

This consists of glycoproteins, manufactured by the enterocytes themselves, which bind certain nutrients (e.g. trace metals and vitamin B_{12}) and also pancreatic enzymes.

Microvillus 'Brush Border'

This contains enzymes responsible for carbohydrate and protein digestion (Fig. 7.6).

Brush Border Membrane.

Solutes cross this membrane barrier by four mechanisms (Fig. 7.7), two depending upon specific carrier systems capable of solute uptake against a concentration gradient.

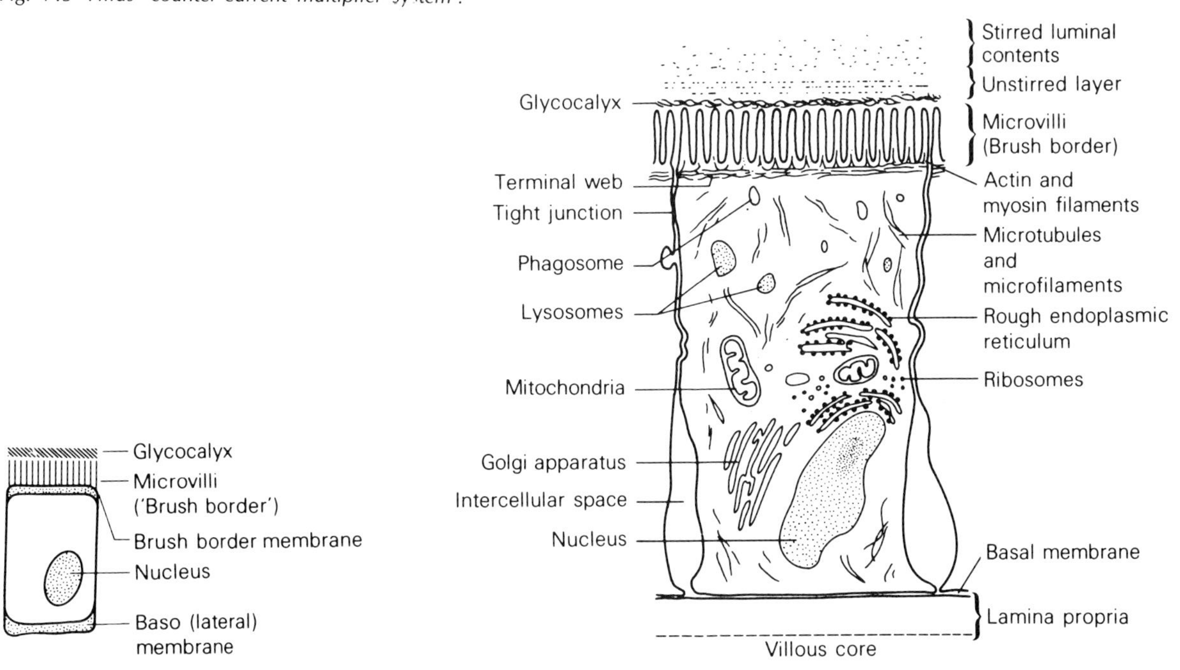

Fig. 7.4 *Basic structure of the enterocyte.*

Fig. 7.5 *Detailed structure of an enterocyte.*

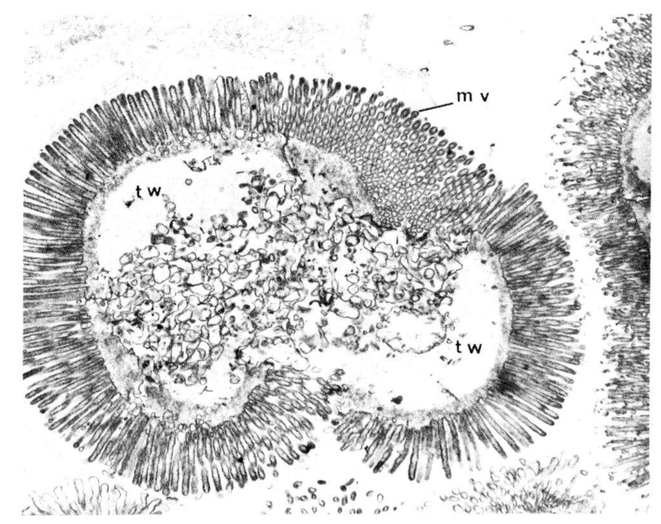

Fig. 7.6 *Electron micrograph of brush borders. mv = microvilli, tw = terminal web.*

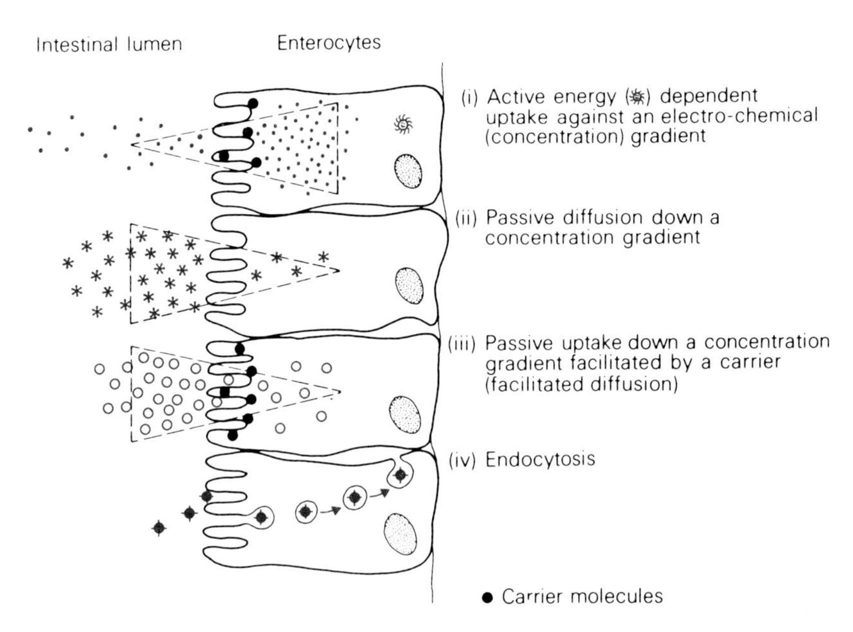

Fig. 7.7 *Mechanisms of nutrient transport.*

Basolateral Membrane

This contains the energy generating enzyme, sodium potassium adenosine triphosphatase (Na-K-ATPase), responsible for active nutrient uptake. This enzyme uses the hydrolysis of ATP to pump sodium into the intercellular space in exchange for potassium, leading to a sodium concentration gradient across the brush border membrane. Carriers for sodium across this membrane also transport nutrients, e.g. glucose, the combined action being termed a 'symport system' (sym, together; port, to carry).

FUNCTION OF SMALL BOWEL

Absorption of Water and Electrolytes

Large volumes of fluid are handled by the gut daily, most of it endogenously produced and most reabsorbed (Fig. 7.8). Water flux is free in the small intestine, both into and out of the lumen. In the duodenum net flux is into the lumen. Most carbohydrate, protein and medium-chain fatty acids are absorbed in the proximal 1.5 m of jejunum, where sodium symport systems are most profuse. Appreciable reabsorption of water and sodium occurs in combination with other solutes such as D-hexoses and L-amino acids.

This mechanism is exploited in the oral treatment of cholera and other choleraic syndromes (see p. 332) by giving large volumes of balanced solutions of saline and glucose or sucrose or by commercial electrolyte solutions such as Dioralyte.

Most of the water reabsorbed by the proximal intestine passes, in fact, *between* enterocytes through the 'tight junctions' (Fig. 7.9). Ions such as

Endogenous secretions	(ml)
Food and drink	2000
Saliva	1500
Gastric juice	2500
Bile	1000
Pancreatic juice	1500
Intestine	1000
Total entering lumen =	9500

Intake: food and drink

2000 ml

Absorption	(ml)
Jejunum	5000–6000
Ileum	2000–2500
Colon	1000–1500

Net loss in faeces = 50–200 ml

Fig. 7.8 *Intestinal water balance.*

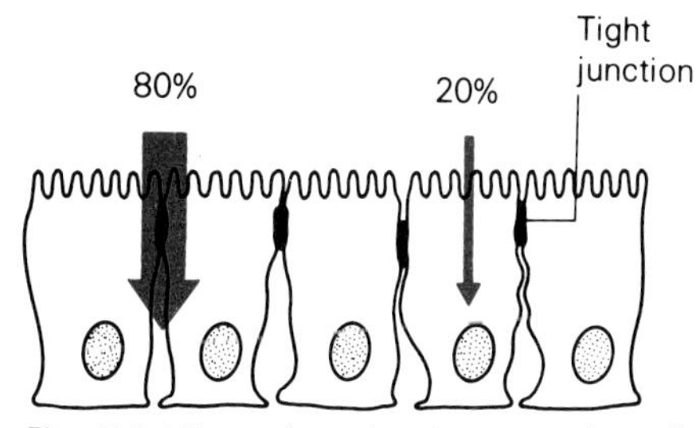

Fig. 7.9 *Water absorption in proximal small intestine.*

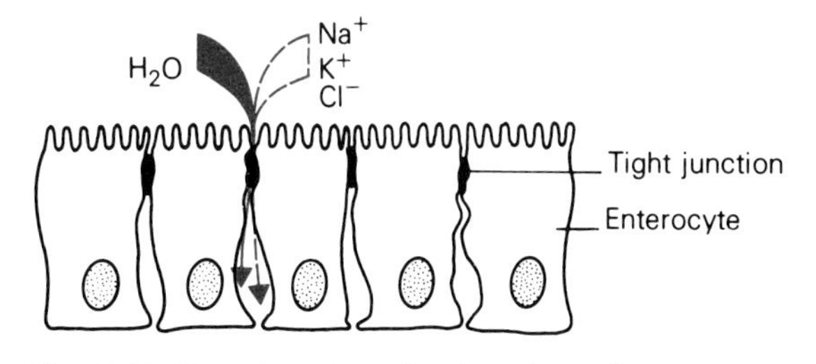

Fig. 7.10 *Electrolyte absorption by solvent drag.*

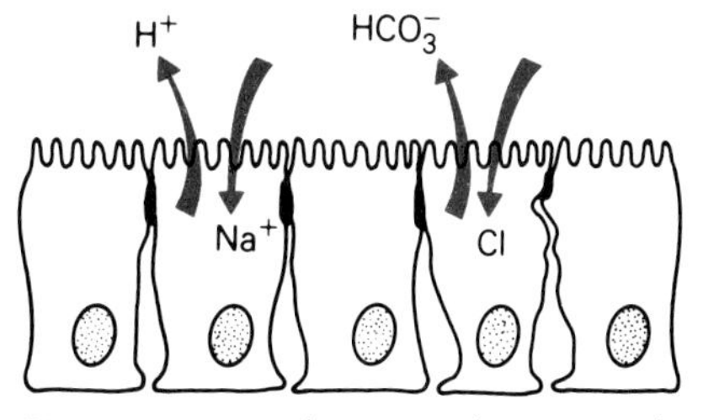

Fig. 7.11 *Ion exchange mechanism in ileum.*

sodium, potassium and chloride are swept in with it (solvent drag, Fig. 7.10). In the distal ileum and colon, single sodium carriers predominate, the tight junctions appear tighter, and only water enters between the cells. Furthermore, in this part of the gut sodium and chloride can enter the enterocytes by a system exchanging hydrogen and bicarbonate ions into the lumen (Fig. 7.11). This system is defective in the extremely rare syndrome of congenital chloridorrhoea, when large amounts of water and chloride are lost leading to dehydration and hypochloraemic alkalosis.

Potassium is passively absorbed in the proximal gut in response to electrochemical gradients and also by paracellular solvent drag, but is secreted by the terminal ileum and colon.

Carbohydrate Absorption

Intraluminal hydrolysis of carbohydrate polysaccharides commences with the action of salivary and pancreatic amylases and is completed by small bowel mucosal oligosaccharidases. Absorption occurs throughout the small bowel via the sodium-linked symport systems. This process is exceedingly efficient; up to 120 g of carbohydrate can be handled in one hour. Consequently man can tolerate quite extensive impairment of the digestive and absorptive mechanisms for carbohydrate.

Congenital defects in the activities of amylase, lactase (see p. 140), and sucrase-α-dextrinase and of the glucose-galactose carriers are rare. Loss of these enzymes is associated more usually with other diseases. Amylase deficiency occurs with pancreatic insufficiency but, if small bowel mucosal function is normal, malabsorption of carbohydrate is rare because of the enzyme's great efficiency. The mucosal oligodisaccharidases and carrier molecules may be defective in mucosal damage sustained with gastroenteritis, gastric hyperacidity, following intestinal surgery, or with enteropathies such as coeliac disease or giardiasis. Lactase is the most susceptible to such insults and is the slowest to recover afterwards; in some instances it never does so (see p. 140).

The symptoms include diarrhoea, abdominal distension, pain, and borborygmi caused by osmotic activity of unabsorbed sugars and their breakdown to hydrogen and carbon dioxide. Fermentation of the saccharides produces volatile organic acids (e.g. lactic, acetic, butyric and proprionic) which are either absorbed by the colon or are passed in the faeces, producing a pH of less than 6.0. The colonic microflora are able to metabolise considerable amounts of carbohydrate and the colon is able to absorb the resultant organic acids and gases. Conversely, in some patients the symptoms are debilitating and the osmotic diarrhoea can cause dehydration with hypovolaemic shock and malabsorption of other essential nutrients.

Absorption of Proteins

Digested protein is either endogenous or exogenous (Fig. 7.12). The process is outlined in Fig. 7.13.

Some protein macromolecules are absorbed intact, perhaps by endocytosis. While this is probably of no nutritional significance, such macromolecule absorption may be of importance in inducing immune tolerance to dietary proteins and in causing immune reactions such as asthma and dermatitis (see p. 17). This is especially relevant in children who may also acquire passive immunity by the absorption of intact immunoglobulins from their mother's milk.

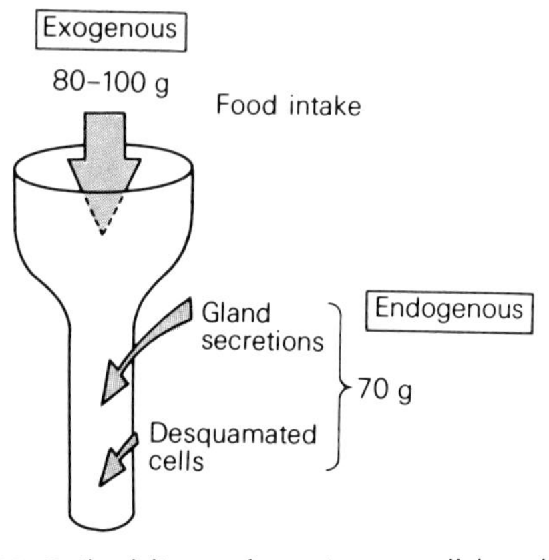

Fig. 7.12 *Daily delivery of protein to small bowel.*

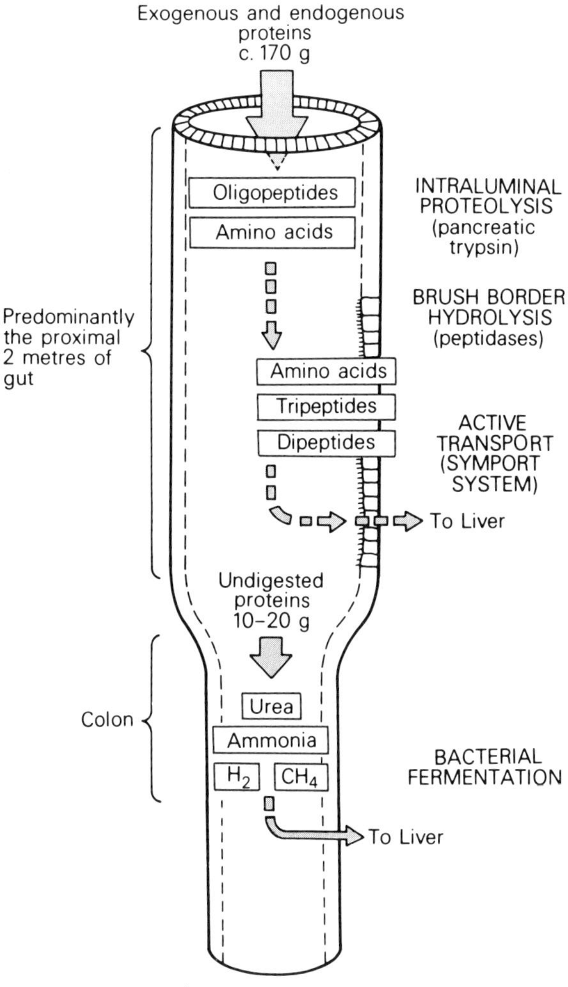

Fig. 7.13 *Protein absorption in gut.*

In some pathological states, protein is lost from the gut, sometimes in quantities large enough to cause considerable hypoalbuminaemia (Fig. 7.14)

Absorption of Fats

To achieve effective intraluminal digestion, lipid droplets need to be broken up, when the surface area available for lipolysis is increased; this is done by the churning action of the gastric antrum and by forceful ejection through the pylorus. The resultant emulsion is stabilised by the bile acids, which aggregate on the surface of the droplets and prevent them from coalescing into larger droplets.

The role of the lingual and gastric lipases may be quite important; they release medium- and short-chain fatty acids which have a carbon chain length of 12 or less and are water-soluble. Thus they are able to diffuse to the mucosa where there are specific Na^+ co-transport mechanisms for their active absorption. Medium-chain triacylglycerols (MCTs) are also taken up actively by the enterocyte, where an intracellular lipase degrades them to glycerol and constituent fatty acids.

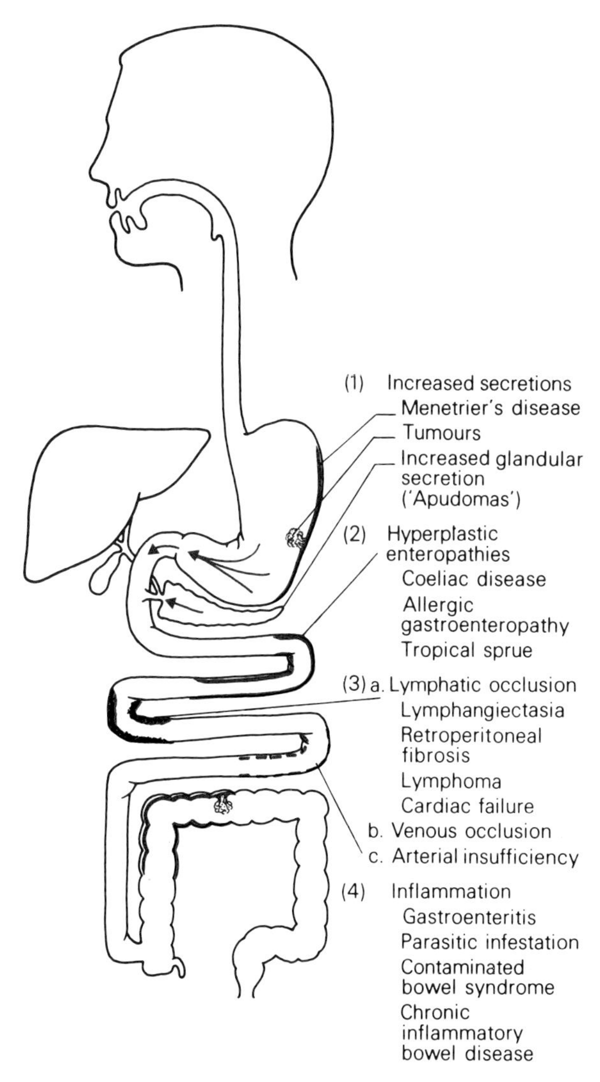

Fig. 7.14 *Some causes and mechanisms of protein-losing enteropathy.*

Bile Salts (see also Chapter 8)

The subsequent digestion and absorption of the hydrophobic lipid is dependent upon the bile salts. These are synthesised from cholesterol, in the liver, and are stored and concentrated in the gall bladder. Bile acids possess a carbon skeleton which is soluble in lipid, and hydroxyl and carboxyl groups which are water-soluble; the water-solubility is enhanced by the conjugation of the carboxyl group with either glycine or taurine to form a bile salt. In short, they are amphiphiles or detergents and this property enables them to 'parcel up' the lipid emulsion and to maintain the products of lipolysis in a water-soluble form. Formation of polymeric aggregates known as micelles is aided by the preliminary concentration of the bile salts in the gall bladder; the intra-intestinal bile salt concentration at which micelles are formed is called the 'critical micellar concentration' (CMC). The CMC is influenced also by the intraduodenal and jejunal pH; if the normally near neutral pH (6.5) of the lumen becomes too acid, the bile salts precipitate out of solution; similarly, if their hepatic production is impaired, the CMC may not be achieved even at physiological pH. In both circumstances lipid digestion is impaired. Another important feature of the action of bile sal' is that they facilitate the intraction of some of the pancreatic lipolytic enzymes – which are water-soluble – with the lipid droplets at the oil/water interface. Pancreatic enzymes and their secretion are discussed on page 102. The micelles diffuse to the mucosa, transporting in their core the residual nonpolar lipids including cholesterol and fat-soluble vitamins. After absorption, lipid molecules are then incorporated into two water-soluble lipoprotein complexes, chylomicrons and very low-density lipoproteins (VLDLs) for passage to the lymphatics. The chylomicrons and VLDLs enter the lacteals through gaps between the endothelial cells. The importance of chylomicrons in the solubilisation and absorption of hydrophobic lipids is illustrated by a rare inherited defect in apoprotein synthesis called abetalipoproteinaemia. Patients with this disorder cannot produce the apoprotein required for the formation of chylomicrons and the enterocytes become engorged with long-chain fatty acid triacylglycerols, and with other hydrophobic lipids.

Although some bile salts are reabsorbed passively along the small intestine, most are reabsorbed actively by specific carriers in the terminal ileum and return via the portal circulation to the liver, where they are taken up by the hepatocytes and are then resecreted. This enterohepatic circulation completes at least two cycles with each meal (Figs 8.9–8.12). If the salvage mechanism is interrupted, e.g. by disease (Crohn's disease) or resection of the terminal ileum, bile salts pass into the

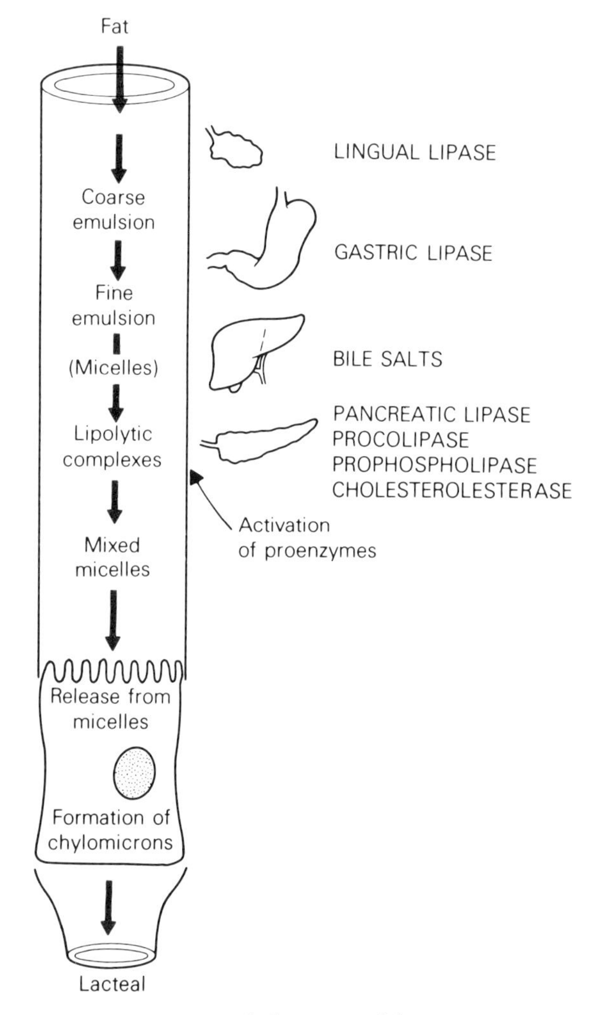

Fig. 7.15 *Digestion and absorption of fats.*

colon and are lost. The liver can increase its synthesis of bile salts 8–10-fold and it can therefore compensate only for the loss of 4–5 g of bile salts daily. Any loss in excess of this depletes the bile acid pool and jeopardises the digestion and absorption of fat and fat-soluble vitamins. Such a patient should be given the bulk of his daily lipid intake and fat-soluble vitamins at breakfast time, i.e. after the gall bladder has had a prolonged period in which to concentrate enough bile salts to achieve the CMC. It is not unusual for patients who have had cholecystectomies, and who cannot therefore preconcentrate bile salts, to have some degree of lipid maldigestion. Fat absorption is summed up in Fig. 7.15.

Patients with gross deficiencies in bile salts or pancreatic lipolytic activity are best managed with special food supplements containing MCT; these are hydrolysed by gastric and lingual lipases to produce water-soluble products which do not require bile salts for their absorption. The fat-soluble vitamins A, D and K may need to be given parenterally, in severe cases.

Absorption of Essential Metals

Metals can be absorbed throughout the small intestine. Active carrier mediated mechanisms seem to exist for the essential trace metals – copper, zinc and iron (Fig. 7.16).

Up to 80% of the daily calcium intake (of approximately 800 mg) is absorbed via mucosal binding proteins, the synthesis of which is regulated by 1,25-dihydroxycholecalciferol. The 1 α-hydroxylation of 25 hydroxycholecalciferol (vitamin D) in the kidneys is regulated by parathyroid hormone (PTH) and is related inversely to plasma calcium concentrations. Calcium is also lost into the intestine, and the resultant net daily absorption is 200 mg; calcium homeostasis is maintained by the adjustment of its excretion in the urine.

Iron is best absorbed in the organic complex haem. Inorganic iron is probably taken up by the duodenum most efficiently as ferrous iron. Gastric secretion facilitates the absorption and this may be achieved by reduction of (ferric) iron in the diet to ferrous iron. Most becomes bound to an intracellular protein, apoferritin, to form ferritin. The release of ferritin iron to the tissues depends on an individual's iron status but it is unknown how this is regulated. Cells loaded with ferritin are unable to absorb further iron and this 'mucosal block' prevents any more uptake of the metal.

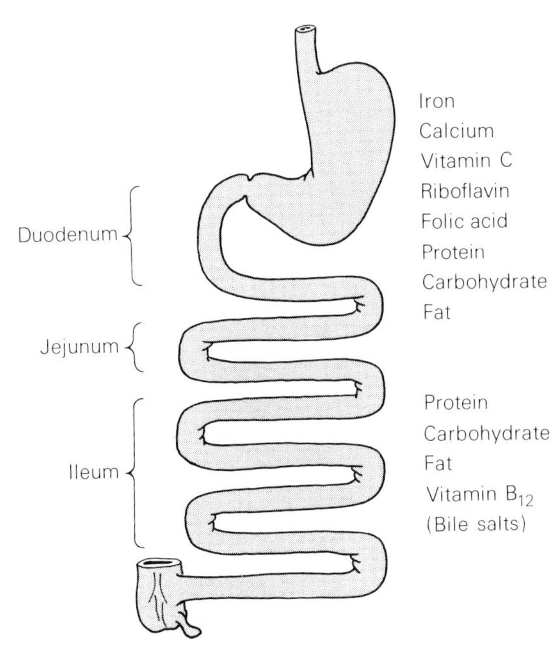

Fig. 7.16 *Sites of absorption of nutrients in gut.*

Absorption of Water-soluble Vitamins

These are probably absorbed by carrier mediated mechanism in the small intestine. The uptake of riboflavine and pyridoxine may be by diffusion.

Dietary folic acid is conjugated with glutamic acid (pteroylpolyglutamate) and hydrolysed at the brush border to a mixture of tri-, di- and monoglutamates, which are thought to enter the enterocyte actively (Fig. 7.17). The tri- and diglutamates are degraded intracellularly to monoglutamate, which leaves the cell by facilitated diffusion. The mucosal hydrolysis and absorption of folate conjugate is especially sensitive to mucosal disease and

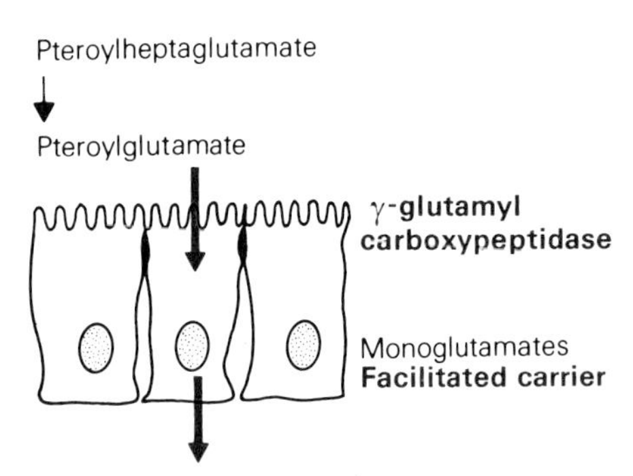

Fig. 7.17 *Absorption of folic acid.*

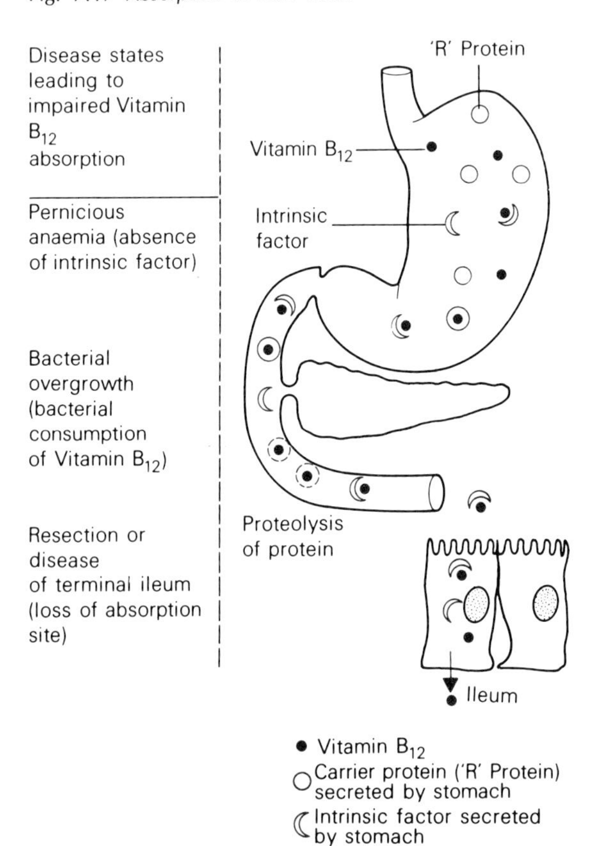

Fig. 7.18 *Disease states leading to impaired vitamin B_{12} absorption.*

the resultant folate deficiency is often the first sign of an enteropathy. Folate deficiency can be screened for by measuring the plasma folate content (usually > 2ng/ml) or, more reliably, the red cell folate content (normally 200–800 ng/l).

The absorption of vitamin B_{12} is susceptible to numerous interferences (Fig. 7.18). Severe impairment of absorption can be present without any deficit being apparent in the plasma concentrations becuase of the large stores of vitamin in the liver. A reliable test of the absorption of vitamin B_{12} is therefore invaluable and it provides, additionally, a valuable means of assessing ileal function (see p. 123).

Ileal Adaptation

Animal experiments have shown that the small bowel has remarkable powers of adapation that come into play in disease states, or after surgical resection (see *massive small bowel resection*, p. 135). There are striking morphological changes, which include dilatation of remaining small bowel and hyperplasia of villi. Even more remarkable are the functional changes that have been demonstrated in humans as well as animals. Following resection of jejunum the ileum will, in time, take over at least some of the functions of the resected bowel and therefore minimise the metabolic consequences. However, there is good evidence that, following resection of ileum or in diseases principally affecting the ileum (see p. 134), the jejunum *cannot* take over the specific functions of the ileum (to absorb vitamin B_{12} and bile salts). In terms of metabolic and nutritional consequences, loss of ileal function (either by disease or surgery) is therefore much more serious than loss of jejunal function.

INVESTIGATION OF SMALL BOWEL FUNCTION

Numerous tests of small bowel function have been devised and used. In practice, since most of them are diagnostically nonspecific and essentially screening tests, most clinicians select a group of tests which are relatively simple and cover the major areas of small bowel function. The selection of tests will vary in different centres according to local interests and expertise. The following is a commonly adopted group.

Lipid Absorption

Faecal fat analysis

The fat excretion is determined on a 3-day collection of stool while the patient is on a normal ward diet, i.e. at least 100 g/day of fat. Normal excretion is less than 54 mmoles/3 days (18 mmol/day).

Butter fat absorption test

A fasting blood sample (t = 0) is taken, after which the patient ingests a standard test meal (0.5 g butter/kg body weight spread on toast). Further blood samples are taken at 90 mins, 120 mins and 150 mins.

A quantitative assessment of the serum chylomicrons provides a measure of fat absorption.

Estimation of serum vitamin A levels.

Serum carotene levels give an indirect measure of vitamin A status.

Carbohydrate Absorption

D-xylose absorption test

D-xylose is a pentose sugar which is normally absorbed rapidly from the small intestine, only slightly metabolised by the body, and exreted rapidly in the urine. It can thus can be used satisfactorily to test monosaccharide absorption.

For this test the patient fasts overnight, empties the bladder in the morning, and drinks 250 ml water containing 25 g xylose. The xylose excreted in the urine in the next 5 hours is measured. Normal persons should excrete more than 40 mmoles in 5 hours. Children should be given a lower dose, e.g. 0.5 g/kg, and with this smaller dose 25% or more of what is ingested should be excreted within 5 hours. It is important to remember that the results of these tests may not be valid if there is significant impairment of renal function.

Increasing use is being made of the measurement of serum levels since this minimises renal effects. Normally, after a 25-mg dose, a serum value at 1 hour of at least 2.5 mmol/l should be obtained.

Lactose tolerance test

Intestinal lactase deficiency can be assessed by giving 50 g lactose orally in 250 ml water and measuring plasma glucose levels at ½-hourly intervals for 2 hours. In subjects with normal lactase activity, the plasma glucose should increase by at least 1.1 mmol/l. A normal glucose tolerance test with an abnormal lactose tolerance test is suggestive of intestinal lactase deficiency. Similar tests can be performed with sucrose, maltose or isomaltose to test for other disaccharidase deficiencies.

Vitamin B_{12} Absorption

For the water-soluble vitamins, the most commonly used test is the Schilling test for vitamin B_{12} absorption. In this test a small (0.5–2μg) dose of ^{57}Co-labelled vitamin B_{12} is given orally, followed 1–3 hours later by a large (1000 μg) intramuscular injection of unlabelled vitamin B_{12} to saturate the liver stores and ensure that all the orally-administered dose absorbed will be excreted and not stored. The radioactivity in the urine excreted in 24 hours is measured. The proportion excreted in the urine is normally more than 12% of the given dose. Pernicious anaemia may be distinguished from other causes of vitamin B_{12} malabsorption by repeating the tests with ^{57}Co-labelled vitamin B_{12} coupled to Intrinsic Factor. By using two separable isotopes of radio-cobalt, both parts of the test can be performed simultaneously.

Bile Salt Metabolism (the ^{14}C GCA breath test)

Of the several conditions resulting in reduced functional bile-salt concentrations, the one most easily investigated is the presence of bacterial colonisation in the intestine. Radiolabelled glycocholic acid (labelled with ^{14}C in the glycine side-chain) is administered orally; samples of ex-

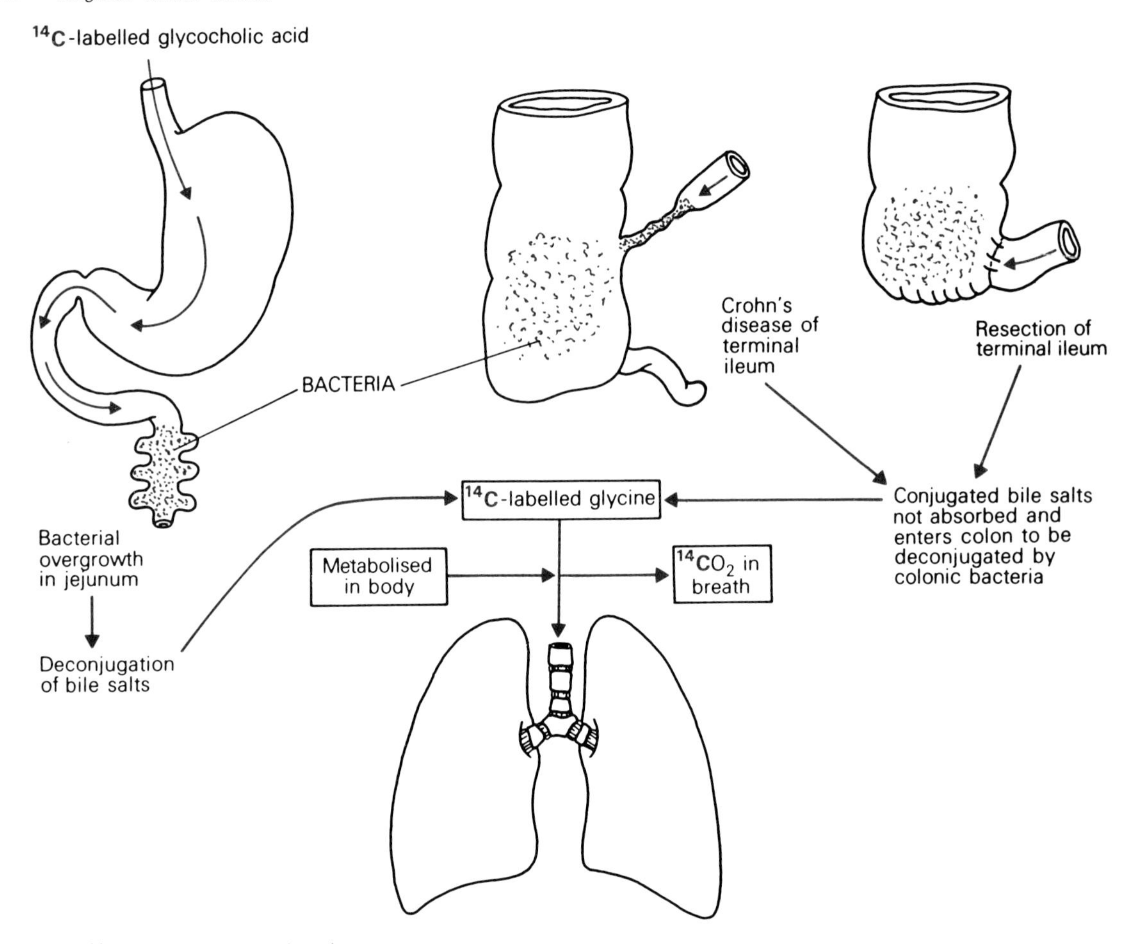

Fig. 7.19 *^{14}C glycocholic acid breath test.*

pired air are collected at hourly intervals for 5 hours and the $^{14}Co_2$ measured. Excessive bile salt deconjugation is shown by increased amounts of radioactivity in the first 3–4 samples. An abnormal result will, of course, also be obtained in destructive disease or following removal of the terminal ileum (where the major part of bile salts are reabsorbed), or in disorders of the bowel causing very rapid transit (Fig. 7.19)

The Hydrogen Breath Test

Hydrogen is one of the gases produced in the intestinal lumen by the bacterial breakdown of carbohydrates. These bacteria are usually only present in the colon and, as most carbohydrates are absorbed from the small intestine, little hydrogen is produced by healthy people. However, when there is malabsorption of any sugar, the colonic production of hydrogen is increased, and after diffusion to the blood stream it appears in the expired air where it can now be easily and cheaply detected by a hydrogen gas-sensing polarographic cell. This non-invasive investigation may be useful in the detection of acquired and inborn (e.g. disaccharidase deficiency) sugar malabsorption.

Investigation of Small Bowel Structure

Radiology

X-ray diagnosis of small bowel disease has already

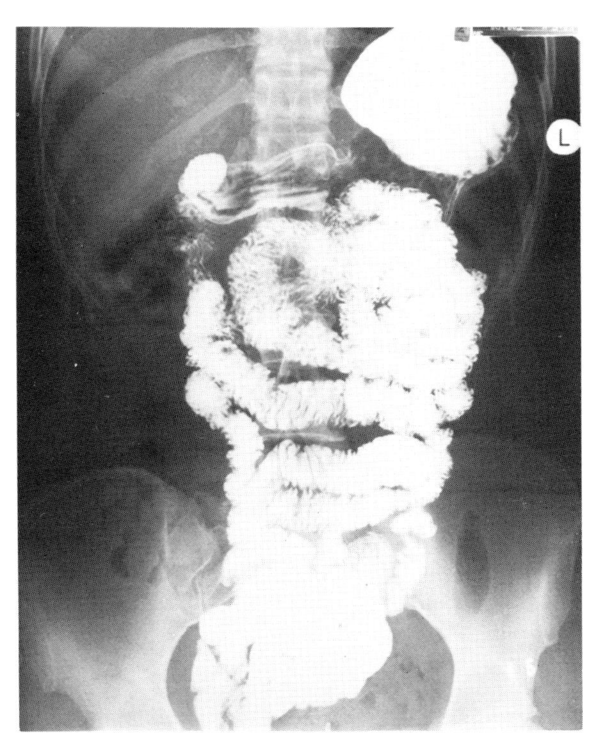

Fig. 7.20 *Norml barium meal and follow-through examination.*

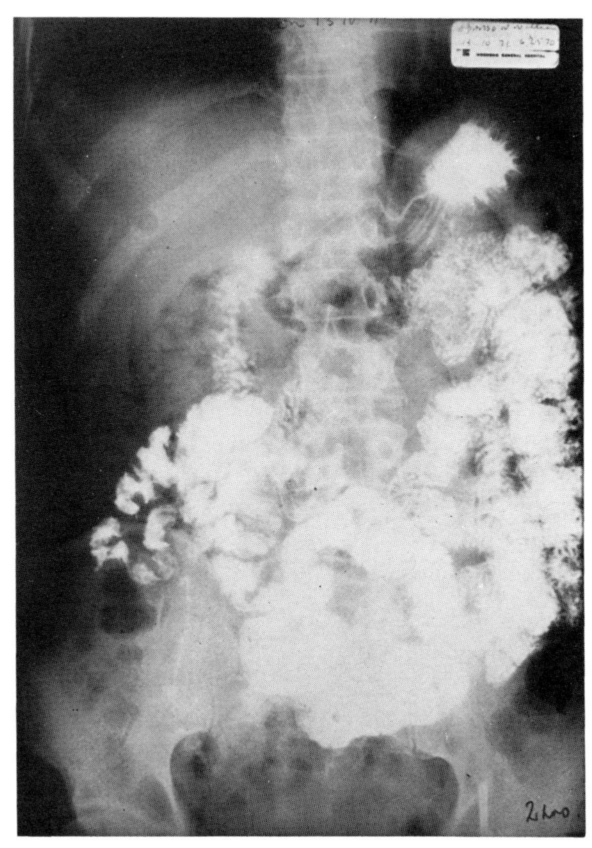

Fig. 7.22 *Nonspecific malabsorption on follow-through examination.*

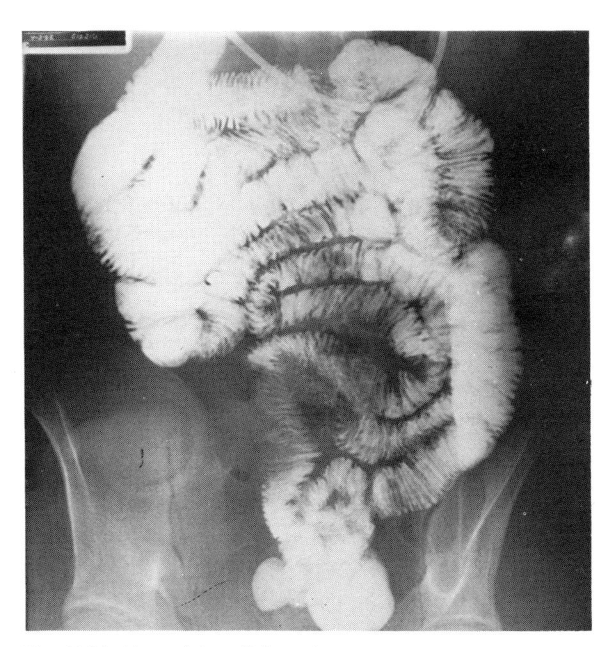

Fig. 7.21 *Normal 'small bowel enema'.*

been referred to in Chapter 3. Barium contrast, either by drinking (Fig. 7.20) or injection via duodenal intubation (small bowel enema; Fig. 7.21) can be used to show:

general nonspecific abnormalities suggestive of malabsorption: clumping and flocculation of barium, dilatation and effacement of the normal feathery pattern (Fig. 7.22)

structural changes in the wall of the small bowel such as strictures, diverticula, polyps, tumours and infiltration.

Mucosal biopsy

Their relative inaccessability has made biopsy of the jejunum and ileum difficult in the past. The distal duodenum can be biopsied under vision with standard endoscopes, and long 'enteroscopes' are available though not in general use. Blind biopsy can be achieved by a variety of mechanical devices, e.g. the multiple biopsy tube devised by Rubin, the pneumatic capsule devised by Crosby and Krugler, and the Watson modification of this. The last named is the standard method in Britain. After checking for normal blood coagulation, the capsule is passed into the upper alimentary tract and guided under x-ray control into the jejunum or allowed to move there passively. By a cunning pressure system (Fig. 7.23), mucosa is sucked into the capsule window or port and a guillotine blade is simultaneously activated to swing across and shave the mucosa. When the capsule is withdrawn, a piece of mucosa is (hopefully) in the capsule. Careful orientation and mounting of the specimen is essential for accurate histopathological assessment, and is generally carried out with the aid of a dissecting microscope.

Aspiration of jejunal juice for microscopy, culture (and biochemistry) can be carried out prior to firing the capsule.

CLINICAL DISORDERS OF THE SMALL BOWEL

Disorders of the small bowel usually present because of poor intraluminal digestion of food substances (Fig. 7.24) as well as malabsorption. The predominant symptoms and signs will depend on the site and the extent of small bowel involvement, but it is important to realise that many pathological processes may have a similar clinical presentation. The resulting complex of signs and symptoms is referred to as a malabsorption syndrome. Although the malabsorption syndrome has an enormous number of potential causes, most are uncommon. Relatively common causes are coeliac disease (gluten-sensitive enteropathy) and Crohn's disease and, less commonly, pancreatic insufficiency (see Chapter 6).

Following the precis of absorptive processes given in the earlier part of this chapter it is conceptually desirable to attempt to classify the causes according to the mechanisms of malabsorption. This has been attempted in Table 7.1. Whilst it is useful in illustrating the multiple

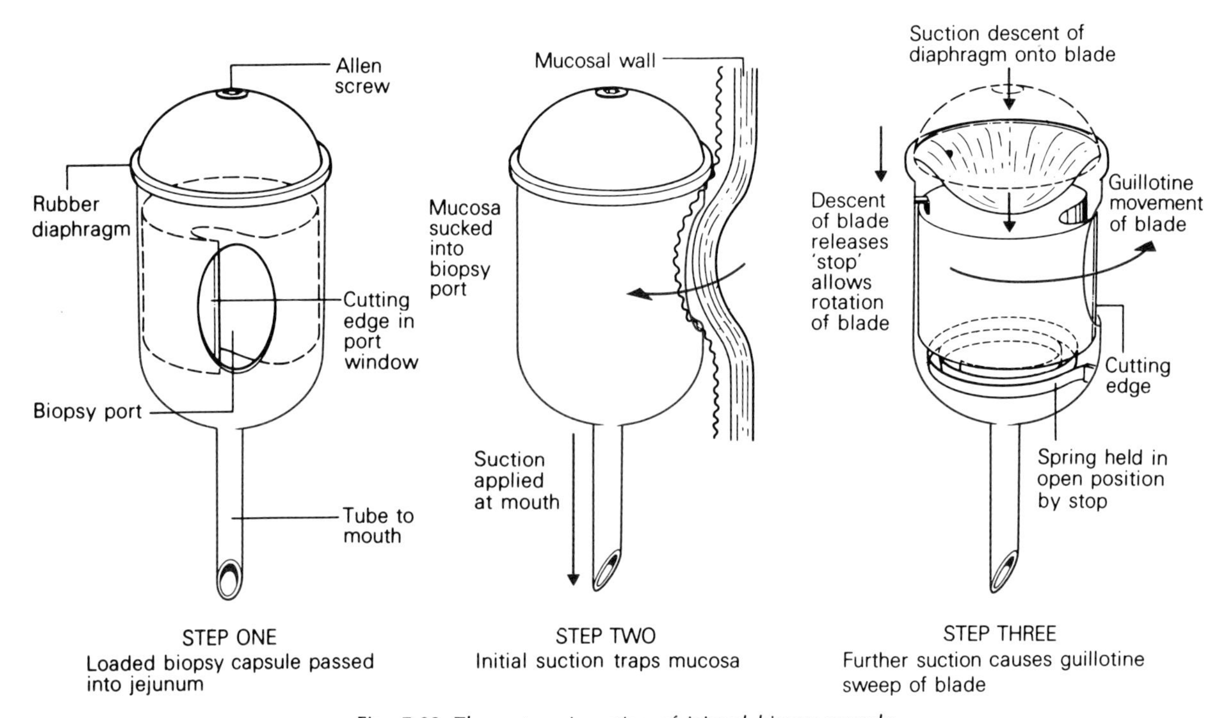

Fig. 7.23 *Three steps in action of jejunal biopsy capsule.*

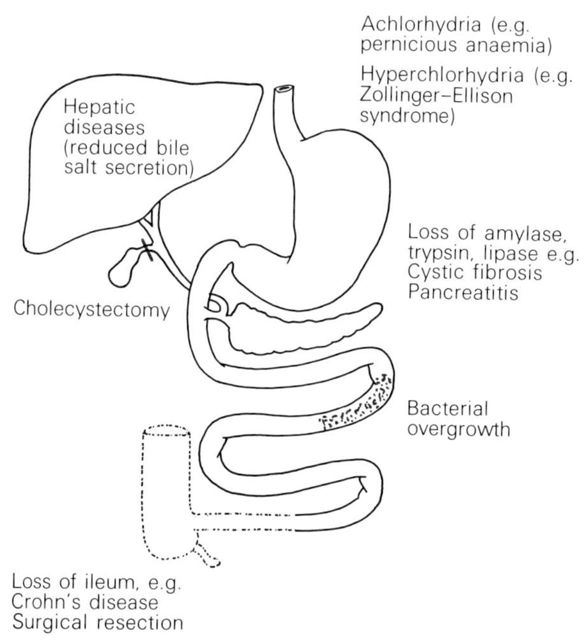

Fig. 7.24 *Common causes of impaired intraluminal digestion.*

possibilities, such a classification is limited by virtue of the fact that in many cases several mechanisms operate. For example, in small bowel Crohn's disease, malabsorption may be due to extensive mucosal destruction, bile salt loss, bacterial overgrowth, or surgical resection. In other patients the mechanism of malabsorption remains obscure.

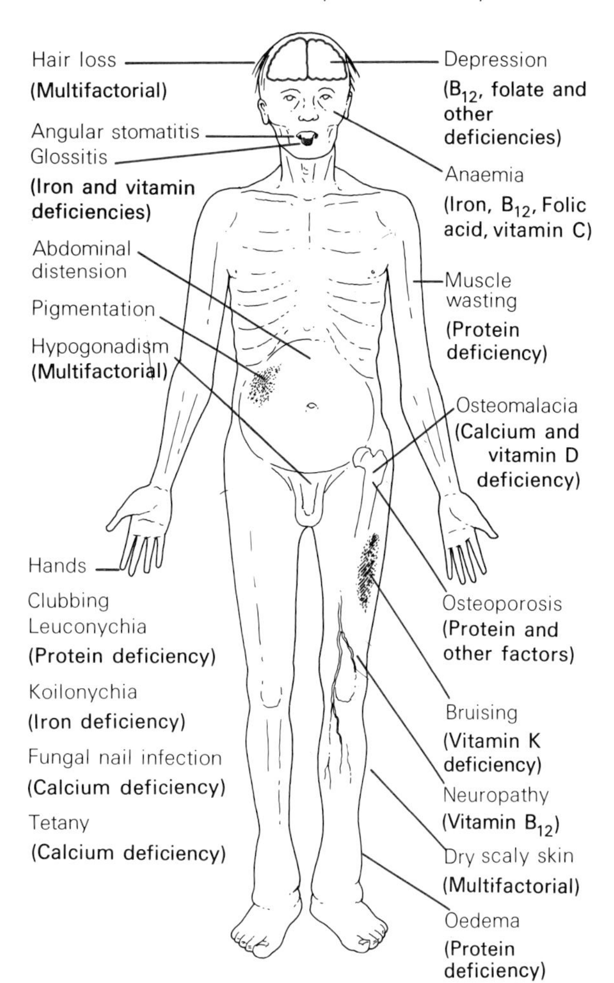

Fig. 7.25 *Clinical presentations of malabsorption.*

Clinical Presentations of Malabsorption

These reflect the nutritional deficiencies present and usually give little clue to the underlying disease process. Possible presentations are illustrated in Fig. 7.25, but the common clinical presentations in the adult are as follows.

Diarrhoea and abdominal discomfort

When steatorrhoea is present, the patient complains of pale, bulky, offensive, frothy stools that often float and also characteristically stick to the lavatory pan. Frequent stools are not a common complaint, and in some patients with proven steatorrhoea the stool may be completely formed and look absolutely normal. Many patients with diseases of the small bowel may never have steatorrhoea. The abdominal discomfort usually complained of is a bloated, distended feeling but occasionally may mimic peptic ulcer disease or irritable bowel syndrome (see Chapter 2). Severe or prolonged steatorrhoea may also produce symptoms caused by loss of fat-soluble vitamins (see p. 121).

Table 7.1
Causes of Malabsorption

Mucosal Lesions	*Iatrogenic*
Gluten-sensitive enterophthy	Radiotherapy to abdomen
Tropical sprue	Drugs
Whipple's diease	Antibiotics
Intestinal lymphangiectasia	purgatives
	PAS
	Surgery
	gastrectomy
	fistulae
	short gut syndrome
Structural Lesions	*Maldigestion*
Crohn's disease	Bile salt deficiency
Gastric surgery	diseases of liver and
Intestinal resection	biliary system
Small bowel malignancy	Pancreatic insufficiency
Ischaemia	Zollinger–Ellison syndrome
Impaired motility and overgrowth	*Biochemical Abnormalities*
blind loops	Alactasia
diverticula	A-β-lipoproteinaemia
fistulae	Hypogammaglobulinaemia
systemic sclerosis	
pseudo-obstruction	
Infection	*Diseases outside alimentary tract*
Acute gastroenteritis	Endocrine
Tuberculosis	Addison's disease
Parasites	thyrotoxicosis
Impaired motility	hypoparathyroidism
	Connective tissue disorders
	Malignant diseases
	Widespread skin diseases
	severe psoariasis
	severe eczema

Anaemia

This may take the form of a microcytic hypochromic anaemia due to iron deficiency, or a macrocytic anaemia due to folic acid or vitamin B_{12} deficiency. Sometimes a mixed anaemia occurs in widespread disorders such as Crohn's disease.

Other nutritional deficiencies

The bone pain of osteomalacia (due to calcium and vitamin D deficiency) is not an unusual presentation, especially in the elderly with long-standing malabsorption. In more acute situations (e.g. after small bowel resection), deficiency of calcium and vitamin D may present as tetany. Vitamin K deficiency may manifest itself with deficient clotting ability; protein loss with oedema of the legs, and weight loss with muscle wasting.

Water and electrolyte depletion

In severe malabsorptive states, water depletion may lead to marked dehydration, and loss of potassium in particular may lead to generalised weakness and malaise.

Malabsorption in infants

In infants the symptoms of malabsorption may

appear soon after the introduction of carbohydrate into the infant's diet at around 3 months. Irritability, loss of interest in feeding, and diarrhoea with pale bulky stools are soon followed by weight loss and general failure to thrive. In contrast to the rather pinched facies and wasted limbs, the abdomen is protruberant, soft and tympanitic. Anaemia may be obvious and muscle tone is poor. If not recognised and the cause treated, then failure to grow is soon obvious and in older children puberty is delayed. Hypoproteinaemia may cause oedema and hypocalcaemia may cause tetany. Rickets may develop. In contrast to adults, megaloblastic anaemia of any severity is uncommon.

Once suspected, the definitive diagnosis must rest on special investigations which usually require hospital attendance. Most patients do not require hospital admission; this is restricted to the minority with severe symptoms, or those who have to travel far.

General Management

Because of the large number of potential causes, the management of a patient with malabsorption syndrome should follow a basic plan such as outlined in Fig. 7.26. The tests of function and morphology usually applied are described above, but those most likely to establish the underlying pathology in the more common causes of malabsorption are also summarised on Fig. 7.26.

Because absorption of drugs takes place largely in the upper small intestine, disease in this area may affect the bioavailability of orally-administered drugs, resulting in treatment failure. It is probable that the small intestine is often

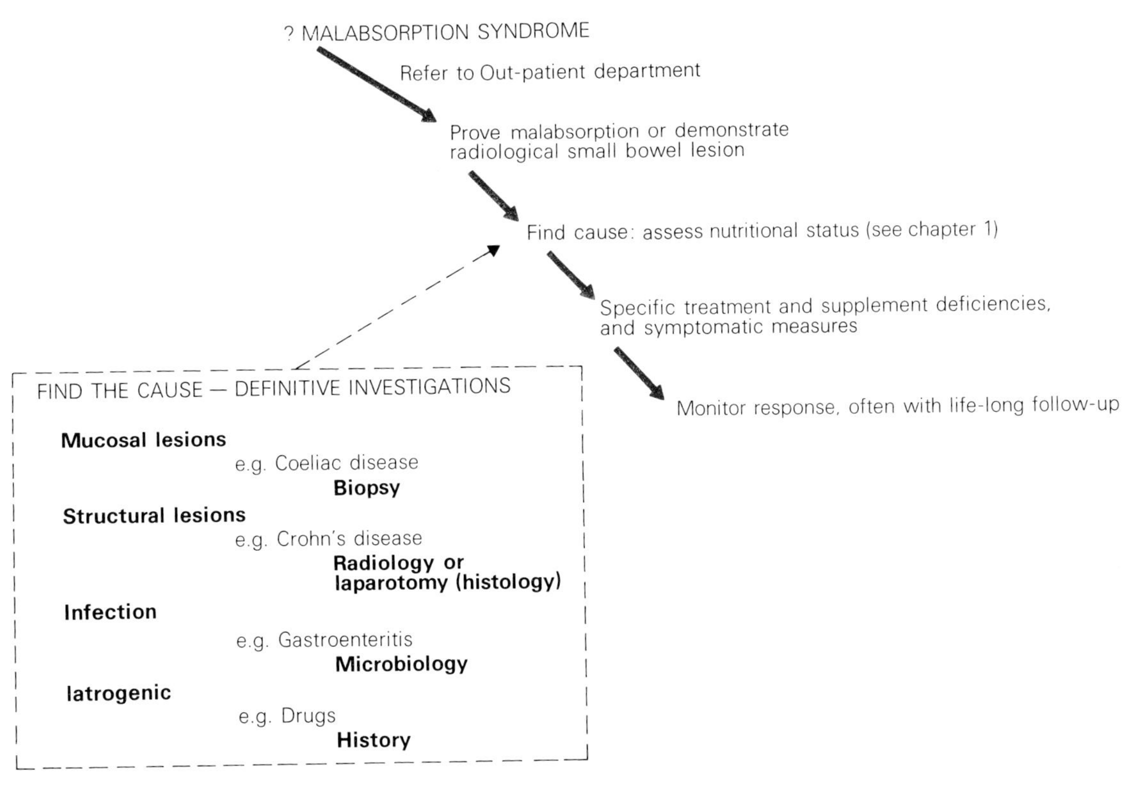

Fig. 7.26 *Plan for the management of malabsorption syndrome.*

secondarily involved, e.g. in cardiac failure (see p. 137).

General Treatment of Malabsorption

Specific treatment is only available for some causes of malabsorption, e.g. coeliac disease.

Nutritional supplements (e.g. iron, folic acid, vitamin C, calcium, vitamin D) may be given by mouth, whilst others (e.g. vitamin B_{12}) must be given parenterally and may have to be given for life. A high-calorie, high-protein diet may also be necessary. When severe malabsorption is present then intravenous fluids supplemented by potassium and other minerals may be necessary.

In many patients with mucosal destruction a secondary alactasia develops, and while the lesion is healing a lactose-free diet may alleviate the symptoms. Medium-chain triglycerides can be absorbed without bile salts, pancreatic enzymes, chylomicron formation or lymphatic transport, and therefore provide a valuable additional nutritional support in those conditions for which there is no specific therapy. In severely ill patients, elemental diets or intravenous feeding (Chapter 1) may be necessary to allow the patient to survive while the small bowel recovers.

Symptomatic therapy, e.g. oral codeine phosphate, may alleviate diarrhoea and abdominal pain. Watery diarrhoea resulting from colonic irritation by unabsorbed bile salts may respond to the bile-salt-chelating effect of cholestyramine given by mouth. In some patients the restriction of dietary fat will reduce diarrhoea.

Specific Disorders Causing Malabsorption

Coeliac disease (gluten-sensitive enteropathy, coeliac sprue, idiopathic steatorrhoea)

Coeliac disease results from a hyperplastic enteropathy induced in a susceptible person by exposure of the small intestinal mucosa to a gliadin component of the protein, gluten, which is found in wheat, barley, rye and oats. It is possible that some other disorders, e.g. cow's milk-sensitivity in children and tropical sprue, may be associated with a temporary sensitivity to gluten, but in coeliac disease the sensitivity is thought to be life-long. It is probable, but not conclusive, that the condition has an immunological basis and mucosal biopsies show increased numbers of lymphocytes in the mucosa, including the surface epithelium (see p. 131).

The incidence of the disorder in the UK is 1 in 2000–6000, but in the west of Eire it is as high as 1 in 300; it can be familial and is more frequent in people with the histocompatability antigens HLA-B8 and DW3. A similar enteropathy is found in the condition 'dermatitis herpetiformis' (see p. 132). Characteristically, the mucosal lesions of gluten-sensitive enteropathies are more severe proximally. Consequently, adaptive changes in the distal small bowel and colon can compensate for the proximal functional defects (see *ileal adaptation*, p. 122) and thus explain the delayed and subtle presentation of the disorder in many adult patients. The severity of the mucosal lesion varies and the essential differences between the normal mucosa and those in gluten-sensitive enteropathy are shown in Fig. 7.27. It is important to realise that the milder histological changes seen in coeliac disease may also occur in a wide variety of other disorders, including many diseases not primarily affecting the small intestine. Although there are other uncommon causes of the absence of villi (e.g. x-ray therapy) in practice it is almost always the result of gluten-sensitive enteropathy.

As with other causes of malabsorption, patients with coeliac disease may present with predominantly abdominal symptoms (distension, discomfort, diarrhoea), nutritional deficiencies (especially iron or folate), general malaise (weakness, tiredness, weight-loss) or any combination of these. About one-third to one-half of adults will have symptoms which can be traced back to childhood. Frequently, coeliac disease is only discovered when it is sought during the investigation of growth retardation or delayed puberty in children, or osteomalacia or isolated nutritional deficiencies (e.g. folate or iron) in adults. Rarely, patients with coeliac disease present as a coeliac crisis with acute dehydration, shock and malabsorption. In

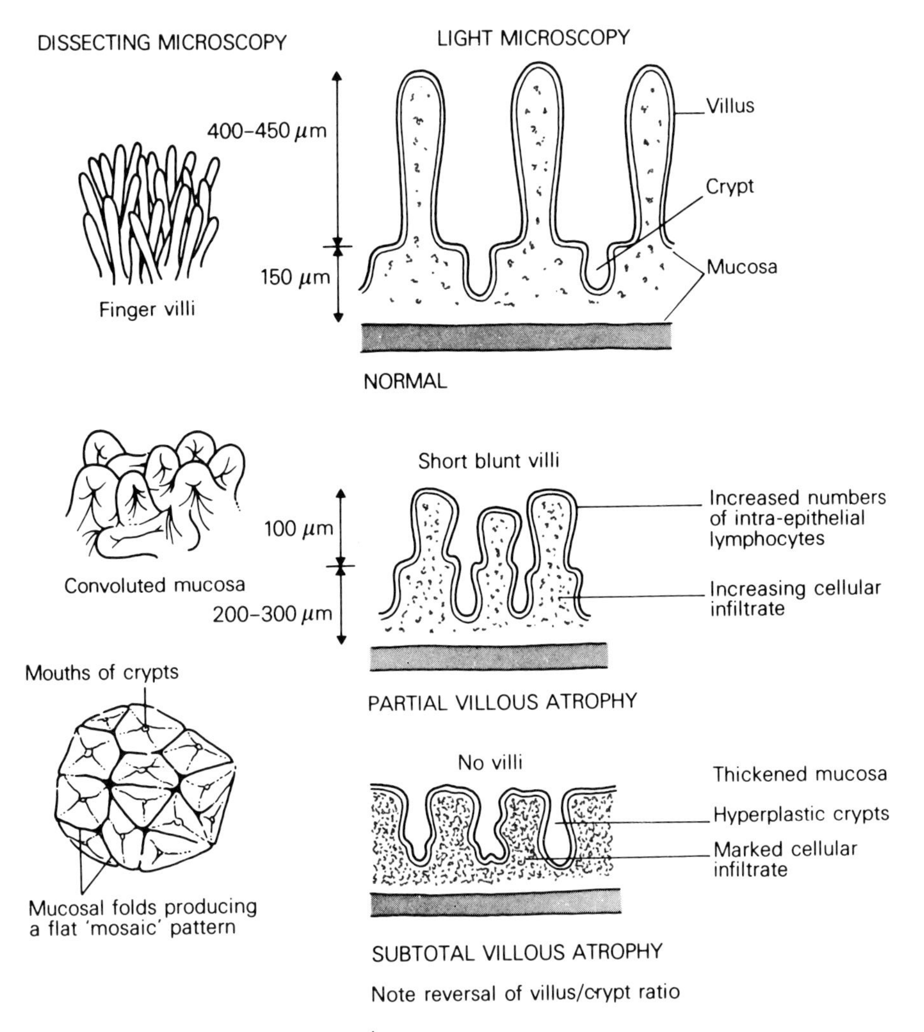

Fig. 7.27 *Mucosal lesion of gluten-sensitive enteropathy.*

these patients small intestinal mucosal ulceration may be present, or associated malignancy (see below) may have developed.

The diagnosis of coeliac disease must be confirmed by jejunal biopsy carried out on at least two separate occasions. The first must show a compatible mucosal lesion and the second a morphological response to gluten withdrawal from the diet. Repeat biopsies must be taken from the same level (checked radiologically) because the lesion is often patchy in distribution and also becomes less severe further down the small intestine. In children, a third biopsy after the reintroduction of gluten (a gluten 'challenge' of at least 10 g per day) is usually advised, since other disorders such as cow's-milk sensitivity may cause diagnostic confusion. In coeliac disease the gluten challenge usually causes a symptomatic relapse and will cause deterioration in the histological appearance.

Once coeliac disease is suspected from the jejunal biopsy, a trial of a strict gluten-free diet is mandatory. This has to be strictly supervised by the gastroenterologist with the close help of a dietitian. The aim is to exclude gluten completely from the diet and this means total life-long exclusion of the protein content of wheat, rye, barley and oats. Rice and maize can be used as substitutes, and soya flour and maize flour can be used in baking. Patients obtain much help and practical advice through the Coeliac Society, whose handbook contains updated lists of safe proprietary foods. It is important to impress on the patient that it is very difficult to ensure a completely gluten-free diet. Many convenience foods contain flour and this may not be declared on the label. It is therefore important that the patient be constantly vigilant. It is easy to forget that gluten may be contained in some items not usually regarded as foods, e.g. sweets, ice cream, some antacids, and communion wafers.

The symptomatic response to a gluten-free diet in some patients is quite dramatic but this must never be allowed to obviate the need for the confirmatory second or third jejunal biopsy. These are usually performed at intervals of three or four months. In some patients the diagnostic morphological improvement in the jejunal mucosa may take up to a year to occur, and during this time it is important that the patient should be encouraged to adhere strictly to the gluten-free diet. In the early stages of treatment it may be necessary to prescribe supplements such as iron or folic acid. It is rarely necessary to prescribe vitamin B_{12} as the lower ileum is only affected in severe cases. In the so-called 'coeliac crisis' the prognosis is poor, and if the patient is to survive he will need urgent intravenous rehydration, corticosteroids and intravenous nutritional support.

'Failure to respond' to a gluten-free diet is usually due to failure, perhaps inadvertent, to keep strictly to the diet. Much less likely causes are the development of secondary pancreatic insufficiency, secondary lactase deficiency, intestinal ulceration (see below), lymphoma, or bacterial overgrowth. If a careful review of the diagnosis confirms coeliac disease, and a careful dietary history suggests patient compliance, then it is worthwhile trying the addition of pancreatic supplements, a lactose-free diet, antibiotics and steroids, either sequentially or together as dictated by the patient's condition. If the patient's condition continues to deteriorate despite these measures, a laparotomy may be needed to diagnose one of the complicating conditions.

Complications of coeliac disease. Unfortunately there is no compelling evidence that strict adherence to a gluten-free diet prevents the development of these fortunately rare but serious complications. Gluten-sensitive enteropathy is a premalignant condition which is associated with increased incidence of carcinoma of the intestinal tract and other parts of the body. After some years lymphoma of the small intestine (usually in the jejunum) may supervene, heralded by loss of response to the gluten-free diet, malaise, abdominal pain, perforation and gastrointestinal bleeding. This is a serious complication which is usually fatal despite surgical treatment, radiotherapy or chemotherapy.

Small intestinal ulceration, sometimes accompanied by the formation of a stricture, is another unusual complication that seems to occur despite treatment with a gluten-free diet. Suggestive symptoms are malaise, fever, abodominal pain, gastrointestinal bleeding and, again, loss of response to a gluten-free diet. Surgical treatment and steroids are usually tried, but the outcome is almost invariably fatal.

Dermatitis herpetiformis

This is a rare disorder characterised by an itchy blistering skin lesion on the shoulders, buttocks, elbows and knees, accompanied in about 90% of patients by a mild patchy enteropathy similar to coeliac disease. The skin lesions respond to the anti-leprosy drug dapsone, but both the skin lesions and those in the small bowel mucosa will respond to a gluten-free diet. Symptomatic malabsorption is rare, but the similarity to coeliac disease is further strengthened by the fact that there is a high incidence of HLA-B8 in dermatitis herpetiformis, even in those without an obvious mucosal lesion. Moreover, lymphoma of the small bowel may supervene in this condition also. The diagnosis is confirmed by biopsy of the skin lesion and demonstration of IgA deposits in the dermal papillae.

Tropical sprue

This malabsorption syndrome occurs in people

living in the tropics (especially India, China and Puerto Rico) or who have even only a brief excursion to these areas. Its cause is unknown and the visit may have been months or years before the onset of symptoms. The condition may be endemic or epidemic, suggesting the possible involvement of some infective agent.

The affected small-bowel mucosa shows features of non-specific partial villous atrophy (rather similar to patients with milder forms of gluten-sensitive enteropathy, and very similar to asymptomatic patients in the tropics) which affects the ileum and usually spares the jejunum. However, since the proximal small intestine cannot compensate for the loss of general or specific ileal function, some patients with tropical sprue present with a more severe illness than those with proximal enteropathies. Malabsorption and subsequent deconjugation of bile salts predispose to steatorrhoea and malabsorption of water and electrolytes. Additionally, a megaloblastic anaemia may develop due to B_{12} or folate deficiency. The disease occasionally resolves spontaneously on return to a temperate climate, but folic acid and tetracycline probably achieve the most rapid remissions. If there is a concomitant deficiency of vitamin B_{12}, this should also be given. Treatment should continue for at least 6 months, and follow-up should continue indefinitely.

Whipple's disease

This is a rare multisystem disorder in which massive deposits of a glycoprotein are deposited in the macrophages of the small bowel, in lymph nodes, and in other tissues. These macrophages have a characteristic foamy appearance on light microscopy, and on electron microscopy it is clear that the glycoprotein deposits are masses of rod-shaped bacilli. This syndrome usually presents in middle-aged white men with a long history of weight-loss, diarrhoea, and migratory polyarthralgia of large joints. Other symptoms, which suggest systemic involvement, include non-specific abdominal pain, fever, lymphadenopathy, skin pigmentation, purpura and oedema. The lungs, heart, and central nervous system may also be involved.

Steatorrhoea is nearly always present, with the usual attendant nutritional deficiencies. The radiological appearances of the small bowel are similar to those in any malabsorptive state. The definitive diagnosis depends on a jejunal biopsy; this shows distended lymphatic spaces, and villi distended by large numbers of foamy macrophages in which glycoprotein is demonstrated by periodic-acid-Schiff (PAS) staining.

Although morphological response is slow, clinical response is rapid to a combination of penicillin and streptomycin for two weeks, followed by tetracycline for one year.

Intestinal lymphangiectasia

This is a rare condition characterised by steatorrhoea. In children, intestinal lymphatic blockage is thought to be congenital; the similar syndrome in adults is usually the result of infection or malignancy. The steatorrhoea is thought to result from obstruction of the lymphatics, and the oedema from loss of protein into the gut when distended lymphatics rupture into the gut lumen. Many patients also have lymphatic abnormalities in the legs contributing to their oedema.

The diagnosis is confirmed by jejunal biopsy which shows dilated lymphatics in the core of the villus. However, as the lesion may not affect all villi, the diagnosis may be missed on a single biopsy. Abnormal lymphangiograms of the legs are very suggestive and it may be possible to demonstrate protein loss from the gut (see p. 119).

Medium-chain triglycerides will replace fat loss very satisfactorily. In some patients it is necessary to proceed to laparotomy and, if necessary, resection of the affected segment of bowel.

Crohn's disease

Possible mechanisms producing malabsorption in Crohn's disease of the small bowel are summarised in Fig. 7.28. The epidemiology, pathology and natural history of Crohn's disease are described in Chapter 10. The most frequent site of Crohn's involvement of the small bowel is the lower ileum, where it results in mucosal destruction and even-

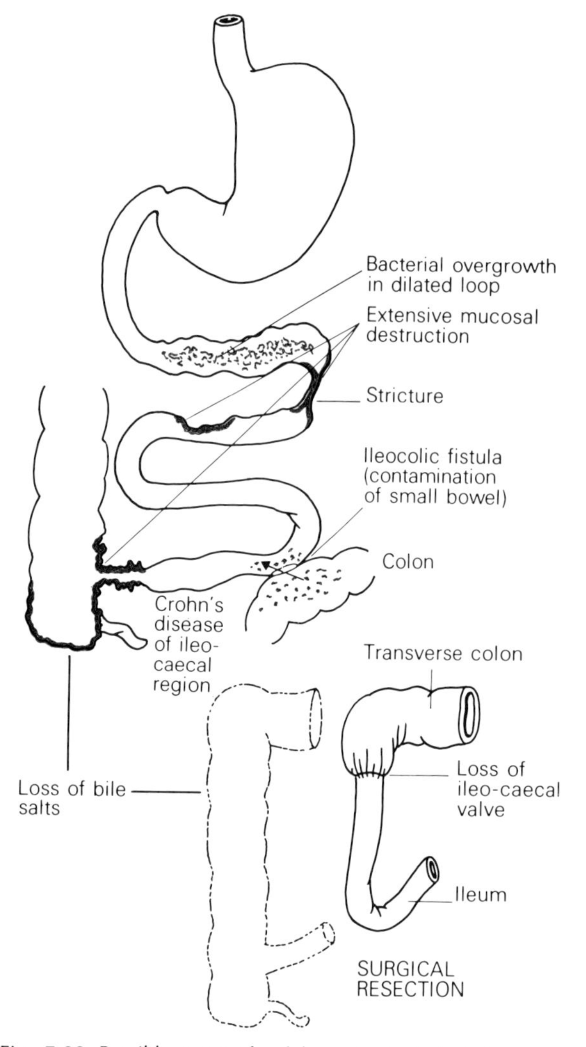

Fig. 7.28 *Possible causes of malabsorption in Crohn's disease.*

tually stricture formation, often with a palpable mass in the right iliac fossa. However, skip lesions throughout the small bowel are common. This disease pattern results in defective absorption of vitamin B_{12} and bile salts in particular (due to involvement of the terminal ileum), and loss of other nutrients to a degree dependent on the amount of mucosal destruction throughout the small bowel. The formation of entero-enteric and enterocolic fistulae and small bowel strictures allow bacterial overgrowth to occur and further promote malabsorption. Surgical resections carried out in the treatment of Crohn's disease necessarily further reduce the absorptive area.

Symptoms and signs vary greatly depending on the site and extent of small bowel involvement. However, common clinical presentation includes diarrhoea, weight loss, low-grade fever, anaemia and a raised erythrocyte sedimentation rate. Sometimes the tenderness in the right iliac fossa may suggest appendicitis, or an appendix abscess. Simultaneous colonic involvement is common; the patient may complain of perianal discomfort and, on examination, may have the typical perianal changes of Crohn's disease (see p. 228). Systemic complication (see Chapter 10) may be obvious.

The biochemical abnormalities are those of any malabsorptive process and will depend on the extent of intestinal involvement. However, B_{12} malabsorption (as shown by a Schilling test) and bile salt malabsorption (as shown by the ^{14}C GCA breath test) are common.

Ideally, the diagnosis is made by histological confirmation. In many patients with small-bowel Crohn's disease this is not possible by direct biopsy from the small bowel, but it is always worthwhile performing rectal biopsy since the suggestive granulomata of Crohn's disease may be present in a biopsy from a rectal mucosa that looks macroscopically normal. Strongly supportive diagnostic evidence may be obtained from a barium study of small bowel showing the typical short segments of small intestinal narrowing (p. 231).

The medical management of small-bowel Crohn's disease is largely supportive. Nutritional deficiencies (e.g. iron, folate and B_{12}) are corrected, and the patient's general state improved by the dietetic measures described under general management. In those patients with severe malabsorption, and with extensive jejuno-ileitis there is some evidence that corticosteroids may help in the acute phase. They do not, however, lessen the need for subsequent surgery. Similarly there is also evidence that azathioprine, a cytotoxic and immunosuppressive agent, will reduce the relapse risk in small-bowel Crohn's disease. Medical management cannot, however, be divorced from surgical treatment. The two must always be considered together as either may be suddenly applicable at any time in what may prove to be half a lifetime of care and management. In general, the indications for surgery are: stricture formation leading to bowel stasis or frank obstruction; the correction of fistulae; and the localised resection of a short segment of symptomatic Crohn's disease. Surgery is best avoided in those in a poor general state with active disease, in those with extensive gut involvement, and in those known to have extensive peritoneal adhesions due to extensive disease or previous surgical resections. Short circuit operations to bypass areas of severe unresectable bowel involvement are rarely necessary and are best avoided.

Gastric surgery

Many mechanisms may contribute to nutritional problems after gastric surgery (Fig. 7.29). A slight increase in faecal fat excretion is common after most forms of surgery for peptic ulcer except highly selective vagotomy. Symptomatic steatorrhoea is, however, unusual and occurs in association with an additional complication, often many years after surgery. Malabsorption of iron alone is not uncommon whilst malabsorption of vitamin B_{12} alone is unusual. Total gastrectomy results in nutritional deficiencies which are often severe.

Once identified, nutritional deficiencies should be corrected. Pancreatic supplements sometimes help even when there is no clear proof of pancreatic insufficiency.

Intestinal resection

Extensive resections of small bowel, especially if involving the lower ileum, lead to severe malabsorption. The most common reasons for massive resection of the small bowel are Crohn's disease, mesenteric vascular occlusion with resultant infarction of bowel, volvulus of the small bowel and, occasionally, incarceration and strangulation of a large section of small bowel in a hernia. The consequences of bowel resection in any individual will depend on the extent of the resection and also

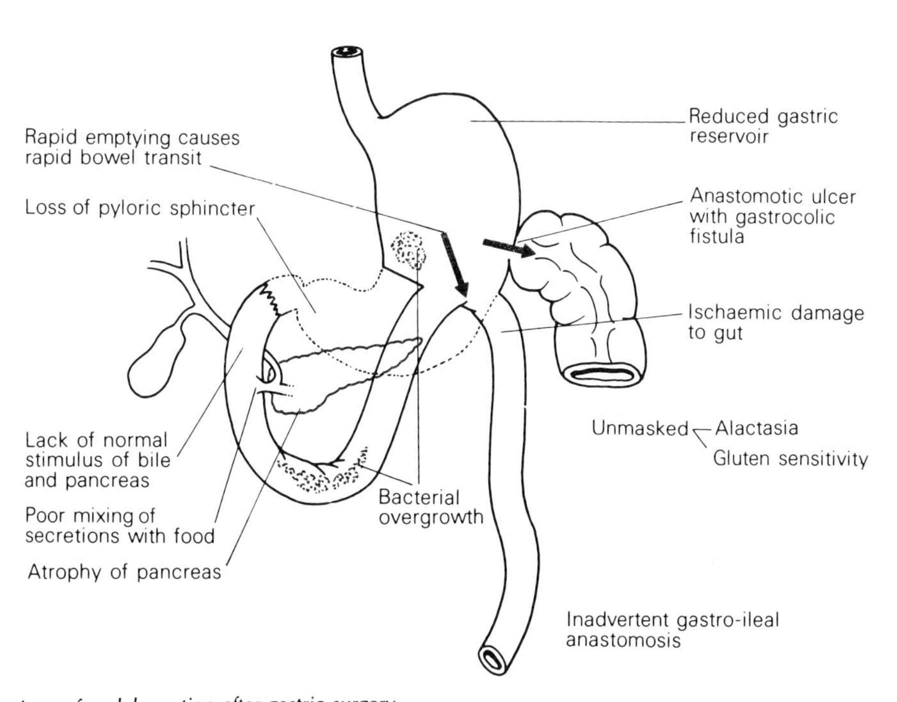

Fig. 7.29 *Mechanisms of malabsorption after gastric surgery.*

the site (proximal or distal small bowel) as well as the condition of the remaining small bowel. The pathogenic mechanisms involved are summarised in Fig. 7.30.

Proximal resections are less serious; the ileum is capable of quite remarkable adaptive changes and compensation for loss of jejunal absorptive capacity. The jejunum adapts less well and cannot take over the specific ileal absorption of vitamin B_{12} and bile salts. Resection of the terminal ileum thus removes the conservation of bile salts, and their deficiency is the most important cause of malabsorption. Unabsorbed bile salts and fatty acids pass into the colon, inhibiting fluid and electrolyte absorption and causing a watery diarrhoea. The latter is often worse in the morning because of the overnight synthesis of bile salts. Colonic absorption of oxalate is increased and this may lead to the formation of urinary oxalate stones. Because of changes in the relative concentrations of bile salts and cholesterol in bile, there is an increased risk of gallstone formation, and because of depletion of the bile salt pool there is decreased micellar absorption of fat. Loss of a

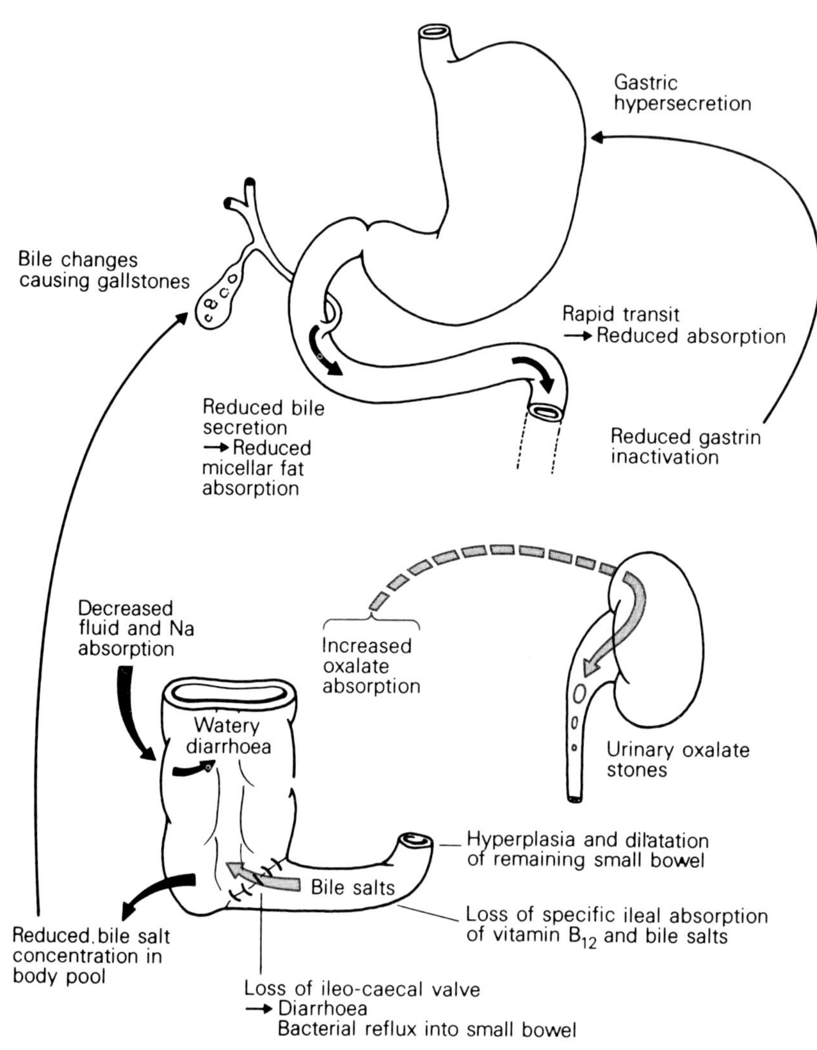

Fig. 7.30 *Pathogenetic mechanisms after extensive small bowel resection, including terminal ileum.*

substantial portion of small bowel mucosa is said to reduce inactivation of gastrin. In approximately 50% of patients with massive small bowel resection there is resultant hypersecretion of acid, leading to peptic ulceration. This is usually transient and settles within a year, and further surgery for peptic ulceration should be avoided.

In the early postoperative period, fluid and electrolyte replacement is important. Having survived the immediate postoperative period, the patient will require long-term care and follow-up. After several months, the remaining small bowel attempts to compensate by dilating and by developing marked hyperplasia of the remaining mucosa. Villi may increase in length by a factor of three or four. Nevertheless, continuing nutrient supplementation and symptomatic measures will be necessary in some patients for life. After extensive distal resection, a low-fat diet and medium-chain triglycerides are usually necessary. Life long vitamin B_{12} treatment will be required. If only a small part of ileum has been resected (one metre or less), the resulting diarrhoea is usually due to colonic irritation and this will normally respond to cholestyramine. Diarrhoea following larger resections of small bowel is due to steatorrhoea, and further depletion of the bile salt pool by giving cholestyramine will merely serve to increase steatorrhoea. Sometimes surgical reversal of a short segment of small bowel will reduce diarrhoea. Gastric surgery should be avoided, and antacids or H_2-receptor antagonists may help. Small frequent feeds of a lactose-free diet and short-term parenteral feeding may help. However, due to adaptive changes, it is remarkable how a patient may be virtually asymptomatic and free of diarrhoea after one or two years. Lifelong follow-up is nevertheless necessary to guard against developing deficiencies.

Small bowel malignancy

The gut may be affected by lymphoma of similar histological type to that occurring elsewhere in the body, although these are nearly always of non-Hodgkin's type. In addition, there are two special types of primary lymphoma of the gut – Mediterranean lymphoma, and α-chain disease.

Patients usually present with a short history of weight loss, abdominal pain, fever, finger clubbing and easily palpable abdominal masses. Gastrointestinal ulceration with bleeding and perforation may occur.

Mediterranean lymphoma occurs in many parts of the world, although initially described in Mediterranean areas, and involves the small bowel diffusely. Diagnosis is usually possible on histological examination of a jujunal biopsy.

α-chain disease is a rare varient of Mediterranean lymphoma. The lesion consists of excess plasmacytoid cells and is characterised by the excessive production of the heavy (α) chain portion of IgA molecules detectable in body fluids or tissues by immunological techniques. Usually confined to bowel, this condition sometimes terminates as disseminated malignancy.

Where possible, for both disorders, curative resection should be attempted. Radiotherapy, chemotherapy and corticosteroids have also been used.

Ischaemia

Chronic and acute intestinal failure secondary to a compromised arterial blood supply to the small intestine is being increasingly recognised, especially in the elderly. Pancreatic exocrine function may deteriorate for the same reason and add to problems of malabsorption. Twenty per cent of the cardiac output is normally carried to the intestine, and this increases two- to four-fold after a meal. If the systemic blood flow is compromised there is no auto regulatory mechanism to maintain this blood flow to the intestinal mucosa; thus in hypovolaemic and haemorrhagic hypotension, ischaemic necrosis of the villous tips ensues, leading in turn to villous atrophy. Thus some villous atrophy can accompany cardiovascular diseases such as hypertension or atherosclerosis, especially if cardiac failure is present. Whereas impaired renal function is frequently considered in these conditions, the fate of the small bowel is often overlooked.

The symptoms of intestinal ischaemia and failure are vague. Many patients have other evidence of circulatory problems. They may initially complain of constipation followed by diarrhoea, and of colicky episodic central abdominal pain after meals which may become so severe that they are afraid to eat. This exacerbates the weight loss secondary to malabsorption. With time, vomiting and episodes of bloody diarrhoea may develop. The latter constitutes as grave an emergency as an acute vascular occlusion.

There are no 'classical' signs of chronic intestinal ischaemia. An epigastric bruit conducted to the right iliac fossa may merely reflect aortic atheroma rather than stenosis of the superior mesenteric artery or one of its major branches. The diagnosis is confirmed by arteriography, usually after other causes of malabsorption have been excluded.

Surgical correction is sometimes possible, either by direct attack on the superior mesenteric artery or by a side-to-side aorto-mesenteric anastomosis.

Impaired motility and bacterial overgrowth

Anatomical causes of impaired motility include surgical blind loops, diverticulosis of small bowel, fistulae and obstruction, and defective motility such as occurs in systemic sclerosis and in the syndrome of pseudo-obstruction (see Chapter 9). In these conditions, and when there is defective immunity, bacterial overgrowth of the small intestine occurs, producing malabsorption (Fig. 7.31).

The proximal small intestine normally has a sparse population of streptococci, lactobacilli,

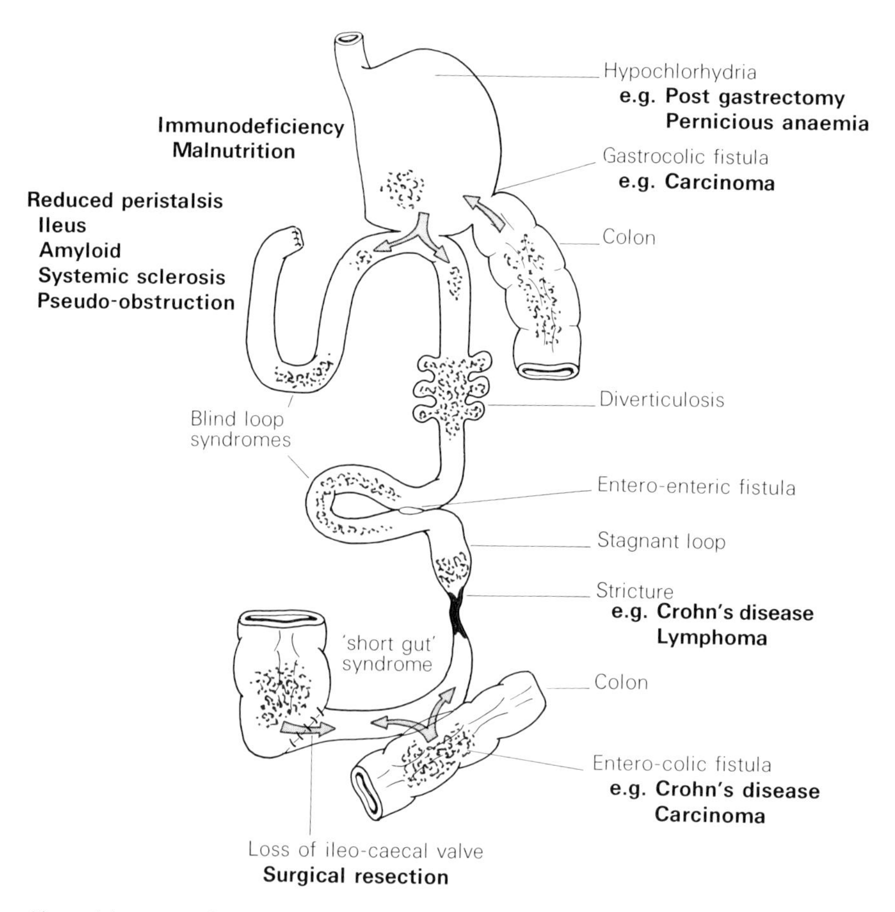

Fig. 7.31 *Causes of bacterial overgrowth of the small bowel.*

some yeasts, staphylococci and a few coliforms. The latter organisms are normally more profuse in the ileum and colon, where the predominant microflora is anaerobic and includes bacteroides, coliforms, lactobacilli, and clostridia. In disease states such as those listed in Fig. 7.31 the distal flora ascends the intestine and produces a number of direct and indirect adverse effects. Bacteria have an adverse effect on bile salts (see ^{14}C GCA breath test), lypolyses, and intraluminal carbohydrate (see p. 118). The contaminating bacteria also produce hydroxyfatty acids which, like unconjugated bile salts, impair colonic uptake of water and electrolytes. As well as this indirect action via effects on lipid and bile salts, bacterial contamination causes a mild enteropathy by direct damage to the intestinal mucosa. Vitamin B_{12} nutrition may also be compromised because bacteria utilise the dietary vitamin and prevent its absorption; folate deficiency is, however, rare in this syndrome, possibly because the bacteria themselves synthesise the vitamin which is then absorbed.

If bacterial contamination is caused by a localised discrete anatomical lesion, it may be eliminated by surgical correction. On the other hand, diffuse lesions (e.g. diverticulosis) will require intermittent courses of broad-spectrum antibiotics (e.g. tetracycline) or metronidazole (especially active against anaerobes such as bacteroides). Cholestyramine may be beneficial if bile-salt-induced diarrhoea is present, but it should be remembered that this resin may interfere with antibiotic function. Nutritional supplements are often needed.

Systemic sclerosis

The small bowel may be involved in this multisystem 'collagen disease' even before the typical skin lesions are present. As well as reduced motility produced by the disease process itself, along with mucosal atrophy and bowel distension, bacterial overgrowth of the small intestine is almost invariable. In addition, the lower end of the oesophagus becomes immobile and reflux oesophagitis may eventually lead to stricture formation (see Chapter 4).

The patient may complain of constipation and dysphagia, and may eventually develop typical steatorrhoea. The presence of Raynauds's phenomenon and the typical skin lesions strongly suggest the diagnosis, which may be confirmed by skin biopsy or a full-thickness surgical biopsy of small bowel which may show submucosal collagen.

Treatment is limited to treatment of bacterial overgrowth, the prescription of supplements, and general supportive measures. Steroids are of no benefit for the skin or gut lesions, and the prognosis is poor.

Radiotherapy

The small bowel is occasionally damaged after radiotherapy (usually to the pelvis), and there is late (after many years) development of colicky abdominal pain and diarrhoea. It is usually possible to demonstrate a stricture radiologically which explains the steatorrhoea that can occasionally be severe. Sometimes surgical resection is needed but this is usually difficult because of adhesions. Attention to nutrition and broad spectrum antibiotic to take care of bacterial overgrowth is usually sufficient.

Drugs and malabsorption

As well as malabsorption syndromes interfering with the bioavailability of prescribed medicines (see above), some drugs can also cause malabsorption, and may affect the absorption of other drugs taken concomitantly. Drugs affecting motility (e.g. propantheline bromide or opiates) may affect absorption by either increasing it or decreasing it, and alcohol may interfere with absorption and exacerbate the nutritional defects of alcoholics (see Chapter 2). Neomycin given long-term to patients with incipient liver failure may cause marked, but reversible, malabsorption – the mechanisms include mucosal damage, precipitation of lipids in the lumen of the gut, and increased bile-salt losses in the faeces. Cholestyramine binds bile salts and may cause malabsorption;

para-aminosalicylic acid and phenindione also may cause reversible malabsorption.

Primary alactasia

Whereas in most parts of the world, lactase levels in the intestinal mucosa diminish through childhood and adolescence and are absent in the adult, lactase persists in people of North European origin. This may represent natural selection; it prevents symptoms in milk-drinking areas and allows increased calcium intake (see Chapter 2).

Most patients are symptomless, but some complain of nonspecific abdominal discomfort and diarrhoea after milk or milk products. The diarrhoea may be episodic and a few patients may have mild steatorrhoea. The diagnosis is suggested by a flat lactose tolerance test (see above) and the development of symptoms during the test, or by means of a positive hydrogen breath test. The diagnosis may be confirmed by demonstrating absence of lactase in a jejunal biopsy. Not all patients who are milk-sensitive have alactasia.

Treatment is by a lactose-free diet. Success is difficult to judge, but in some patients the improvement is dramatic.

Secondary alactasia. Alactasia, with lactose intolerance, may occur in association with a wide range of diseases of the small bowel (e.g. infection, Crohn's disease) and may be transient. Usually other mucosal enzyme levels are also low, and the importance of this phenomenon in adults is highly debatable.

Hypogammaglobulinaemia

This is a rare condition in which gastrointestinal symptoms are common. The condition is characterised by defects in immunoglobulins. Large lymphoid nodules are diffusely scattered throughout the small intestine of some of these patients. Disaccharidase deficiency is common, and may explain diarrhoea. Many have giardia or bacterial infestation of the intestine, and these improve dramatically when treated with metronidazole or broad spectrum antibiotics. In some, there is marked mucosal atrophy of the small bowel with marked reduction in plasma cells in the lamina propria, and there are reports of improvements on a gluten-free diet. Weight-gain and increased growth in children may follow injection of gamma globulin or infusion of fresh frozen plasma.

8

Diseases of the Liver and Biliary System

Hepatobiliary disorders are very common. It is estimated that 200 millions in the world carry the hepatitis B virus; about 200 millions suffer from hepatic schistosomiasis; primary liver cancer is one of the commonest tumours in the world; 20% of all Britons have gall stones; cirrhosis is now the fourth commonest cause of death in males in the USA.

In Britain the major clinical problems are:

- the diagnosis and management of clinical jaundice and the recognition of extrahepatic (surgically correctable) obstruction
- the elucidation of gall-bladder-associated pain and 'dyspepsia'
- determination of the significance or importance of abnormalities in so-called 'liver function tests'.

MECHANISMS OF DISEASE

The liver is remarkable in three respects, which affect its response to insult.

Firstly, it has enormous reserve functional capacity. It can be largely replaced by tumour and yet function adequately. Advanced but compensated cirrhosis may be accompained by few if any clinical signs or biochemical abnormalities. Prolonged extrahepatic obstruction may be tolerated well for weeks before liver failure occurs.

Secondly, the liver has the greatest powers of regeneration of any body tissue. Surgical removal of a lobe is followed by rapid return to normal structure. Regeneration is the hallmark of the end-state of injury, i.e. cirrhosis.

Thirdly, the liver's function is more diverse than that of any other organ. Liver failure may be expressed primarily as jaundice, fluid retention and ascites, bleeding, or encephalopathy, or any combination of these.

STRUCTURE OF LIVER AND BILIARY TRACT

Anatomy

The liver weighs 1 500 g and is by far the largest solid intra-abdominal organ. Figure 8.1 shows that the liver is almost all contained within

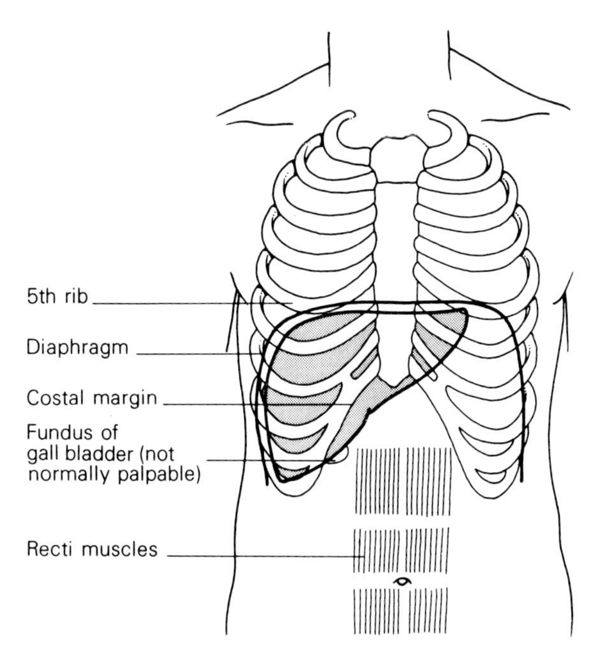

Fig. 8.1 *Anterior surface markings of the liver.*

the lower part of the right rib cage. The edge of the normal liver may sometimes be felt emerging from beneath the costal margin during inspiration on palpation lateral to the right rectus abdominis muscle. If the liver edge is felt one or two finger-breadths inferior to the costal margin it may not be abnormally enlarged, but three or more finger-breadths raises suspicion of abnormal enlargement. Emphysema may cause the liver to be pushed downwards. The upper border may be percussed in the 4th or 5th intercostal space at the anterior axillary line. The texture of the liver may also be assessed as its edge rolls on to the palpating fingers in deep inspiration, and the abnormal hardness of cirrhosis or malignant infiltration may be apparent. In the midline, the liver is covered by the thick recti abdominis muscles and its edge cannot easily be felt, though a mass in the left lobe of the liver may be palpable in the epigastrium.

The liver may be divided into two true anatomical lobes of roughly equal mass and with independent blood supply and biliary drainage in an antero-posterior plane, running from the gall-bladder fundus inferiorly to the left margin of the inferior vena cava superiorly (Fig. 8.2). This has an important bearing on operations to remove part of the liver, which may be indicated for tumour and occasionally for trauma. Large liver resections may temporarily compromise liver function, but the liver has the capacity to regenerate to its original mass over several months.

Blood Supply

In the resting state, the liver receives a large blood supply of approximately 1500 ml/min from two sources: the hepatic artery (25%) and the portal vein (75%). Portal blood supply, though partially oxygen depleted, is the more important. The portal vein is formed by the confluence of superior mesenteric and splenic veins and runs upwards and to the right, posterior to the common bile duct and the hepatic artery, and within the free edge of the lesser omentum (Fig. 8.2). Below the porta

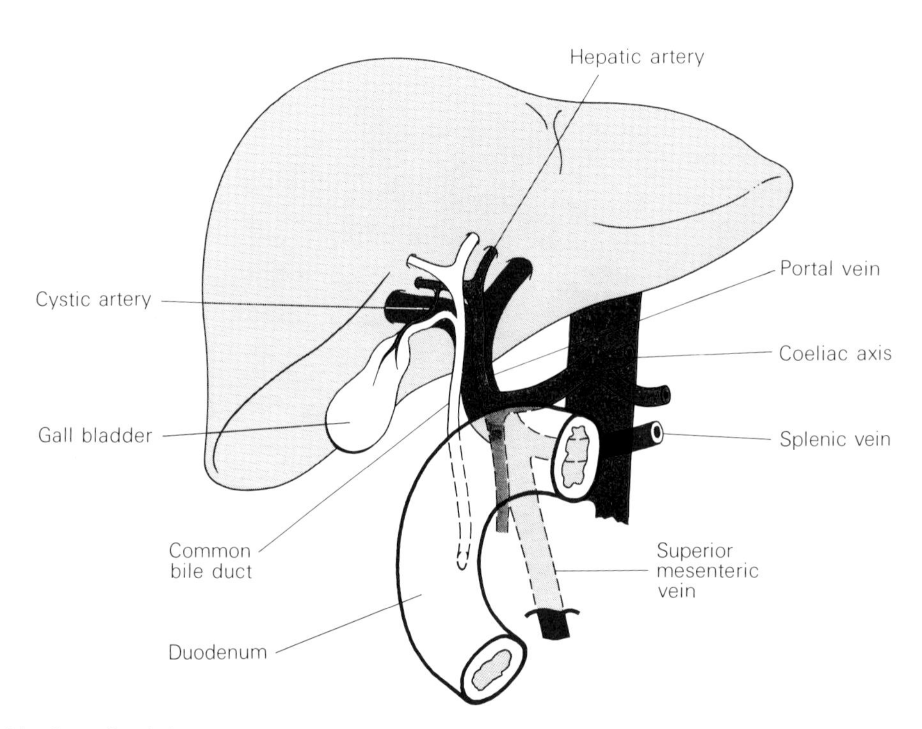

Fig. 8.2 *The blood supply of the liver and gall bladder.*

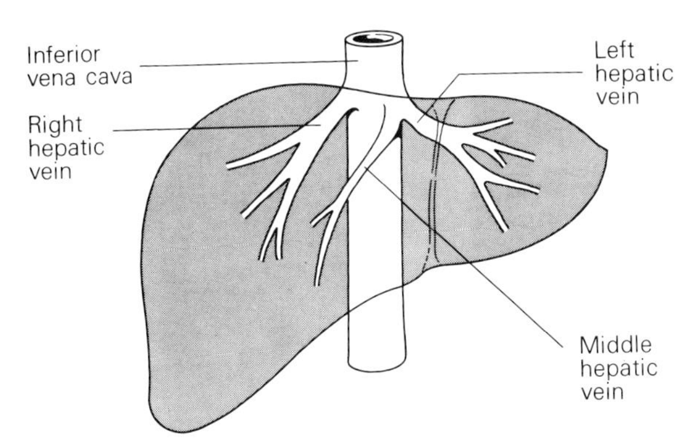

Fig. 8.3 *Venous drainage of the liver.*

hepatis, the portal vein and the inferior vena cava run close together for a few centimetres. The portal blood may be diverted into the systemic circulation in the operation of porta-caval anastomosis. The convenient close disposition of the portal vein and hepatic artery makes it clear that the total inflow of blood into the liver may be temporarily interrupted by a soft atraumatic clamp (or by finger and thumb) applied across the free edge of the lesser omentum, which will control desperate blood loss from traumatic rupture of the liver.

Venous blood drains from the liver into the inferior vena cava through three main hepatic veins (Fig. 8.3) and the liver is suspended by these large venous attachments to the vena cava and by adjacent peritoneal reflections.

Internal Structure

The right and left hepatic arteries divide into short segmental branches and thence into an arborisation, in which they are closely accompanied in triads by corresponding branches of the portal venous system and by radicles of the bile duct system. These triads are ensheathed in a connective tissue framework continuous with the external capsule of the liver (Glisson's capsule) underlying the mesothelial cells of the peritoneal covering and form the portal tracts (Fig. 8.4). The liver substance consists of fenestrated plates of hepatocytes, seen in histological sections as rows of cells radiating out from a central venous radicle to form a roughly hexagonal liver lobule at each corner of which lie the portal tracts containing small branches of the hepatic artery, the portal vein, and a bile ductule ensheathed by a small amount of connective tissue. The hepatocyte plates are separated by blood sinusoids lined by fenestrated endothelial cells showing intercellular spaces. Plasma escapes through these fenestrations and spaces to bathe the hepatocytes. Some of the cells lining the sinusoids (Kupffer cells) are capable of phagocytic activity and form part of the reticulo-endothelial system. The bile canaliculi are channels formed by matching grooves in adjacent hepatocytes. Tight cell junctions isolate the canaliculi from the plasma-filled perisinusoidal intercellular space (Fig. 8.5). Anastomosing canaliculi form the finest biliary ductules, which drain into the larger ducts in the portal tract.

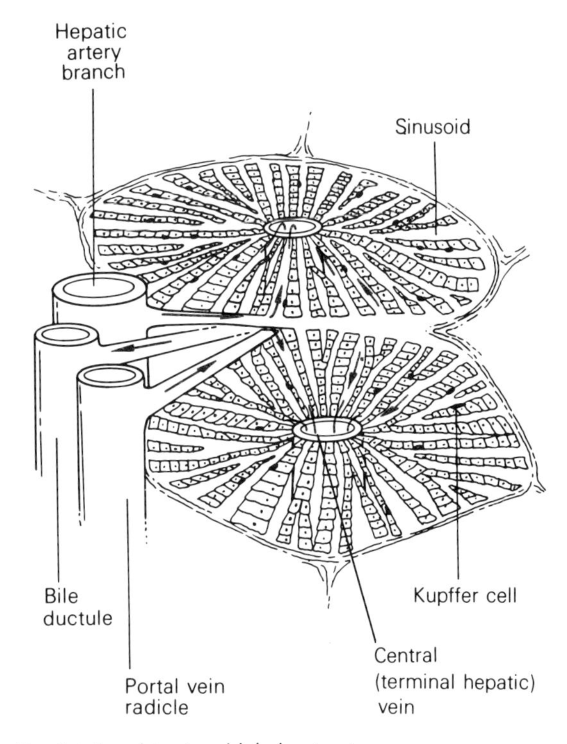

Fig. 8.4 *Portal tract and lobular structure.*

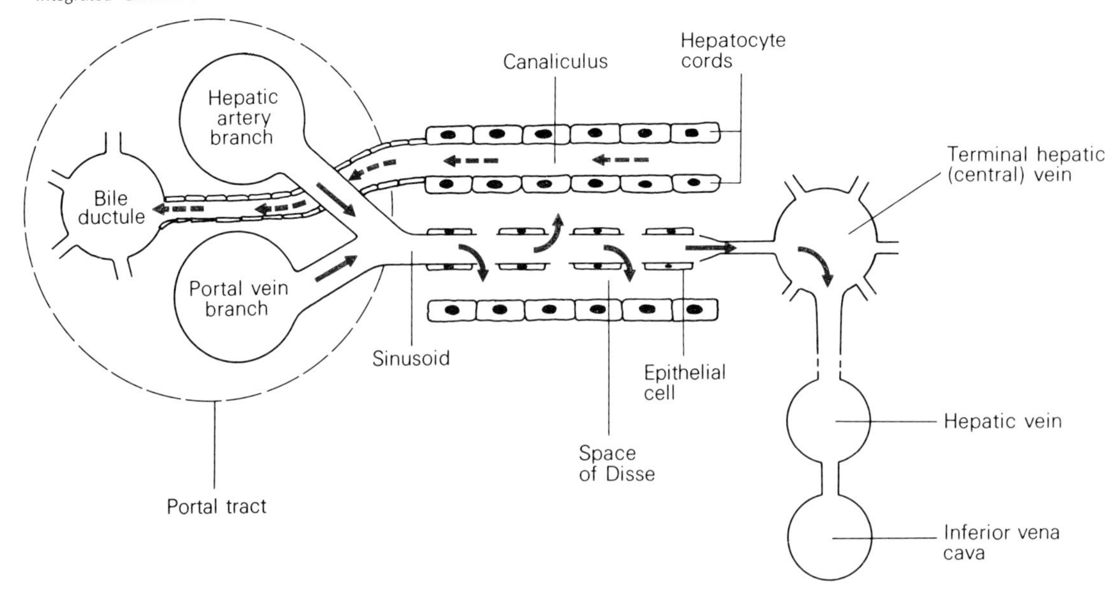

Fig. 8.5 *Schematic representation of the internal structure of the liver.*

The Gall Bladder and Bile Ducts

The gall bladder is not normally palpable, but the distended fundus may be felt near the tip of the ninth costal cartilage in obstruction of the cystic duct or common bile duct. The peritoneum covering the undersurface of the liver passes smoothly over the gall bladder, which may be partly embedded within the liver substance; acute cholecystitis may therefore be associated with a localised peritonitis. Anatomical variations of the biliary tree are fairly common and, during cholecystectomy, the anatomy must be carefully defined before division of the cystic duct is begun lest the common bile duct be damaged.

The walls of the bile ducts contain only small amounts of smooth muscle. The lower end of the common duct and the main pancreatic duct most often share a common opening (the ampulla of Vater), and are surrounded by a complex sphincter (the sphincter of Oddi).

Nerve Supply of Liver and Biliary Tract

The liver and biliary tract are supplied with both parasympathetic and sympathetic fibres, carried around the hepatic artery from the coeliac plexus. The preganglionic parasympathetic fibres reach the plexus in the vagal trunks. Preganglionic sympathetic cell bodies are in the 7th–9th thoracic segements and reach the coeliac plexus via the sphanchnic nerves. Afferent pain fibres from the liver and biliary tract probably run in the sympathetic nerves.

CELLULAR FUNCTION AND DYSFUNCTION

The liver is the most important metabolic organ in the body. Its normal functions are extremely complex and still only poorly understood. They can be summarised as follows (Fig. 8.6 a and b):

Metabolic Functions

Carbohydrate metabolism

The liver is essential for glucose homoeostasis and maintenance of blood sugar. Extensive liver resec-

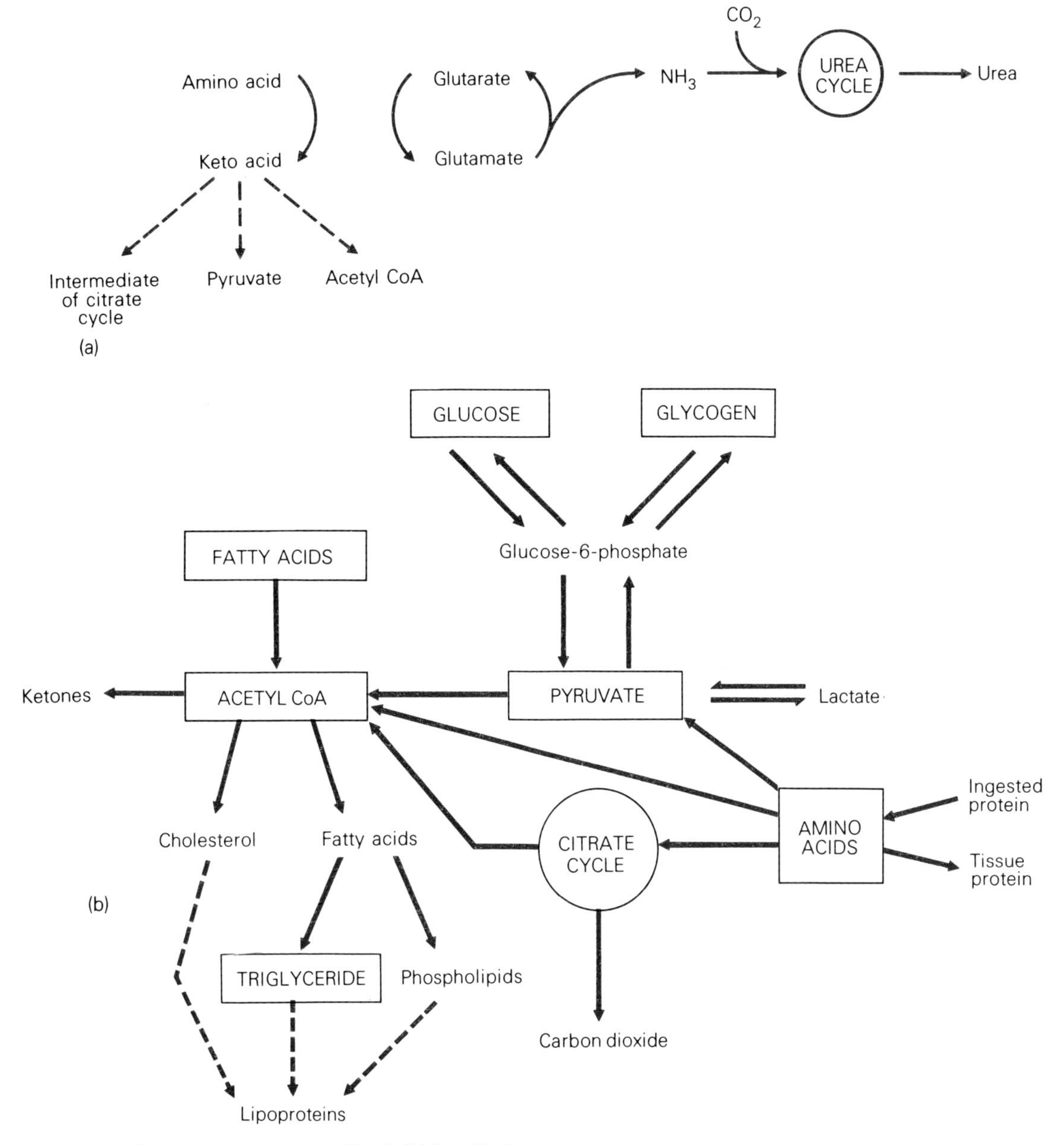

Fig. 8.6 *(a) Synthesis of urea (greatly simplified). (b) Simplified overview of the interrelationship of carbohydrate, lipid and amino acid metabolism in the liver.*

tion and severe liver failure lead to profound hypoglycaemia. After carbohydrate ingestion and glucose uptake, the liver stores of carbohydrate in the form of glycogen are increased by glycogenesis. There may also be glycolysis and disposal of glucose via the hexose monophosphate shunt. During fasting, blood glucose is maintained by gluconeogenesis and glycogenolysis. In prolonged starvation, some degree of adaptation occurs in tissues, including even brain, with increasing reliance upon ketones as the primary fuel.

Carbohydrate (glucose) intolerance is a common feature of chronic liver disease. A variety of mechanisms may be involved, including an increase in peripheral insulin resistance, impaired insulin action, and circulating insulin antagonists. There may be, furthermore, increased levels of diabetogenic hormones, including growth hormone, cortisol, and glucagon.

Elimination of nitrogenous wastes and formation of urea

Products of protein digestion are taken via the portal vein to the liver and metabolised. Amino acids are transaminated and then the carbon skeletons are metabolised by several pathways (including the Krebs citrate cycle; Fig. 8.6a). The amino groups are converted, via glutamate and ammonia, to urea. Failure of these processes, either because of cellular dysfunction or because of shunting of portal blood flow from the liver (directly into systemic circulation), leads to brain toxicity and neuro-encephalopathy, although the actual toxic substance is unknown.

Lipid metabolism and cholesterol synthesis

Cholesterol, synthesised from acetyl CoA in the microsomal fraction of the hepatocytes, is a constituent of cell membranes and a precursor of steroid hormones and bile acids. Cholesterol may occur free or esterified with long-chain fatty acids. Triglycerides, esters of glycerol and fatty acids, are convenient energy stores. Phospholipids (such as lecithin), which are complex lipids found in cell membranes, are also formed in the liver.

Lipid transport across membranes in the body is facilitated by carrier lipoproteins, produced in liver. These are of several groups: α-globulin-associated (high density) lipoproteins; β-globulin-associated (low density) lipoproteins; and very low density lipoproteins. Characteristic changes in lipoprotein patterns may occur in hepatobiliary diseases. Chronic cholestasis leads to accumulation of abnormal lipoproteins and excess cholesterol. Deposition xanthomas may be seen in the skin. Changes in cell membranes may occur and are seen most readily in the erythrocytes (target cells and burr cells: Fig. 8.7).

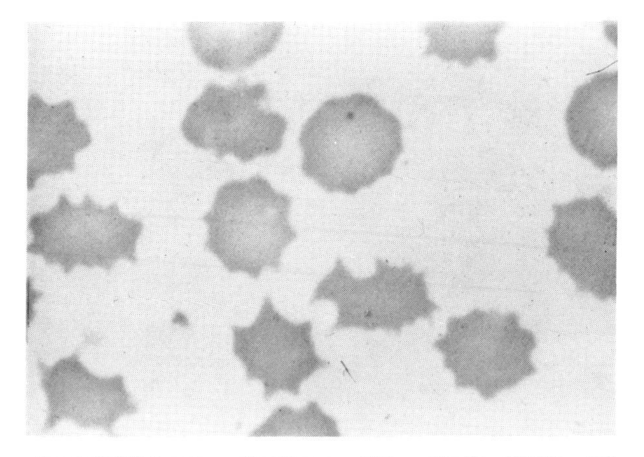

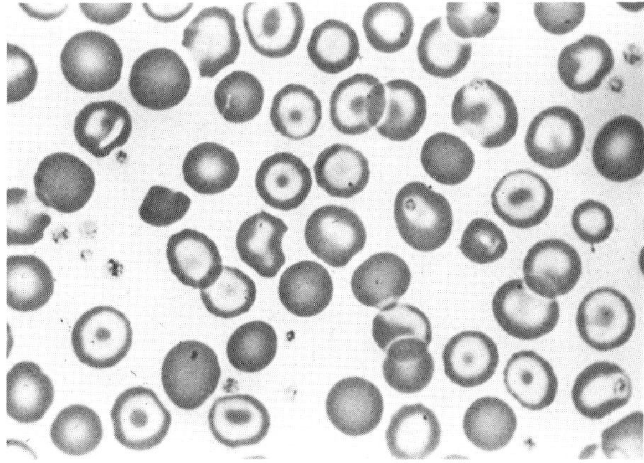

Fig. 8.7 *Red blood cell changes in liver disease.*

There is a complex interrelationship between carbohydrate, protein, and lipid metabolism in the liver, with the key 'link' substances being pyruvate and acetyl CoA (Fig. 8.6b).

Formation and elimination of bile salts

Two primary bile salts, cholate and chenodeoxycholate, are formed in the hepatocytes from cholesterol. Before excretion, their solubility is increased by conjugation with glycine or taurine. These salts are altered by intestinal bacteria to produce the secondary bile salts, deoxycholate and lithocholate. Deoxycholate is reabsorbed to reenter the bile, but lithocholate is less soluble and is excreted in the faeces (Fig. 8.8).

Bile salts are detergents and their function is to facilitate absorption of lipids. In aqueous solution

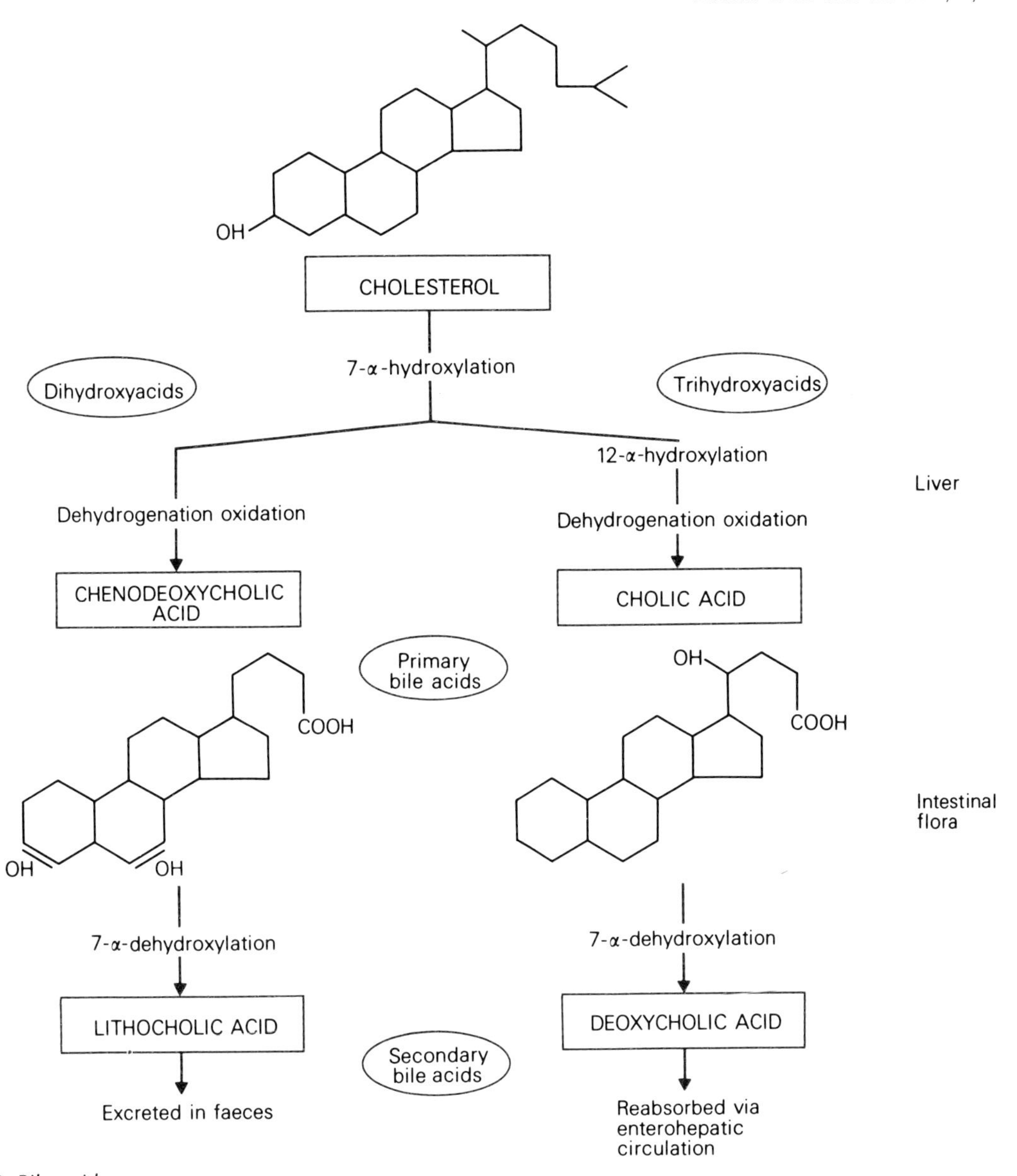

Fig. 8.8 *Bile acids.*

they aggregate into groups of several molecules called micelles (see p. 120). Micelles can incorporate lipids and remain in aqueous solution. Lecithin and cholesterol are transported in bile within the micelles. Bile salts, lecithin and cholesterol make up about 90% of the solids in bile and the remainder consists of bilirubin, fatty acids, and inorganic salts (Fig. 8.9).

Bile salts participate in fat absorption in the small bowel and are reabsorbed partly by passive transport in jejunum but mainly by an active transport system in the distal ileum, so that about 95% of the secreted bile salts are returned to the liver in the portal venous blood. The entire bile-salt pool of 2.5–4 g circulates twice through the enterohepatic circulation during each meal, and no less than 6–8 cycles are made each day. About 10–20% of the bile-salt pool is lost daily in

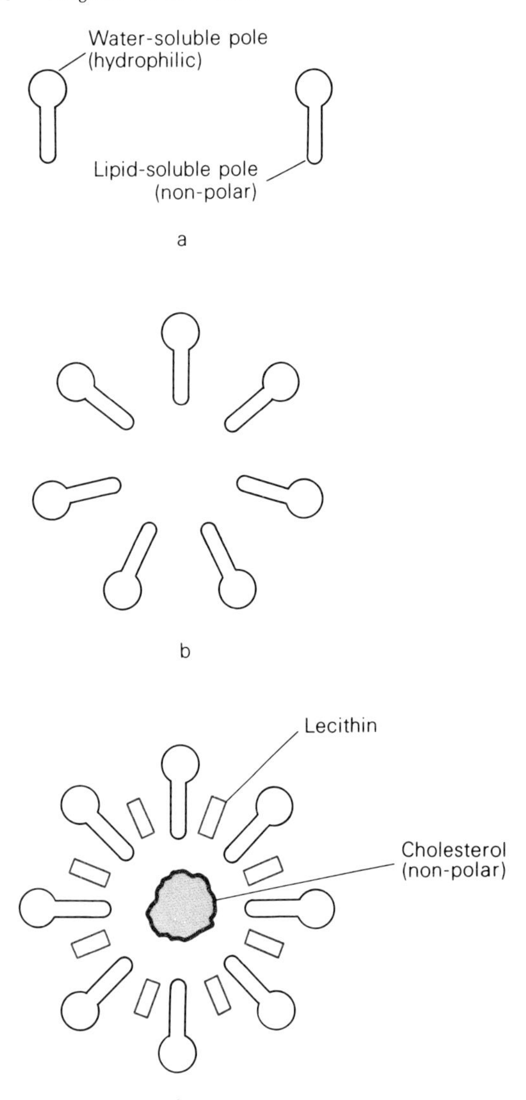

Fig. 8.9 *Bile salt micelles. (a) Bile salts. (b) Bile salt micelle. (c) Mixed ('functioning') micelle.*

the faeces and is restored by hepatic synthesis (Fig. 8.10).

Degradation of hormones

Insulin, glucagon, glucocorticoids, thyroxine and growth hormone are all metabolised in the liver. The precise causes of some of the clinical features of liver failure such as palmar erythema,

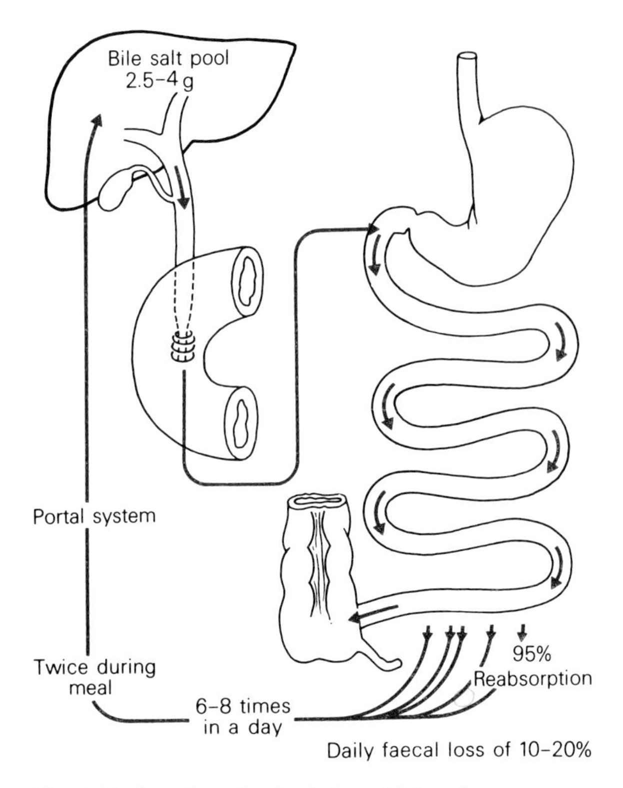

Fig. 8.10 *Enterohepatic circulation of bile salts.*

spider naevi, female hirsutism, and gynaecomastia and testicular atrophy in the male, are still unclear, but changes in oestrogen metabolism, androgen metabolism and relative concentrations of albumin and sex-hormone-binding globulin are all involved.

Excretory Functions:

A major function of mammalian livers is to convert insoluble, non-polar substances into an excretable polar form for elimination (Fig. 8.11).

Excretion of bilirubin (Fig. 8.12)

Bilirubin is formed predominantly from breakdown of haemoglobin of effete red cells in the reticulo-endothelial system, although about 15% arises from myoglobins, cytochromes, and catalases. The ring protoporphyrin of haemoglobin is

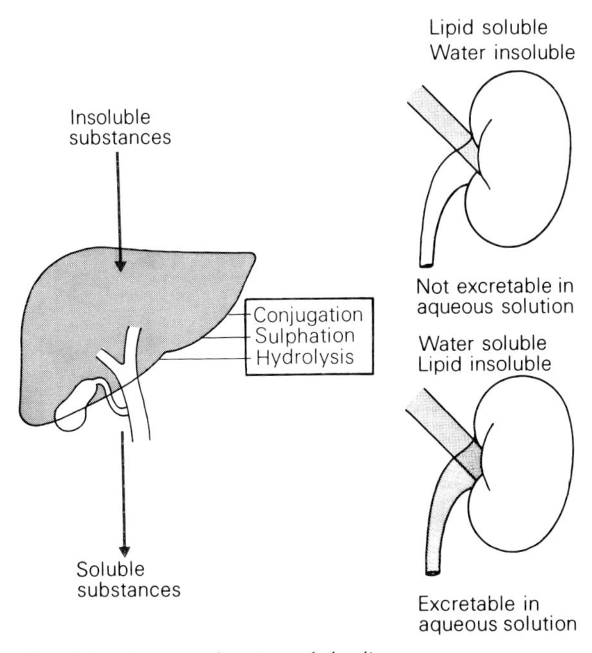

Fig. 8.11 *Excretory function of the liver.*

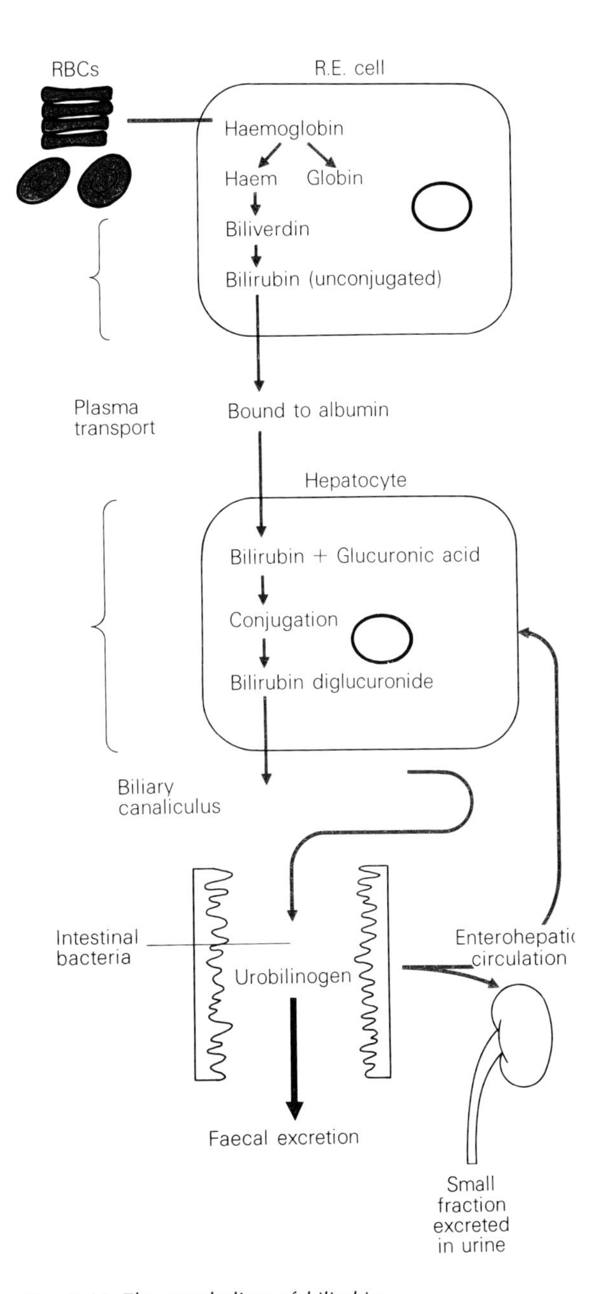

Fig. 8.12 *The metabolism of bilirubin.*

broken open at the alpha-methene bridge by haem oxygenase to form a tetrapyrrhol compound – biliverdin – which is then oxidised to bilirubin. Being very insoluble in water (though soluble in lipid), bilirubin is transported to the liver attached to albumin, from which it breaks loose in the sinusoids to be taken up into the liver cells. Transporter substances, Y and Z proteins, carry the bilirubin to the endoplasmic reticulum for conjugation, first to monoglucuronide and then to diglucuronide, by the action of the enzyme bilirubin – UDP – glucuronyl – transferase. These steps are impaired in the benign genetic abnormality called Gilbert's disease, and also in the neonate (especially when premature) in so-called 'physiological jaundice'. The water-soluble, polar, conjugated bilirubin is then actively secreted into the canaliculus and thence eliminated into the intestine in bile. This step is apparently both rate-limiting and 'fragile' – being readily impaired in viral infections, hypoxaemia, septicaemia, and severe surgical trauma (leading to so-called intrahepatic cholestatic jaundice). 'The contraceptive pill' and 17-alkyl substituted steroids may also impair bilirubin excretion.

In the gut, bacterial action converts bilirubin conjugates by a series of steps to urobilinogen (stercobilinogen). A little is reabsorbed and taken up by the liver but this enterohepatic circulation is only important when the system is overloaded (as in haemolysis), or when liver re-uptake is impaired by mild liver disease. In these situations, urobilinogen is readily detected in the urine using Ehrlich's aldehyde reagent.

Mild recurrent jaundice occurs in several situations. Excess breakdown of red cells (haemolysis) arises from a large number of causes; if mild, it may cause no jaundice, but even if severe it seldom raises the bilirubin above 4 or 5 times normal. Because the bilirubin is insoluble (unconjugated) and protein-bound, the jaundice is acholuric, i.e. without bilirubin escaping into the urine. Gilbert's disease is a common minor abnormality leading to mild or recurring unconjugated hyperbilirubinaemia in up to 3–4% of the population. It is familial. Being totally benign, its recognition is important in order to prevent meddlesome investigation or surgical interference. Bilirubin has a predilection for collagen, hence the deposition in skin and sclerae. Clearance of bilirubin from skin and sclerae may therefore lag behind changes in plasma bilirubin concentrations.

Organic anions

Some of these are endogenous, e.g. steroid hormones, and some exogenous, e.g. insoluble drugs. An example is the cholecystographic

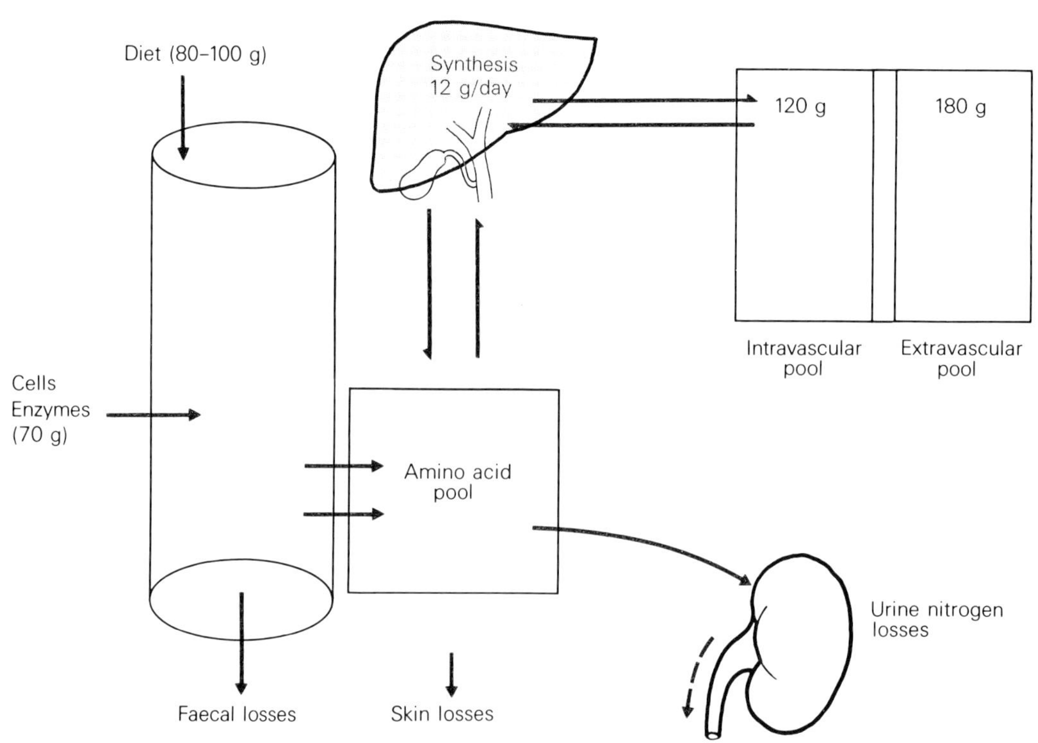

Fig. 8.13 *Simplified scheme of protein/nitrogen turnover in the body.*

group of dyes. These share the same metabolic pathway as bilirubin, and this is the reason why oral and intravenous x-rays are impracticable when the bilirubin is raised. If the bilirubin cannot move through the pathway then neither can the contrast dyes in sufficient concentration to produce pictures.

Manufacturing Functions

Protein production is a prime liver function; all the circulating proteins apart from gamma globulin are made in the liver.

Albumin is required for two main functions:

– maintenance of plasma colloid osmotic pressure
– transport of insoluble plasma constituents.

The normal liver manufactures some 10–12 g of albumin daily but this forms part of a large continuous turnover within an exchangeable pool of some 300 g (Fig. 8.13). The normal half-life of albumin is about three weeks. Synthesis is impaired in liver diseases, in fever, and in cachexia. Albumin levels are usually well maintained in the early stages of biliary obstruction. Apart from impaired formation, there are other important causes of a low plasma albumin (Fig. 8.14).

Hypoalbuminaemia is therefore associated with movement of fluid into extracellular spaces and the formation of oedema. Since portal pressure may be raised in many forms of chronic liver disease (see p. 92), there is a special predilection for fluid escape from the peritoneal vessels and hence ascites. Handling of and response to drugs (e.g. corticosteroids) may be abnormal. Most drugs are protein-bound and, because binding is unpredictable, the response will also be unpredictable. This means that drug-prescribing in liver disease requires care.

Carrier proteins. The liver also produces specialised carrier proteins including glycoproteins, haptoglobins, transferrins, and caeruloplasmin. Immunoglobins which are not produced in liver tend to rise in liver diseases. However the term 'albumin: globulin ratio', once widely used, has no physiological significance or practical value.

Coagulation factors. All the proteins concerned with blood coagulation, with the exception of Factor VIII, are produced in the liver, i.e. fibri-

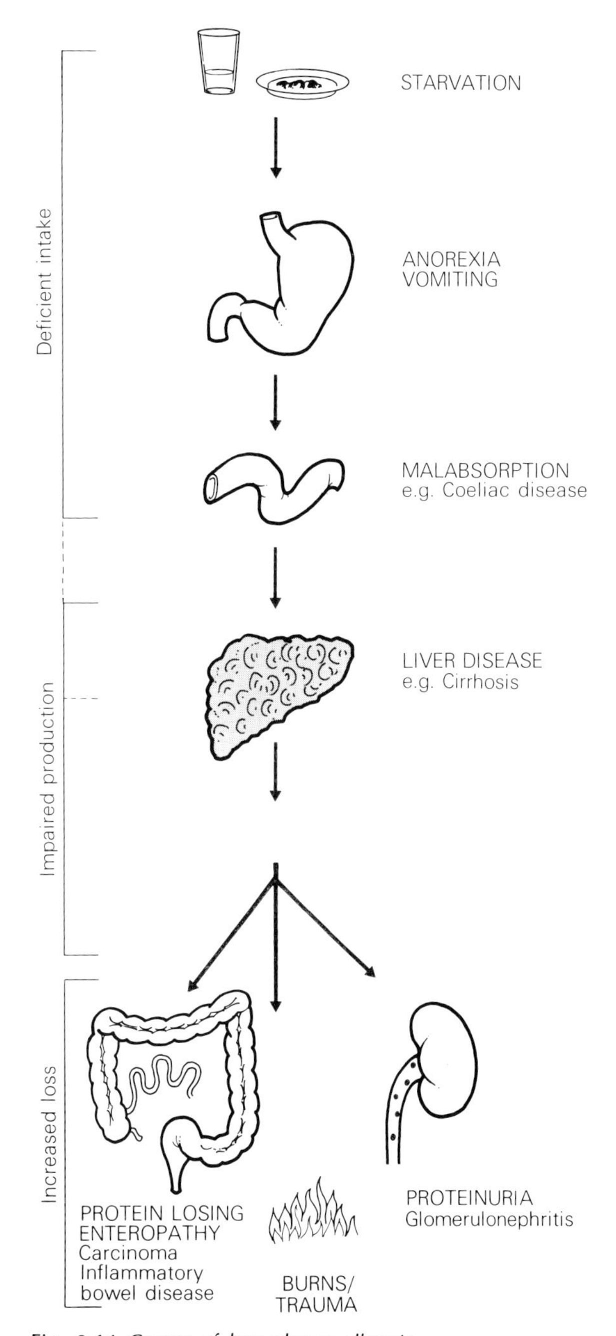

Fig. 8.14 *Causes of low plasma albumin.*

nogen, prothrombin, factors II, V, VII, IX, X, XI, XII, and XIII.

Bile Flow

Bile is a dilute aqueous solution produced at an approximate rate of 0.5–1.5 litres per day. Active secretion of bile salts by the hepatocytes into the biliary canaliculi is the main determinant of bile flow, and water and electrolytes (mainly Na^+) follow passively along osmotic and electrical gradients. The lipids lecithin and cholesterol also enter the canaliculi according to variations in bile salt secretion. The ductular cells secrete a fluid rich in HCO_3 (Figs 8.15, 8.16).

Bile flow is augmented during a meal by increased turnover of bile salts in the enterohepatic circulation.

Bile is stored in the gall bladder, where it undergoes approximately a ten-fold concentration. Bile flow into the duodenum is regulated by hepatic secretion, by gall bladder contraction, and by the bile-duct sphincter (Fig. 8.17). During fasting the pressure in the common bile duct is 5–10 cm water, and bile is diverted into the gall bladder. After a meal, the gall bladder contracts, mainly as a result of the humoral action of the hormone cholecystokinin-pancreozymin, which is released from the duodenal mucosa by intraluminal fat and lipolytic products. At the same time the sphincter relaxes and bile squirts into the duodenum as the ductal pressure rises to 15–20 cm water, and intermittently exceeds sphincteric resistance.

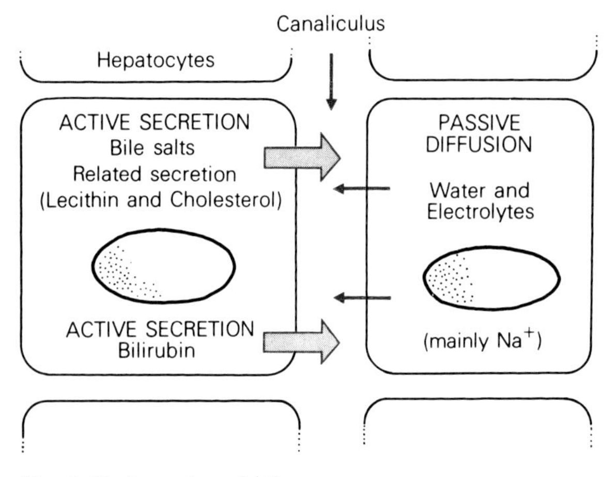

Fig. 8.15 *Formation of bile.*

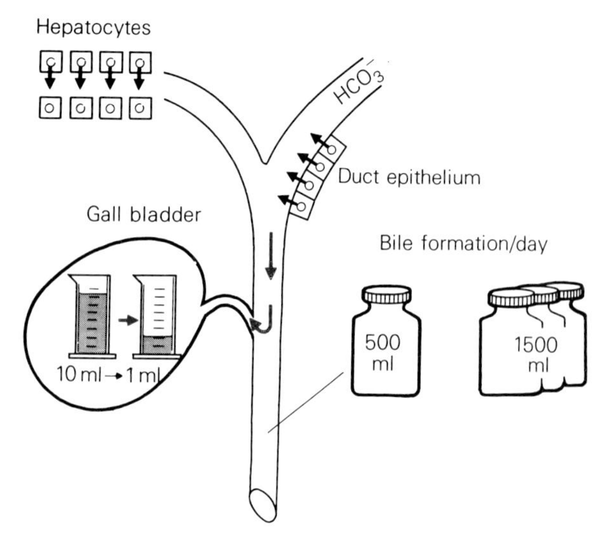

Fig. 8.16 *Concentration of bile.*

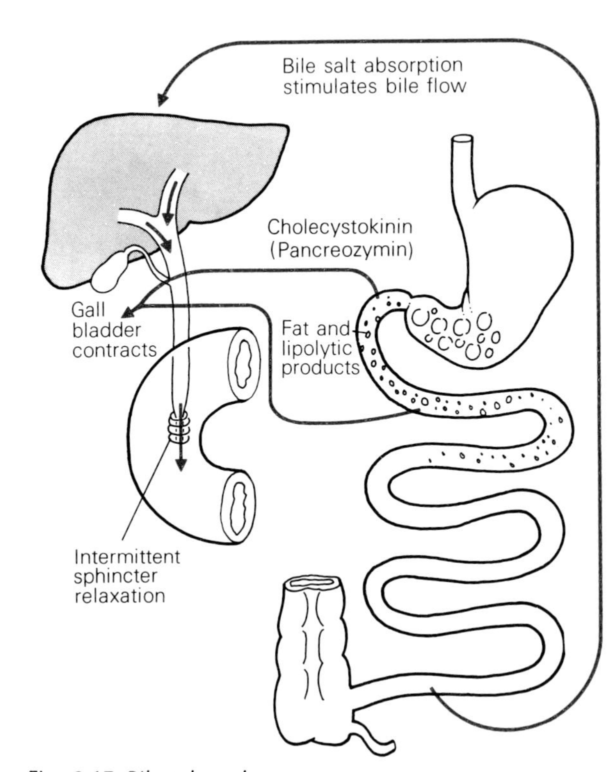

Fig. 8.17 *Bile salt cycle.*

PATTERNS OF CELLULAR INJURY AND RESPONSE

Although numerous insults lead to liver damage, the pathological responses are few but distinctive.

Cell Damage or Necrosis

This means damage to or death of hepatocytes, and may be:

a. scattered or 'spotty' (e.g. in mild virus and toxic hepatitis)
b. confluent and massive (e.g. in fulminant viral hepatitis or paracetamol poisoning)
c. focal (e.g. in centrilobular hypoxaemia in heart failure).

Microscopically, cells are swollen (ballooned) and may contain hyaline material. Following injury, fat may be deposited. Severe necrosis is followed by architectural collapse (and the liver is then clinically small). The causes are many (Fig. 8.18), and include:

hypoxaemia due to circulation insufficiency as in trauma or cardiac failure
metabolic disorders notably iron deposition (haemochromatosis) and Wilson's disease
physical injury such as hyperthermia and radiation
biliary obstruction (a relatively late effect)
industrial toxins such as trichlorethylene and carbon tetrachloride
dietary toxins including fungal poisons (such as aflatoxin found in spoiled grain, i.e. grain

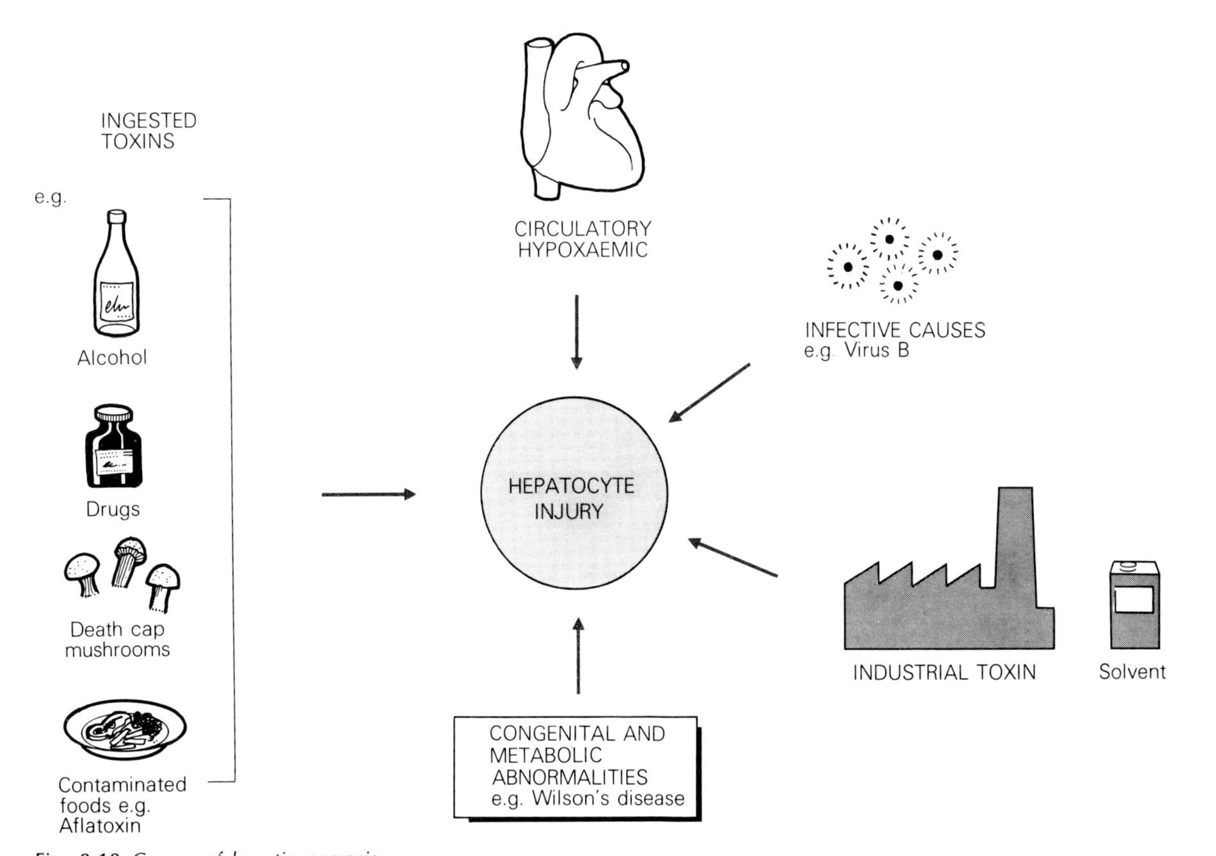

Fig. 8.18 *Causes of hepatic necrosis.*

infected with the fungus *Aspergillus)* and, notably, ethyl alcohol
pharmacological agents such as paracetamol and halothane
infective agents: viruses such as hepatitis B (HBV)
bacteria such as *E. coli*
protozoa such as schistosomiasis.

If the noxious insult ceases the liver can, because of its remarkable regenerative capacity, recover completely, sometimes leaving scarring of little clinical importance. Prognosis therefore depends primarily upon the patient's survival of the episode of hepatic failure. This highlights the importance of the development of a satisfactory support system for life-threatening acute hepatic

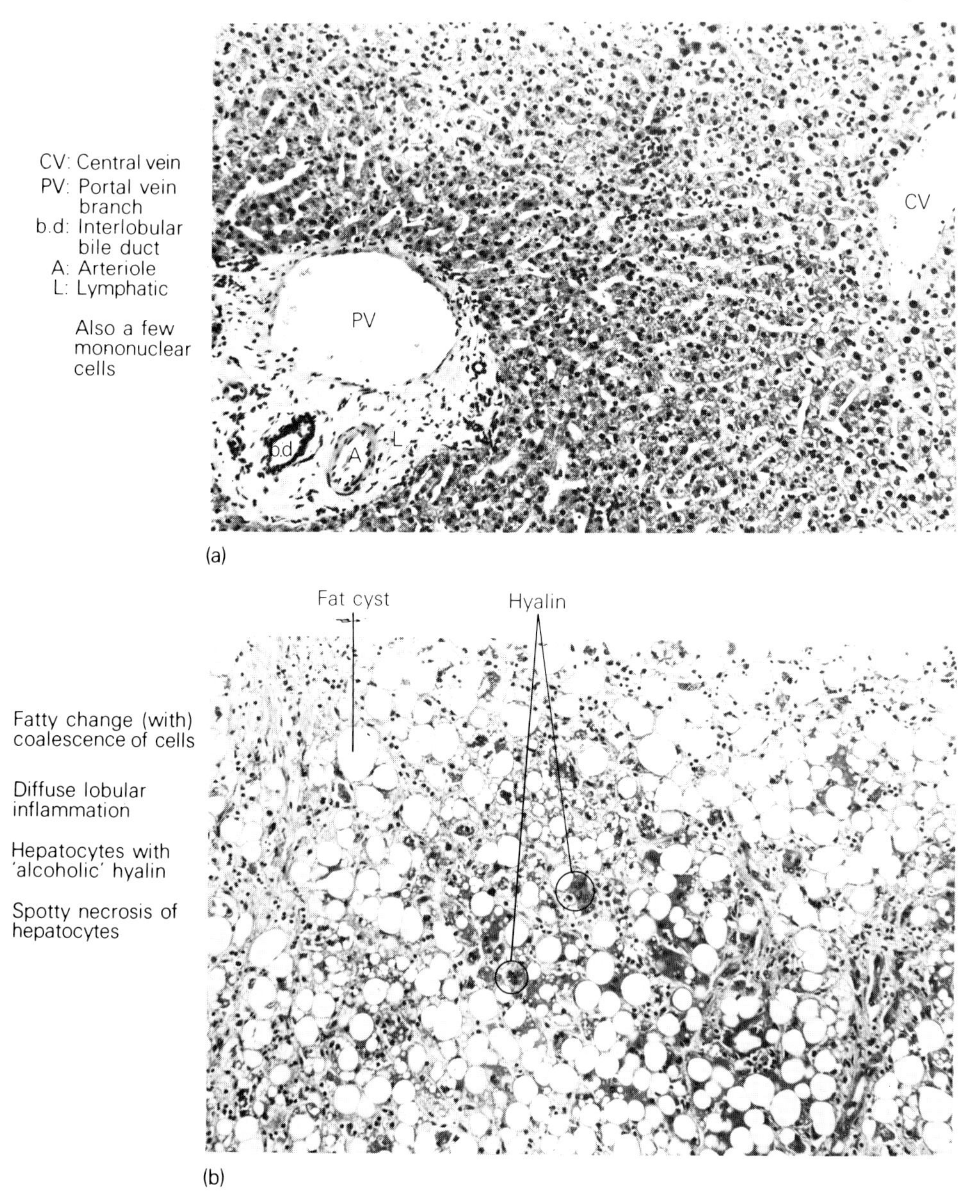

Fig. 8.19 *(a) Normal adult liver (M = × 100). (b) Acute alcoholic hepatitis with necrosis (M = × 100).*

failure—as yet beyond our reach. If the injury continues or is repeated (as for example in alcohol abuse), important permanent effects may occur, recovery is incomplete, and irreversible histological change (cirrhosis) follows (Fig. 8.19).

Hepatitis

This is said to occur where injury stimulates an inflammatory reaction. The reaction may be focal, generalised, or located around the portal tracts. The common causes are: viral infection, alcohol, certain drugs, autoimmune reactions, septicaemia, and ascending biliary infection. The hepatitis may be acute or chronic. It may have distinctive histological features, e.g. fat and Mallory's hyaline (both of which are suggestive, but

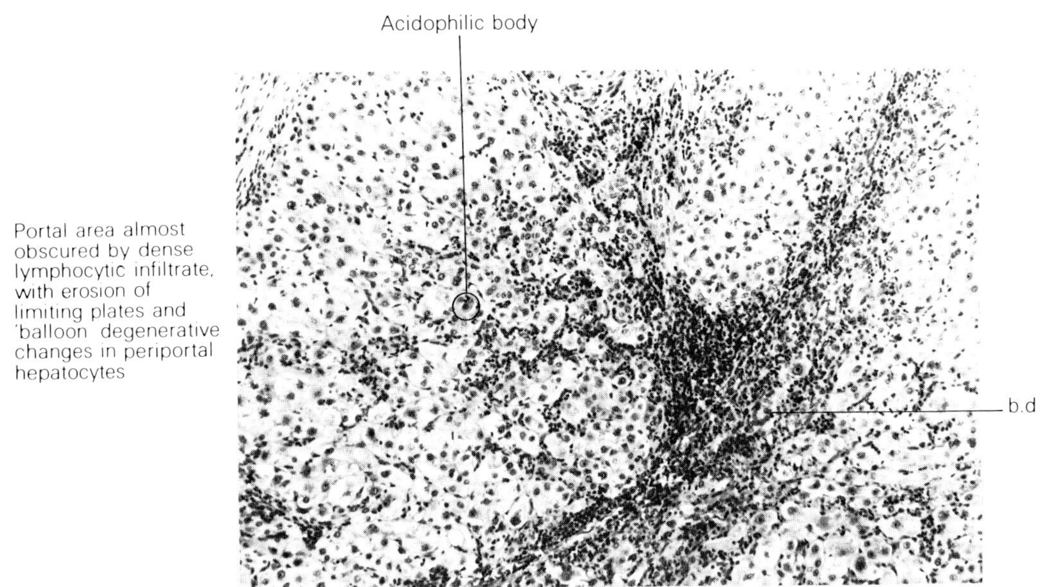

Fig. 8.20 *Chronic active hepatitis (M = × 100).*

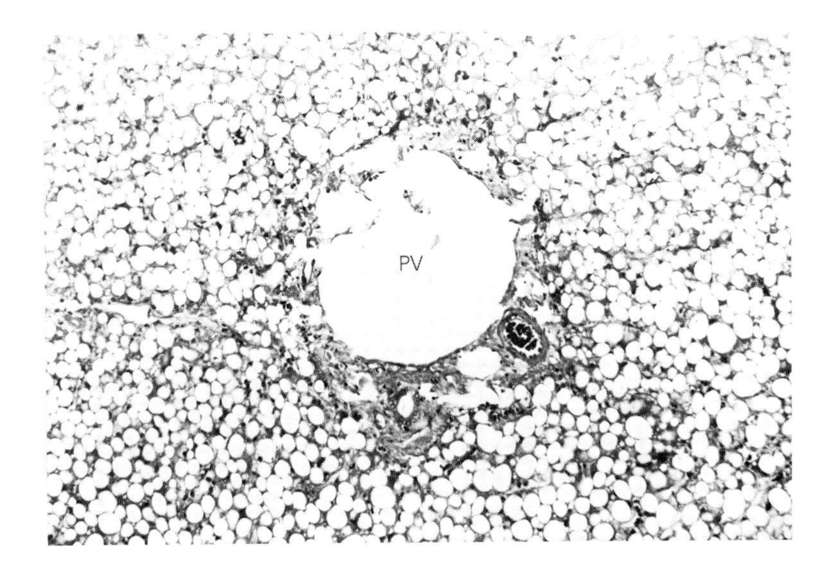

Fig. 8.21 *Alcoholic fatty liver (M = × 100).*

not conclusive, of an alcoholic aetiology). Hepatitis may be accompanied by or followed by fibrosis, suggesting early progression to cirrhosis (Figs 8.20, 8.21).

Cirrhosis

This is an end-stage and essentially irreversible reaction to necrosis and hepatitis (Figs 8.22, 8.23). It is characterised by:

- fibrosis and distortion of the normal liver architecture
- regeneration with new nodule formation
- disturbance of vascular supply with intrahepatic shunting.

The nodules may vary in size:

- In *micronodular cirrhosis* they are small and regular and, in general, this is the hallmark of continuing activity. The liver tends to be clinically enlarged.
- In *macronodular cirrhosis* they are coarse and irregular and the disease is usually burnt-out. The liver tends to be small and contracted and clinically impalpable.
- *Mixed intermediate forms* may occur.

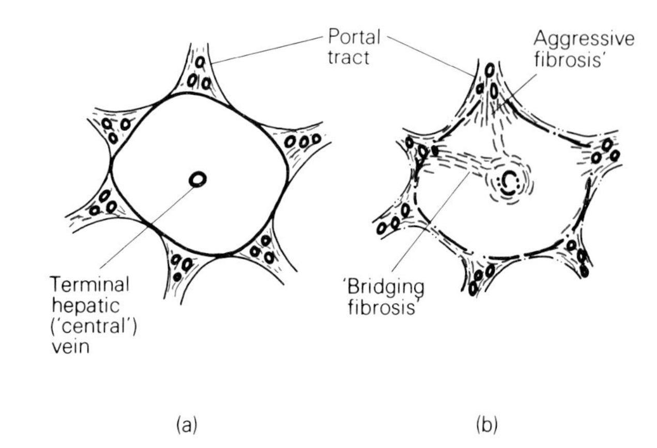

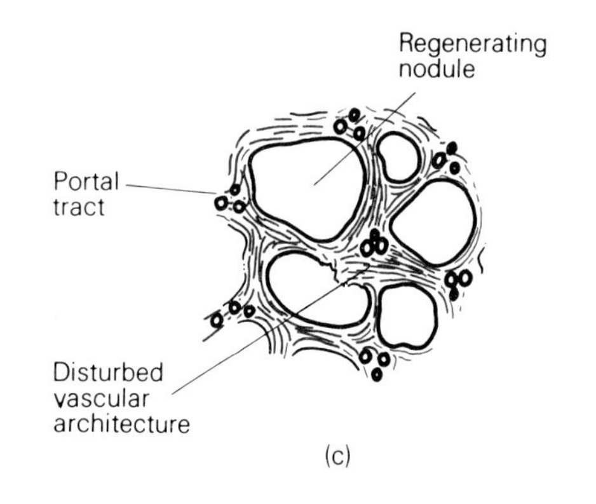

Fig. 8.23 *Development of cirrhosis. (a) Normal liver. (b) Early cirrhosis. (c) Established cirrhosis.*

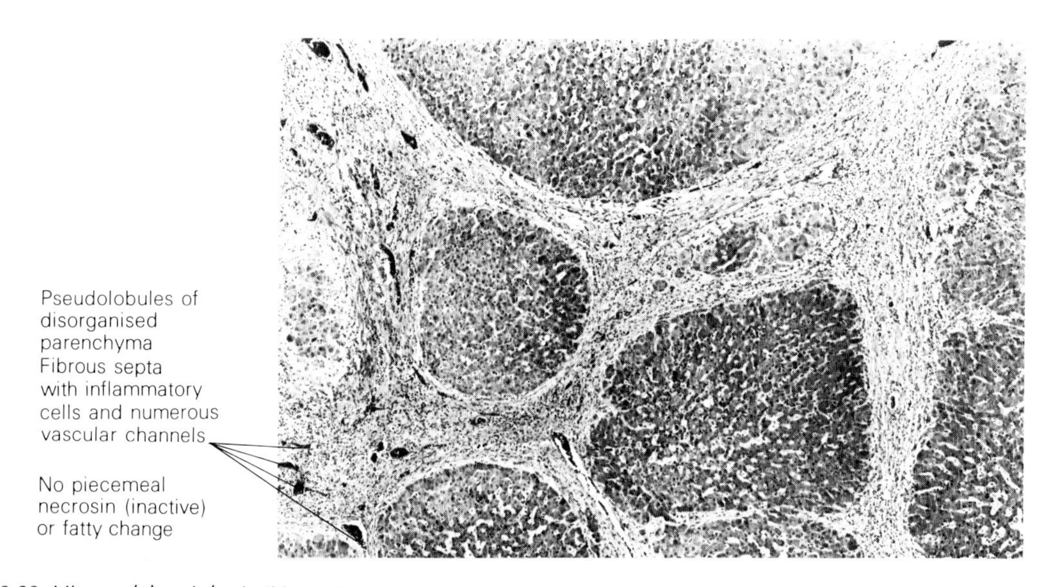

Fig. 8.22 *Micronodular cirrhosis (M = × 100).*

Since portal hypertension is a common accompaniment of cirrhosis, splenomegaly is common. It is important to recognise, however, that portal hypertension may also occur in non-cirrhotic conditions such as hepatitis with predominant centrizonal inflammation (e.g. alcoholic hepatitis), in veno occlusive disease, portal vein thrombosis, and granulomatous liver disease.

The reason why some patients with necrosis and hepatitis progress to cirrhosis and others do not is unknown, although disturbed immune reactions probably play some part.

Markers of immunological reaction such as circulating autoantibodies (humoral immunity) and lymphocyte cytoxicity (cell-mediated immunity) are common in some forms of chronic liver disease, including chronic active hepatitis (p. 163), alcoholic hepatitis (p. 160) and primary biliary cirrhosis (p. 163). It is not clear yet whether all these are simply secondary or epiphenomena (as some undoubtedly are) or whether they truly represent the mechanism of perpetuation of injury. A number of plausible theories to explain the latter have been put forward. Genetic influences play some part (in these so-called autoallergic diseases) as evidenced by increased frequencies of certain human leucocyte antigen (HLA) phenotypes. In chronic hepatitis there is also a common association with multisystem involvement (renal disease, pulmonary disease, colitis, arthritis).

SPECIFIC DISEASE PROCESSES

Viral Hepatitis (see p. 348).

Hepatitis is common in association with many virus infections, including infectious mononucleosis (glandular fever), yellow fever, rubella, herpes simplex and cytomegalovirus. However, by convention, the term 'viral hepatitis' is applied to three forms:

Virus A disease ('infectious hepatitis', HAV)
Virus B disease ('serum hepatitis', HBV)
Virus non A non B disease (2 or more viruses).

Both HAV and HBV are worldwide and responsible for vast numbers of infections and, especially in the case of HAV, for epidemics. HAV is

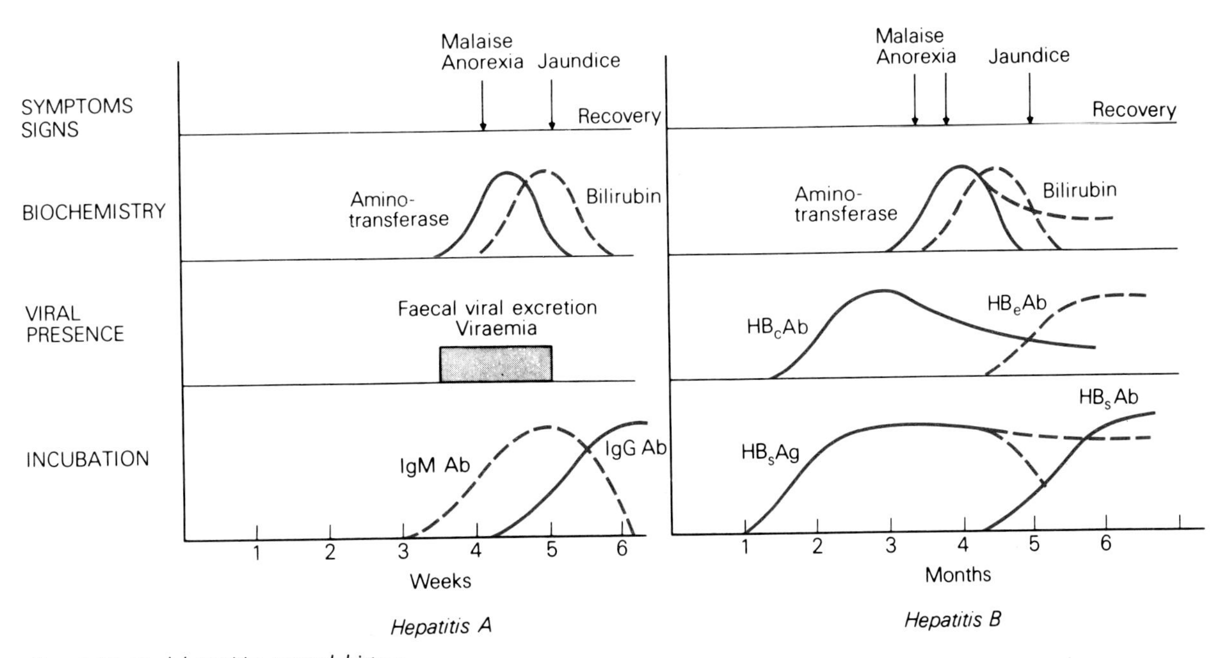

Fig. 8.24 *Viral hepatitis: natural history.*

common in schools and institutions and may also be a food-borne infection, whereas HBV is more sporadic and transmitted mainly parenterally or by close contact with body fluids (e.g. transfusions, dental treatment, tattooing, sexual and homosexual acts, drug abuse). Both are transmissible by either parenteral or faecal/oral routes. Patients with depressed immunocompetence (e.g. renal unit patients) are especially susceptible. In some outbreaks, their medical and nursing attendants have had depressingly high mortality.

The response to both HAV and HBV infection is most commonly a self-limiting, unpleasant but not life-threatening, acute hepatitis. A short (3- or 4-day) prodromal phase of profound malaise, anorexia and nausea, during which the transaminases are high and the urine contains both bilirubin and urobilinogen, is followed by jaundice and then a gradual improvement over 2–3 weeks, with eventual complete recovery (Fig. 8.24). Vague symptoms of malaise, pains, and fat intolerance, and sometimes modest rises of transaminase, may persist for weeks or months but are not important in themselves.

Variants of the classic acute hepatitis include:

severe abdominal pain (traditionally assumed to be due to capsular distension) simulating an acute surgical abdominal emergency.
marked and prolonged cholestasis simulating extrahepatic obstruction
anicteric disease – probably recognised as 'gastroenteritis'
meningism
fulminant hepatic failure.

These variants present considerable diagnostic challenge. A laparotomy in a patient with unrecognised hepatitis is dangerous for both patient and staff.

Diagnosis

Fortunately, diagnostic markers are now available for both HAV and HBV:

HAV: A specific IgM antibody; it rises to reach a peak about 2–3 weeks after the onset of symptoms. Disappears in 3 months.
Antigen in stool early in course of disease.
HBV: Surface antigen (HBsAg) rises early in acute attack. Indicates infection (including a continuing carrier state).
Surface antibody (HBsAb) rises late and indicates immunity.
Core antibody: high titre indicates continuing viral replication.
E-antigen: rises early in acute attack. Persistence indicates continuing chronicity and connotes increased infectivity of blood.
E-antibody: indicates relative lack of infectivity.
Delta antigen: indicates the presence of a separate infective agent complicating HBV and dependent upon simultaneous HBV presence to produce infection.

Management

This is simple in uncomplicated acute hepatitis, since no measures are of proven benefit. There is no evidence that either bed rest or dietary modification have any influence on the clinical course.

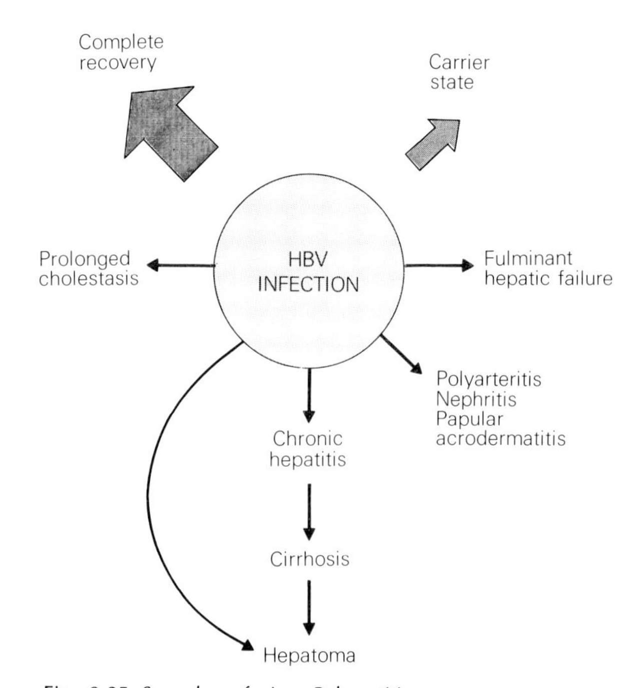

Fig. 8.25 *Sequelae of virus B hepatitis.*

Nevertheless, bed rest is probably wise while transaminases are very high and the patient feels unwell. Alcohol is usually prohibited for six months. Fat-free diets are widely suggested but unnecessary; the patient will limit his fat intake if it nauseates. A high-calorie/protein diet is advisable as soon as appetite resumes. Hepatitis may be prevented, or an attack attenuated, by the use of gamma globulin – standard human gamma globulin provides approximately six months' protection in the case of HAV. Specific high-titre antibody is available for HBV. Active immunisation with a specific hepatitis B vaccine is now possible.

Patients with active HAV may be kept in semi-isolation in their own homes. Since HBV has a considerably higher mortality, greater care is needed and isolation in an infection unit is preferable where possible. Special precautions for dealing with blood sampling, intravenous infusion, operative procedure, and removal of excreta, are now laid down in most hospitals.

Sequelae of hepatitis (Fig. 8.25)

While HAV is always self-limiting and never leads to chronic disease, this is not true of HBV. In addition to acute hepatitis, response to HBV infection includes:

1. *The chronic carrier state,* or *failure to clear the virus;* with persistence of surface antigen in the bloodstream for months, years or life. 'Carriers' in the community, though clinically well, do represent some hazard to others, especially hospital staff dealing with them and their blood, since they have low-grade infectivity. The presence of the E-antigen is associated with risk of infection; its absence suggests the risk is very small. The carrier frequency is less than 1% in most Western countries; but higher in Africa and Asia (15% in Taiwan and Singapore). Screening (for HBsAg) is routine for blood donors, antenatal patients and renal patients.
2. *Chronic hepatitis* (usually HBsAg positive). The pathological changes may be those of a chronic persistent hepatitis, with a good outcome, or a chronic aggressive hepatitis, with eventual progression to cirrhosis. No treatment is as yet known to prevent this progression. Treatment with antiviral agents such as arabinosides has been tried with limited success.
3. *Primary liver cell cancer* (see p. 170).
4. *Extrahepatic complications.* These include:
   glomerulonephritis
   polyarteritis (multisystem necrotising vasculitis)
   polymyalgia rheumatica.

Alcoholic Liver Disease

Along with virus hepatitis, alcoholic damage constitutes the greater part of liver disease in the world. As consumption of alcohol rises so will liver damage, and there is a consistent relationship. About one-quarter to one-third of heavy drinkers will develop cirrhosis over some ten years; many others will show fatty change or hepatitis. What is intriguing and, as yet, unknown, is why some heavy drinkers apparently escape irreversible disease. The overall problem of alcoholism is vast; it costs the United States over 113 000 million dollars yearly in medical costs, accidents, crime, and industrial losses.

Pathogenesis

The pathogenesis of alcoholic liver disease (ALD) reflects the predictable toxicity of alcohol (ethanol). Controlled experiments in volunteers and primate models (baboons) show consistent microscopic changes induced by heavy drinking – notably fatty deposition – regardless of the type of alcoholic beverage or of nutritional intake. These findings suggest also that malnutrition is not a major factor in pathogenesis.

Ingested alcohol must be metabolised – only traces of it are excreted (in breath and urine) – and this metabolism occurs almost exclusively in hepatocytes. The process of conversion is shown in Fig. 8.26.

This process generates reducing power in the form of NADH. Furthermore, alcohol is burned preferentially as a fuel in place of other nutrients,

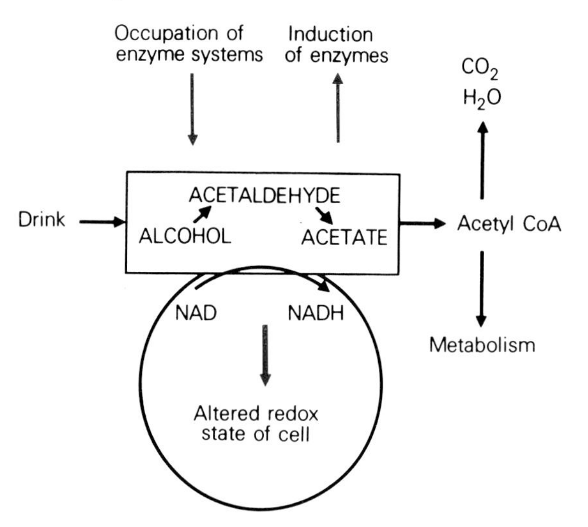

Fig. 8.26 *Metabolic consequences of ethanol (alcohol) ingestion.*

but the calories produced (7 kcals/g of ethanol) are empty and nutritionally poor. As the alcohol load increases, the ability of the mitochondria to cope with the hydrogen ions is exceeded, the Redox state of the cell alters, and most of the cell's vital metabolic functions may be disrupted. Acetaldehyde is a more chemically-active molecule than ethanol and its accumulation may be more toxic to the cell than the ethanol itself. Damage to cell membranes and microstructures is followed by necrosis and, in some instances, by a full-scale hepatitis. Cirrhosis is an end-stage phenomenon, just as in other forms of liver damage, but it is possible that with alcohol there is a specific stimulation to fibrogenesis by liberation of 'collagen stimulating factors'. Laying down of collagen around cells and in the spaces of Disse encourages self-perpetuation by strangling the nutritional supply of the hepatocytes. Disorders of immune reaction, especially cell-mediated immunity, are common in hepatitis and cirrhosis (but not fatty liver) and there is some evidence that Mallory's hyaline – a newly-formed protein aggregation in some liver cells – acts as an antigenic stimulus. But it is not known how important these findings are in pathogenesis.

Forms of alcoholic disease

These include:

a. *Hepatomegaly* due to swollen liver cells stuffed with accumulated export protein. It is an almost universal finding in heavy social drinking but of little clinical significance.

b. *Fatty liver,* which is highly chracteristic and strongly suggests alcoholic aetiology. Other causes of fatty liver include diabetes, gross obesity and malnutrition. Fibrosis may also be seen.

c. *Alcoholic hepatitis,* which may be acute, with jaundice, fever, leucocytosis, abdominal pain, ascites, tender hepatomegaly, and even portal hypertension. Distinction from extrahepatic ·obstruction and cholangitis may be difficult, and liver biopsy – if coagulation will permit – can be diagnostic.

Alcoholic hepatitis may also be chronic, with tender hepatomegaly and often a paucity of other signs. Symptoms, if present, may simply reflect the alcoholism (anxiety, tremulousness, tachycardia, confusion, convulsions, amnesia episodes) or the alimentary effects of alcohol (anorexia, nausea, vague abdominal pains, and diarrhoea). Mortality may be as high as 30%.

d. *Cirrhosis.* In the earlier stages of the disease, this is micronodular, the liver being enlarged, firm, with 'hob-nail' surface, and often containing fat. Episodes of hepatitis with jaundice may supervene. Later in the disease, often with lessening of drinking, the liver shrinks to a macronodular cirrhosis. Although it takes some ten years to develop a cirrhosis in men (and somewhat less in women, who appear more susceptible), the disease may only present at that stage with some complication such as variceal haemorrhage or ascites.

e. *Hepatoma* a late complication of cirrhosis in perhaps 15% of cases. It should be suspected when pain is a prominent feature, or when a palpable lump appears.

Management and prognosis

These hinge upon abstinence. Numerous studies

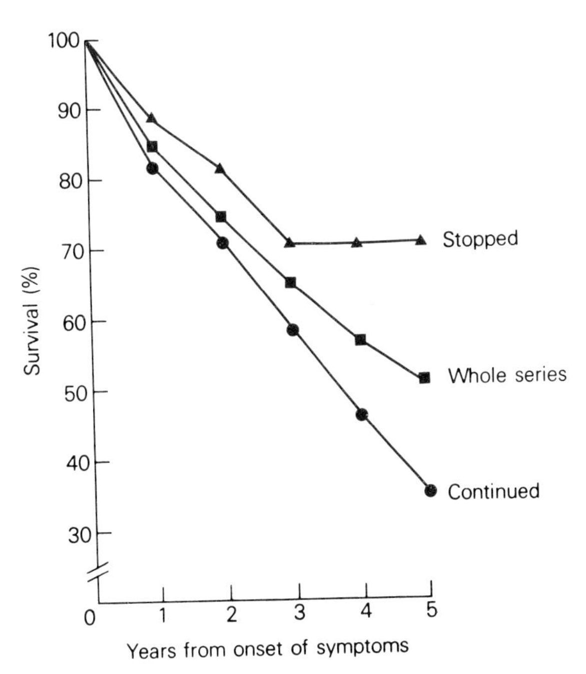

Fig. 8.27 *Survival in alcoholic liver disease.*

attest the considerably improved prognosis, even where cirrhosis has already developed (Fig. 8.27).

No treatment is known to prevent progression. Corticosteroids have been used in acute alcoholic hepatitis with mixed results. Supportive measures include intravenous polyvitamin preparations, high-protein diet and correction of complications. Patients with advanced liver disease are notoriously susceptible to opportunistic infection such as septicaemia, infected ascites and tuberculosis.

Drug- and toxin-induced disease

Many drugs which are non-polar and insoluble depend upon the liver for their excretion, and this may explain the frequency of hepatoxicity. The mechanisms of drug toxicity are complex and ill-understood. The major groupings include:

a. Direct toxic effect (producing necrosis) which tends to be dose-related.
b. A hypersensitivity reaction which is not dose-related.

The pathological reaction varies from a picture closely resembling acute (viral) hepatitis to a predominantly cholestatic form (when extrahepatic obstruction may be simulated). Intermediate forms also occur.

Important examples of drug-induced liver disease are as follows:

Hepatocellular necrosis

Paracetamol: fatal necrosis can follow as little as 15 g, liver failure becoming manifest in 2 – 3 days. n-acetyl cysteine and methionine may be effective if given within 10 hours of ingestion (Fig. 8.28).

Carbon tetrachloride: jaundice, bleeding and renal failure usually appear about 48 hours after exposure. Marked centrilobular necrosis and fatty change is seen.

Hepatitis

These are usually hypersensitivity, unpredictable, reactions.

Halothane: occurs rarely and usually following several exposures over a short time (four weeks). The picture resembles viral hepatitis. About 40% of icteric cases die.

Isoniazid: usually occurs after some 3 months of treatment, and is more common in 'fast acetylators'. The picture resembles viral hepatitis.

Cholestatic reaction

Here the picture is one of obstructive jaundice with little or no hepatitis. It is commonly a hypersensitivity reaction.

a. *Chlorpromazine:* along with similar phenothiazine drugs, shows a hypersensitivity reaction; even a single tablet may cause jaundice. It is said to occur in 1–2% of patients treated with the drug. Most cases get better.

b. *Sex hormones,* especially 17-alkyl-substituted

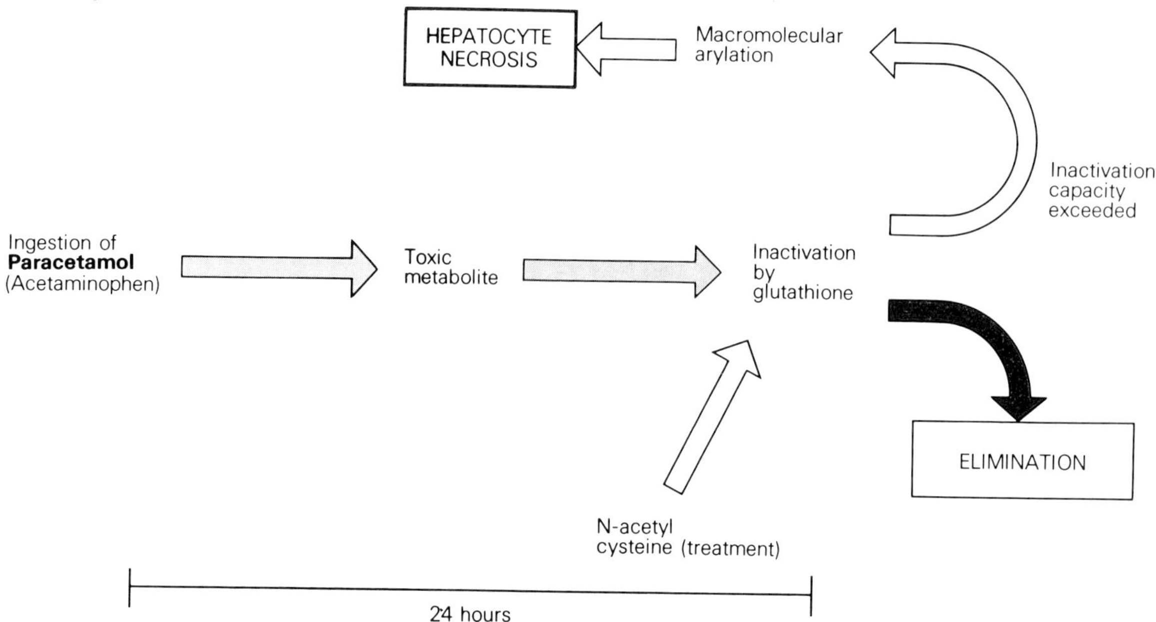

Fig. 8.28 *Paracetamol toxicity.*

compounds. The reaction is usually dose-related and improves on cessation. Jaundice associated with 'the pill' is rare, but relatively common in Chile and Scandinavia.

c. *Erythromycin estolate* causes a hypersensitivity cholestatic hepatitis with rash, arthralgia and fever, and eosinophilia. Other drugs with similar risk are *chlorpropamide, cotrimoxazole, nitrofurantoin* and *chlordiazepoxide*.

Steatosis (fatty liver)

Tetracycline especially in high doses intravenously, and in pregnant women, may cause severe fatty liver associated with hepatorenal failure. There is a high mortality.

Chronic active hepatitis (and cirrhosis)

Methyldopa, isoniazid, perhexilene and possibly *aspirin* have been implicated in causing an aggressive hepatitis. Withdrawal of the drug in most cases leads to dramatic improvement, but occasionally there is progression to cirrhosis.

Hepatic fibrosis

Arsenic and *vinyl chloride* in industrial exposure may both cause fibrosis and portal hypertension, and may also lead to tumour formation.

Hepatic tumours

Cyclical oestrogens may cause benign adenomas or hepatomas. Presentation may be with pain, hepatomegaly or serious intraperitoneal bleeding; it usually follows years of treatment. Arsenic, thorotrast and vinyl chloride are also associated with liver tumours.

Budd–Chiari syndrome

This is a rare condition in which the hepatic veins are occluded by thrombus (see Fig. 14.14). Any cause of venous thrombosis may be responsible and cases following cyclical oestrogens have been reported. The liver is large, tense and painful, and portal hypertension is a consequence. Survival is uncommon.

Auto-allergic Liver Disease

In this group of diseases, chronic active liver inflammation is associated with antibody markers of autoimmunity and disturbed immunoglobulin levels. Characteristically there is an inexorable progression to cirrhosis. The reaction may primarily affect liver cells (parenchyma – chronic active hepatitis) or intrahepatic bile ducts (primary biliary cirrhosis).

Chronic active (aggressive) hepatitis

This affects all ages, but commonly young females. The liver shows both lobular and portal tract inflammation with lymphocytes and plasma cells, piecemeal necrosis, and the early development of fibrosis. Many patients have the HLA B8 genotype. Smooth muscle antibodies are usual and in some cases a positive antinuclear factor (ANF) and lupus erythematosus (LE) cell phenomenon is seen (so-called 'lupoid hepatitis'). The level of IgG may be elevated.

Clinical features. The patient usually presents with insidious onset of malaise, anorexia and abdominal discomfort followed by jaundice. In young people the onset may be quite sudden with the rapid development of ascites. Sometimes jaundice is early and the picture may be confused with that of acute viral hepatitis.

Associated phenomena include joint pains and skin rashes and there is a well-recognised association with glomerulonephritis, thyroiditis, fibrosing alveolitis and non-specific proctocolitis.

Differential diagnosis. When the LE cell phenomenon is positive in the blood, the distinction from systemic lupus erythematosus can be difficult, but in CAH the liver disease dominates the picture and determines the prognosis. The diagnosis should always be established with liver biopsy. Other conditions which have a similar histological picture of aggressive hepatitis include:

Chronic virus hepatitis (B and non-A, non-B). The hepatitis B surface antigen is usually positive in chronic HBV (there is no satisfactory marker yet for H, non A, non B, V). The response to treatment with immunosuppressives such as steroids, is less clear than in Lupoid hepatitis and they could even worsen the condition.
Alcohol.
Drugs, e.g. methyldopa.
Wilson's disease (p. 164).

Course and treatment. Most patients show an inexorable course to cirrhosis. Corticosteroids (prednisolone orally) seem to be effective in slowing this progression, reducing the mortality and improving symptoms such as pain and jaundice. Treatment may be required for several years and, when stopped, relapse may occur. Progress is monitored by 'liver function tests' and also by liver biopsy about once a year. Biopsy is necessary because the biochemistry can be normal or near normal even with quite active disease. Side-effects with steroids are common, e.g. facial mooning, hypertension, dyspepsia and bone collapse, and may cause problems in management. Dosage may be reduced by adjunctive treatment with azathioprine.

Primary biliary cirrhosis (PBC)

This rare, slowly progressive disease, most common in middle-aged females, is characterised by chronic non-suppurative intrahepatic destructive cholangitis. There are characteristic histological changes occurring in four stages over some 10 years, the last being an established cirrhosis. Although not specific, the antimitochondrial antibody (AMA) test is positive in over 95% of cases and the IGM level is usually raised.

Clinical features. The onset is insidious and jaundice is almost always a late sign. Pruritus is common and may be the first symptom; it can be very severe and intractable. Some patients are picked up in the presymptomatic phase by the finding of an unexplained raised alkaline phosphatase or a positive AMA. Pigmentation and xanthomas and xanthelasmas (due to hyperlipidaemia), especially around the eyes and joint surfaces, are common. There may be an associated 'sicca syndrome' – dry mouth (xerostomia) and dry eyes (xerophthalmia). Diarrhoea is common and may be due to malabsorption caused by diminished bile salt secretion into the gut. Malabsorption of vitamin D and calcium leads to bone thinning and consequent pains. Liver failure and variceal haemorrhage are late features.

Differential diagnosis. The most important differential is extrahepatic obstruction and this must be carefully excluded, preferably by ERCP (see p. 173). Biliary calculi may, of course, coexist with PBC.

Treatment is mainly supportive. No drugs have been clearly shown to alter the prognosis although azathioprine and penicillamine have been used. Cholestyramine (Fig. 8.29) relieves the itch but aggravates the malabsorption. Calcium combined with vitamin D has been shown to prevent troublesome bone disease. This can be given orally as a combined BPC preparation; in severe cases, a monthly injection of vitamin D – 100 000 units intramuscularly, is necessary.

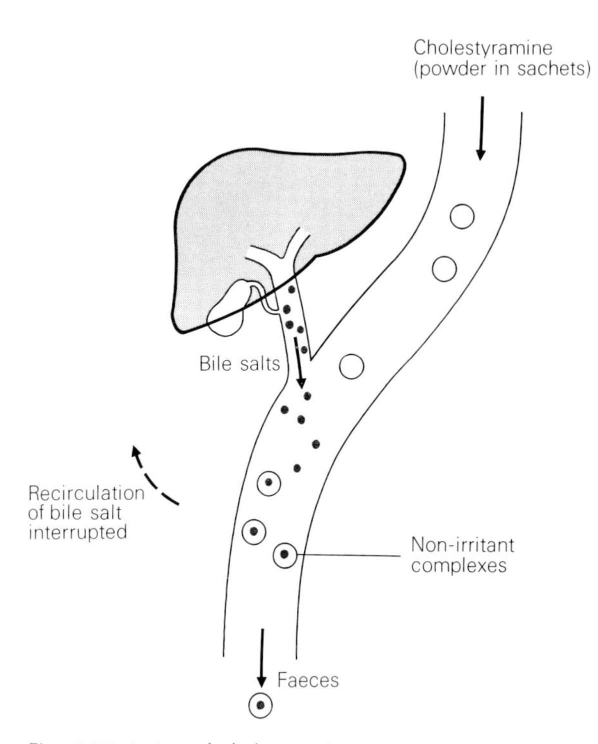

Fig. 8.29 *Action of cholestyramine.*

Metabolic Liver Diseases

These are, in the main, genetic anomalies and as such are rare.

Deficiency of alpha-1-antitrypsin

This is probably the commonest metabolic cause of neonatal hepatitis, and leads to cirrhosis in early childhood. It is also associated with early onset of panacinar emphysema. Partial deficiency may predispose to liver damage from other causes.

Wilson's disease

This is important because it is treatable (Fig. 8.30a). It should be considered in all young patients with chronic hepatitis or cirrhosis. Brownish corneoscleral rings (Kayser – Fleischer rings) should be sought in the eyes (preferably by slit-lamp examination) and estimation of caeruloplasmin, serum copper, and urinary copper should help to clinch the diagnosis. Treatment is by early, prolonged and careful use of penicillamine.

Galactosaemia

Galactosaemia should be picked up at neonatal screening; appropriate treatment avoids development of cirrhosis.

Haemochromatosis

Iron deposition in the liver with fibrosis and cirrhosis is either a primary defect of iron metabolism with increased intestinal uptake or secondary to iron overload (more strictly haemosiderosis), e.g. as occurs in multiply-transfused patients. The primary disease is associated with slatey-grey pigmentation of the skin, pancreatic impairment with diabetes ('bronze diabetes') and cardiac involvement with cardiomyopathy and heart failure (Fig. 8.30b). Arthritis and hypogonadism are common. The liver is invariably large and firm and the diagnosis is readily confirmed on biopsy. Treatment is reasonably effective; iron stores are gradually depleted by repeated venesection every two weeks or so for 2–3 years. Fibrosis, and even cirrhosis, may revert on this treatment. Hepatoma is a complication.

Indian childhood cirrhosis

This is of unknown cause but bears some striking histological resemblance to alcoholic liver disease in adults. It is common in the Indian subcontinent.

Reye's syndrome

A rare and curious disease of childhood, with

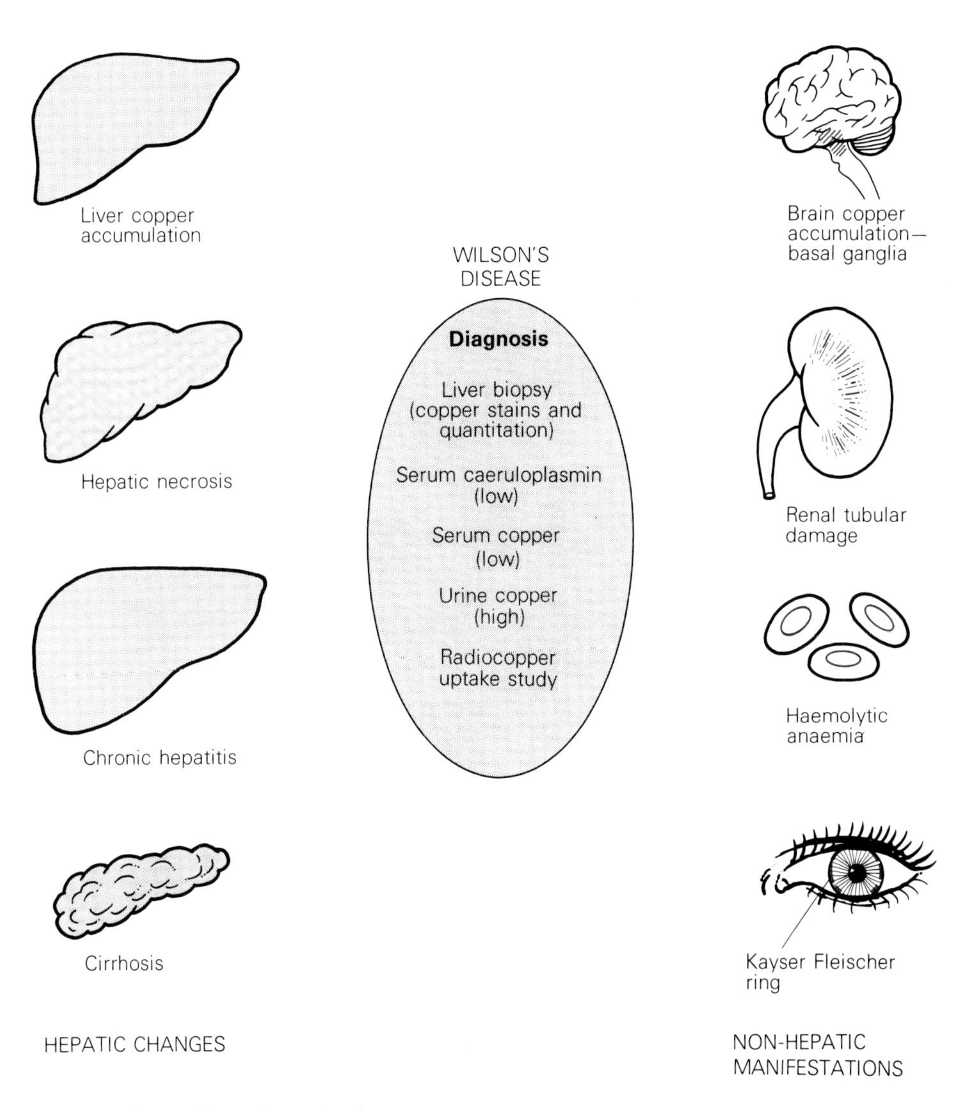

Fig. 8.30 *(a) Wilson's disease (hepatolenticular degeneration).*

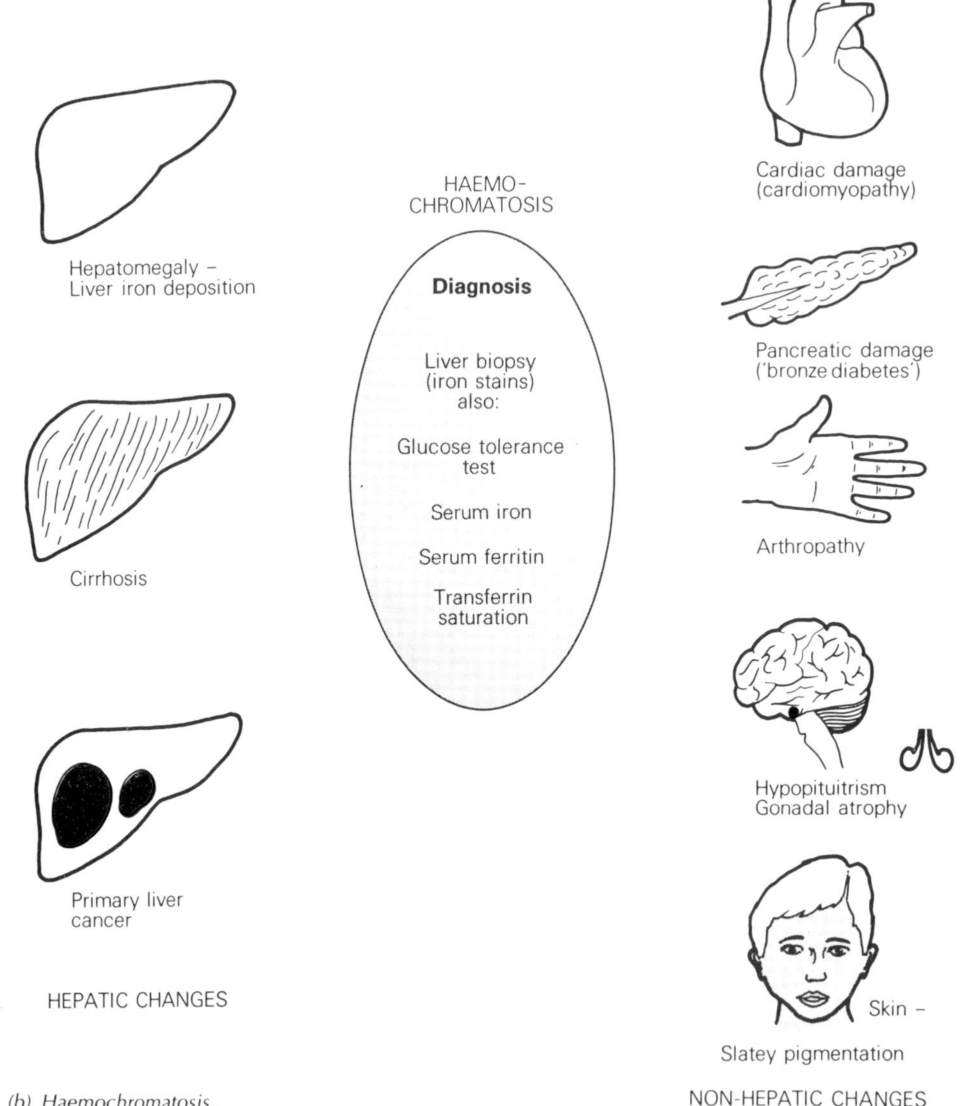

Fig. 8.30 *(b) Haemochromatosis.*

marked encephalopathy, serious metabolic disturbances (notably hypoglycaemia), and fatty infiltration of the liver. The cause is unknown but both toxins (including mycotoxins and aspirin) and infective agents have been implicated. The treatment is supportive and the mortality is high.

Others

Tyrosinosis, porphyria and some storage diseases (e.g. glycogen storage disease) may be associated with cirrhosis, as also Sickle Cell Disease and *Fibrocystic Disease* (p. 109).

ABNORMALITIES OF BILE COMPOSITION

Gallstone Formation

There are three major constituents of bile that are involved in the formation of cholesterol gall stones: cholesterol, lecithin (and other phospholipids), and bile salts. Basically, cholesterol and lecithin are insoluble in water and depend on bile salts to keep them in solution by the formation of macromolecular complexes termed micelles (Fig. 8.9). Bile salts have the remarkable property that one pole of the molecule is hydrophilic and the other hydrophobic. These molecules aggregate with their hydrophilic aspect to the outside and the hydrophobic pole to the centre, where a tiny droplet of cholesterol can be held in solution. Phospholipids aggregate within and stabilise the micelle.

Retention of bile cholesterol in solution therefore depends on a delicate balance between these three principal constituents, and normally a large excess of bile acids and lecithin ensures the solubility of cholesterol. If the cholesterol concentration rises, or the bile salt content falls, then the risk of cholesterol precipitating out of solution rises and the bile is said to be *lithogenic* (Fig. 8.31)

Obesity is associated with an excess of cholesterol in bile.

Oestrogens are believed to reduce hepatic bile acid production, and this probably accounts for the greater frequency of cholesterol stones in women, and for the recent increase in the occurrence of stones in young women taking the contraceptive pill.

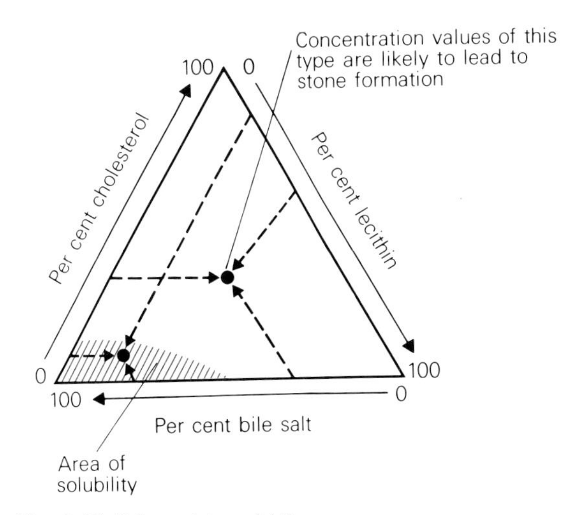

Fig. 8.31 *Lithogenicity of bile.*

Diet appears to play an important part in stone formation; wherever people eat much refined carbohydrate food, of high caloric value, then gallstones are common – i.e. throughout the Western world. Curiously, starvation appears to produce a rise in the cholesterol content of bile as does the use of diet high in unsaturated vegetable oils and low in cholesterol.

The role of infection in the formation of gallstones is not considered to be so important as it used to be. The general belief is that most stones are formed without the assistance of infection, although it is well known that some stones form around clumps of bacteria and fibrin. Probably infection most often occurs in a gall bladder which already contains stones.

Types of stone

There are three types of gallstones.

Pigment stones which account for 10–15% of all stones, are especially associated with conditions causing haemolysis – they are found in about 50% of patients with congenital spherocytosis. They are multiple, small, irregular, brown concretions composed of calcium bilirubinate and bile acids, and are usually radiolucent. Pigment stones are especially common in the Far East and make up a high proportion of stones forming in the bile ducts after cholecystectomy.

Pure cholesterol stones account for about 10% of all gallstones; and when small they are bright yellow in colour and are composed of a fused collection of spheres (spheroliths) to make a 'mulberry' stone (Fig. 8.32). As they grow, fresh layers are deposited on the original small collection of spheroliths so that the stone becomes smooth and rounded: on section, concentric rings

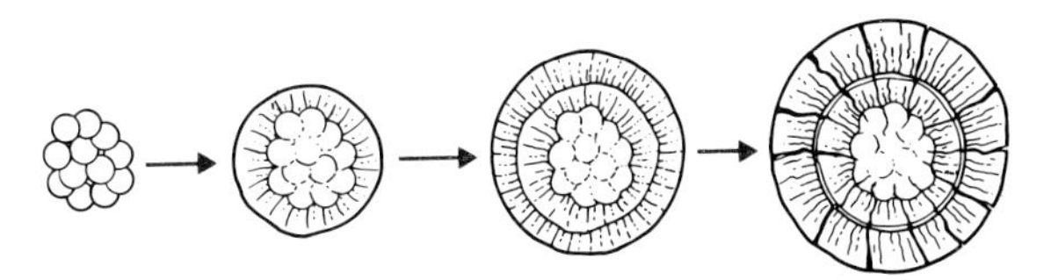

Fig. 8.32 *Formation of a cholesterol stone.*

with radiating fissures are seen. These stones, of more-or-less pure cholesterol, may attain a size of 2–2.5 cm, are often single, and are radiolucent.

Mixed stones are by far the commonest, and vary in appearance and composition. Cholesterol is the principal constituent, with a variable admixture of bile pigment, calcium carbonate, phosphate and glycoprotein. In appearance, they are most often multiple, yellow or brown stones, with faceted surfaces where one calculus has formed in contact with others. They range in size from a few millimetres to 2–3 cm, and are often lying in thick 'biliary mud'. If the calcium content is relatively high they will be radio-opaque.

Clinical pathology of gallstones

Gallstones are very common in Western countries, especially in North America and Australasia, where as many as 20% of the population over the age of 40 are believed to have them.

In many of these people, the gallstones remain totally asymptomatic, or 'silent', and are discovered by chance – when an abdominal x-ray is taken (10% of gallstones are radio-opaque), at laparotomy, or at autopsy.

Presumably everybody's gallstones are 'silent' for a time, during formation and growth, and the stage at which they produce symptoms appears to be entirely fortuitous. They may present in a number of ways (Fig. 8.33). Probably the majority cause acute attacks of pain, known as biliary colic, when a stone migrates into the cystic duct. If a stone becomes impacted in the neck of the gall bladder, with superadded infection, the patient suffers acute cholecystitis. In many patients the presence of stones in the gall bladder, perhaps accompanied by low-grade infection, produces the grumbling 'dyspepsia' of chronic cholecystitis. If a stone migrates from the gall bladder into the common bile duct (choledocholithiasis) it may, if small, be passed down and through the ampulla of Vater, probably with an attack of biliary colic and temporary elevation of aspartate transaminase and alkaline phosphatase. Some 15% of patients with stones in the gall bladder also have stones in the bile ducts, which may number from one to over 100. Impaction of a stone in the ampulla will produce calculous obstructive jaundice, which may or may not be painful. However, the presence of stones in the common bile duct does not necessarily produce jaundice because the stones may float up and down, without causing obstruction. Their presence may or may not produce symptoms but patients in this situation are particularly liable to the serious complication of *cholangitis,* i.e., an acute infection of the bile with intestinal bacteria which produces a rapid and grave form of septicaemia. Bile itself is bacteriostatic and normally sterile. How it becomes infected is not yet clear but presumably intestinal organisms pass up the portal vein and into bile. If foreign bodies, in the form of stones, are present then such organisms have a focus around which to multiply; when stones are removed from the common duct, about 65% of cases show infected bile.

The presence of more-or-less silent stones in the gall bladder over many years is (rarely) associated with the eventual development of carcinoma of the gall bladder. If a large stone develops in the gall bladder it may produce pressure ulceration of the wall of the gall bladder and of the adjacent duodenum to produce a cholecyst-duodenal fistula. If the stone passes through this fistula and migrates down the intestine it may impact, usually in ileum, to produce gallstone obstruction.

There is an important association between gallstones and the occurrence of acute pancreatitis (p. 104).

Non-infective cholangitis

Cholangitis is usually infective in nature and secondary to biliary obstruction. A rare condition – primary sclerosing cholangitis – is an occasional cause of slowly-progressive cholestasis leading to liver damage and, ultimately, death. Fibrosis is extensive, and may involve both the intrahepatic and extrahepatic biliary tree. In up to one-half of these patients there is also inflammatory bowel disease – usually nonspecific proctocolitis – but the nature of the relationship is unclear. The cholangitis may antedate the appearance of the bowel disease.

Two-thirds of patients present with pruritus and then jaundice. Weight-loss is common and fever

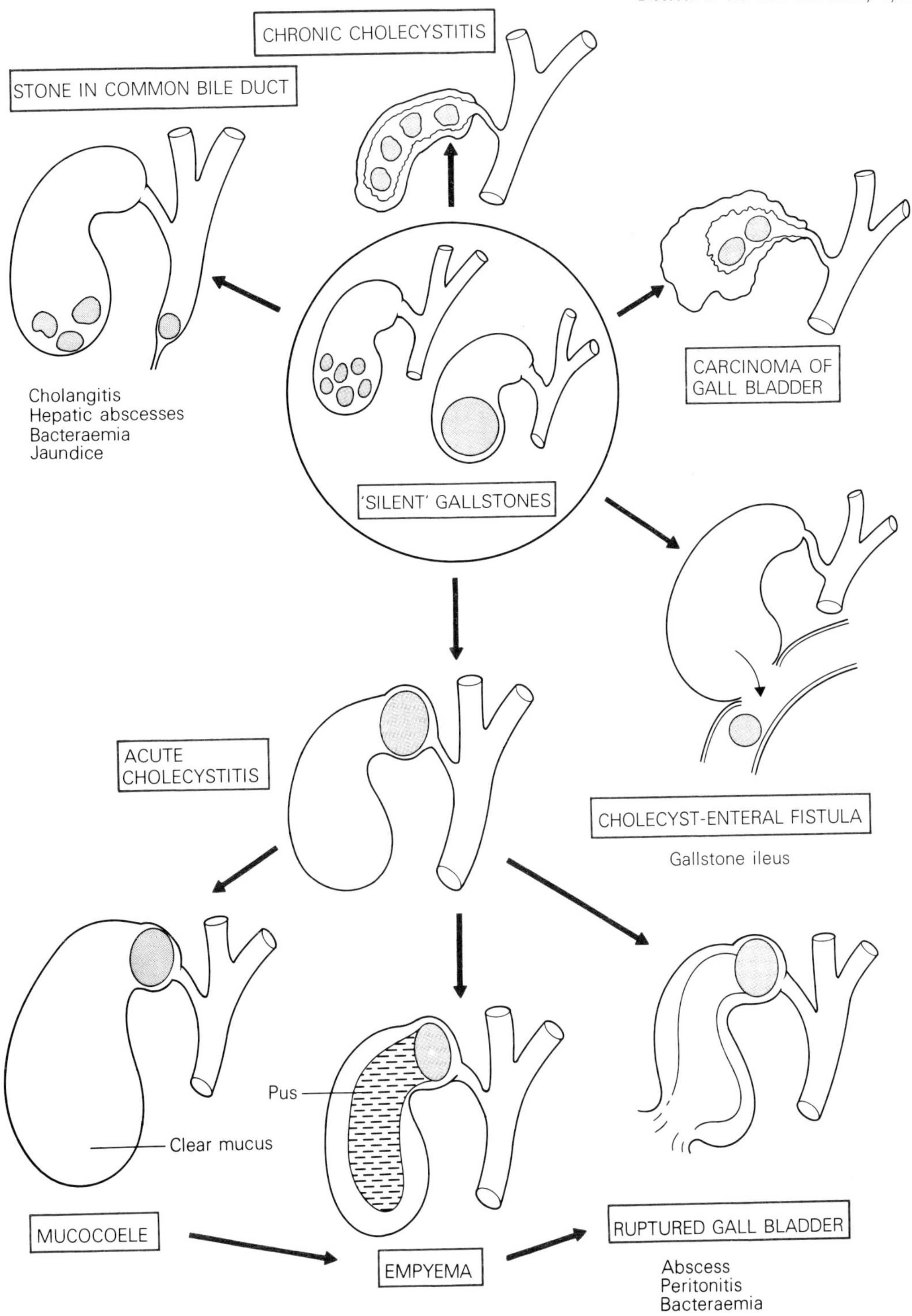

Fig. 8.33 *Presentation of gallstones.*

occurs in about one-third, making distinction from obstructive cholangitis more difficult. The diagnosis is made by demonstration of the typical narrowing and beading of the biliary tree as seen on ERCP or PTC (p. 173) and may be confirmed histologically. The distinction from bile-duct carcinoma can be difficult, even at laparotomy.

There is unfortunately no satisfactory treatment, medically or surgically. Removal of the diseased bile duct and enteroanastomosis may be possible; some temporary relief of the effects of biliary obstruction can be achieved by intraduct stenting with a fine polythene cannula (Fig. 8.49e).

ONCOGENESIS

Although uncommon in Britain, primary liver cancer is overall one of the world's most frequent tumours (Table 8.1). Hepatocellular cancer (PHC: hepatoma) is the main variety, but cholangiocarcinoma, fibrosarcoma, angiosarcoma and a number of benign tumours are all seen.

There is compelling evidence that hepatitis B virus (HBV) is a prime cause of hepatoma. Evidence comes from:

1. Geographic studies. Hepatoma is common in areas where HBV is also common.
2. Epidemiology. For example, the observed risk of hepatoma in Taiwanese men with past HBV infection (proven with markers) is 220 times the risk in similar men without HBV. Similar evidence occurs in other areas (see p. 28).
3. Comparative pathology. American woodchucks with a closely similar hepatitis virus infection die with hepatic tumours.
4. Molecular biology. Studies strongly suggest that integration of virus DNA into host hepatocyte DNA presages the onset of hepatoma.

Table 8.1
Annual Incidence of Primary Liver Cancer (per 100 000 males)

UK	3.0
USA	2.7
South Africa	14.2
China	17.0
Mozambique	98.2

It is certainly possible that other environmental factors either alone or in combination with HBV are important. Mycotoxins, especially aflatoxin from the fungus *Aspergillus flavus* which contaminates grain, have been shown to produce tumours in experimental animals. Alcohol may be important. Infection with the oriental liver fluke, *Clonorchis sinensis,* in the Far East predisposes to both hepatoma and cholangiocarcinoma, the latter accounting for up to 20% of all malignant tumours in China.

The use of some drugs is associated with tumour. The liver may convert some non-carcinogenic agents into carcinogenic metabolites. The prolonged use of oral contraceptives is associated with benign adenoma and hepatoma.

Workers exposed to vinyl chloride have developed fibrosis and angiosarcoma.

Hepatoma complicates most forms of cirrhosis – especially alcoholic cirrhosis and haemochromatosis (about 15% of cirrhotics die with the cancer). Cirrhosis is not, however, a necessary precursor to tumour.

Tumours may be single and massive, or multifocal and nodular. Cholangiocarcinoma may arise in cuboidal epithelium anywhere in the intrahepatic or extrahepatic biliary tree. It may complicate cysts and is occasionally associated with proctocolitis.

Primary Liver Tumours

Diagnostic features

Primary liver tumours tend to present in one of four ways:

Right upper quadrant pain, anorexia, weight loss
Sudden onset of ascites (possibly due to invasion and thrombosis of the portal vein)
Pain, a palpable lump, or general deterioration in a patient with pre-existing cirrhosis
Sudden intraperitoneal haemorrhage.

The serum alpha-feto-protein, as detected by radioimmunoassay, is positive in up to 99% of hepatomas.

Management and course

Death usually occurs within months of diagnosis. Resection may be possible with unifocal tumours and should certainly be attempted in young patients without cirrhosis. Some extenuation of the disease may be achieved by treatment with doxorubicin (Adriamycin).

Bile Duct Tumours

Diagnostic features

Wholly intrahepatic cholangiocarcinomas behave like hepatomas. Tumours of the extrahepatic bile duct present with progressive, usually painless, obstructive jaundice.

Ultrasonography will usually show dilatation of the ducts proximal to such an obstruction and percutaneous transhepatic cholangiography (PTC, p. 173) is the simplest way of demonstrating the lesion and establishing the site of the tumour. PTC is unlikely to fail in the presence of dilated extrahepatic ducts but if it does then endoscopic retrograde cholangio-pancreatography (ERCP, p. 173) may be diagnostic. PTC has greatly simplified the diagnosis of hepatic duct tumours in the hilum of the liver which may be difficult to detect at laparotomy.

Management

Bile-duct tumours are often slow-growing, which makes surgical removal attractive. In the hilum of the liver, operability largely depends on the absence of portal vein invasion. In this site, resection – though only possible in a minority of patients – is the ideal treatment, with restoration of continuity by anastomosing the proximal hepatic ducts to an isolated loop (Roux loop) of jejunum. If resection is not possible, palliation may be achieved by prosthetic intubation; recently, local irradiation of such tumours from within has been described, the radiation source being accurately placed within the tumour through a transhepatic tube.

Tumours arising at the termination of the common bile duct (ampullary) are less aggressive than those arising in the head of the pancreas and lend themselves to radical excision by the operation of pancreatico-duodenectomy, with about 40% 5-year survival (see p. 183).

TECHNIQUES FOR INVESTIGATING HEPATOBILIARY DISEASE

Although clinical skills remain paramount, extremely sophisticated diagnostic techniques are now available. See also Chapter 3.

Definition of Structural Change

This depends upon radiographic, radionuclide and ultrasonic techniques.

Plain x-rays

These may show liver size, gas or cysts within the liver or biliary tract, calcification in liver or pancreas, and the radio-opaque 10% of gall stones. Ascites may also be suggested on plain x-rays (Fig. 8.34).

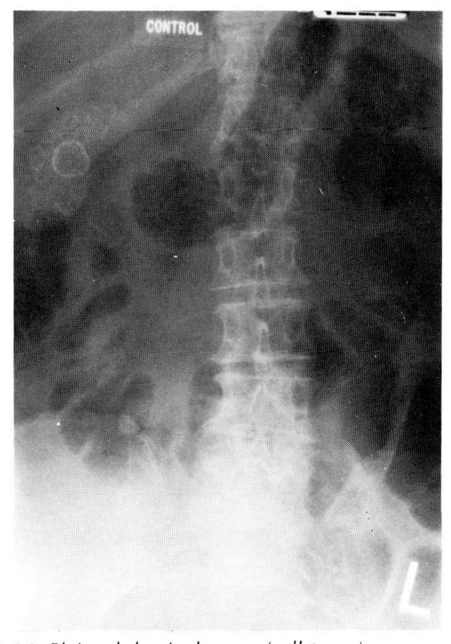

Fig. 8.34 *Plain abdominal x-ray (gallstones).*

Computed axial tomography (Fig. 8.35)

CT gives a good all-round picture of the liver and pancreas and may show dilated ducts, cysts and tumours well.

Biliary contrast radiology

Oral cholecystography (OCG) (Fig. 8.36). After a plain film, an OCG is the next investigation for right upper quadrant pain and intermittent jaundice. Opacities may fail to occur if the bilirubin exceeds twice normal. If liver function is normal, and the tablets have been taken and absorbed, a 'non-functioning' gall bladder strongly suggests gallstones. The gall bladder is encouraged to contract with a fatty meal, and this allows some

a

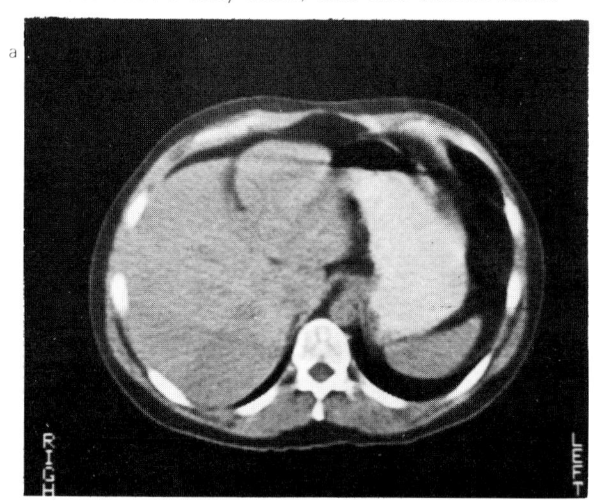

b

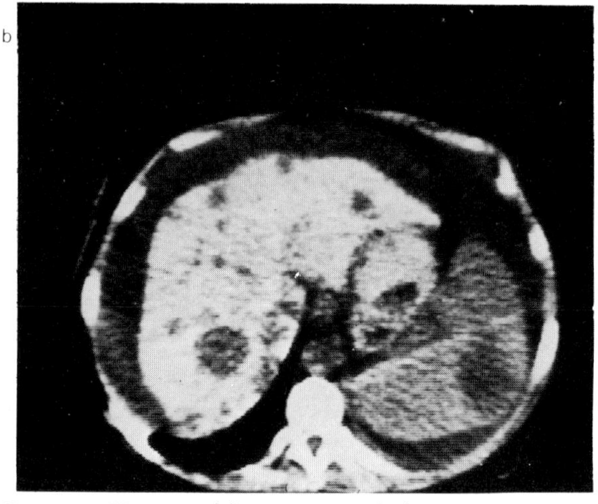

Fig. 8.35 *CT scans of liver. (a) Normal. (b) Metastases.*

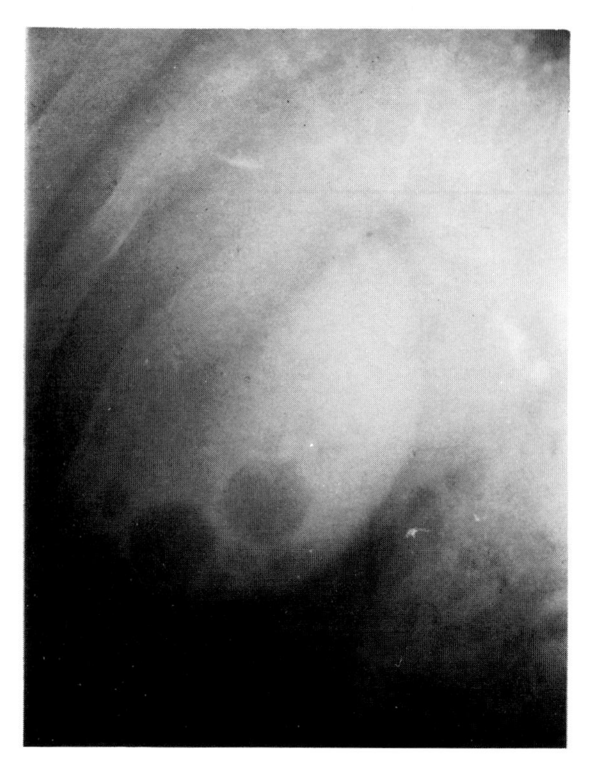

Fig. 8.36 *Oral cholecystogram showing stones.*

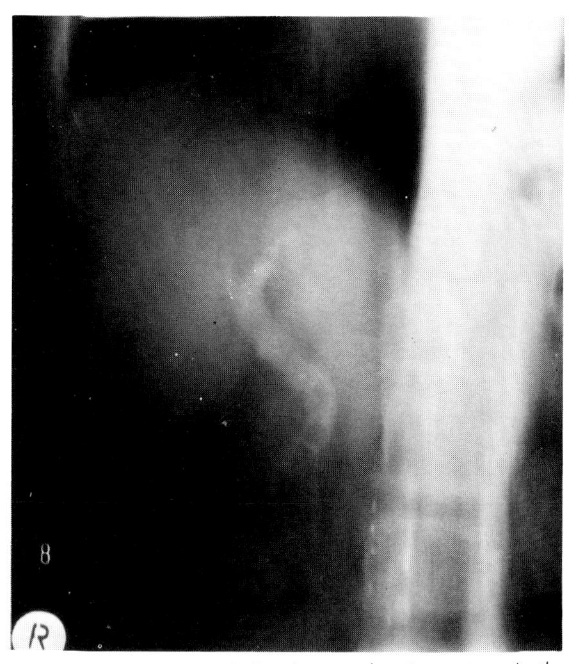

Fig. 8.37 *Intravenous cholangiogram showing a stone in the common bile duct.*

assessment of gall-bladder function and may increase the pick-up of small stones. A 'normal' OCG does not exclude gallstones.

Intravenous cholangiography (IVC) (Fig. 8.37). Intravenous iodopamide (Biligrafin) is excreted by the liver cells in sufficient concentration (assuming normal hepatic function) to outline the bile ducts and, in the absence of cystic duct obstruction, to outline the gall bladder. The degree of opacification does not approach that of cholecystography and an intravenous cholangiogram is not an alternative method of investigating the gall bladder. Tomography is an essential part of the study, but even so there is a 15–20% incidence of false negative results and stones can be missed. Nonetheless a positive result is helpful in forecasting the need to explore the duct system. Fatal allergic reactions can occur. Its main use is in suspected common duct stones and postcholecystectomy pain.

Direct injection contrast radiography. This is necessary in the investigation of prolonged jaundice in order to outline the biliary tree. It takes three forms:

a. *percutaneous transhepatic cholangiography (PTC).* This is accomplished using a fine 'skinny' needle, and is simple and relatively safe. As with liver biopsy (see p. 178), coagulation defects will preclude its use. Leakage is unusual but may occur when obstructed ducts are demonstrated. The needle is directed into the liver under x-ray control, while contrast is gently injected. Dilated ducts are surprisingly easy to 'hit' (Fig. 8.38).
b. *endoscopic retrograde cholangiography (ERC (P)).* Endoscopic cholangiography can be more time-consuming and demands more skill but gives excellent pictures of the common ducts and also allows the papilla of Vater to be inspected and the pancreatic duct to be cannulated. A fine-bore cannula is threaded down a fibre-optic endoscope emplaced in the duodenum and manoeuvred into the punctum of the papilla. Cholangitis is a rare complication. It may be carried out even when coagulation is impaired (Fig. 8.39).
c. *operative and postoperative T-tube cholangiography.* The duct system may be visualised at operation by injection of contrast material through a cannula placed in the cystic duct. This technique is used as a routine to search for stones and confirm that all have been removed (Fig. 8.40).

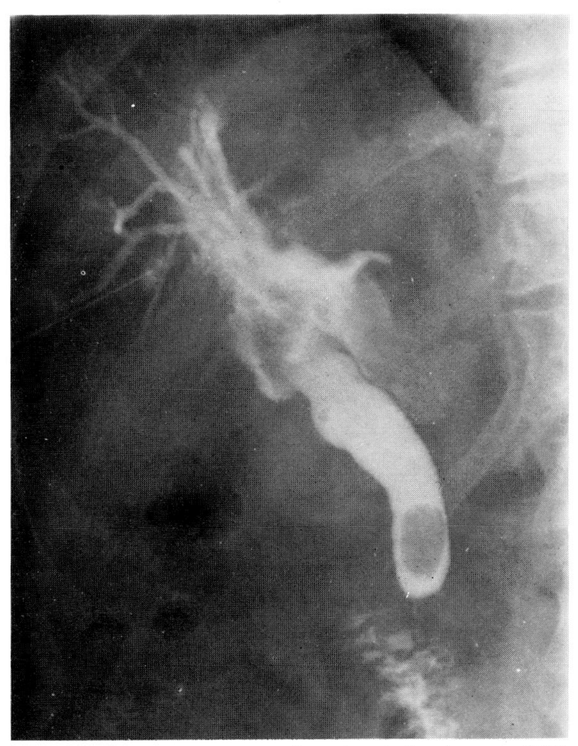

Fig. 8.38 *Percutaneous transhepatic cholangiogram (PTC) showing dilated duct (caused by stone in common bile duct).*

Vascular contrast radiology

Information on the size, shape and anatomy of the liver can be obtained by selective arteriography. It may be helpful in the elucidation of space-occupying lesions, showing tumour 'blushes' or avascular spaces, and in assessing operability. A transfemoral Seldinger technique is used to cannulate the coeliac axis.

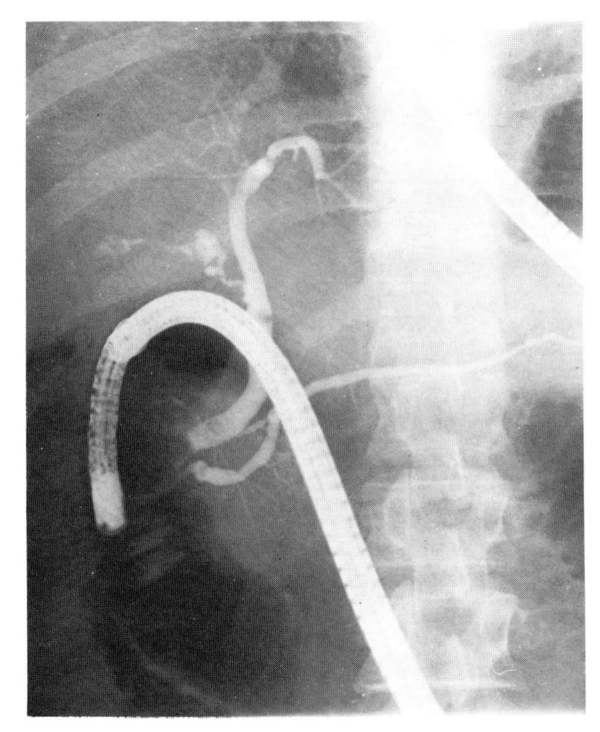

Fig. 8.39 *ERCP. Stones in common bile duct.*

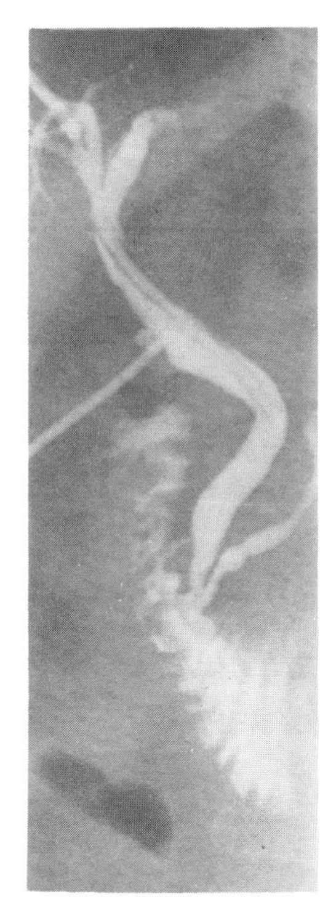

Fig. 8.40 *Normal T-tube cholangiogram.*

Venography may be achieved either by splenic puncture (splenic portography), cannulation of the vestigial umbilical vein, by direct liver puncture, or from the venous phase after contrast injection into the superior mesenteric artery.

Radionuclide imaging

Scintiscanning is widely used, and is simple, safe, relatively cheap and reasonably accurate for assessing liver size and shape, the presence of filling defects, and in some techniques biliary flow.

If the non-radioactive carrier is a 'foreign' particle (e.g. sulphur colloid), the Kupffer cells will pick it up and 'light up' all the functioning liver (scintiscanning). Alternatively if the carrier is an excreted anion (e.g. Rose Bengal or HIDA), excretion through the biliary tree can be imaged (cholescintigraphy). In each case the commonest radioisotope used is Technetium 99.

Radiogallium may be used where lymphoma or abscesses are suspected and radio seleniomethionine when a primary liver cancer is suspected.

Ultrasonic scanning

This carries the greatest potential. It is simple, painless, cheap, non-invasive and very accurate (especially with newer grey-scale techniques) but it is heavily dependent upon operator skill and quality of interpretation. It is the primary investigation in the jaundiced patient, when dilated ducts should be detected in up to 97% of cases with obstruction. It is also relatively accurate in picking up gallstones, especially when cholecystography is negative, and is useful in primary liver disease, especially cystic lesions. Being non-radiographic, it can safely be used in pregnancy (Figs 8.41, 8.42, 8.43).

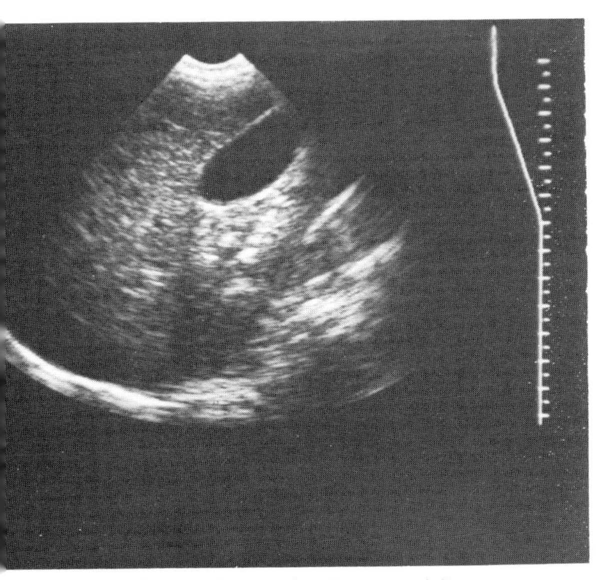

Fig. 8.41 *Ultrasound scan showing normal liver.*

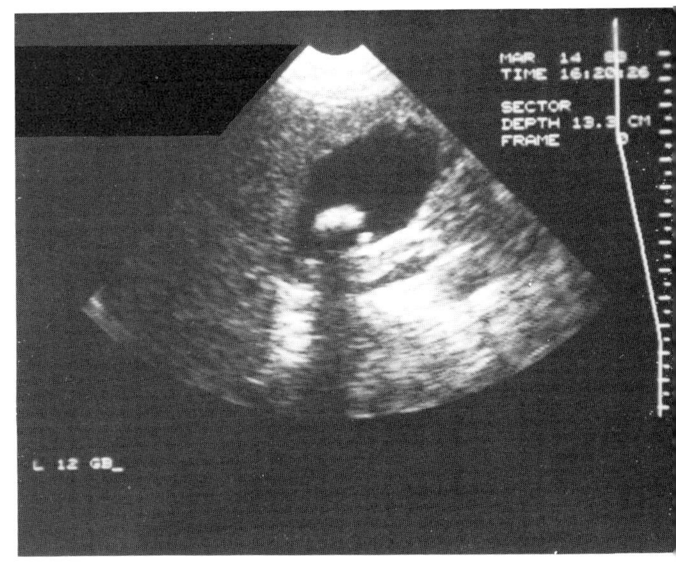

Fig. 8.42 *Ultrasound scan showing stone in gall bladder.*

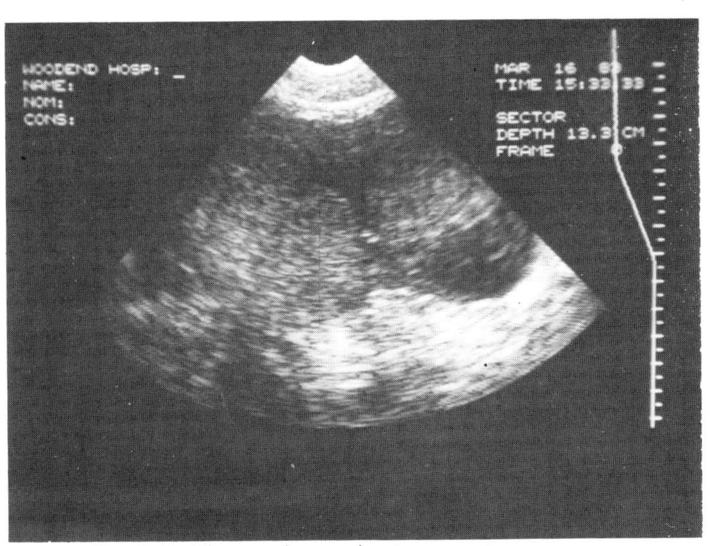

Fig. 8.43 *Ultrasound scan showing metastases.*

Tests of Cellular Injury and Dysfunction

There is some overlap of biochemical tests reflecting injury or dysfunction. So-called 'liver function tests' are useful in drawing attention to or confirming the hepatobiliary origins of the patient's problem and in monitoring progress but they have serious limitations in differential diagnosis and should always be used in conjunction with clinical and other diagnostic information.

Enzymes of parenchymal injury

Transaminases (aminotransferases) reflect liver and other tissue damage especially in cardiac and skeletal muscle. Alanine transaminase (ALT; serum glutamic pyruvic transaminase, SGPT) is more specifically related to liver damage, but it is not more sensitive than aspartate transaminase (AST; serum glutamic oxaloacetic transaminase, SGOT), and the latter is more generally used. Very high levels (over 1000 units) are found in hepatic necrosis, e.g. severe hepatitis, and occasionally in hepatic venous congestion. More modest elevations are not very helpful diagnostically. Transient elevations may occur in biliary colic and cholecystitis. Elevation due to cardiac infarction is usually obvious from the history and electrocardiogram. Normal or near-normal values can occur in cirrhosis.

Numerous other enzymes (e.g. lactic dehydrogenase, ornithine carbamoyl transferase) have been used in laboratories with special interests, but are not widely applicable. LDH isoenzymes are highly specific.

Enzymes of induction

Gamma glutamyl transpeptidase (GGT) is a sensitive enzyme now widely used as a screening test and, in conjuction with alkaline phosphatase, to establish the hepatic origin of the latter, with which it rises in concert. Some drugs, and particularly alcohol, cause modest to major rises in GGT (50–500 units).

'Duct' enzymes

Alkaline phosphatase (AP) is an important enzyme of several origins but is normally mostly derived from biliary ductular epithelium. Modest rises (up to twice normal) are common; they often reflect liver damage and may be difficult to interpret. Elevations in excess of 2–3 times normal occur in biliary tract obstruction and tend to rise along with bilirubin and GGT. Intrahepatic (non-surgical) cholestasis tends to be associated with minimal rises only. Space-occupying lesions – primary and secondary tumours and abscesses – can cause very high levels of AP (in excess of 6 times normal). Isoenzymes of AP occur in other tissues and can be separated by electrophoresis:

placenta (high AP is normal in pregnancy)
bone (elevations in fractures, bone secondaries, sarcoidosis, osteomalacia and Paget's disease) and in children with active growth
intestinal mucosa.

Bilirubin

Mild elevations of bilirubin (up to 4–5 times normal) may reflect increased production (haemolysis), impaired transport or conjugation (e.g. Gilbert's disease), or mild cellular damage.

Significant rises reflect a failure of excretion, i.e. either intrahepatic or extrahepatic cholestasis. Almost all will be conjugated bilirubin and will therefore be soluble in water and excreted in urine. Tests to split bilirubin into direct reacting (conjugated) and indirect (unconjugated) are largely a waste of time and money except in cases of mild recurring jaundice, and in neonatal jaundice.

High bilirubin levels occur in drug-induced and cholestatic viral hepatitis. In established liver disease, e.g. chronic hepatitis or cirrhosis, high levels denote a poor prognosis. Biliary obstruction may produce rapid rises in bilirubin, often progressive in carcinoma and fluctuant in stones and cholangitis.

Bilirubin is one of the best and most reliable 'function' tests, but it may be normal in quite advanced disease (e.g. cirrhosis, multiple secondaries). Other exogenous anions of similar metabolism, notably bromsulphthalein (BSP), have been used as sensitive tests of dysfunction but they are not generally applicable now.

Protein synthesis

Albumin tends to be low where protein synthesis is impaired or protein lost, e.g. cirrhosis, malignant disease (See Fig. 8.14). The plasma albumin may also be low in a variety of non-alimentary systemic disorders, e.g. severe infections.

Prothrombin time (PT) is a sensitive and useful indicator of hepatic function. In simple obstructive jaundice, prolongation may be rapidly reversed with parenteral vitamin K. In drug damage and hepatitis a lengthening or very prolonged PT suggests a poor prognosis.

(For haemostasis in liver disease see p. 191).

Other tests of protein abnormality, such as thymol turbidity, are no longer of any practical value.

Specific Disease Indicators

These are numerous and related to specific processes. They tend therefore to be highly discriminant. The most important are:

Viral markers

These are many but the single most important is hepatitis B surface antigen and, in view of the implications of a diagnosis of hepatitis B, should be done routinely in all jaundiced patients and in cases of chronic liver disease and unexplained hepatomegaly (see p. 158).

Tumour markers

A positive alpha-feto-protein test strongly suggests primary hepatoma.

Immunological markers

Mitochondrial antibodies are markedly discriminant for primary biliary cirrhosis (positive in 98% cases) and therefore useful.

Smooth muscle antibodies suggest chronic active hepatitis, but are not specific.

Histological Diagnosis

Ultimately a histological diagnosis should preferably be made in most cases (with exception of gallstone disease and the relief of extrahepatic obstruction).

Biopsy is possible by:

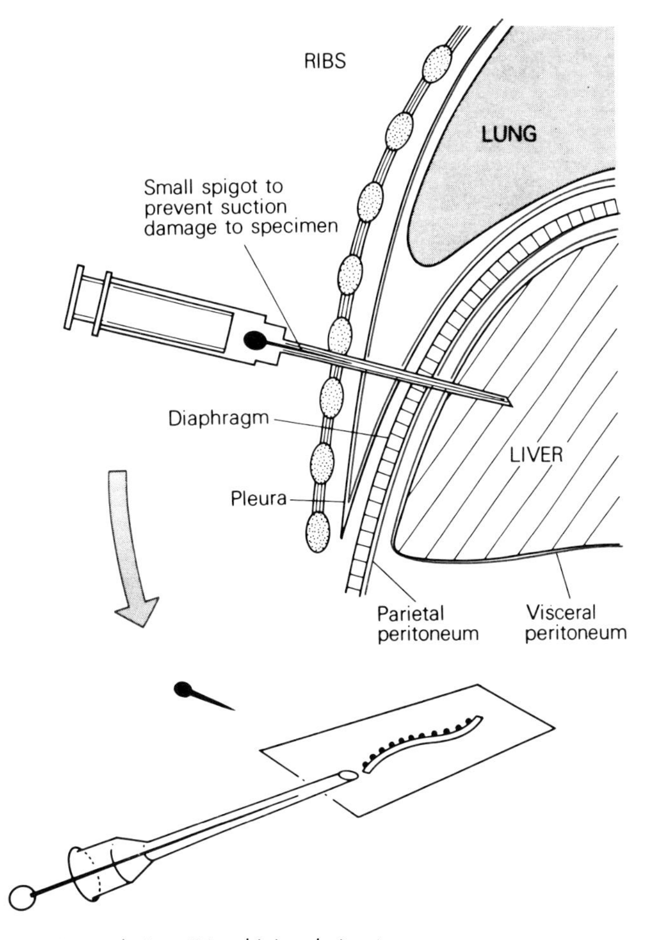

Fig. 8.44 *Needle biopsy with aspiration technique (Menghini technique).*

i. Blind puncture using an aspiration (Menghini) or cutting (Trucut Vim) needle (Fig. 8.44).
ii. Directed biopsy during inspection of the liver at laparoscopy or by ultrasound or CT screening.
iii. Open biopsy ('wedge' biopsy) at laparotomy.

Needle biopsy is simple, generally safe in experienced hands, and very useful. Blood clotting must be satisfactory (prothrombin ratio not more than 1:3, platelet count greater than 80–100 000) and the patient capable of cooperating. After local anaesthetic the patient holds his breath while the needle is advanced via the 8th or 9th intercostal space. Serious complications include bleeding, biliary leakage, and pneumothorax, but are rare in experienced hands. Biopsy is contra-indicated where hydatid or angioma is suspected. Laparoscopy (peritoneoscopy) has the advantage of direct vision of the liver surface and permits target biopsy of specific areas but, with the increasing diagnostic accuracy of imaging techniques, is not often necessary.

Biopsy, of course, requires skill in interpretation. Some conditions are associated with problems of sampling error. In addition to diagnosis, biopsy may be used to monitor treatment and progress (e.g. in chronic hepatitis).

CLINICAL PRESENTATION AND MANAGEMENT OF HEPATOBILIARY DISEASE

This section attempts to convey the economical and clinical reasoning process that leads to diagnosis and to management in patients who present with clinical features of liver or biliary tract disease.

Jaundice (Fig. 8.45)

A patient with haemolytic anaemia may develop a mild degree of clinically apparent jaundice from excess circulating unconjugated bilirubin, but jaundice is seldom the presenting feature. Therefore jaundice as a presenting clinical sign will almost always be a feature of hepatobiliary disease. In jaundice, diagnostic logic is primarily directed towards establishing whether or not the cause is post-hepatic, i.e. extrahepatic obstruction (EHO) which, in direct contrast to other forms of jaundice, is usually an indication for operation. During the past few years the differentiation of EHO from other causes of jaundice has been made much easier by the imaging technique of ultrasonography, which does not involve ionising radiation and has no known biological side-effects. Although this technique has greatly simplified the diagnosis of EHO, it does not supplant clinical diagnosis based upon history-taking and clinical examination.

Clinical features

The first diagnostic indicator is the patient's age. A child or teenager with jaundice is likely to have viral hepatitis and may give a history of contact. An aged patient is more likely to have EHO.

The presence or absence of abdominal pain antedating the onset of jaundice is an important diagnostic feature. Servere pain suggests EHO and usually means obstruction by stone or by pancreatitis. Pain together with fluctuating intensity of jaundice strongly suggest EHO due to stones. Insidious, progressive jaundice especially in the aged is suggestive of malignant obstruction. However, drug-induced cholestasis is similar, and it is essential to define drug exposure in every patient with jaundice. The alcoholic may deny or minimise his or her intake but it may be obvious from the demeanour, facies, palmar erythema and tremor.

Thus, these simple facts lead meaningfully towards or away from a diagnosis of EHO. Pruritus, which is probably attributable to bile-salt accumulation in the skin, is a feature of obstructive jaundice but does not differentiate EHO from intrahepatic cholestasis. Weight loss with progressive jaundice usually suggests malignant obstruction. However, cholangitis, usually secondary to stones but with fluctuating jaundice and fever, is

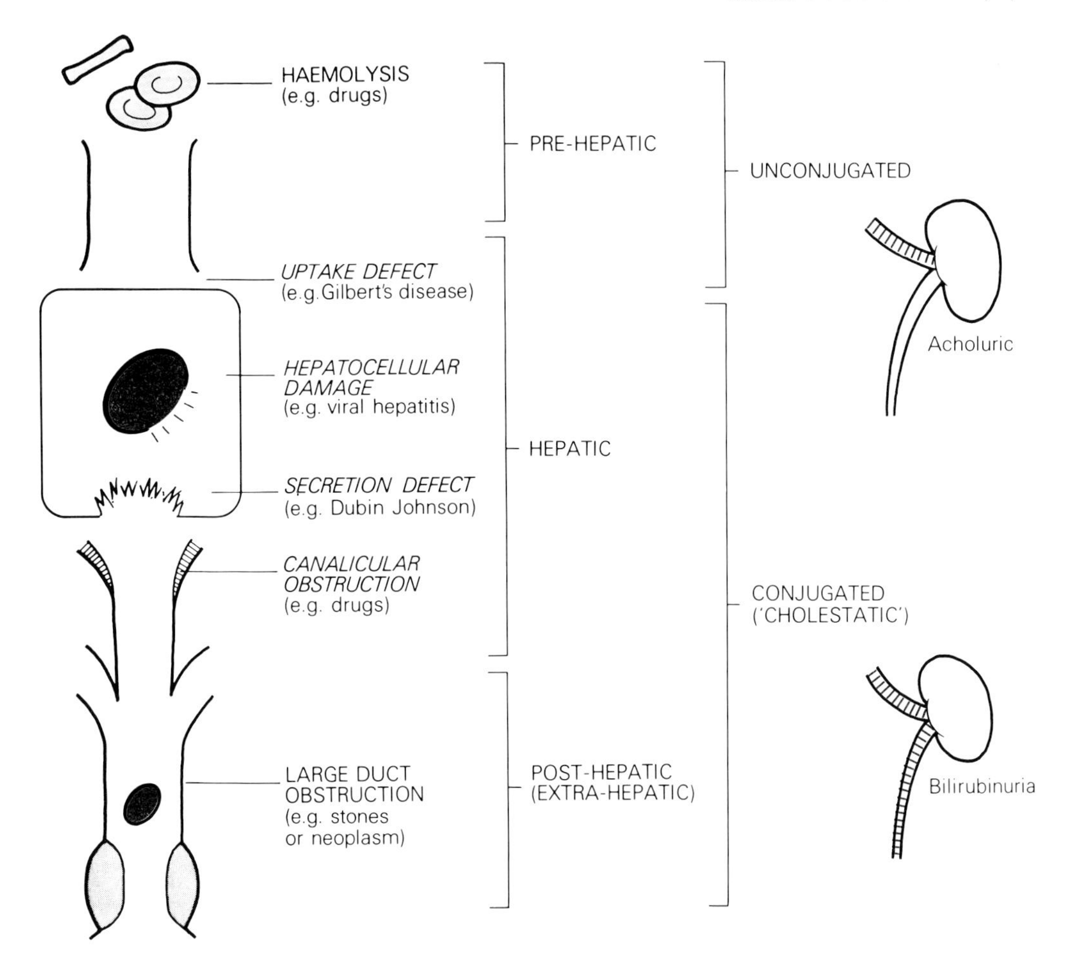

Fig. 8.45 *Classification of jaundice.*

also associated with weight loss, at times profound.

On general examination of the patient, the degree of jaundice is first apparent. Deep jaundice, in which the skin is orange-yellow or (later) greenish, is an indication of EHO. Severe pruritus may be evidenced by scratch marks on the skin. Mental impairment or mild personality change suggests hepatocellular jaundice. Foetor and flapping tremor are signs of impending hepatic coma (see p. 195). Stigmata of chronic liver disease, e.g. vascular spiders (Fig. 8.46), palmar erythema, white nails, gynaecomastia and loss of secondary sexual hair, are looked for. In alcoholics these stigmata may include parotid enlargement and Dupuytren's contracture. The neck should

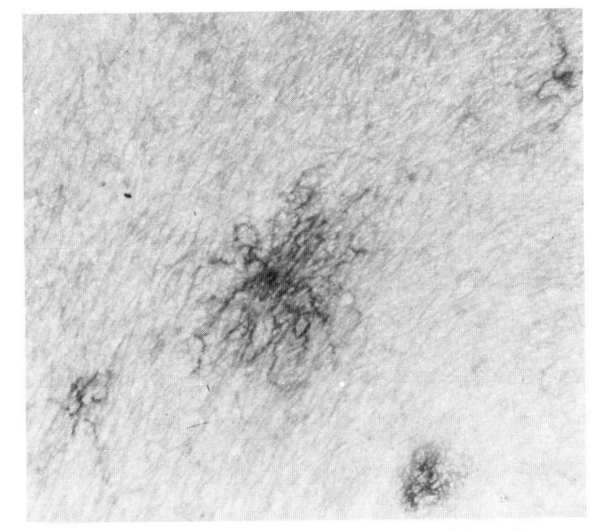

Fig. 8.46 *Spider angioma in skin of patient with liver disease.*

always be carefully felt for the presence of lymphadenopathy.

Useful diagnostic information is likely to come from abdominal examination. Ascites may be due to cirrhosis or to metastatic malignant disease of the peritoneum. The whole of the abdomen is palpated but attention is focused on the right upper quadrant. In EHO the liver is almost always palpably enlarged with a smooth blunt edge; failure to feel it makes the diagnosis doubtful. The gall bladder is much less constantly distended and more difficult to feel. It may lack distensibility as a result of fibrosis associated with chronic cholecystitis or, even when distended, may be hidden by the liver edge. If the fundus of a distended gall bladder can be felt, this suggests malignant obstruction (Courvoisier's rule, Fig. 8.47). If the liver is large and grossly nodular, extensive hepatic metastatic cancer is almost certain. In hepatitis the liver edge is tender.

Rectal examination must not be overlooked since, in disseminated intra-abdominal malignant disease, pelvic peritoneal deposits resulting from transcoelomic spread are often palpable; their detection indicates the advanced nature of the disease. In an aged jaundiced patient with a hard knobbly liver and palpable pelvic metastatic disease, the diagnosis of advanced malignant disease is a clinical certainty even in the outpatient clinic and admission to hospital for investigation is both needless and useless. Jaundice is, however, a late feature of metastatic disease. It requires clinical experience to make such a decision, and otherwise jaundiced patients do require in-patient investigation.

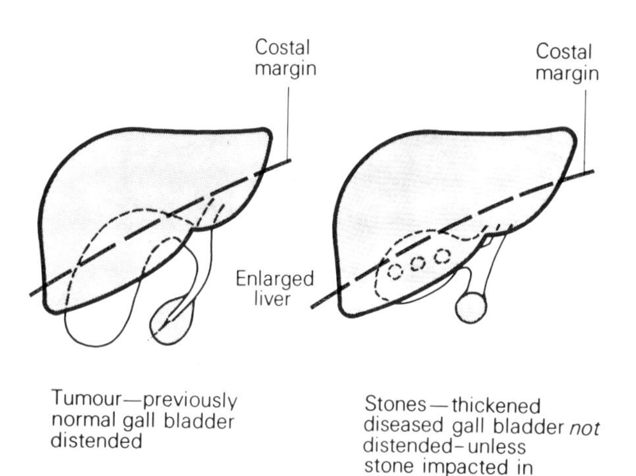

Fig. 8.47 *Courvoisier's rule.*

Pale, acholic faeces obtained at rectal examination suggests biliary obstruction but does not differentiate intrahepatic cholestasis from EHO. Occult blood in the faeces raises suspicion of ampullary cancer or of alimentary cancer with jaundice attributable to metastatic disease.

Further investigation

Urine. The simplest and first investigation is examination of the urine. Bilirubinuria is present in both hepatocellular and obstructive jaundice, but absent in haemolytic jaundice. In complete obstruction, usually due to malignant disease, bile does not enter the gut and therefore urobilinogen is absent from the urine. In haemolytic jaundice, excess urobilinogen is present in the urine and the faeces are dark in colour.

Biochemical abnormalities (see p. 175). Serum biochemical tests are of limited value, but the serum bilirubin level is a useful measure of increasing or decreasing depth of jaundice. A low serum albumin and a high globulin level is suggestive of chronic hepatocellular disease.

Haematological abnormalities. In obstructive jaundice, the absence of bile salts in the gut results in impaired fat absorption and may therefore lead to deficiency of the fat-soluble vitamin K, which is necessary for prothrombin synthesis. Such deficiency may be detected by prolongation of the prothrombin time and may be evidenced by a bleeding tendency. Parenteral administration (usually intramuscular) of vitamin K_1 will result in correction of the abnormality in obstructive jaundice but is of little benefit in hepatocellular jaundice, in which liver-cell synthesis of prothrombin is impaired.

Immunological abnormalities (see p. 163). Hepatitis antigens (see p. 158). Antimitochondrial antibody (see p. 163).

Plain x-rays. A chest film is taken to exclude primary or secondary tumours. Plain x-ray of the right upper quadrant is diagnostically essential to pick up the 10% of stones which are opaque.

Special investigations. Clinical assessment, together with the above simple investigations, will often lead to a clinical diagnosis and a firm opinion on the likelihood of EHO. The appropriate and simple confirmatory investigation is an ultrasonic scan of the liver and biliary tree. In EHO dilated intrahepatic and extrahepatic bile ducts are reliably visualised though differentiation between calculus and malignant obstruction is less reliable. The abnormal texture of the cirrhotic liver may also be apparent on ultrasonography.

If dilated ducts are not seen, and the clinical diagnosis is viral hepatitis or drug-induced jaundice, the patient will usually improve over the course of a week or two and further investigation may be unnecessary. In a patient with advanced cirrhosis complicated by jaundice, the diagnosis is usually obvious; if possible, this diagnosis should be confirmed by biopsy.

In patients thought not to have EHO, in whom jaundice deepens rather than improves over 2–3 weeks, and where the diagnosis remains uncertain, further investigation is necessary. Ultrasonography should be repeated. If still negative, the duct system may be visualised by injection of radiographic contrast material directly into the ducts either by percutaneous transhepatic cholangiography (PTC) or endoscopic retrograde cholangiopancreatography (ERCP). PTC is the simpler procedure and, even when the duct system is not dilated, it is possible to visualise it in most patients. If the duct system is dilated, PTC succeeds in over 90% of patients and determines the site of obstruction: failure of PTC makes dilated

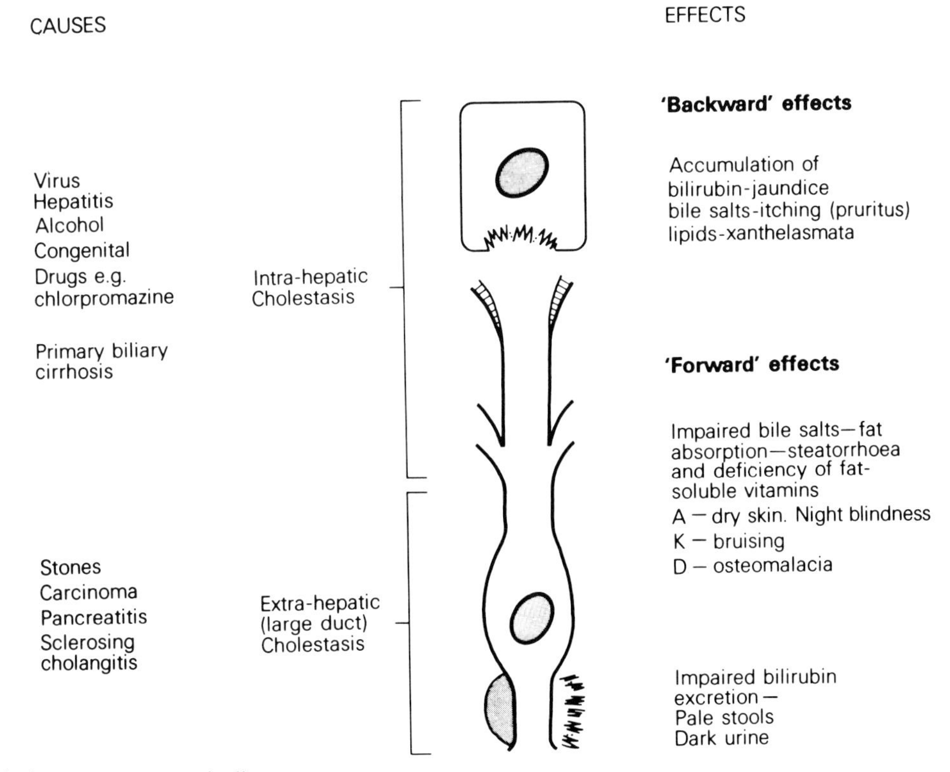

Fig. 8.48 *Cholestasis – causes and effects.*

ducts unlikely but should this still be considered possible, ERCP is indicated. Before the development of these important and effective techniques such patients underwent diagnostic laparotomy but nowadays this procedure, potentially hazardous in the presence of deep long-standing jaundice and impaired liver function, is almost never necessary.

If the diagnosis is still elusive and EHO is ruled out, percutaneous needle biopsy of the liver is indicated. Figure 8.48 shows causes and effects of cholestatic jaundice.

Management of extrahepatic obstruction

The diagnosis of EHO will usually have been made, early in the course of jaundice, by clinical assessment, and will have been confirmed by ultrasound. If the duration of jaundice is short, and the clinical presentation together with the ultrasound findings is that of stone in the common bile duct, either passage or disimpaction of the stone may occur, with spontaneous relief of the jaundice. Thus, if the diagnosis is calculous obstruction, operation may be delayed in the hope of spontaneous improvement. If liver function returns to normal, further investigation by cholangiography and cholecystography will be possible. When jaundice is lasting and progressive, however, unless there is evidence of advanced disseminated malignant disease, early surgical relief of the obstruction is indicated. Operation should be preceded by PTC, which may confirm the diagnosis and define its site as well as (often) clarifying the nature of the obstruction. This is helpful in forecasting the complexity of the operation and the likely time required. PTC should be 'covered' by a prophylactic broad-spectrum antibiotic since, in the presence of infected bile, there is a risk of bacteraemia. If the prothrombin time is prolonged, vitamin K_1 is given intramuscularly for some days beforehand, and the patient should be well hydrated, if necessary by intravenous fluid.

The aims of the operation are:

to relieve the obstruction,
to eradicate the disease (if possible), and
to minimise the risks of doing so.

In the simple example of stone or stones in the common bile duct, the gall bladder is removed, the duct is incised and the stones cleared (Fig. 8.49a). It is important to make sure that the papillary region is normal and to be as certain as possible that all the stones have been removed. This may be confirmed by intraoperative x-rays taken after injection of contrast material into the duct system. In the presence of multiple small stones it is wise to carry out choledochoduodenostomy (Fig. 8.49b). After exploration of the common bile duct it is customary to guard against the possibility of bile leakage by inserting a latex T-tube, which drains bile to the exterior. T-tubes are removed at about 2 weeks and further contrast x-rays are taken before doing so to re-confirm the absence of residual stones (Fig. 8.40). The need for T-tubes after duct exploration is debated.

Biliary obstruction caused by localised tumour in the ampullary region or in the adjacent head of pancreas is best treated by radical excision (pancreaticoduodenectomy: Whipple's operation – Fig. 8.49c). This is one of the major abdominal operations and involves excision of the distal stomach and the whole of the duodenum, together with the head of the pancreas and the distal common bile duct. The mortality rate of such procedures approaches 10% but the cure rate for periampullary carcinoma is about 40%.

If the obstructing tumour at the lower end of the common duct is inoperable or associated with metastatic disease, the obstruction may be bypassed to relieve the jaundice (Fig. 8.49d). This is most satisfactorily achieved by anastomosing the fundus of the gall bladder to an isolated limb (Roux loop) of jejunum.

Tumours involving the common hepatic duct are best removed if they have not invaded the portal vein, and continuity is restored by bringing a Roux loop of jejunum to the hilum of the liver for anastomosis to the proximal hepatic ducts. If such tumours are inoperable because of local invasion, the duct lumen may be reestablished by dilatation and a silastic tube may be inserted to maintain luminal patency. It is now possible to intubate malignant strictures of the biliary tract percutaneously or endoscopically (Fig. 8.49e) and this

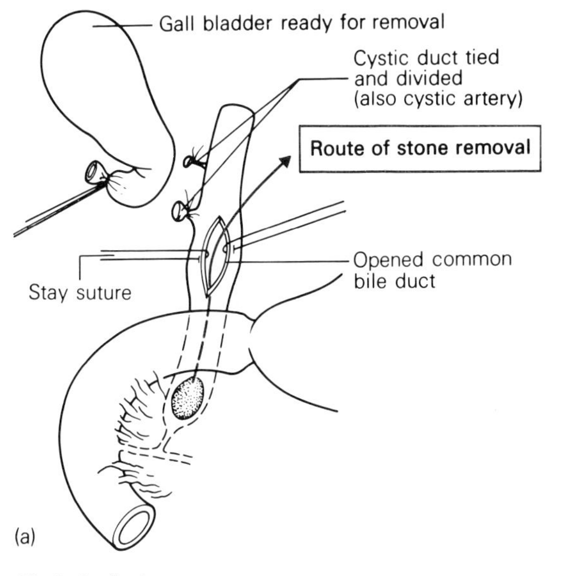

Choledochotomy

Choledochoduodenostomy

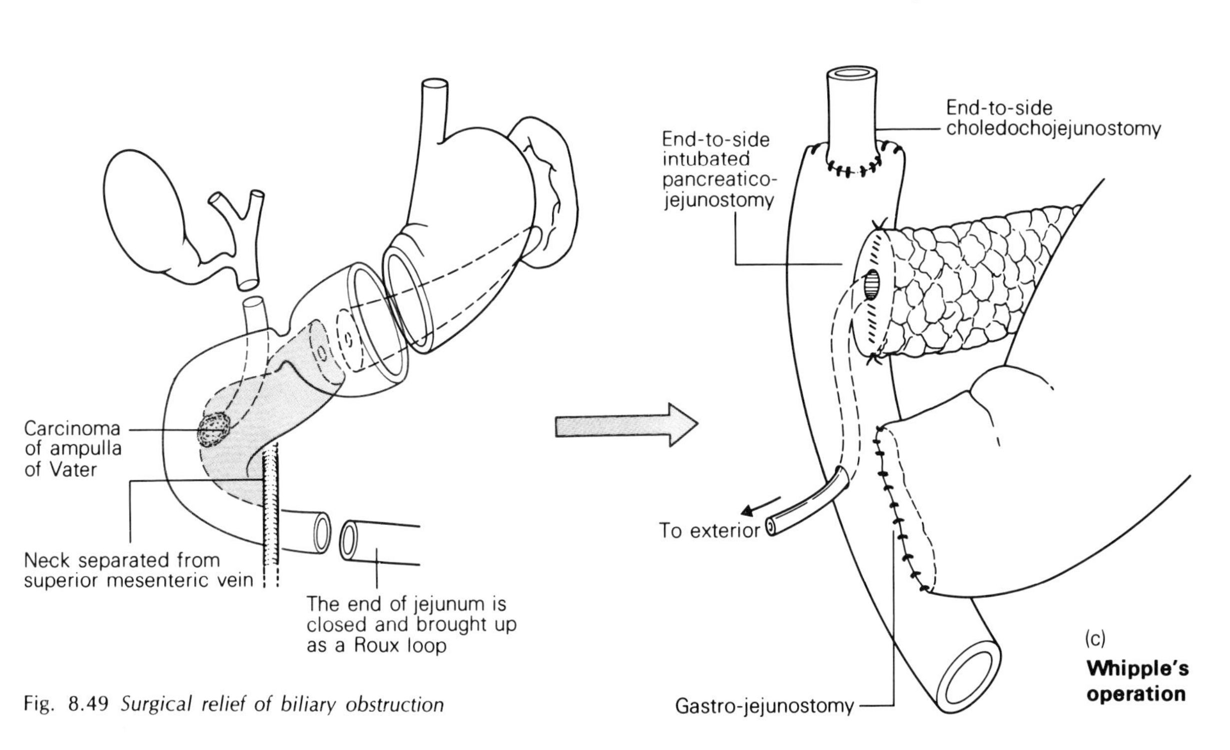

Fig. 8.49 *Surgical relief of biliary obstruction*

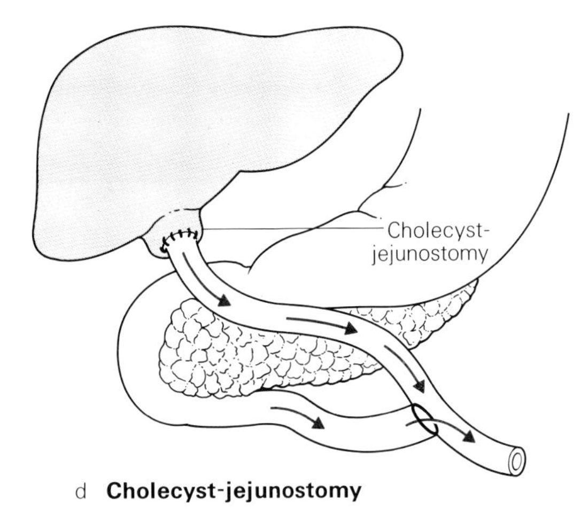

d **Cholecyst-jejunostomy**

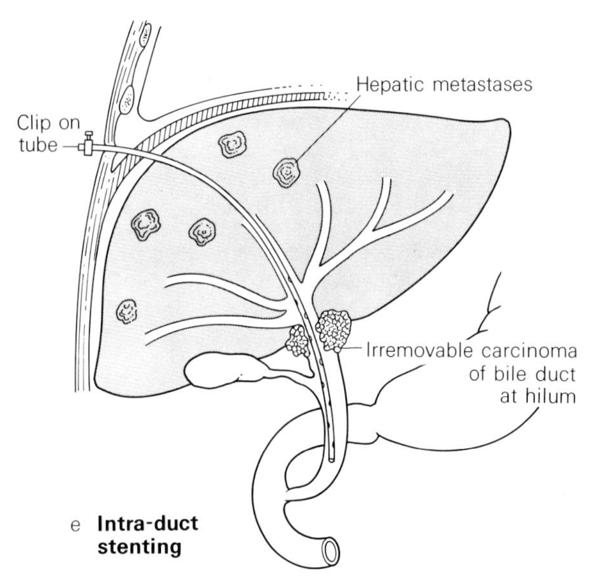

e **Intra-duct stenting**

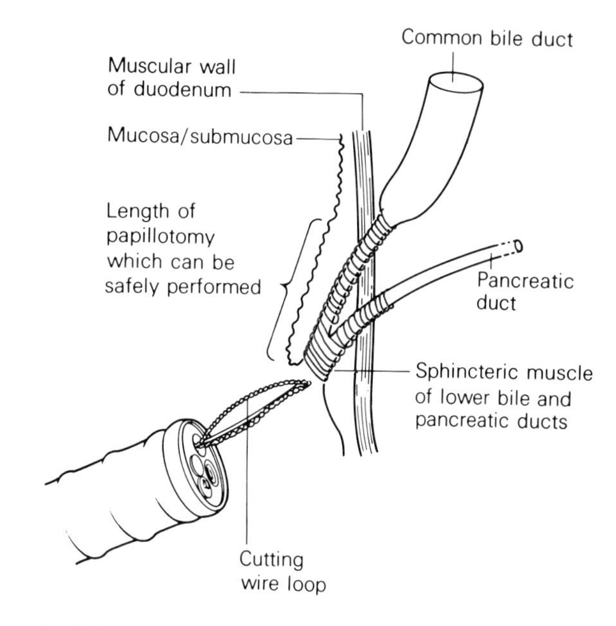

f **Endoscopic sphincterotomy and stone removal**

Fig. 8.49 *Surgical relief of biliary obstruction.*

improves the quality of life by relieving jaundice and pruritus.

It is also possible to perform sphincterotomy and removal of common duct stones via the fibre-optic endoscope (Fig. 8.49f).

Hazards of operation in deeply jaundiced patients. The risks of defective haemostasis, though rare, are real and require attention. Similarly, wound healing may be impaired and so wound closure must be technically sound. The major hazards are infection and acute renal failure. In biliary obstruction due to stones, infected bile is common (much less so in obstruction due to tumour). There is therefore a risk of bacteraemia and endotoxaemia during operation, and of wound contamination with subsequent wound infection . These risks are minimised by prophylactic antibiotic (e.g. gentamicin or cefotaxime) immediately before and during operation.

The precise explanation for the development of the syndrome of acute renal failure (ARF) in relation to jaundice and operation is not known. A majoı factor is diminished glomerular filtration and renal hypoperfusion, which can be forestalled by good peri-operative hydration and maintenance of a high rate of urine flow.

Jaundiced patients must be catheterised and have their hourly urine flow measured during the first 48 hours after operation. Urine flow during operation is augmented by intravenous mannitol. Hourly urine volume must be watched critically after operation; if this falls below 28 ml/hr it indicates a falling GFR – urine flow will usually improve on plasma-volume restoration by intravenous colloid (usually plasma protein solution). Occasionally, when urine flow fails to improve on colloid infusion, it will improve after Mannitol.

Hepatic failure is a remote risk of operation in a jaundiced patient.

Pain Originating in the Liver and Biliary Tract

Precise explanations of the mechanisms underlying the production of pain from disease of the liver and biliary tree cannot be given but various types of pain can be categorised and logically explained to become a basis for clinical diagnosis.

Pain arising in the liver

This is usually felt as a dull ache in the right upper abdomen and over the rib cage. Such pain (which can sometimes be severe) is thought to be produced by rapid distension of the liver capsule, as may occur in viral hepatitis or acute congestive cardiac failure. Focal disease such as liver abscess or tumour may also produce discomfort. Pain is, however, not necessarily a feature of these conditions and, in malignant disease, whether primary or secondary, pain is a late development and usually indicates advanced disease. If an inflammatory or neoplastic process in the liver extends to involve the parietal peritoneum over the undersurface of the diaphragm then pain may be referred, via phrenic afferents, to the right shoulder tip (see p. 34).

If a focal abnormality is suspected, a raised alkaline phosphatase level is supportive and ultrasound is usually diagnostic.

Pain arising in the biliary tract

This is experienced very much more often than liver pain. The various patterns of pain that stem from the biliary tract are almost all due to the presence of gallstones but , very infrequently, the gall bladder may be responsible for pain in the absence of stones. A tumour at the lower end of the common bile duct may also obstruct the termination of the main pancreatic duct to produce pain from pancreatitis as well as obstructive jaundice, a combination that may suggest gallstone obstruction. Thus not all malignant obstruction of the bile duct is painless.

Gallstone-related pain

Gallstones may remain 'silent' for years. When they are responsible for pain, the mechanisms are uncertain but it is assumed that migration occurs into sites where the stones interfere with gall-bladder emptying or ejection of bile through the duodenal papilla. Pain may be explained on the basis of inappropriate rise of pressure within the gall bladder and resultant distension. The character of the pain depends on whether the obstruction is intermittent or lasting, and whether bacterial inflammation complicates it. Similar severe pain may also result from intense muscle spasm independent of gall-bladder obstruction. The bile ducts contain little smooth muscle in their walls except within the complex sphincter arrangement at the lower end of the common bile duct (sphincter of Oddi), and the most severe biliary pain is logically explicable on the basis of muscle spasm in that area. Such pain is usually called 'biliary colic', but this term is inaccurate since the pain may not be 'colicky'.

Biliary Colic. This is one of the most severe types of abdominal pain. It begins fairly abruptly, most often in the epigastrium rather than in the right upper quadrant, radiates through to the tip of the right scapula, builds up to a level of severe, steady intensity and usually lasts a matter of hours. It is often associated with nausea, vomiting, sweating and restlessness. The patient is unable to continue whatever task he or she was engaged in and will usually call out the family doctor. Relief often requires a potent analgesic such as pethidine and the patient is left with an aftermath of upper abdominal discomfort during the following day or two. Gallstone-induced pain of this type is explained either by acute obstruction of the cystic duct or by transient impaction of a stone at the lower end of the common bile duct with resultant severe muscle spasm: it is not possible to distinguish between the two simply from analysis of the pain. Whilst the pain of biliary colic is fairly characteristic, it can be confused with other important conditions, such as myocardial infarction, and acute pancreatitis.

On examination there is little to be found except some tenderness under the right costal margin: rarely, the gall bladder may be palpable. Recovery is usually rapid. Figure 8.50 illustrates diagnosis of biliary pain.

The appearance of bile in the urine, or disturbances of liver function tests, in association with biliary colic, strongly suggests a stone in the common bile duct. Continuing impaction of a stone at the lower end of the duct will lead to obstructive jaundice.

Biliary colic with jaundice (Fig. 8.51). The development of jaundice due to impaction of a stone is not necessarily an indication for early operation, because such stones may pass on into the duodenum, or they may disimpact upwards. In the acute obstruction phase, when no contrast radiography is possible, ultrasonography can be of great help in showing dilatation of the bile ducts, and the obstructing stone. If the jaundice resolves, intravenous cholangiography becomes possible.

Operation to remove the stone or stones in the duct is usually an elective procedure. An operative cholangiogram is done to show the position and number of stones, which are then removed, along with the gall bladder in which they have grown.

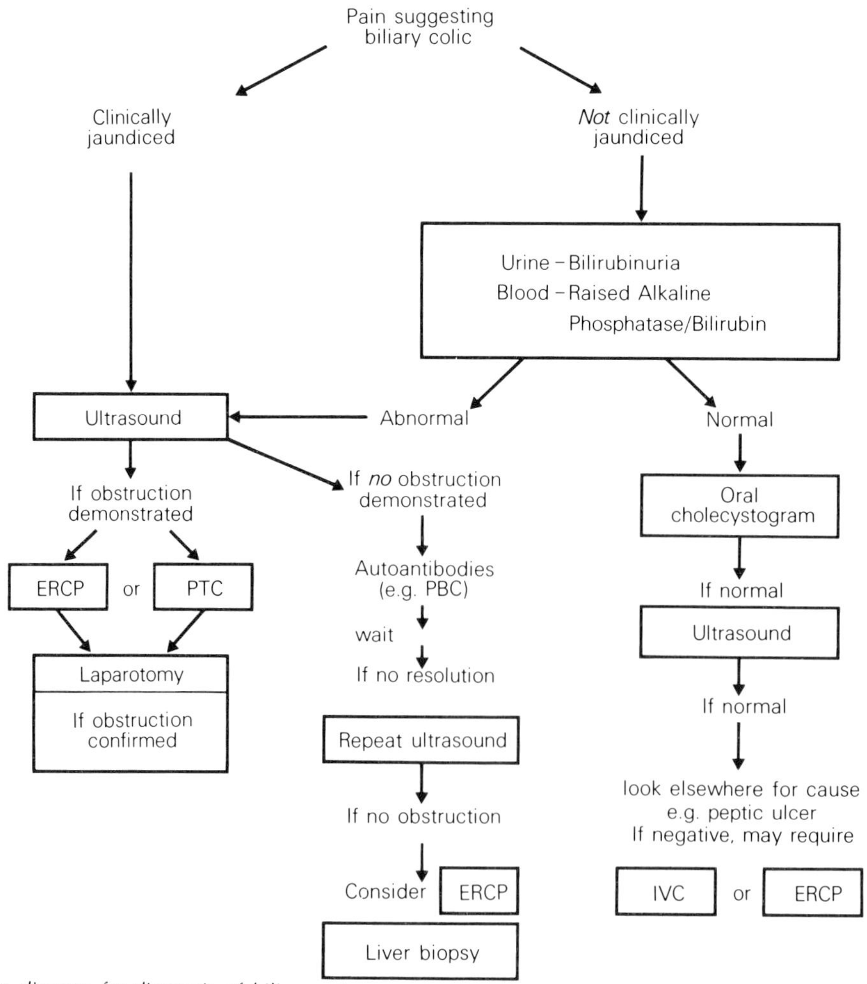

Fig. 8.50 *Flow diagram for diagnosis of biliary pain.*

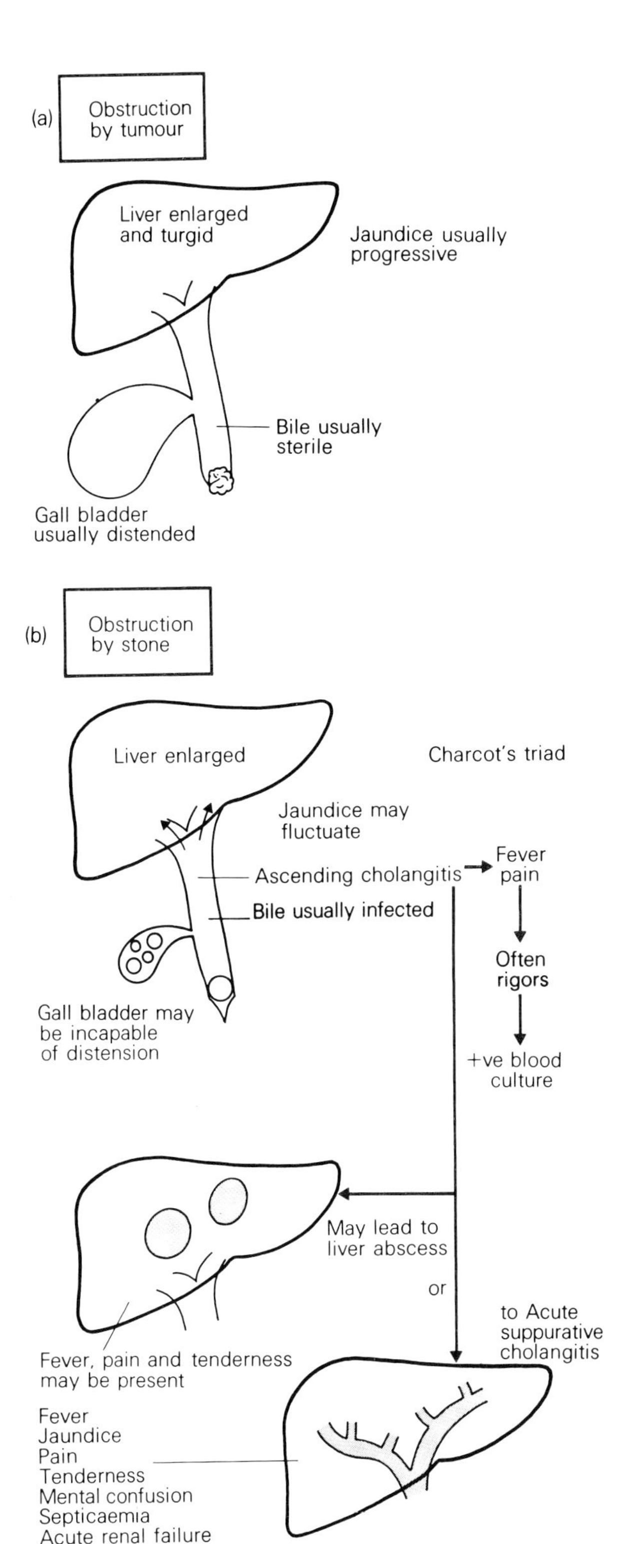

Fig. 8.51 *Clinical presentation of obstruction and infection.*

The indications for early operation are:

continued impaction with progressively deepening jaundice
superimposition of acute suppurative cholangitis.

Patients may present, years after cholecystectomy, with a stone in the commmon bile duct which was either overlooked at the original operation or which has subsequently formed (primarily) within the duct. In some centres where the technique has been developed it is possible to manage these patients by incising the papilla with a diathermy wire loop passed through a duodenoscope (endoscopic papillotomy, Fig. 8.49f) and thereafter extracting the stone or stones using an ingenious spiral wire basket which is expanded inside the duct to enmesh the stone and withdraw it. A proportion of these stones are quite large, however, and require operative removal.

Acute cholecystitis. Stones in the gall bladder must, for most of the time, remain mobile and relatively asymptomatic. When an attack of biliary colic occurs, a stone may impact at the neck of the gall bladder or in the cystic or bile duct but, when the attack passes off, the stone either disimpacts and falls back into the gall bladder, or is forwarded down the ducts, sometimes passing through the ampulla of Vater.

When, however, a stone at the neck of the gall bladder (Hartmann's pouch) fails to disimpact and remains stuck in that position, one of two things may happen:

1. If the bile is sterile, the mucus secreted by the gall bladder mucosa slowly accumulates to produce a mucocoele (Fig. 8.33).

2. If the bile is infected at the time of impaction, suppuration occurs within the obstructed gall bladder to produce acute obstructive cholecystitis. The gall-bladder wall becomes acutely inflamed and tension within the gall bladder rises as a purulent exudate forms. In about 70% of such patients the increasing expansion of the gall-bladder wall allows the stone to drop back into the gall bladder; the mucopurulent contents can then drain down the cystic and bile ducts and the attack comes to an end.

If, however, the stone remains stuck at the junction of gall bladder and cystic duct, the gall bladder distends with pus to form an empyema. If the infection is a virulent one, this process is likely to go on to patchy mural necrosis, gangrene and perforation: this may in turn produce either a generalised peritonitis or a localised abscess around the gall bladder (Fig. 8.33).

Acute cholecystitis may supervene upon an episode of biliary colic, but it more usually develops as a continuous pain, less intense than that of biliary colic, localised in the right upper quadrant. The pain may radiate round the right lower rib cage and upwards towards the scapula. Systemic effects of sepsis are present and inflammation of the visceral surface and the overlying parietal peritoneum results in local tenderness and signs of parietal peritoneal irritation, e.g. local muscle rigidity and percussion tenderness (more coarsely elicited by rebound tenderness). Nausea and vomiting are frequent, and x-rays may show local dilatation of small bowel. Most patients with acute cholecystitis will improve rapidly on a regime of temporary nasogastric tube aspiration, intravenous fluids, and antibiotics, because these give time for disimpaction of the stone to occur. Elective cholecystectomy may be planned 6–8 weeks later. Such patients are, however, exposed to the risks of failure and the complications outlined earlier. They may also suffer a subsequent acute episode while awaiting elective operation. Therefore the benefits of early operation – not as an emergency, but within days of admission to hospital – are increasingly appreciated and this policy is also economical of hospital resources and shortens the duration of illness. If early operation is intended, accurate diagnosis is essential: this has been greatly simplified by ultrasound, which can clearly demonstrate the oedematous wall of the gall bladder, together with the contained stones.

These patients must be closely observed because, although resolution of an attack of acute cholecystitis often occurs, in some cases an empyema forms. It is vital to recognise that persistent pain and fever, with tenderness and guarding over the gall bladder, is an indication for urgent operation: the gall-bladder wall is tense, and is often ischaemic, but emergency cholecystectomy is generally followed by a quick recovery.

Chronic cholecystitis. Most gall bladders which have contained stones for many months or years show signs of chronic inflammation in the wall. There is no certainty whether the inflammation preceded and encouraged stone formation, or whether the stones provided the conditions favourable to the establishment of infection. In no more than 20% of such gall bladders will bile show an active infection. It is common to find a rather shrunken, white, thick-walled gall bladder, containing many faceted stones, that has clearly contained little or no bile for a long time.

The typical symptom complex in such patients is one of recurrent biliary pain, often after eating fatty foods. Nausea, together with a feeling of gaseous distension, and frequent eructation, is associated with the pain. Typically the patient avoids foods with a high fat content such as fried food, eggs, cream, cheese, chocolate and pork. Such an association may, however, be absent and quite often patients avoid fats solely because they have been advised to do so by their general practitioner. The pain is explained on the basis of disturbance of gall-bladder emptying, with temporary obstructive features and inappropriate increase in intraluminal pressures, but without complete obstruction to the outflow of bile from the gall bladder. There is seldom any clinical abnormality on examining a patient complaining of such symptoms, but there may be deep tenderness over the gall bladder fundus, which is most easily elicited in deep inspiration (Murphy's sign).

Acalculous cholecystitis. There are some patients with typical symptoms of gall-bladder disease in whom a cholecystogram and ultrasonography apparently show no evidence of stones. Very occasionally, the cholecystogram shows the appearance of adenomyomatosis (cholecystitis glandularis proliferans), in which there is glandular proliferation (Rokitansky–Aschoff sinuses) within the gall bladder wall to produce the appearance of pseudodiverticula.

There remain patients with apparently typical

symptoms in whom throrough investigation of the gall bladder is completely negative, yet symptoms are so troublesome as to justify laparotomy (exploratory operation) and removal of the apparently-normal gall bladder. When the gall bladder is opened after excision, it may contain fine biliary debris or its wall may show cholesterol deposition within the mucosa (cholesterolosis). Associated mucosal inflammation with the superimposed pale flecks of cholesterol gives the appearance of 'strawberry gall bladder'. The outcome of such operations cannot be guaranteed though symptoms are certainly relieved in some patients.

Medical treatment of gallstones. It is possible to dissolve small cholesterol (non-opaque) stones in a functioning gall bladder by the administration over many months of the bile salts chenodeoxycholic acid or ursodeoxycholic acid, which desaturate the bile with respect to cholesterol and slowly dissolve the stones. Such medical treatment of gallstones is presently unattractive; it has no effect on secondary structural abnormalities on the gall bladder and, on cessation, the bile reverts to its supersaturated quality. It may, however, be considered in the occasional patient who is unfit for surgery and who has non-opaque stones in a functioning gall bladder. In an aged patient with infrequent mild symptoms, avoidance of fats may give sufficient symptomatic relief, and the patient may feel happier to avoid operation.

Cholecystectomy. In every patient in whom a decision to remove the gall bladder has been taken, the possibility of stone or stones in the duct system must be considered. The likelihood is increased by a history of jaundice, when it is wise to visualise the duct system before operation by intravenous cholangiography. The operation of cholecystectomy is usually a straightforward and relatively minor procedure, but care must be taken to define the anatomy of the cystic duct and artery because variations from normal are common and failure to define them may result in serious injury to the duct system or right hepatic artery. During operation it is increasingly accepted that routine intra-operative x-ray of the duct system (operative cholangiogram) is wise and this is done by injection of contrast material through the cystic duct. The presence or suspicion of stone in the duct system is an indication for duct exploration.

Liver Enlargement

Liver enlargement may be found in patients who present with the associated upper abdominal discomfort or with associated features of general ill health, or may be an entirely incidental and unexpected clinical finding.

In infancy, the liver is normally readily palpable. It may be enlarged as a result of rare abnormalities such as glycogen storage disease, or the rare primary malignant tumour, hepatoblastoma. In young adults in Western countries, the commonest cause of liver enlargement is alcohol abuse. The possibility of primary hepatic cell malignancy (hepatoma) must be considered. In women of child-bearing age, the rare benign conditions of hepatic adenoma and focal nodular hyperplasia may be asymptomatic, or be discovered because of the complication of haemorrhage into the liver substance or into the peritoneal cavity.

In later life, hepatomegaly is commonly due to alcohol and malignant disease. Metastatic disease is much more common than primary malignancy, but the rapid development of liver enlargement in a cirrhotic patient suggests hepatoma. Other causes include cardiac failure, leukaemia and myelofibrosis.

The cause of liver enlargement will often be apparent from clinical assessment, especially if there are other features of cardiac failure or if the spleen is also large. In addition, the large hard knobbly liver of extensive metastatic disease is often readily appreciated. If the liver is enlarged in isolation from any other clinical abnormality, and without characteristic features of metastases, the first investigation should include a chest x-ray to exclude primary or secondary tumour in the lungs, followed by liver scanning techniques. Ultrasound should be very accurate in defining abnormalities within the liver and, even if no focal abnormality is found, percutaneous needle biopsy may be diagnostic. If metastatic disease is confirmed, this is generally an indication to cease further investigation in the humane recognition that the patient can only at present be offered symptomatic treatment.

If a localised liver mass is apparent on ultrasound it will also be possible to define whether it is cystic or solid. Liver cysts and abscesses may be aspirated percutaneously under ultrasonic direction and isolated solid masses may similarly be biopsied. Suspected hydatid cyst (p. 352) is a clear contra-indication to aspiration because of the risk of spillage of fluid with dissemination, as well as the possibility of anaphylactic reaction to cyst contents. Calcification suggests hydatid, and a specific complement fixation test is available. A solitary tumour mass, whether it be primary or secondary, requires that the possibility of treatment by liver resection should be considered. In that case, further information on the disposition of the mass in relation to the principal plane separating the liver lobes may be gained at laparoscopy, which also facilitates target biopsy. Information on the disposition of the mass in relation to the hepatic vasculature is gained by hepatic arteriography and by portal phlebograms obtained during the venous phase after superior mesenteric arteriography (Fig. 8.52).

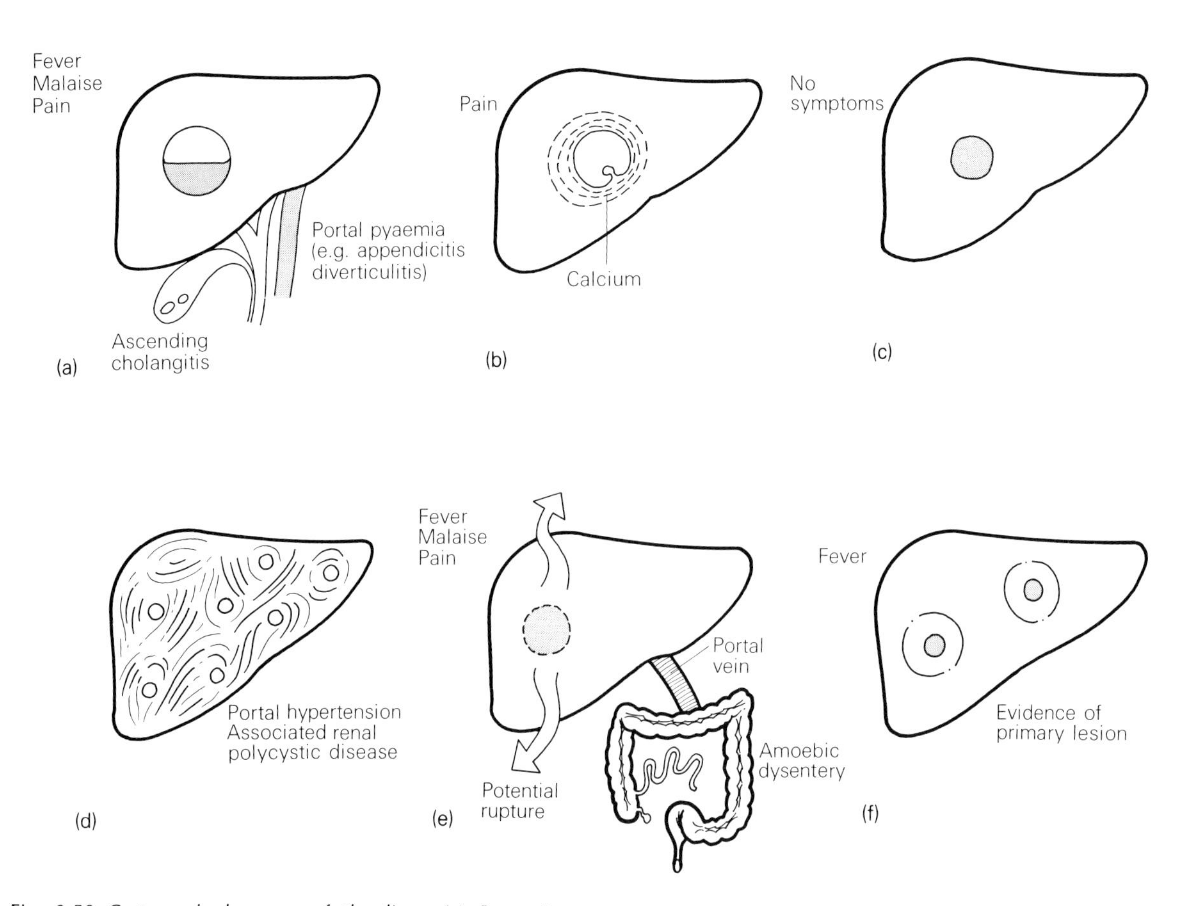

Fig. 8.52 *Cysts and abscesses of the liver. (a) Pyogenic abscess. (b) Hydatid cyst. (c) Solitary cyst. (d) Fibro-polycystic Disease. (e) Amoebic abscess. (f) Secondary tumour with necrosis.*

Haemorrhage

General disturbances of haemostasis

Bleeding is the commonest mode of death in liver failure. A bleeding diathesis is common in liver disease and in prolonged biliary obstruction, although in the latter it is usually rapidly reversible since it is mainly due to vitamin K malabsorption.

Coagulation problems are summarised in Fig. 8.53.

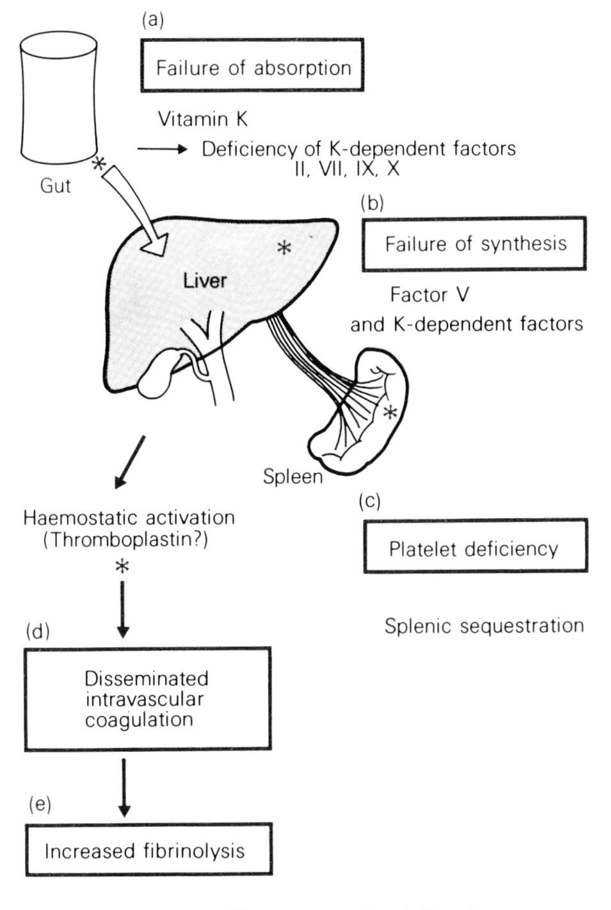

Fig. 8.53 *Coagulation problems in liver disease.*

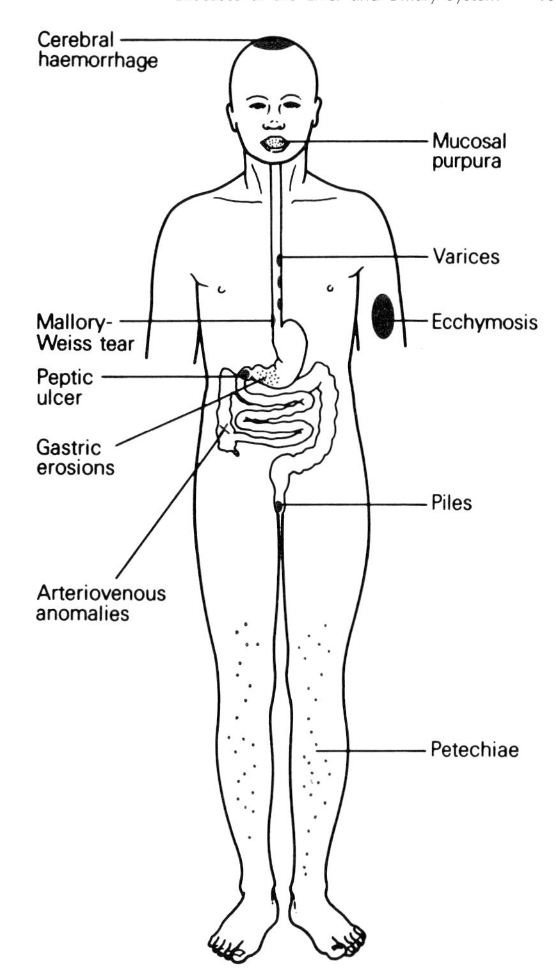

Fig. 8.54 *Bleeding sites in liver disease.*

Bleeding may be into skin (petechiae, ecchymoses) and mucous membranes, or (rather rarely) into serosal spaces, joints, and brain (Fig. 8.54).

There is a strong predilection for bleeding into the alimentary tract, for several reasons:

- vomiting and retching producing a Mallory – Weiss tear of oesophageal mucosa
- gastric erosions, of uncertain causation, are relatively common
- bleeding from coexistent peptic ulcer
- portal hypertension with oesophageal and gastric varices

Alimentary haemorrhage is a major problem with high mortality. Management is detailed in Chapter 14; only specific points relative to liver disease are mentioned here.

Estimation of haemoglobin, prothrombin time, and platelet count are baseline information in all liver-disease patients. Where bleeding is evident or major, and intervention is therefore planned, a full 'clotting screen' with estimation of other coagulation parameters (such as thrombin clotting time) is advisable to reveal the rare patient with a clotting abnormality despite a normal prothrombin time.

In emergency, the freshest blood possible should be used and 10 mg of vitamin K given slowly intravenously (pure vitamin K deficiency may be corrected within several hours). Factor concentrates and platelet infusions may be required where bleeding continues or where operation or biopsy is necessary in patients with defects. In emergency, two units of fresh frozen plasma may be given. Hypocalcaemia is a potential risk in patients requiring large volumes of citrated blood.

Portal hypertension

Portal blood-flow (1500 ml/min) constitutes about 75% of total hepatic blood supply. Rise in portal pressure results from obstruction at one of three sites (Figs 14.13, 14.14, 14.15).

a. In the portal vein (*Prehepatic*). This is usually thrombus due to infection in the neonatal period or secondary to encroachment upon the vein by hepatic tumours.

b. In the liver (*Hepatic*)
   cirrhosis
   schistosomiasis
   congenital hepatic fibrosis
   central vein sclerosis (as occurs in acute alcoholic liver disease)
   the reason for the rise in pressure in this group is not clearly understood.

c. In the hepatic venous drainage (*Posthepatic*)

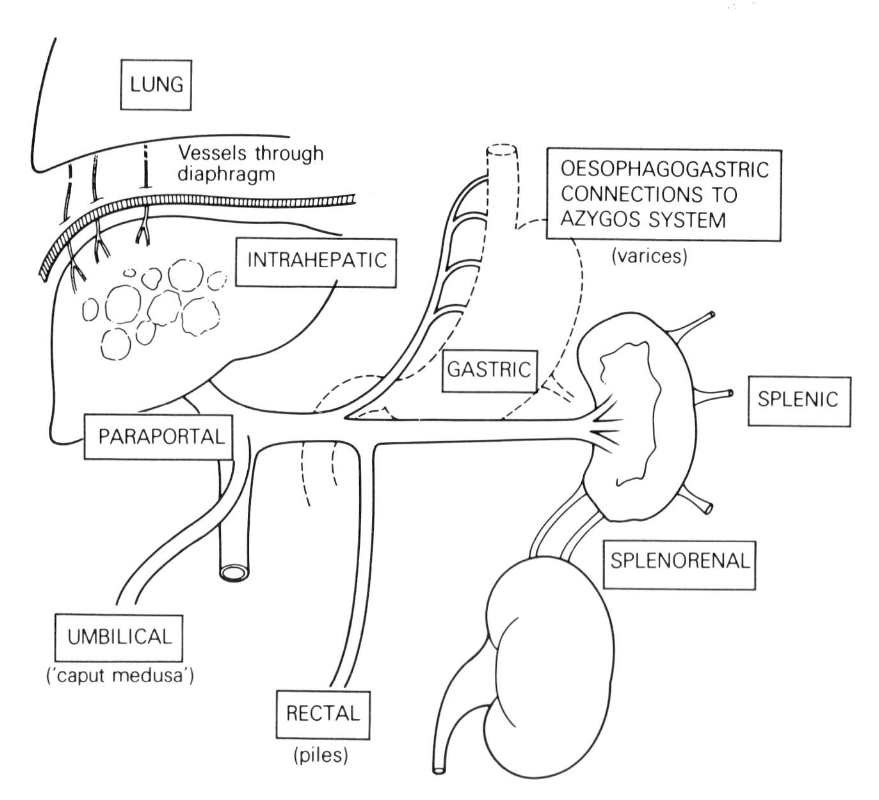

Fig. 8.55 *Portasystemic connections.*

hepatic vein occlusion (Budd–Chiari syndrome)
constrictive pericarditis, e.g. tuberculosis
severe right-heart failure, predominantly tricuspid incompetence.

Increase in pressure leads to opening up of dormant anastomotic channels (Fig. 8.55). As sources of haemorrhage, only the oesophagogastric channels are of clinical significance because they cause severe and continuing bleeding into the alimentary tract. Bleeding from other anastomotic sites is rarely troublesome.

Dilated veins may be evident on the abdominal wall (Fig. 8.56). The radiating leash of veins from the umbilicus (caput medusa) beloved of textbook writers is only rarely seen. The spleen is invariably enlarged: this leads to hypersplensim with a low white-cell count and thrombocytopenia.

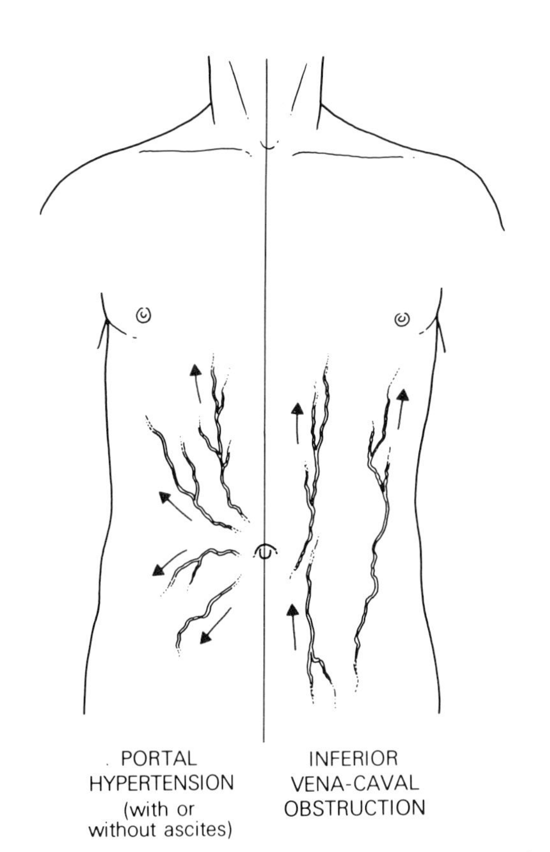

Fig. 8.56 *Distended abdominal wall veins. Arrows show direction of flow.*

Portal hypertension (and varices) may remain dormant for many years and the reason why bleeding from varices suddenly occurs is often obscure. A superimposed hepatitis in the alcholic cirrhotic (following a drinking bout) may rapidly raise portal pressure still further. Trauma from sharp food or coughing and retching is probably a factor in some. Aspirin and other analgesics have been implicated.

The portal venous system can be demonstrated by injection of dye into the spleen (splenic portogram) or by selective arteriography and venous phase films. Alternatively, filling may be achieved by injection into the liver itself or the vestigial umbilical vein (see p. 174). This is a prerequisite if shunt surgery is being contemplated.

Intrahepatic diversion of blood away from functioning parenchyma is an important feature of cirrhosis. Hence, sudden decompression of portal hypertension, as happens in

a devastating bleed and fall in blood volume
a surgically-created 'additional' shunt,

further insults an already-compromised blood supply and may precipitate liver failure. This is why shunt surgery in cirrhotics tends to stop bleeding from varices but does not extend life. Surgical shunts are being done less often now, and are reserved for special problems in patients with well-preserved liver function (e.g. congenital hepatic fibrosis).

Details of the management of variceal bleeding are given in Chapter 14.

Abdominal Distension (Ascites)

In liver disease, abdominal swelling reflects ascites together with the gaseous bowel distension that commonly accompanies it. Intestinal obstruction may be simulated. Tense ascites may be confused with gross bladder enlargement and also with a large ovarian cyst, although in these the maximum girth is lower abdominal and the flanks are resonant (see p. 39).

Ascites (Greek, askos: a bag), the accumulation of peritoneal fluid, has many causes broadly divisible into two groups:

Exudates Protein greater than 3 g/100 ml.	1. Infections	Tuberculous Pneumococcal
	2. Malignancy	Peritoneal Secondaries
	3. Pancreatic disease	
	4. Chronic venous congestion	Congestive cardiac failure Constrictive pericarditis Budd – Chiari syndrome (Hepatic vein thrombosis)
Transudates Protein usually less than 3 g/100 ml	1. Hepatic disease	Cirrhosis
	2. Hypoproteinaemia	'Nephrotic syndrome' 'Protein-losing enteropathy'

Other rare causes of ascites include biliary leakage and uropathic ascites in neonates.

The mechanism of ascites in liver disease involves a combination of hypoalbuminaemia and portal venous obstruction, together with rather ill-understood functional renal disturbances (Figs 8.57, 8.58). Escape of lymph from the liver surface also occurs. Sodium is avidly retained and the whole body sodium increased even though the serum sodium may actually be low, due to haemodilution and redistribution.

Onset of ascites may be either insidious and gradual or sudden. Sudden appearances of ascites suggests one of two situations. Firstly, there may

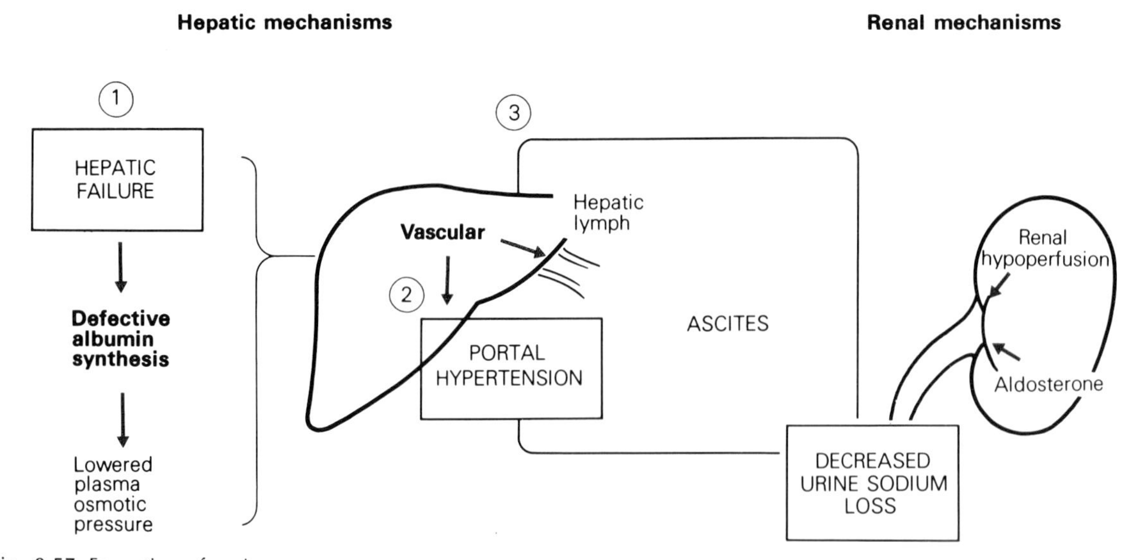

Fig. 8.57 *Formation of ascites.*

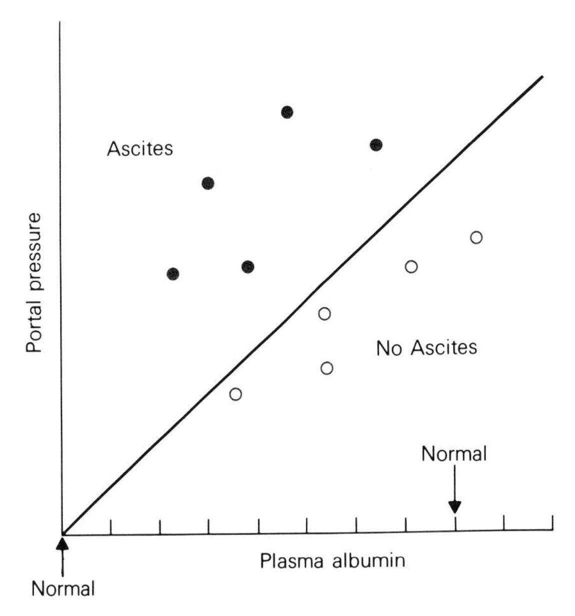

Fig. 8.58 *Relation between plasma albumin and portal pressure.*

be an acute rise in portal pressure, as in portal or hepatic vein thrombosis, and the fairly rapid occlusion of the central (terminal hepatic) veins that occurs especially in acute alcoholic hepatitis. Secondly, there may be an expisode of acute liver impairment following haemorrhage, hypoxia or septicaemia. Pain suggests a primary liver tumour involving the portal vein but it also occurs in acute occlusion of the hepatic outflow veins (Budd–Chiari syndrome).

Clinical signs include dullness in the flanks (in mild ascites) and shifting dullness and a fluid thrill (in tense ascites). The umbilicus is everted and existing hernias are exaggerated. It may be possible to ballotte the liver, i.e. to feel the liver 'hit' the fingers on quick gentle pressure. Similarly, malignant masses may be palpable. Rectal and vaginal examinations should be carried out to exclude pelvic disease. Pleural effusions are common in liver disease but also occur in other forms of ascites. Venous distension and acute new striae may be evident in the abdominal wall.

Management of hepatic ascites. Diagnostic paracentesis, tapping of a little fluid (30–50 ml) with syringe and needle, should *always* be done. Occult opportunistic infection is common in cirrhosis. The fluid should be sent for microscopy and culture and for estimation of albumin content. 'Therapeutic' paracentesis should *never* be done: it may precipitate liver failure and acute sodium and albumin depletion and is only of temporary benefit. An occasional exception may be made in a severely discomforted patient with end-stage liver disease or malignant disease.

Salt restriction is the sheet anchor of therapy. 'No added salt' may be adequate: in refractory cases, restriction to a strict 20–25 m mol/24 hours may be necessary. Salt substitutes can help to make this diet less objectionable. Potassium-sparing diuretics are especially valuable, since hypokalaemia is common in cirrhosis. Furthermore, hypokalaemia is aggravated by thiazides and frusemide and tends to precipitate encephalopathy. Spironolactone, 100–400 mg daily, is the drug of choice; its disadvantages are its high cost, the 4–5 day delay in action, and its tendency to produce gynaecomastia. Amiloride is an alternative. Treatment can be commenced with spironolactone. If this fails, a small increasing dose of thiazide or loop diuretic may be added.

In the very rare really resistant case, ascites may be recycled into the circulation either by intravenous infustion or via a special surgically-emplaced shunt (Leveen shunt).

Correction of ascites should not be too vigorous. Removal is largely for comfort and cosmetic reasons: overall, liver function is not improved and may indeed be worsened.

Hepatic Encephalopathy

This neuropsychiatric complication of liver disease is a major, though relatively uncommon, manifestation of liver failure. It also arises when there is substantial portasystemic diversion of blood and is therefore a common complication of shunt operations. The mechanisms are unknown. One possibility is the absorption of 'toxic' substances in the gut, (from protein digestion) which either bypass the liver because of shunting, or which the failing liver cannot degrade, or a combination of both. Postulated substances have included ammonia, amines, and free fatty acids (Fig. 8.59). An attractive theory, but one for which the evidence is thin, suggests the formation of false neurotransmitter substances, e.g. octopamine and phenylethanolamine, in the brain, which block receptor sites in neurotransmission.

The nature of the syndrome depends upon whether the failure is acute (see p. 198) or chronic, i.e. superimposed upon preexisting liver disease.

Chronic Encephalopathy (precoma)

This condition occurs episodically in patients with chronic liver disease, especially those with a great deal of naturally-occurring portasystemic shunting or with surgically-constructed shunts. Precipitating factors include superimposed hepatitis (as may happen following an alcoholic binge), infections, a gastrointestinal bleed, and electrolyte disturbance (hypokalaemia from diuretic use). In very susceptible patients, use of a sedative drug, constipation, or even a high protein meal may be sufficient to precipitate encephalopathy.

Clinical features. These include insidious personality changes and intellectual impairment in long-standing disease. In acute exacerbations there may be irritability, euphoria, inappropriate social behaviour, apraxia (inability to construct shapes or to follow a trail-making test), ataxia, dysarthria and a slow jerking flap on the outstretched fingers ('flapping tremor', asterixis). Eventually, drowsiness, stupor and coma supervene. Neurological changes may occasionally be severe and include paraplegia and quadriplegia. A character-

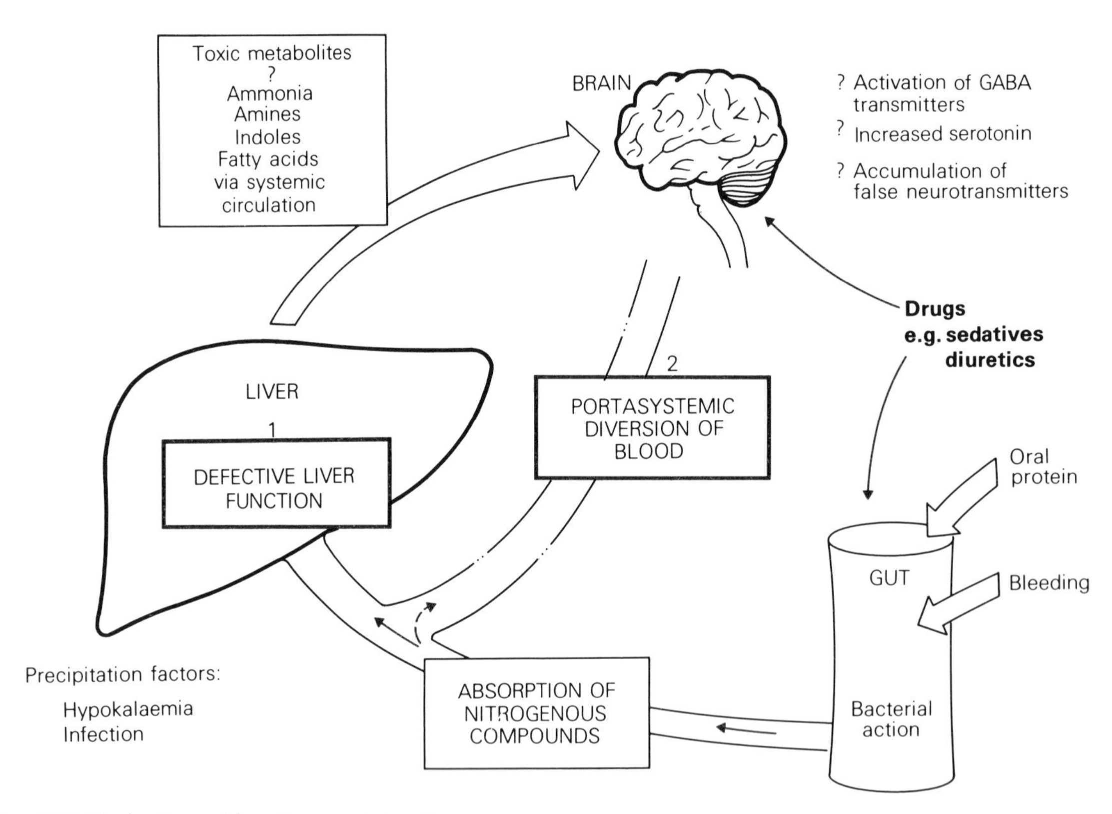

Fig. 8.59 *Mechanisms of hepatic encephalopathy.*

istic musty smell in the breath (foetor hepaticus) may be noted.

Laboratory investigation. The diagnosis is principally clinical, and tests are not of great help. The blood ammonia is commonly, though inconsistently, elevated. The electroencephalogram shows slowing of the dominant rhythm, but this can occur in any toxic encephalopathy. The CSF glutamate is usually elevated.

Differential diagnosis. Clearly, other forms of nervous system catastrophe need to be excluded. In alcoholic cirrhosis an important consideration is trauma leading to subdural haemorrhage and, where doubt exists, a CT brain scan is a useful test. Alcohol withdrawal syndrome and Wernicke's encephalopathy may also cause diagnostic confusion or, indeed, may coexist with hepatic precoma (Fig. 8.60).

Management. The first principle of treatment is to eliminate a precipitating cause such as infection, haemorrhage or hypokalaemia.

The second principle of treatment is to reduce the degree of assimilation of nitrogenous compounds by lowering oral protein intake (reducing the diet to 30–40 g protein daily) and by clearing the gut of protein (e.g. blood from bleeding in the upper alimentary tract) by magnesium sulphate enemas. Nitrogen uptake can further be reduced by suppression of normal colonic bacterial flora

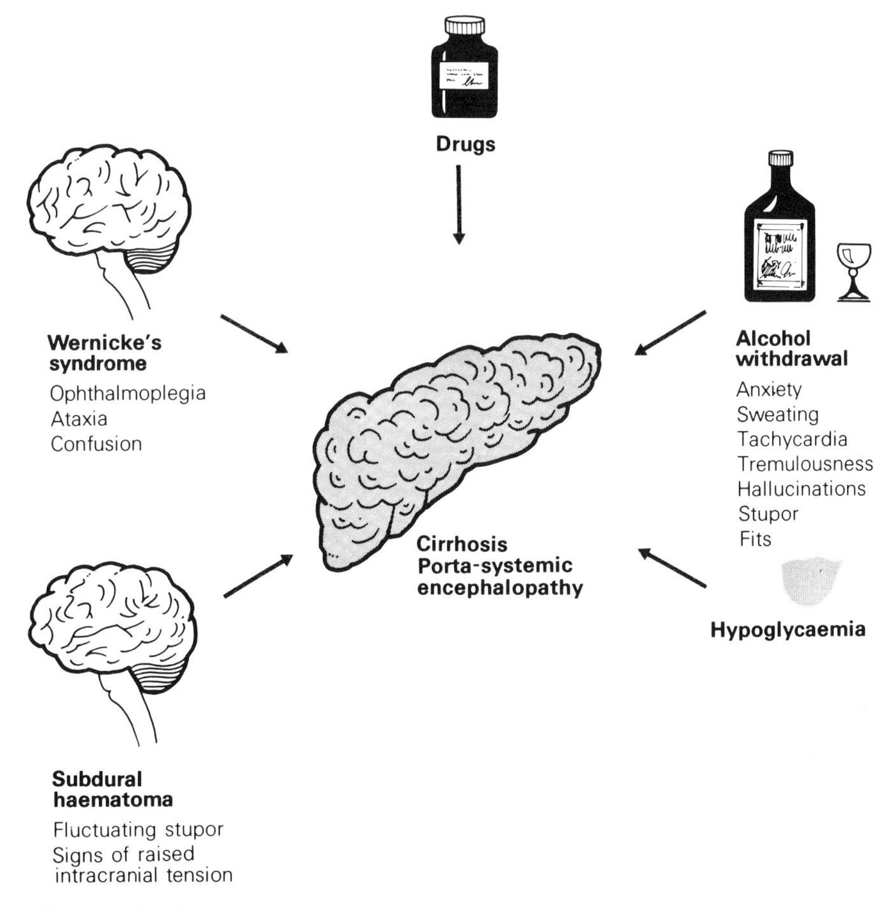

Fig. 8.60 *Differential diagnosis of hepatic precoma.*

with a poorly-absorbed antibiotic such as neomycin. Lactulose, a non-absorbed sugar, also helps by encouraging overgrowth of saccharolytic bacteria to the exclusion of peptide-splitting bacteria. It also acts as a mild osmotic laxative and is safe for use over long periods of time.

The third principle of treatment is the avoidance of aggravating factors such as sedative drugs, fluid overload and electrolyte imbalance.

Rarely, surgical exclusion of the colon or colectomy has been performed in chronic disabling intractable encephalopathy.

Fulminant Hepatic Failure

This devastating and highly mortal disease of rapid onset is fortunately rare. The causes include:

- viral hepatitis (mainly HAV and HBV)
- drugs – the best-known example is paracetamol (acetominophen) (see p. 161)
- poisoning, e.g. with the death cap mushroom, *Amanita phalloides*
- acute fatty liver of pregnancy
- Reye's syndrome (see p. 165)

The liver usually shows widespread necrosis, with collapse of the reticulin framework (and, in consequence, the liver is small). Sometimes fatty change is extensive. Cerebral oedema is common and may be a cause of death. Renal failure, alimentary haemorrhage, and pancreatitis are other potentially fatal complications.

Clinical features. Signs of impending encephalopathy may supervene upon an otherwise unremarkable case of acute hepatitis. Vomiting, abdominal pain, drowsiness, confusion and tremor are ominous developments. Alternatively the encephalopathy may occur with such rapidity that jaundice is minimal or absent and the diagnosis may be unsuspected until a massive rise in transaminases is discovered. Widespread haemorrhage is common and the prolongation of prothrombin time is a useful index to progress and prognosis. Extensive neurological signs may develop, with spasticity, decerebrate rigidity and fits. Recovery from Grade IV (unresponsive) coma is exceedingly rare.

Laboratory investigations. The most useful tests are transminases, prothrombin time, bilirubin and electrolytes; hypokalaemia and a remarkably uncorrectable hyponatraemia are common. Intractable hypoglycaemia is an important feature.

Management. The principles outlined above (chronic encephalopathy) also apply to acute encephalopathy. In addition, since fulminant failure has such a poor prognosis, intensive and highly-skilled medical and nursing management are essential if survival is to be achieved. Regular monitoring of vital signs, central venous pressure, fluid balance, neurological status, blood sugar, urea and electrolytes and acid–base balance are all essential. Risk of hypoglycaemia is reduced by giving 10% dextrose intravenously. Cimetidine or ranitidine may reduce the risk of alimentary haemorrhage. Fresh frozen plasma may help. Corticosteroids do not seem to be of value.

Since recovery from acute hepatic failure commonly means that the liver returns to virtual normality, it is clear that temporary support, if it can be achieved, is vital. Several methods have been tried, including exchange transfusion, haemodialysis, charcoal column haemoperfusion, pig-liver perfusion and cross-circulation. Current interest centres on haemodialysis (with polyacrylonitrile membranes) and charcoal columns but these techniques, especially the latter, are only available in specialist centres.

Renal Failure in Liver Disease

Renal failure is a common accompaniment of both acute hepatic failure and advanced chronic hepatic decompensation. Its cause is unknown but both depressed renal perfusion and altered intrarenal haemodynamics are important. The kidneys are microscopically normal. A rising urea and creatinine with a falling sodium in an oliguric patient is an ominous sign. Despite measures to improve perfusion (e.g. albumin infusions) and induce diuresis (e.g. mannitol), the prognosis is usually poor. The term 'hepato-renal syndrome' has been applied to this situation, but is a loose term probably better avoided. The renal changes complicating obstructive jaundice have been discussed on p. 184).

Rarely, the kidney is involved directly in the injurious process damaging the liver, e.g. in carbon tetrachloride poisoning.

9

Diseases of Colon and Rectum

The obvious difference in length and shape between the small and large intestines reflects their different functions. Normal nutrition depends on the existence of an adequate length of small bowel but, if colonic disease dictates that the whole of the colon and rectum is removed, the patient can still enjoy normal health: what is lost is the specific function of the large bowel to dehydrate, store and evacuate faeces.

ANATOMY

Considerable areas of the ascending and descending colon, and of the rectum, are extraperitoneal. The blood supply to the colon comes from both superior and inferior mesenteric arteries and there is a good anastomosis between the two areas of supply. There is also a useful contribution to the rectum from the middle and inferior rectal arteries (Fig. 9.1). The lymphatic channels and nodes follow the course of the arteries.

The colonic wall is made up of several layers, including the lamina propria with its epithelial lining, the muscularis mucosa, submucosa, two layers of smooth muscle, and a serosal layer. The epithelium dips down into the lamina propria at frequent intervals to form mucosal crypts (Fig. 9.2). The bases of the crypts almost make contact with the muscularis mucosa. The crypt openings on the surface of the colon can be clearly seen by

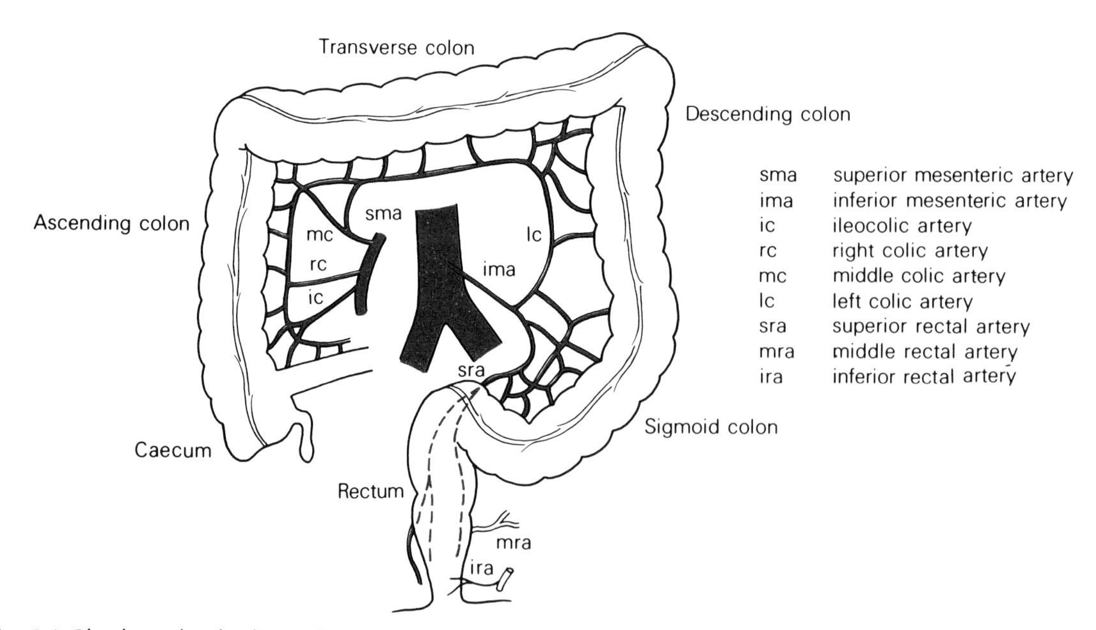

Fig. 9.1 *Blood supply of colon and rectum.*

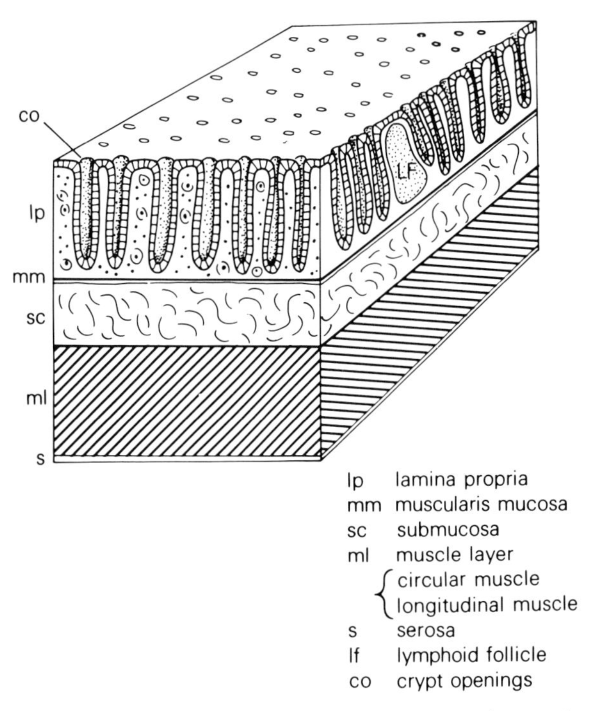

Fig. 9.2 *Schematic representation of histology of normal colon.*

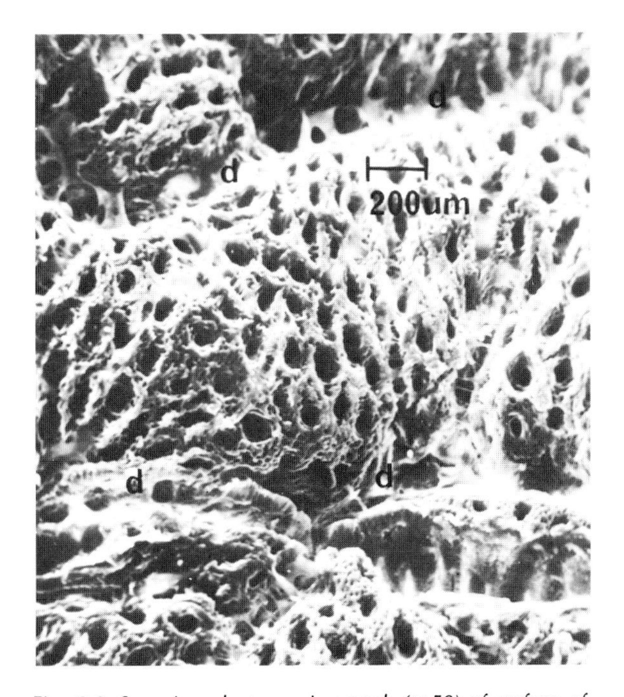

Fig. 9.3 *Scanning electron micrograph (× 50) of surface of large-bowel mucosa, showing the crypt openings.*

surface microscopy using a scanning electron microscope (Fig. 9.3). Numerous goblet cells allow copious secretion of mucus. Within the lamina propria are a variety of cell types, including macrophages, plasma cells, lymphocytes and mast cells. Some disturbance of the immunological capability of these cells may be an important factor in some diseases of the colon. Lymphoid follicles are also prominent in the lamina propria.

PHYSIOLOGY

Whereas peristaltic activity is more-or-less constant in the small bowel, two separate types of movement can be distinguished in the colon. Segmentation produces mixing of the contents, whereas propulsion is a mass movement which on three or four occasions in the day (generally after a meal) propels faeces down the colon.

Transit through the small bowel takes 4–5 hours but on average it takes a further 12–18 hours for faeces to travel from caecum to rectum.

About 1.5 l of liquid chyme passes through the ileocaecal valve each 24 hours, but only about 100–200 g of stool is evacuated, of which 60–80% is water. On a typical Western diet a daily stool weight in excess of 300 g would be consi-

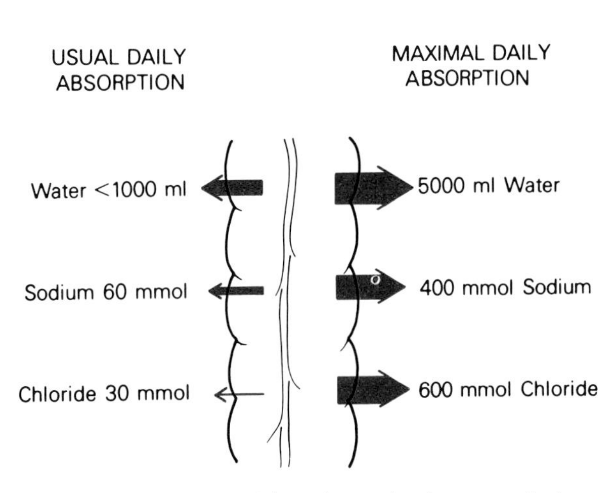

Fig. 9.4 *Spare capacity of the colon to absorb water and salt.*

dered pathological unless exceptional quantities of dietary fibre were being eaten, i.e. diet influences the volume of undigested or partially digested cellulose in the faeces and, therefore, the actual bulk of the stool passed. Only 1 in 100 Western citizens have fewer than three bowel movements per week or more than three per day.

The colon functions at far below its maximum capacity (Fig. 9.4) and can compensate for considerable small-bowel malabsorption of water and electrolyte. Sodium absorption involves an active transport process. Some calcium is absorbed in the colon, assisted by vitamin D.

The usual colour of stools is derived from bile pigments.

Dietary Fibre

This is plant-derived material comprising non-starch polysaccharides (NSP) such as cellulose. Associated with NSP in plant cell walls is a non-carbohydrate polymer, lignin, which increases the rigidity of the cell wall. Whereas these substances are resistant to digestion by human intestinal enzymes, they are metabolised to differing extents by the intestinal microflora; for example, pectin and hemicellulose can be degraded totally, cellulose partially, and lignin virtually not at all.

In the large bowel, the anaerobic microflora metabolise fibre to gases (CO_2, H_2 and CH_4) and to short-chain organic acids, all of which can be absorbed and then metabolised systemically. The short-chain fatty acids from fibre in a typical Western diet provide less than 10% of the daily energy requirements, but the higher fibre intakes in African and Asian diets contribute proportionately more to the energy balance.

The availability of fibre as a metabolisable substrate in the colon stimulates growth of the microflora. The subsequent excretion of this bacterial load constitutes the major component of the faecal bulking caused by fibre. Increased faecal bulk decreases intracolonic pressure and intestinal transit time, and so increases the frequency and ease of defaecation. In general, unrefined cereal foods are more effective faecal bulking agents than fruit or vegetables. This point is exploited in the use of wheat bran in the management of constipation, diverticular disease (p. 216) and irritable bowel syndrome (p. 8).

The average fibre content of a Western diet is 20 g per day, compared with 130–150 g per day in some areas of Africa. These regional and cultural differences have been linked with the varied incidence of diseases of the large bowel and this is further considered in Chapter 2.

Bacteriology

There is usually a bacterial population in the lower ileum, but it is in the colon that the intestinal microflora flourish, anaerobes (such as *Bacteroides fragilis*) outnumbering aerobes by 1000 to 1. Faecal bacteria assist in the metabolism of bilirubin and bile acids and in the synthesis of vitamins K, B_{12}, thiamin and riboflavin. The bacterial content of faeces, along with desquamated cells and secretions, contribute at least half of the protein (> 10 g) and fat (> 7 g) found in stools (see Fig. 15.1).

Intestinal Gas

The presence of intestinal gas can be a source of discomfort. The healthy adult has 30–300 ml of gas in the gut at any one time. Much of this is acquired by air swallowing and in food; an egg, for example, contains 80% by volume of air.

Excessive eructation (belching) is commonly due to behavioural problems such as excessive air swallowing or to consumption of antacids or carbonated drinks which release carbon dioxide in the stomach. Gastric and intestinal stasis and bacterial overgrowth allow the production in the small bowel of unusual gases which may cause foul eructations.

The volume and composition of flatus depends on the amount of unabsorbed carbohydrate, lipid and protein presented for fermentation by the colonic microflora, and upon the predominant bacterial type. Nitrogen and carbon dioxide are the predominant gases, with very little oxygen; the amount of hydrogen and methane varies according to diet.

NEOPLASIA OF THE LARGE BOWEL

New growths of the colon and rectum arguably represent one of the most important groups of the neoplastic diseases, for the following reasons:

Carcinoma of the large bowel is the second commonest malignant neoplasm of Western communities.

In contrast to the commoner malignancies of the respiratory tract, colorectal cancer is responsive to timely surgery, with corrected five-year survival rates (among those suitable for radical surgery) of 70–80%.

The benign colonic neoplasms are known to be premalignant, so their diagnosis and removal is of special importance.

Forty per cent of all large bowel neoplasms occur in the rectum (Fig. 9.5) and at least one-third of these are palpable on rectal examination; about half of all neoplasms are visible through the sigmoidoscope (Fig. 9.6). There is therefore an excellent opportunity to reach a definitive diagnosis at the first visit to the surgery or out-patient clinic.

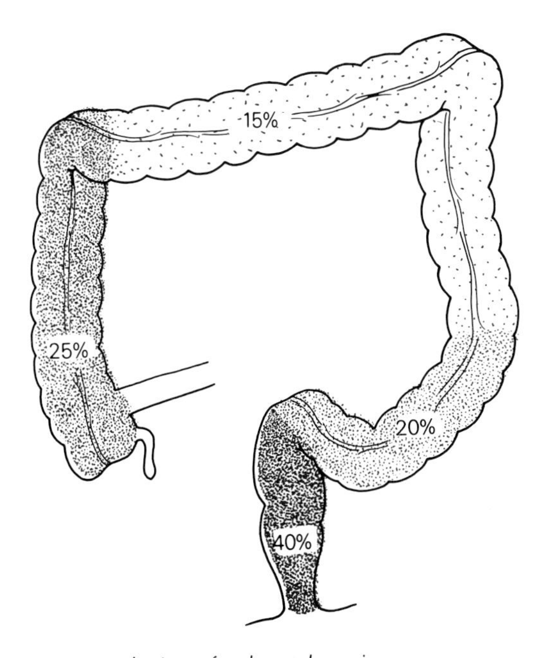

Fig. 9.5 *Distribution of colorectal carcinomas.*

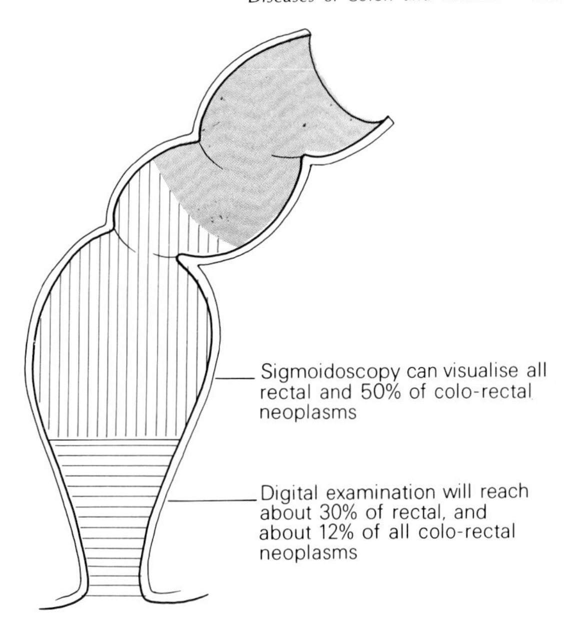

Fig. 9.6 *Outpatient diagnosis of colorectal neoplasms.*

Aetiology

In spite of a great deal of investigation, the cause of neoplastic change in the large bowel is unknown. Like colonic diverticulosis, this is a disease of Western civilisation (see p. 28). In common with other malignancies, environmental factors seem to be more important than genetic influences: several studies have shown that, when communities migrate from an area of low incidence to an area of high incidence, they assume the higher risk of developing a neoplasm.

Roughly equal numbers of men and women are affected. At the time of diagnosis, two-thirds are over 65 years of age and 30% are over 75.

Predisposing Conditions

Familial factors

Despite the fact that environmental factors may be more important than genetic ones in the development of carcinoma of the colon, two distinct groups of patients have emerged who are genetically predisposed to developing carcinoma of the large bowel.

Familial polyposis coli. This disorder is inherited as an autosomal dominant trait. The incidence in the general population is one per 10 000. The total number of adenomas varies from 100 to 10 000 in each colon affected (Fig. 9.7). The adenomas tend to appear in adolescence and early adulthood and the risk of carcinoma developing in the untreated patient is around 90% at the age of 40 years. More

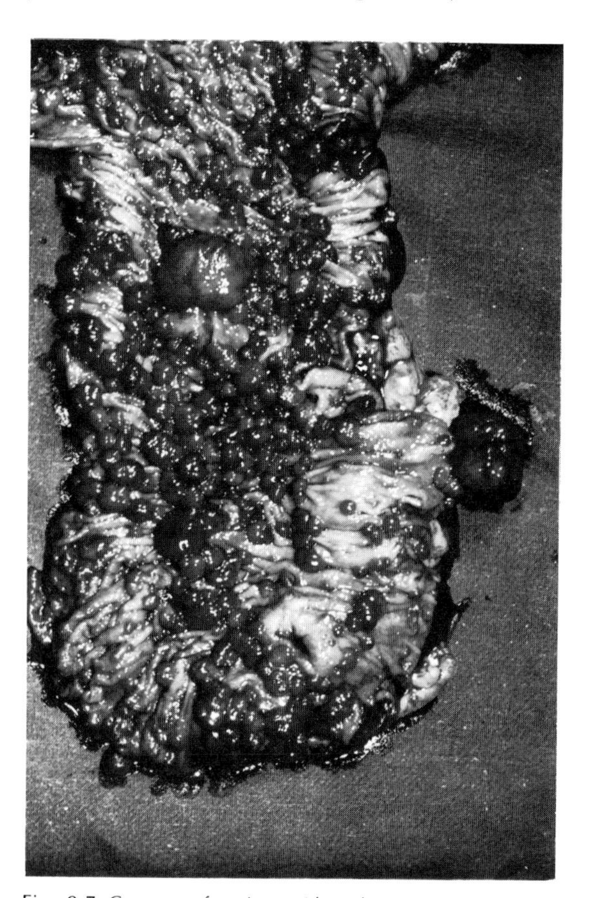

Fig. 9.7 *Caecum of patient with polyposis coli.*

recently, it has been discovered that some of these patients have polyps elsewhere in the gastrointestinal tract, particularly in the stomach. Gardner's syndrome is a variant of familial polyposis in which the occurrence of multiple colonic adenomas is associated with multiple osteomata, dental abnormalities, and soft-tissue tumours, including desmoids.

Familial large bowel cancer. Between 4–8% of patients with large bowel cancer, while not having familial polyposis, have a close relative who has had carcinoma of the colon. There are certain characteristics which are peculiar to patients who are so affected. They tend to be younger at the age of onset, and there is a higher incidence of multiple primary tumours and proximal colon cancer. The mode of genetic transmission is not known, and environmental factors may be important.

Inflammatory bowel disease

There is an increased incidence of carcinoma of colon among patients with inflammatory bowel disease, particularly nonspecific proctocolitis (NSP) (see p. 232).

Pathology of Large-Bowel Tumours

Adenomas of large bowel

Adenomas are common in the large bowel of the middle-aged and elderly. This is particularly true in countries where the incidence of large-bowel cancer is high. In a series of post-mortem examinations from the USA, 38% of males over the age of 55 had one or more adenomas present in the large bowel. Several kinds of adenomas are found in the large bowel which are of clinical importance.

1. The tubular adenoma is a deeper red colour than the surrounding mucosa. It may be situated at the end of a mucosal stalk (when it is called a polyp), or it may be sessile. The surface is criss-crossed by intercommunicating clefts (Figs 9.8 and 9.9).

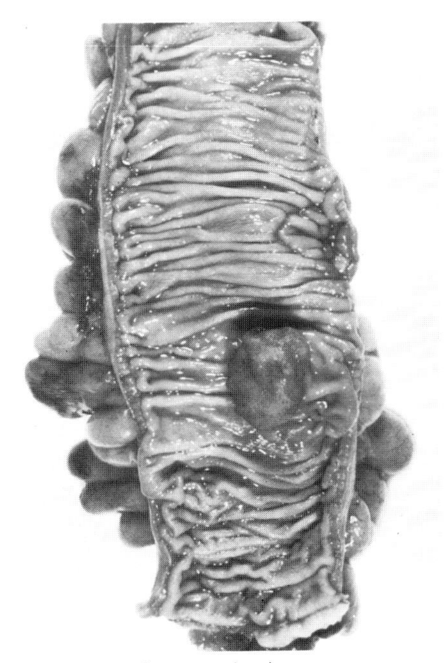

Fig. 9.8 *Tubular adenoma of colon.*

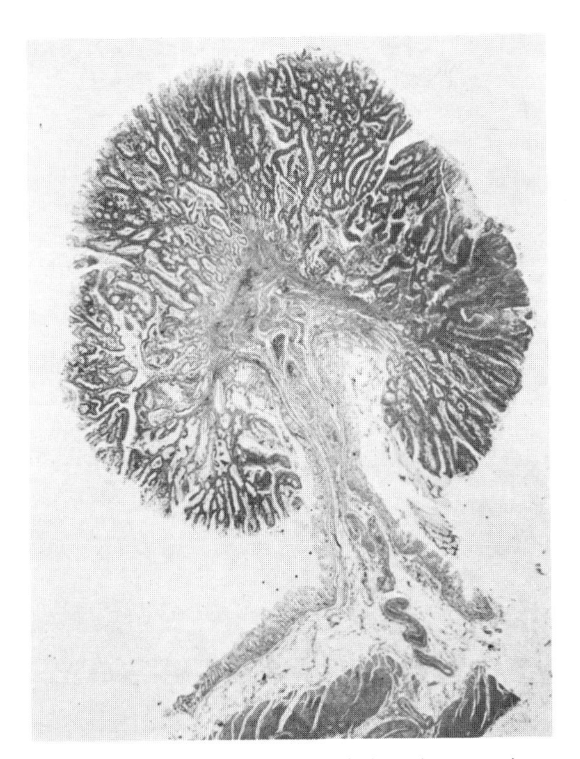

Fig. 9.9 *Longitudinal section of tubular adenoma, showing stalk.*

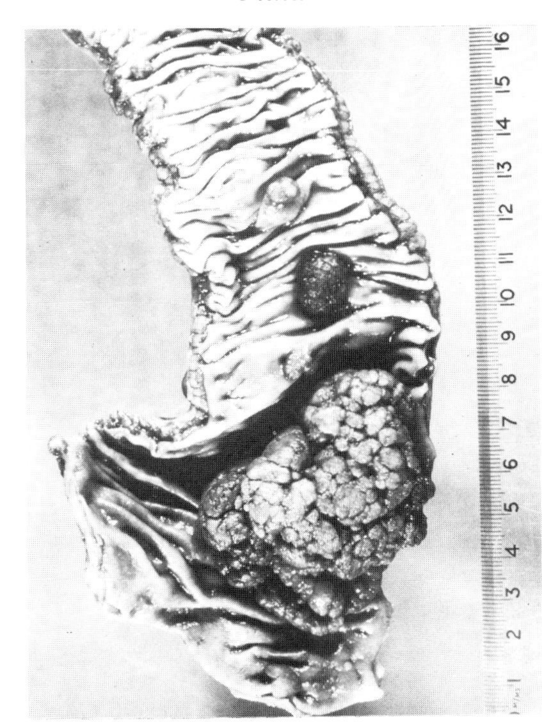

Fig. 9.10 *Villous adenoma of rectum.*

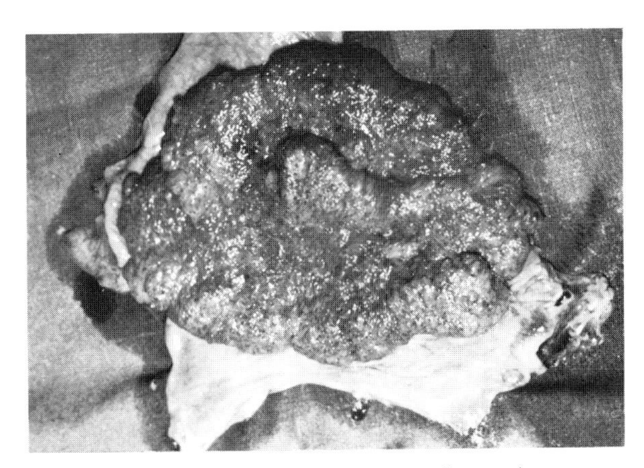

Fig. 9.11 *Extensive villous adenoma/papilloma of rectum.*

2. The villous adenoma tends to be sessile, involves an area of mucosa of varying extent, and consists of numerous fronds of tumour (Fig. 9.10). The distribution of these tumours is mainly in the rectum and sigmoid colon. A villous lesion, if untreated, may eventually grow to involve most of the rectum in a circumferential manner (Fig. 9.11).

3. The tubulo-villous adenoma consists of a

varying proportion of both tubular and villous elements (Fig. 9.12).

Adenomas may be graded as showing mild, moderate or severe dysplasia on the basis of nuclear changes such as loss of polarity, stratification, and an increased number of mitoses, and also on the appearance of the glandular architecture. If these changes occur superficial to the muscularis mucosa then there is no risk of metastatic spread since there are no lymphatics present in the lamina propria. Only when tumour growth breaches the muscularis mucosa does the lesion become an invasive carcinoma (Fig. 9.13).

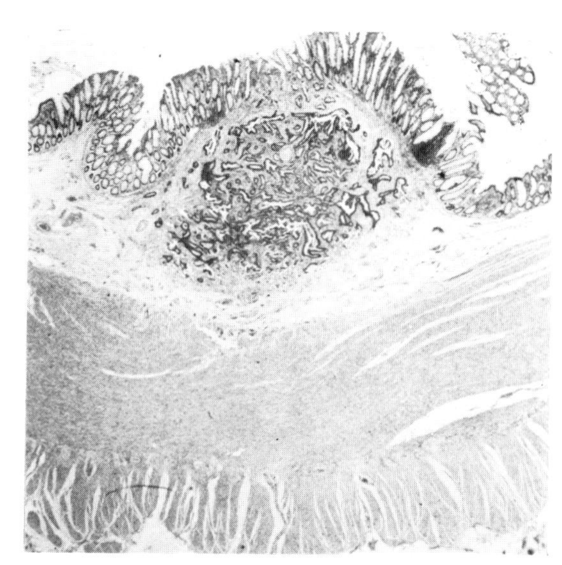

Fig. 9.13 *Section showing early invasive carcinoma of colon.*

The adenoma–carcinoma sequence

It is now generally believed that carcinomas of the large bowel arise from a preexisting adenoma. The evidence for this hypothesis is convincing.

If the age incidence of patients with adenomas and carcinomas are plotted, they run parallel, but adenomas occur 5 years earlier than carcinomas (Fig. 9.14). About one-third of all operative specimens of colonic cancer show additionally one or two adenomas. When two or more cancers coexist, then 75% of specimens will also show the presence of adenomas. Adenomas are commonest in the distal colon and rectum, where carcinomas are also most common. If the size of adenomas is recorded and compared with their histology, only 1% of adenomas less than 1 cm in diameter will show invasive changes; in adenomas of 1–2 cm diameter, the percentage is 10%; and when the adenoma is over 2 cm in diameter then adenocar-

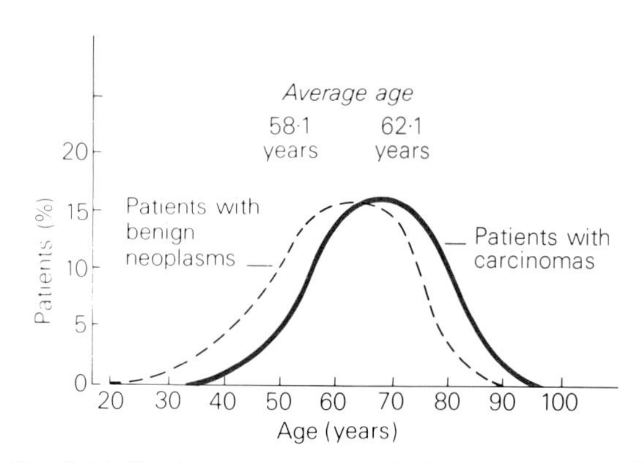

Fig. 9.14 *Graph comparing age at which patients present with adenomas and with carcinomas of the colon (after Morson and Dawson).*

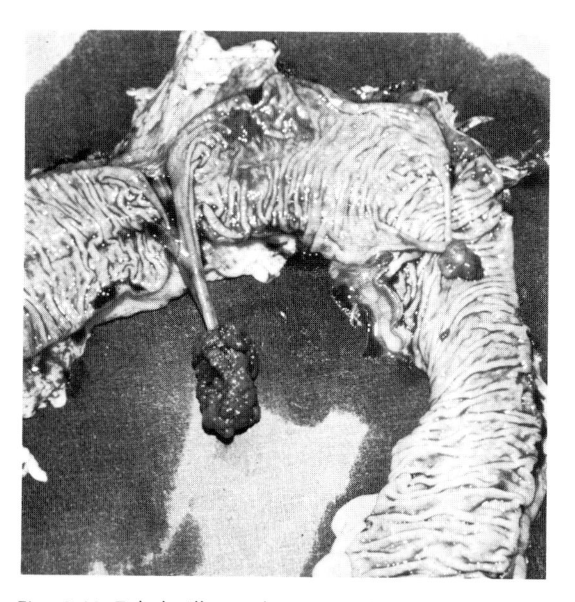

Fig. 9.12 *Tubulovillous adenoma, with a long stalk.*

cinomatous change is seen in 46%. Only 5% of tubular adenomas show carcinomatous change, compared with 41% of villous papillomas, but adenomas are eight times more common and so are of equal importance.

Spread of large-bowel carcinoma

As a carcinoma grows, it spreads along and around the bowel wall; in many tumours, this tendency to spread circumferentially produces narrowing of the bowel (annular carcinoma). Hence it is common for large bowel tumours to produce a degree of intestinal obstruction (Fig. 9.15). Polypoidal or ulcerating carcinomas (Fig. 9.16) are also found.

Spread of carcinoma through the wall of the bowel is also important because cancer cells on the peritoneal surface of the bowel may disseminate across the peritoneal cavity, or cause direct invasion of adjacent structures.

The eventual prognosis of large-bowel cancer has been shown to correlate well with the Dukes' staging system, which indicates the extent to which the tumour has spread through the wall of the bowel and whether lymph nodes in the mesentery are involved (Fig. 9.17). It is clear from

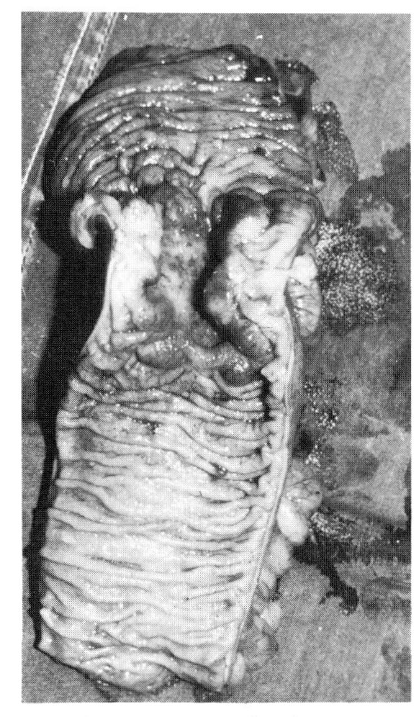

Fig. 9.15 *Annular carcinoma of colon.*

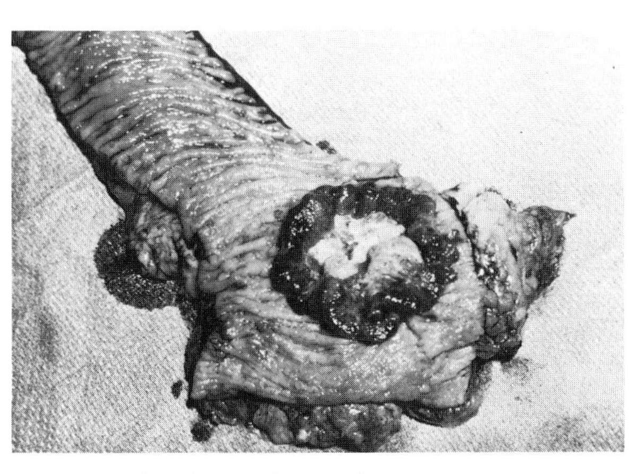

Fig. 9.16 *Ulcerating carcinoma of rectum.*

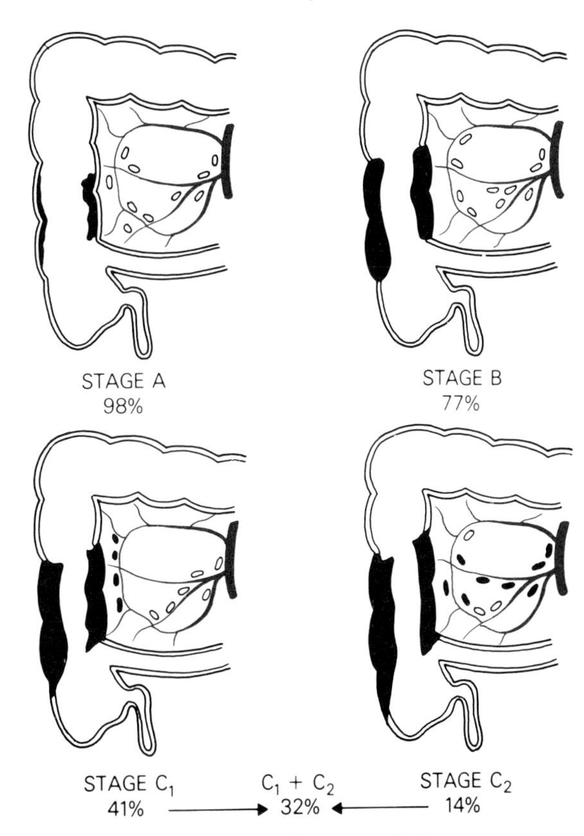

Fig. 9.17 *Dukes' staging of the spread of colorectal carcinoma.*

the survival figures that radical surgery in patients with stage A and B carcinomas offers good prospects of survival and, even at stage C, one-third of patients survive for more than five years. The finding of cancer emboli in the veins draining the tumour is a grave prognostic sign, as is the extension of the neoplasm to the peritoneal surface of the colon, opening the way to trans-coelomic spread to the omentum and other serosal surfaces. Where there is spread via the portal vein to the liver, the outlook is very poor.

Presentation of Large-Bowel Tumours

Neoplasms of the large bowel predominantly affect the elderly – 70% occur in patients over 65 years of age. However, a small but very important proportion arise in young people, and a colorectal carcinoma can be seen in the early twenties.

The incidence is roughly equal in males and females.

Adenoma

Commonly the lesion is asymptomatic and is noted incidentally on sigmoidoscopy or barium enema, but some patients will have symptoms appropriate to the site and the size of the lesion. Occasionally they can give rise to alteration in bowel habit, or cause colic when intussusception takes place. In the left colon the most common symptom is rectal bleeding. Most villous adenomas arise in the rectum and sigmoid colon and, if they are large, the main complaint may be passage of large quantities of clear mucus per rectum with some blood, which can occasionally cause dehydration and electrolyte depletion.

Carcinoma (Fig. 9.18)

Right colon carcinoma. It is vital to recognise that it is common for patients with a carcinoma of caecum or ascending colon to present with the entirely nonspecific symptoms of iron-deficiency

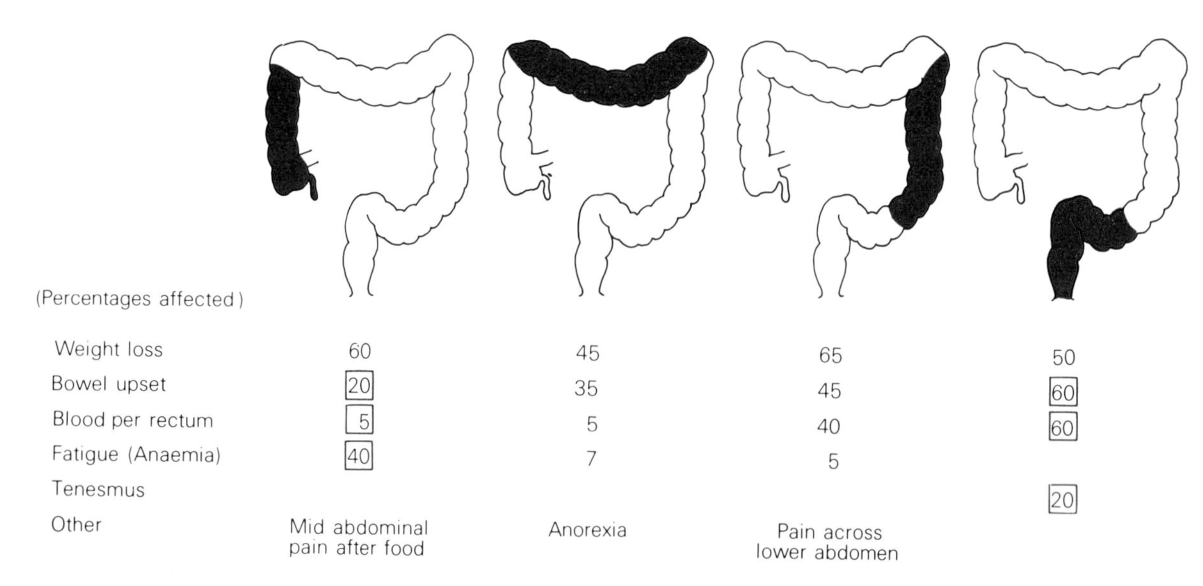

Fig. 9.18 *Frequency of symptoms of carcinoma in proximal, transverse and distal colon, and in the rectum.*

anaemia. The unexpected occurrence of anaemia should always raise the possibility of an occult colonic carcinoma, which is more likely to be in the proximal than in the distal colon. Weight loss and central abdominal pain are relatively frequent, but rectal bleeding is uncommon. A mass is palpable in the right side of the abdomen in 50–60% of patients.

Left colon carcinoma. The more distal the site of the carcinoma, the more likely is it that there will be disturbance of bowel habit, and recognition of blood in the stools. Some carcinomas of the transverse and sigmoid colon are palpable through the abdominal wall.

Rectal carcinoma. A majority of patients present with disturbance of bowel function, a feeling of incomplete evacuation (tenesmus), and frank rectal bleeding. It is not possible to distinguish between the type of bleeding from a carcinoma low in the rectum and the bleeding produced by haemorrhoids: physical examination is essential.

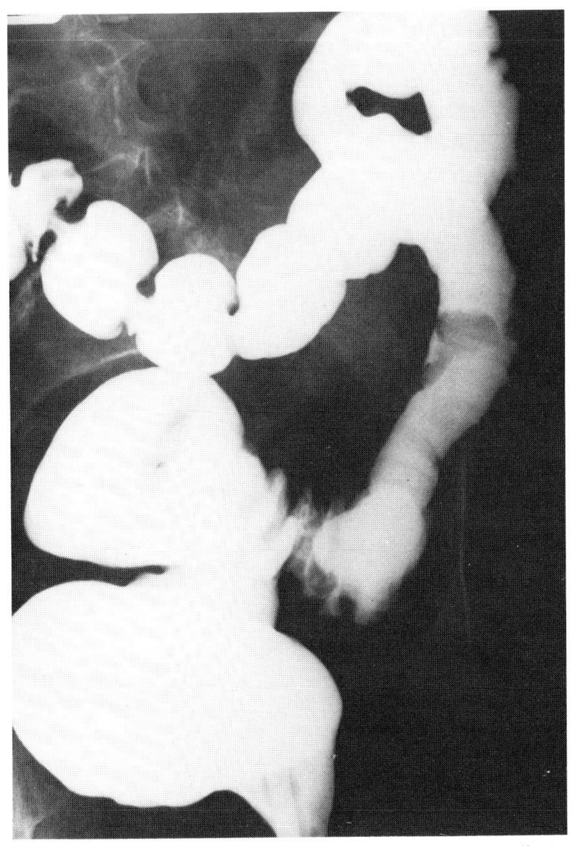

Fig. 9.19 *Barium enema, showing adenoma on stalk in descending colon.*

Diagnosis of Large Bowel Tumours

Adenomas

Some adenomas may be diagnosed on digital examination or sigmoidoscopy, or small quantities of blood can be seen on normal rectal mucosa of many patients with polyps in the distal large bowel: this sign should make the clinician insist on a double contrast enema, with colonoscopy if appropriate.

Adenomas of the colon may be seen in a double contrast barium enema, when they appear as filling defects coated with a thin layer of barium (Fig. 9.19).

Carcinomas

The diagnosis of carcinoma of the large bowel may be made by digital examination of the rectum, sigmoidoscopy, barium enema examination, or colonoscopy. *Digital examination* is of particular value in diagnosing rectal carcinoma, and in about 30% of rectal carcinomas the diagnosis can be made in this way: it is also possible to make a fairly accurate assessment of the extent and degree of local spread of the tumour.

Sigmoidoscopy is necessary in all patients with large-bowel symptoms. Not only is it possible to visualise rectal lesions directly but in some patients a considerable portion of the sigmoid colon may also be examined, particularly if the flexible fibre-optic sigmoidoscope is used. The tumour is easily recognised by its raised lower edge, which is a darker red or purple colour compared with normal mucosa. The tumour bleeds easily, which may make further visualisation difficult. A portion of the tumour edge is always removed with biopsy forceps for histological examination.

Barium enema examination is the next examination if the diagnosis is still in doubt. The classical appearance of a colonic carcinoma on barium enema is of a shouldered stricture with an 'apple-core' appearance (Fig. 9.20). The tumour is usually short and a varying degree of obstruction of the lumen is found. Smaller, earlier neoplasms are liable to be missed on conventional barium enema examinations, so that the double contrast barium enema is increasingly used. The radiologist can visualise a small tumour producing a filling defect on one wall of the colon. Particular care is needed to identify caecal carcinoma and, in a suspicious case, a negative enema report should be interpreted with caution.

Colonoscopy, which allows direct visualisation and biopsy, is being used increasingly in selected patients for the diagnosis of large-bowel neoplasms. Indications for colonoscopy include:

suspicion of a stricture on barium enema
examination and removal of polyps seen on barium enema
the presence of blood on normal rectal mucosa with a negative barium enema
unexplained diarrhoea.

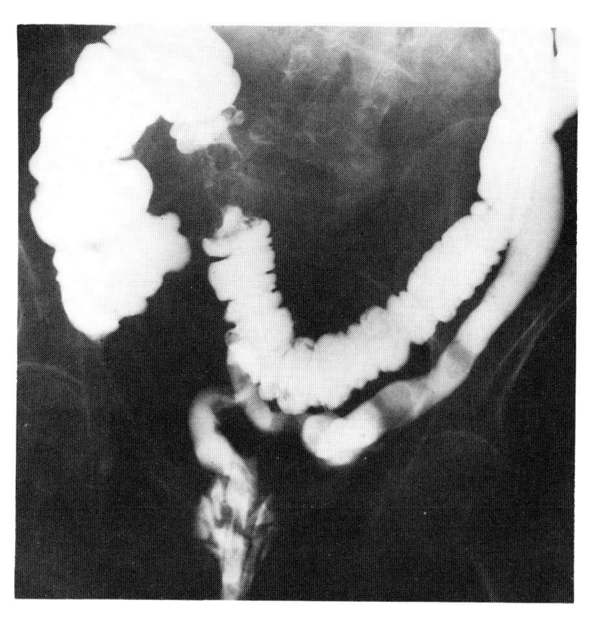

Fig. 9.20 *Barium enema showing typical 'apple-core' filling defect in transverse colon.*

It is also of value in the surveillance of patients with long-standing colitis who are at risk of developing carcinoma.

Differential Diagnosis

Many conditions must be considered, inflammatory bowel disease (see p. 221) and diverticular disease (see p. 214) being the most frequent possibilities. Amoebiasis must not be forgotten in patients from appropriate countries. In the distal colon and rectum, gynaecological disease such as carcinoma of the ovary or cervix, or endometriosis, must be considered. It must never by forgotten that the patient with haemorrhoids or an anal fissure may also have a rectal carcinoma.

Treatment

Preoperative assessment

In addition to making a correct diagnosis, it is important to assess and prepare the patient carefully before operation.

The results of liver function tests, especially a raised serum alkaline phosphatase, may suggest the presence of liver metastases, and scanning of the liver may support this suspicion. However, this should not generally discourage laparotomy because these investigations are occasionally misleading. Pulmonary metastases are not often seen, but a chest x-ray must be obtained.

Intravenous pyelography, with or without cystoscopy, is used in patients with bulky pelvic turmours to demonstrate any involvement of the urinary tract.

Colorectal surgery is extensive, and demanding on the patient, so it is important to correct anaemia before operation and to improve, where possible, any cardiac or respiratory disease.

Preparation for surgery

Surgery for carcinoma of the colon and rectum may require either temporary or permanent colostomy. This must be explained to the patient, emphasising the efficacy of modern appliances and the importance of radical surgery. The stoma therapist (a specially trained nurse) is an important member of the surgical team, before and after operation.

To obtain good results from surgery, with low rates of infection, the bowel must be properly prepared by mechanical cleansing. Although there is no agreement at present on preoperative use of antimicrobials, there is convincing evidence of the value of antibiotics given intravenously during operation.

Surgical technique

Principles of resection. The first task on opening the abdomen is to determine whether the carcinoma is resectable, i.e. whether it can be removed. Resectability does not mean that the tumour is potentially curable: this depends on whether (a) the carcinoma can be completely removed without leaving adjacent infiltrated tissue, and (b) there is no apparent distant spread to the liver or other parts of the abdominal cavity. The diligent surgeon will make considerable efforts to remove colorectal tumours because if they are not resected they cause distressing symptoms: furthermore, even though hepatic metastases are found at laparotomy, a number of patients live 2–3 years in reasonable health after resection of the primary lesion. Over 90% of patients have a resectable tumour and, in about two-thirds, the carcinoma is potentially curable.

In a patient without signs of local or distant spread, a radical resection is performed. The tumour is resected together with a wide margin of adjacent tissue and, if necessary, adjacent adherent structures such as small bowel or the uterus. All possible infiltrated lymphatics are removed by a planned excision of the vascular tree supplying the affected bowel. The extent of the common resections is shown in Fig. 9.21 a–d.

Anastomotic technique. Once the resection is complete, the aim is to restore continuity of the bowel by end-to-end anastomosis. In most circumstances the two ends of the large bowel are sutured together after bowel resection is complete. The principles which govern the technique have now been well worked out. Blood supply to both ends of the bowel must be adequate and this usually necessitates having a pulsating mesenteric artery adjacent to the line of section of the bowel. The mucosa of both ends of bowel must be inverted for adequate healing to take place (Fig. 9.22).

A single or double-layered hand-sutured anastomosis gives satisfactory results, and recent experience with circular anastomosis stapling instruments has shown this method to be of some value in making anastomoses low in the rectum. Spillage of faecal material at the time of anastomosis is avoided because it is thought to increase the risk of dehiscence of the anastomosis, and also makes postoperative intra-abdominal and wound infection more likely.

Defunctioning colostomy. In elective colonic surgery, a defunctioning colostomy (Fig. 9.23) is rarely necessary except when extraperitoneal anastomoses are performed low in the pelvis, where the incidence of leakage from the anastomosis is higher. If the anastomosis is judged to be at risk at the time of operation, a defunctioning colostomy can be made by bringing out a loop of transverse colon through the abdominal wall. The colostomy is then opened and sutured to the skin. Isolation of the anastomosis from the faecal stream assists healing and usually the colostomy can be closed after six weeks.

Abdominoperineal excision of the rectum. This procedure is indicated when a rectal tumour lies so low that adequate clearance below it cannot be achieved without removing the anal canal. It is less commonly employed than previously, since surgeons are prepared to make anastomoses low in the rectum using the abdominal approach, either by hand-suturing or stapling instruments. Alternatively, the colo-anal anastomotic technique is used, in which the anastomosis is performed through the dilated anal canal.

Abdominoperineal excision of the rectum is

(a)

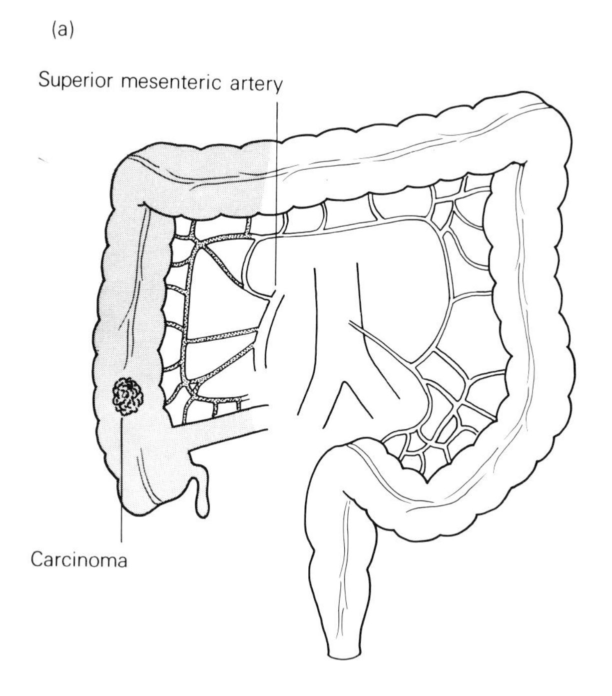

(c)

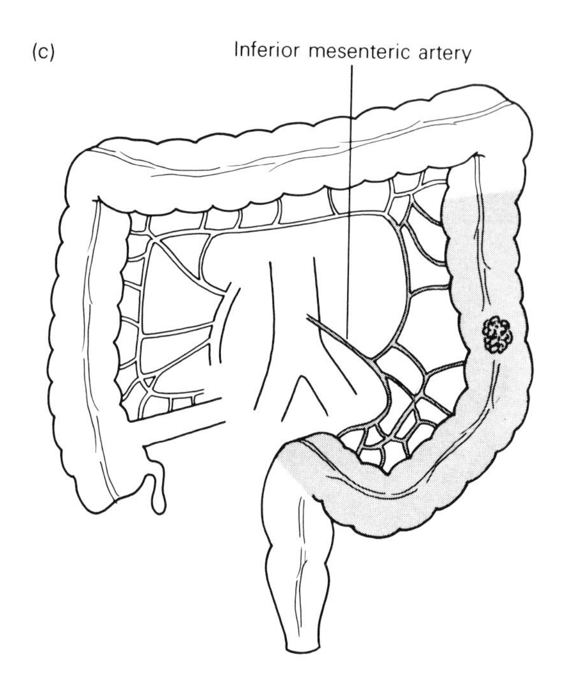

(b)

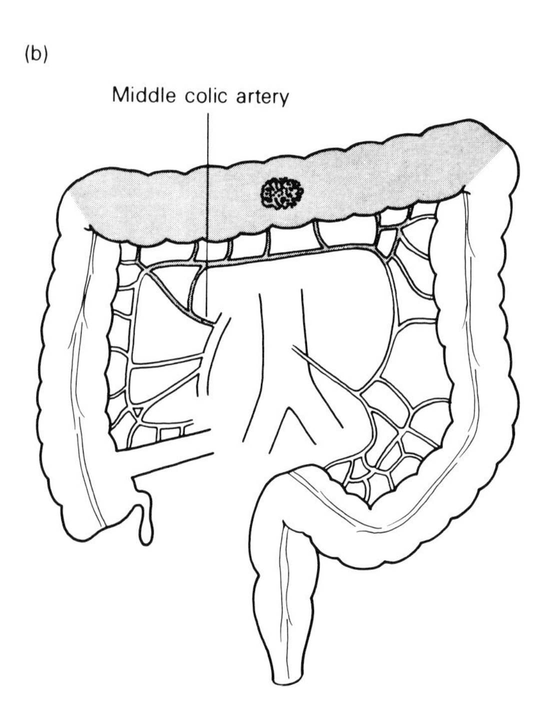

(d)

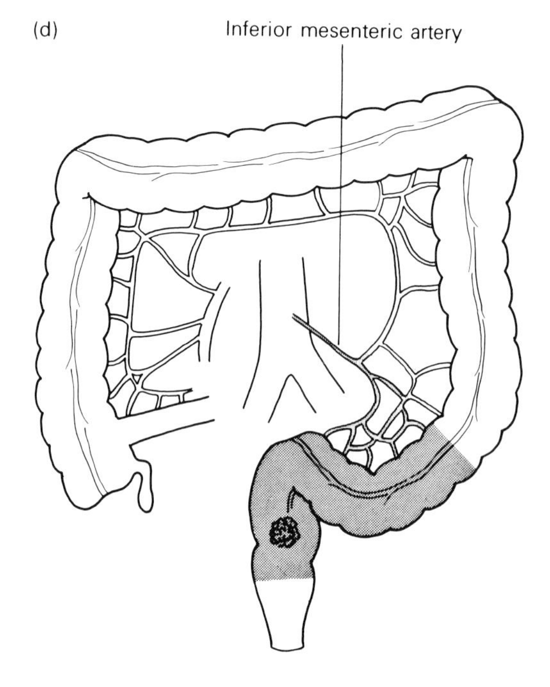

Fig. 9.21 *Extent of resection for colorectal carcinoma. (a) Right hemicolectomy. (b) Transverse colectomy. (c) Left hemicolectomy. (d) Anterior resection of rectum and sigmoid colon.*

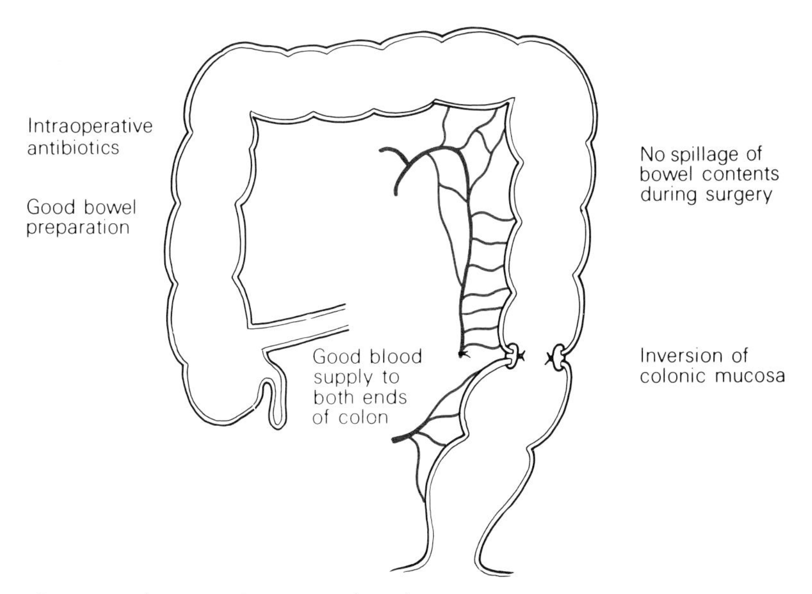

Fig. 9.22 *The principles of large bowel anastomosis.*

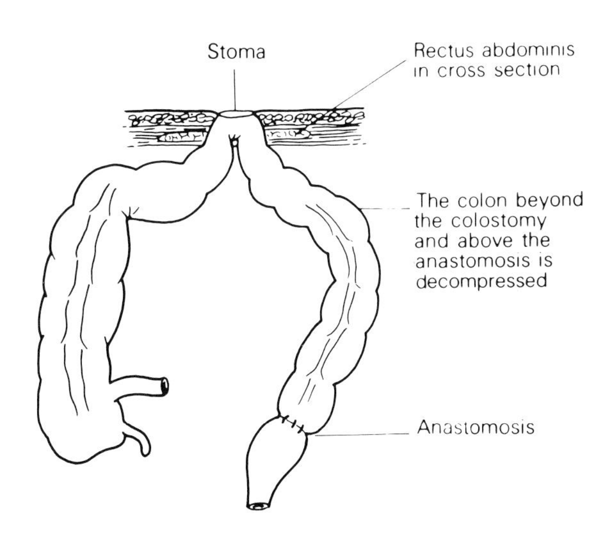

Fig. 9.23 *Defunctioning transverse colostomy.*

usually performed using two teams, one operating in the abdomen and the other at the perineal end. The sigmoid colon is divided, after the inferior mesenteric artery is ligated, and the rectum and meso-rectum, together with the anal canal and sphincters, are removed (Fig. 9.24). The sigmoid colon is brought out, at a carefully-chosen site, into the left iliac fossa as a terminal colostomy, and the pelvic peritoneum and perineal wounds are sutured. A urinary catheter is left *in situ* for several days because post-operative pain and possible damage to the pelvic autonomic nerves can precipitate urinary retention.

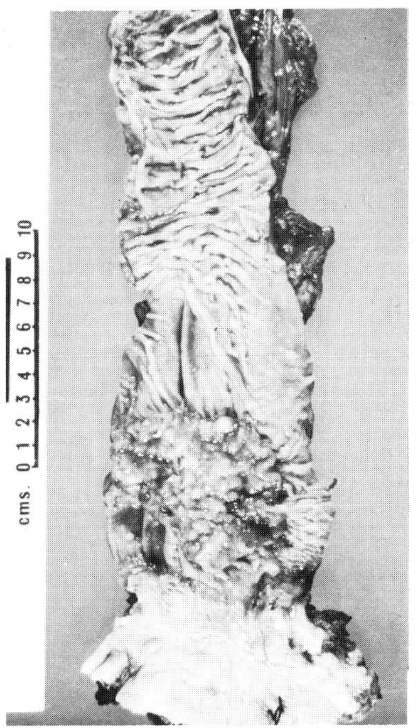

Fig. 9.24 *Abdominoperineal excision: the carcinomatous ulcer is seen lying just above the dentate line, and the perianal skin.*

Stoma care

A number of patients with a rectal carcinoma will require total excision of the rectum and so will be left with a permanent sigmoid colostomy. This produces fairly solid stools and most patients wear an adhesive bag over the stoma, changing it regularly. Some patients choose to perform a washout each day so that the colostomy should remain inactive for the rest of the day, and then it is sufficient to wear only a pad over the stoma. Either way, with good instruction and supervision by trained nurses, it should be possible for the patient to lead a completely normal life with a colostomy.

Prognosis

The most serious aspect of colorectal cancer is that, at the present time, about 40% of all patients presenting are already incurable by current methods of treatment. This emphasises the importance of prompt and thorough investigation of all suspicious symptoms, but in some patients – especially the young – colorectal neoplasms are aggressive and have already metastasised before causing appreciable symptoms. So far, screening programmes to secure earlier diagnosis have not proved their worth.

Among the 60–70% of patients who have a radical resection with the hope of cure the outlook is much better. Survival is naturally limited in a predominantly elderly population, but 75% of them can expect to live as long as their contemporaries. Prognosis is clearly related to the extent of spread of the tumour at the time of the operation (Fig. 9.17), and the grade of histological activity. Patients who present with obstruction or perforation have a poorer prognosis.

Management of Recurrent Large-bowel Carcinoma

Diagnosis of recurrence of colonic carcinoma is often difficult to make. The history and examination will be helpful in locating the site of recurrence in some patients but often, by the time symptoms are present, the disease is so far advanced that further therapeutic efforts are of limited value. Carcinoembryonic antigen (CEA) may be of value in the follow-up of patients with colon carcinoma. Although this blood-borne tumour marker is not specific for colon cancer it has been found that, in patients who have had a positive test and have had radical surgery for colon cancer, the test becomes negative. If the test becomes positive some time later during follow-up, it is very likely that recurrence of disease is the explanation.

Site of recurrence

Patients who have anterior resection for rectal or sigmoid carcinoma should be followed up by sigmoidoscopy every six months for five years, to look for anastomotic recurrence of tumour. Masses may be palpable on abdominal examination but isotope and ultrasonic scanning of the liver, bone scans and CT scanning all have a role in the diagnosis of recurrent colonic cancer. Once a colorectal cancer has occurred, there is a definite risk of another developing, at a different site (metachronous recurrence).

Treatment of recurrent disease

Patients who have recurrence of tumour at the site of a previous anastomosis should have further resection if this is possible. If recurrence of tumour is confined to one lobe of the liver or lung, then resection of the affected lobe is very occasionally possible.

If recurrent tumour occurs in bone then palliative radiotherapy is worthwhile to relieve pain. Chemotherapy, immunotherapy and radiotherapy are sometimes useful in relieving symptoms in patients with widespread recurrent disease, but these measures are not of value in bringing the disease under control.

DIVERTICULAR DISEASE OF THE COLON

This is a common condition in which the colon,

usually the sigmoid area, acquires outpouchings of the mucosa, which protrude through weakened areas of the muscular wall. By the age of 60 about one-third of individuals living in North America and Northern Europe have acquired such diverticula but in only a small minority (5–10%) will they produce symptoms.

It is generally believed that relative absence of roughage from the diet accounts for the high incidence of diverticular disease in the Western world and the rarity of diverticula in Third World countries: it is noticeable also that African and Asian citizens who move to live permanently in the West are also subject to diverticular disease (see p. 28).

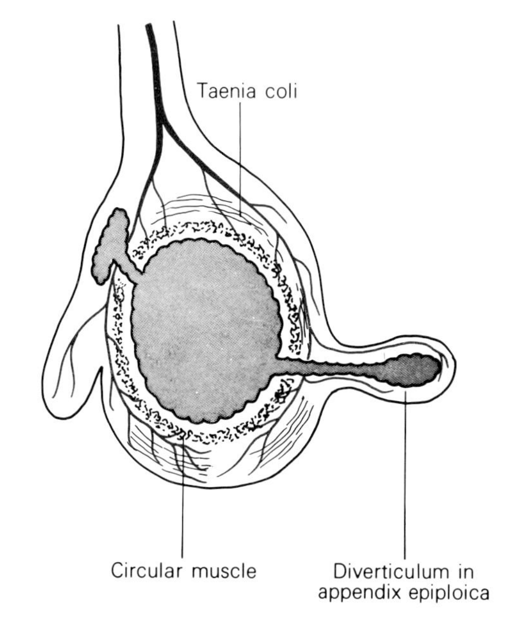

Fig. 9.25 *Site of formation of diverticula of the colon.*

Definitions

A *diverticulum* of the colon is a protrusion of mucosal lining through a defect in the muscle coat.

Diverticulosis denotes the presence of asymptomatic diverticula.

Diverticular disease is present when the patient has symptoms from diverticula which are not complicated by inflammatory sequelae.

Diverticulitis refers to any inflammatory complication of diverticula in the colon.

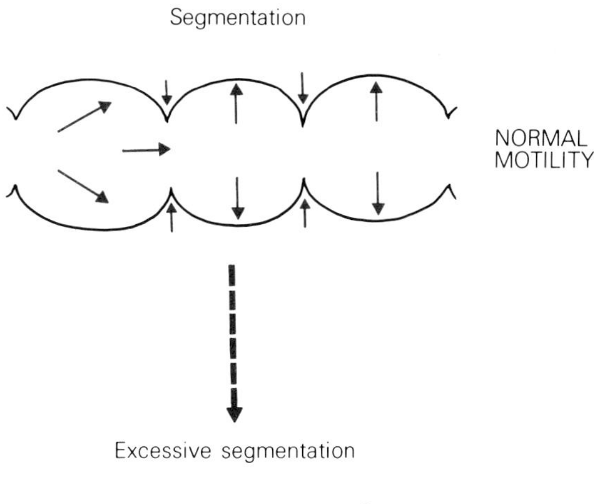

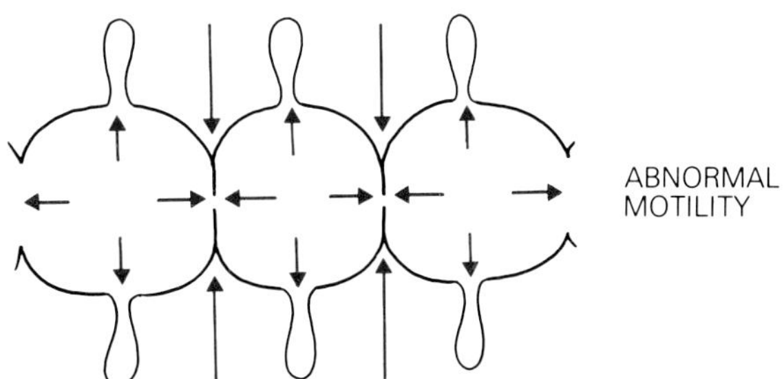

Fig. 9.26 *Aetiology of diverticulosis of colon.*

Anatomy and Pathophysiology

Diverticula are most often seen in the sigmoid colon between the taenia coli, usually at the point of weakness created by a segmental blood vessel piercing the muscular wall to enter the submucosa (Fig. 9.25). Increased segmentation is thought to produce a series of small 'bladders', in each of which very high intraluminal pressures (exceeding 50 mm Hg) can be developed. Over long periods this sort of abnormal muscular activity gradually produces outpouchings of mucosa at the weak points in the muscular wall (Fig. 9.26). The most striking feature of surgical resection specimens is the remarkable hypertrophy of the muscular wall of the colon, affecting both taenia coli and the circular muscle. It is believed that the bulky stools in the distal colon of individuals eating a high-fibre diet may reduce the excessive segmentation activity.

In a minority of patients a more diffuse form of diverticulosis, spread through the colon, is seen. These patients are appreciably younger, suggesting that a genetic factor could be important in the aetiology. The rectum is never involved in diverticular disease.

There is no doubt that vigorous muscular contraction can in itself be painful because specimens of sigmoid colon, resected for pain, often show muscular hypertrophy but no histological evidence of inflammation. The cause of true diverticulitis remains unknown: possibly it is due to a small perforation of a diverticulum subjected to high pressure, or to suppuration behind an impacted faecolith.

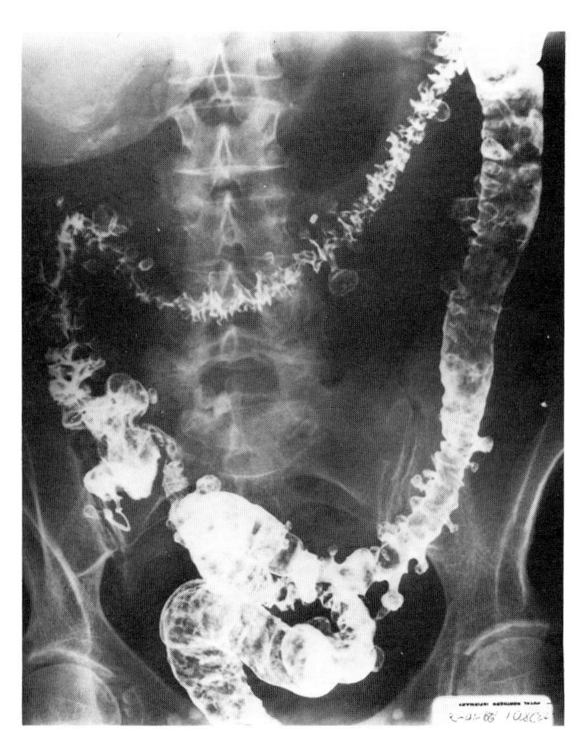

Fig. 9.27 *Barium enema showing generalised colonic diverticulosis.*

Clinical Manifestations

Only a minority of patients with diverticula will have symptoms. Vague symptoms such as flatulence and other abdominal symptoms may be related to this problem, but more specific symptoms are passage of small hard stools ('sheep droppings'), and pain across the lower abdomen or in the left iliac fossa. This pain may be continuous or may come on after meals due to an exaggerated gastrocolic reflex. Rectal bleeding is a very rare symptom of diverticular disease. Abdominal examination in these patients will often reveal a tender thickened area of sigmoid colon palpable in the left iliac fossa.

Sigmoidoscopy is essential to rule out rectal disease. Much spasm and oedema is seen at the rectosigmoid junction, making it difficult to enter the sigmoid; only occasionally are the mouths of diverticula visible. Similarly, circular muscle spasm makes colonoscopy difficult. Barium enema is the most useful examination in making a diagnosis (Fig. 9.27).

Treatment

Patients may respond to a high-residue diet, the most popular way being to give wheat bran in one of its forms: it can be mixed with other foods to make it more palatable. Anti-cholinergics such as propantheline, or smooth muscle relaxants such as mebeverine, may be of value. If the pain is severe, analgesics may be required, but opiates (including codeine) should be avoided since these drugs increase intracolonic pressure and theoretically expose the patient to the risk of perforation of a diverticulum. Only rarely will the patient require surgery for the pain of uncomplicated diverticular disease but, if it is necessary, resection of the sigmoid colon with end-to-end anastomosis is the treatment of choice for this condition.

Complications of Colonic Diverticula

Acute diverticulitis and pericolic abscess

A diverticulum may become infected because of

obstruction and ulceration of the neck of the diverticulum, giving symptoms in the left iliac fossa similar to appendicitis. The inflammation may resolve within a few days or may progress to involve a significant portion of the sigmoid colon. If resolution does not take place, pus collects around the colon producing a pericolic abscess which causes pain and pyrexia and, occasionally, urinary frequency. Treatment consists of observation in hospital, with oral fluid restriction, intravenous antibiotics (e.g. gentamicin and metronidazole), analgesia for pain, and regular examination of the abdomen to detect evidence of spread of the inflammation. Most patients will settle using this regime. A barium enema must be done a few weeks later to check the accuracy of the diagnosis, because it can be difficult (if not impossible) to distinguish complicated diverticular disease from carcinoma. If colonic diverticula are found, the patient can be commenced on a high-residue diet. Rarely, surgery will be necessary for a pericolic abscess which does not resolve.

Peritonitis due to perforated diverticulum of sigmoid colon

This condition is most often found in the elderly patient. The patient complains of severe abdominal pain, often commencing in the left iliac fossa, and there may be referral to the shoulders. On examination there are signs of shock, and abdominal examination will show signs of local or general peritonitis. An erect film of the chest sometimes reveals gas under the diaphragm but the plain film of the abdomen may not be helpful.

Treatment consists of urgent resuscitation of the patient with a view to laparotomy. If pus is present in the peritoneal cavity, and the inflamed area in the colon is reasonably well sealed, drainage of the abdomen with lavage of the peritoneal cavity with antibiotic solution and administration of intravenous antibiotics may be all that is required (see Chapter 13, p. 286). If, on the other hand, there is faecal contamination of the peritoneal cavity, most surgeons advocate excision of the perforated area of the colon with formation of a colostomy above the resected area. The rectal stump can be oversewn (Hartmann's resection: Fig. 9.28) but, if the perforation is high in the sigmoid colon, the affected area should be exteriorised as a double-barrelled colostomy (Fig. 9.29). In addition to this, the peritoneal cavity should be thoroughly lavaged with antibiotic solution, and intravenous antibiotics are also given for several days. the bowel is re-anastomosed six months later.

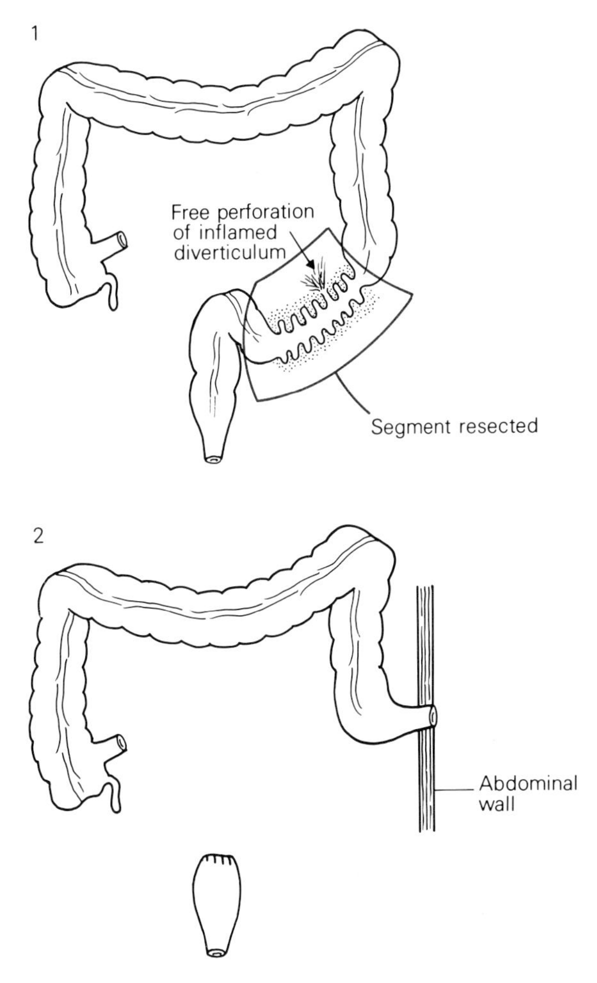

Fig. 9.28 *Hartmann's resection.*

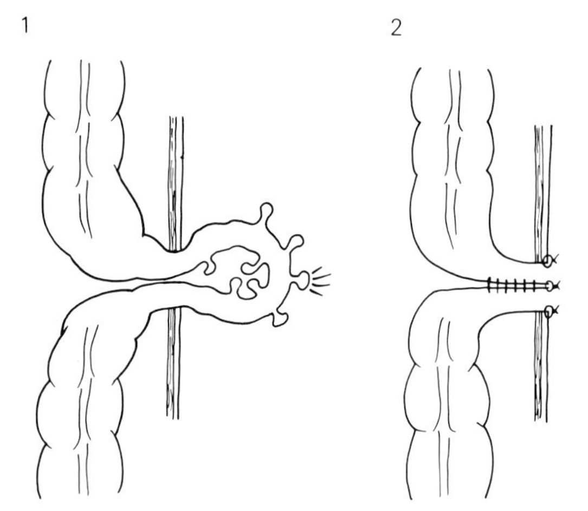

Fig. 9.29 *Paul–Mickulicz resection (double-barrelled colostomy).*

Fistula formation

If an abscess which has formed around the colon discharges into a structure adjacent to it, a fistula may be formed into the vagina, bladder, small bowel or, very occasionally, on to the skin.

The most serious of these complications is colovesical fistula. The urine becomes infected and wind (pneumaturia) and/or faeces is present in the urine. It is important to differentiate diverticulitis from carcinoma as a cause of this problem by barium enema, sigmoidoscopy, colonoscopy and cystoscopy, but this can be difficult. In either case, treatment consists of surgery, with removal of the colonic lesion and the affected area of bladder, primary or secondary anastomosis of the two ends of the large bowel, and closure of the bladder defect. Colovaginal fistula is almost equally distressing and requires a similar operation to separate vagina from diseased colon, which is then resected.

Haemorrhage

Bleeding is an uncommon but serious complication of diverticular disease (p. 309). If the blood-loss is small, a conservative attitude to treatment may be used. If blood-loss is severe then laparotomy may be necessary. Colonoscopy may be useful preoperatively to determine the site of bleeding but if blood-loss is severe this may be difficult. Selective arteriography of the superior and inferior mesenteric arteries can give very useful information on the site of bleeding. If surgery is necessary then resection of the appropriate area of colon is the method of choice. If the site of bleeding is uncertain, total colectomy with ileorectal anastomosis may occasionally be required.

ISCHAEMIC DISEASE OF THE COLON

Spontaneous ischaemia of the oesophagus, stomach and duodenum is virtually unknown. On the other hand ischaemic damage to the small bowel and colon have become increasingly recognised as clinical conditions in recent years.

The presentation of ischaemic damage to the colon is often less dramatic than small bowel ischaemia. One of two clinical pictures tends to emerge in the patient with ischaemia of the large bowel. When only the mucosa of the bowel is affected and the outer coats of the colon remain viable, a reversible condition called transient ischaemic colitis is the outcome. If, on the other hand, the whole thickness of the colonic wall is

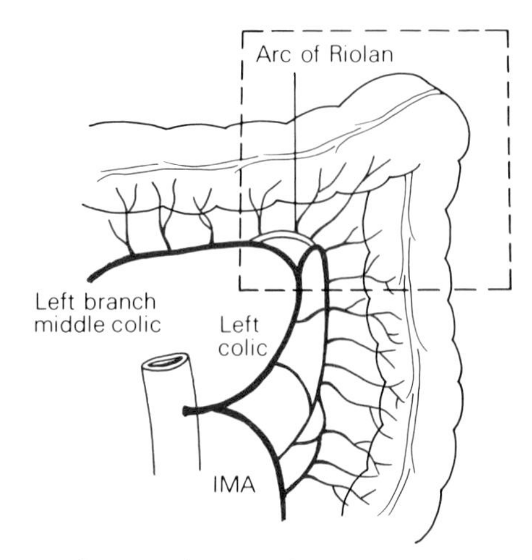

Fig. 9.30 *The critical area of blood supply at the splenic flexure.*

completely bereft of its blood supply, gangrene of the colon supervenes, with serious consequences if not treated surgically.

The precise cause of spontaneous ischaemia of the colon is unknown but the fact that it most often occurs at the splenic flexure area in elderly patients may give a clue to the aetiology. The splenic flexure area is the junctional area of blood supply from superior and inferior mesenteric arteries. In a minority of patients, the anastomosis between superior and inferior mesenteric arteries is poorly developed (Fig. 9.30) so that if one of the colonic arteries, affected by atheroma, is the site of a thrombosis it is this junctional area which tends to show ischaemic damage first of all.

Transient Ischaemic Colitis

In a typical case, a middle-aged or elderly patient complains of severe left-sided abdominal pain associated with diarrhoea and passage of dark red blood per rectum. There may be tachycardia and fever and on abdominal examination tenderness is generally found over the affected colon, without signs of peritonitis. Sigmoidoscopy does not usually show anything except some blood flecks on a normal mucosa; but on plain x-ray of the abdomen, narrowing of the gas shadow at the splenic flexure as a result of oedema of the mucosa is a common finding. An emergency barium enema examination will confirm the narrowing and the typical 'thumb-printing' appearance due to submucosal haemorrhage in the distal transverse colon or upper descending colon (Fig. 9.31). If colonoscopy is performed, the mucosa is a blue-purple colour and the colonic lumen is narrowed. The mucosa is friable and ulceration may be seen, depending on when the colonoscopy is performed. These patients require close observation in hospital but usually settle down over a few days.

Acute Gangrene of the Colon

This occurs in a minority of patients. It may result from ligation of the inferior mesenteric artery during surgery on the abdominal aorta, or due to accidental damage to the mesocolon in blunt or penetrating abdominal trauma. More typically, an elderly patient, already known to have cardiac disease, complains of sudden severe abdominal pain and rapidly shows signs of peripheral circulatory failure with clinical evidence, on abdominal examination, of peritonitis. Very prompt resuscitation is needed with intravenous fluids (including colloid). Intravenous antibiotics, e.g. combined gentamicin and metronidazole, should be administered and, as soon as the patient is fit for surgery, laparotomy is undertaken. The affected segment of colon at operation often has a green or black appearance and perforation of the organ may already have occurred. This segment of colon must be resected back to viable tissue, but if there is evidence of peritonitis no attempt should be made to anastomose the two ends of bowel at this stage.

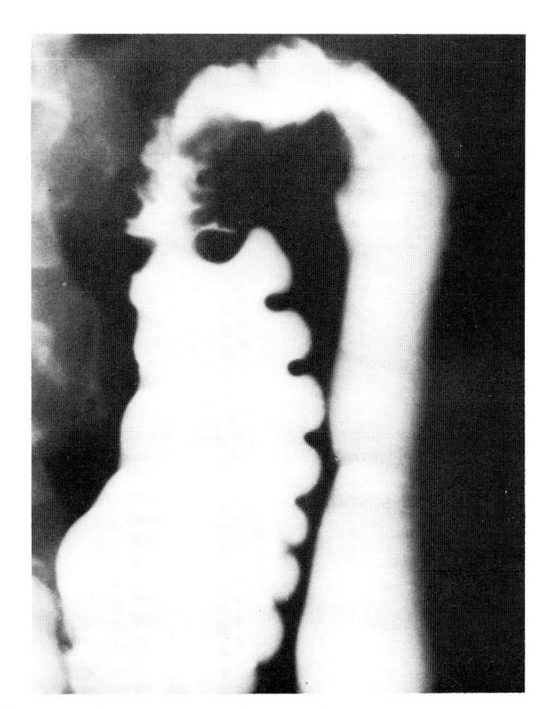

Fig. 9.31 *Barium enema showing changes (thumb printing) of ischaemic colitis at the splenic flexure.*

The two ends of colon can be brought out on to the abdominal wall as stomas and an anastomosis between the two ends of the colon should be delayed for several months. This serious condition carries a high mortality rate.

MEGACOLON

This term embraces a number of clinical conditions in which the diameter of the colon is markedly increased. The main presenting features of megacolon include prolonged constipation and abdominal distension.

Hirschsprung's Disease (see p. 265).

Most patients present as neonates or in the first year or two of life, but a few are diagnosed much later when they are adult. The usual history is of life-long severe constipation and varying abdominal distension. Such a patient can present with a sudden increase in the degree of abdominal distension which demands urgent colostomy to forestall respiratory failure. The best definitive operation in the adult has proved to be Duhamel's procedure (p. 268).

Chagas Disease

This is seen most commonly in South America. It is an acquired aganglionosis due to infestation with *Trypanosoma cruzi*. This affects the distal large bowel (and also the oesophagus), and ganglionic degeneration takes place slowly. When the degree of constipation and distension is intolerable, it is reasonable to attempt surgical treatment. Duhamel's operation is the procedure of choice.

Idiopathic Megacolon

Most patients in the UK who present with acquired megacolon suffer from an idiopathic condition. There is often a history, dating back to early childhood, of constipation and distension, and, unlike patients with Hirschsprung's disease, the rectum is capacious and full of faeces. It is important, nevertheless, to differentiate between short-segment Hirschsprung's disease and acquired idiopathic megacolon by doing a rectal biopsy. Surgical treatment for acquired megacolon is not usually recommended. The aim of treatment is to completely empty the over-distended rectum and to keep it empty. High-fibre diet, judicious use of laxatives, and proper toilet training are the most useful aspects of management of this difficult problem.

PNEUMATOSIS CYSTOIDES INTESTINALIS

In this rare condition, nitrogen-filled cysts are present in the mucosa and submucosa of the intestines. Their aetiology is unknown, but there is an association with chronic obstructive lung disease, peptic ulcer, and gastric cancer.

Although usually found by chance on sigmoidoscopy or radiography, when these cysts are large or diffuse they may give rise to obstruction, or to malabsorption syndrome.

Surgery is usually not required because the cysts tend to resolve, sometimes with high-flow oxygen therapy for 4–5 days.

10

Inflammatory Bowel Disease

INTRODUCTION

Inflammatory bowel disease (IBD) is now recognised as one of the most serious non-malignant disorders involving the gastrointestinal tract. In its most severe form it is responsible for 250–300 deaths each year in England and Wales, many of these in young people. For those not so severely affected, IBD causes much chronic disability, with a continuing cycle of relapse and remission and, in a number of patients, requires major surgery, with a permanent stoma, for its control.

Two major forms of IBD are recognised: non-specific proctocolitis (NSP), which is more generally but less accurately called ulcerative colitis, affecting the large bowel only; and Crohn's disease (CD), which can affect any part of the gastrointestinal tract from the mouth to the anus. In about 10% of patients, features of both diseases are seen and classification is difficult.

Unlike many other inflammatory conditions of the intestine (Table 10.1), the cause of IBD is as yet unknown. Many hypotheses have been suggested, including infection by transmissible agent, an immunological disorder, food allergy, and even psychosomatic influences: these are more fully considered on page 31.

The incidence of the inflammatory bowel disorders is thought to be on the increase. In recent detailed surveys in the Grampian region of Scotland this appears to be true for NSP (Fig. 10.1) but not for CD (Fig. 10.2).

The age distribution of both diseases is similar

Table 10.1
Differential Diagnosis of Inflammatory Bowel Disease

	Mainly Small Bowel	*Small and Large Bowel*	*Mainly Large Bowel*	*Ano-Rectal*
Specific infective causes	Cholera Yersinia Giardiasis	Tuberculosis Necrotising enterocolitis Enteric group of fevers Staphylococcal enterocolitis Campylobacter	Bacillary dysentery Amoebiasis Schistosomiasis Trypanosomiasis (Chagas' disease) Pseudomembranous enterocolitis	Syphilis Gonorrhoea Lymphogranuloma venereum
Other specific conditions	Coeliac disease Whipple's disease	Irradiation 'Irritable bowel' Eosinophilic gastroenteritis Crohn's disease Drug-induced diarrhoea	Diverticular disease Ischaemic colitis Ulcerative colitis *or* Non-specific proctocolitis	Crohn's disease 'Solitary ulcer'

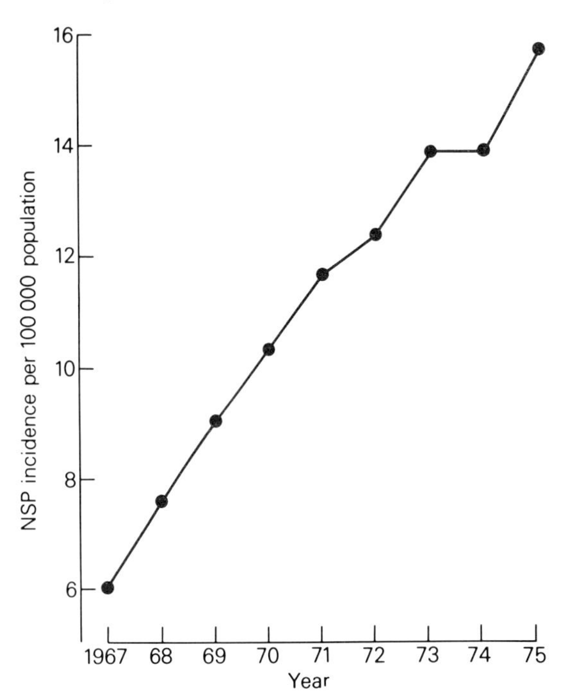

Fig. 10.1 *Incidence of NSP in North East Scotland per 100 000 population.*

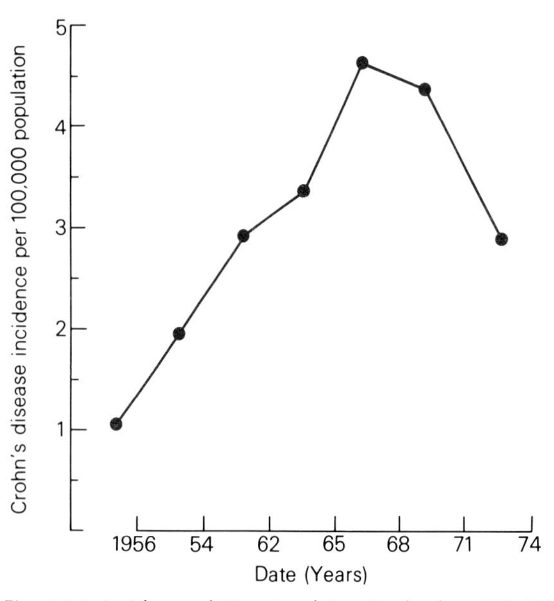

Fig. 10.2 *Incidence of CD in North East Scotland per 100 000 population (from Kyle and Stark, 1981).*

and bimodal, showing peaks in young adult life and in older age groups.

PATHOLOGY

Non-specific Proctocolitis

The principal naked-eye feature is that the disease is confined to the large bowel. In about two-thirds of patients (Fig. 10.3) only the distal large bowel is affected; when disease is confined to the rectum, it is known as proctitis, and when part or all of the sigmoid is involved it is termed proctosigmoiditis. Disease may remain confined to these areas for years, or there may be gradual extension to proximal parts of the colon. Alternatively inflammation may, from the start of the illness, be either extensive or affect the whole of the colon.

Non-specific proctocolitis is essentially a disease of the mucous membrane and in proctitis the mucosa is typically red, oedematous and granular, and bleeds easily when touched. Ulceration is unusual in the rectum, but is typical of more extensive disease. The clinical severity of NSP can, in fact, best be judged (as in burns of the skin) by the extent and depth of the ulcerative process, and in severe disease long strips of mucosa, 1–1.5 cm wide, are shed over considerable distances, exposing the muscular layer of the bowel wall. In the most severe examples (Fig. 10.4) almost all mucosa may be lost, leaving only a few islands of oedematous mucosa, which are known as mucosal islands. The exposed muscularis becomes covered with granulation tissue and it is the sero-sanguinous exudate from this raw surface that causes the hypoproteinaemia and anaemia characteristic of severe attacks. Occasionally the ulcerative process penetrates further and perforation of the colon occurs. Extensive ulceration in the transverse colon may be complicated by wide atonic dilatation – 'toxic megacolon' (see p. 231). 'Pseudo-polyps', or inflammatory polyps, form in about 20% of patients with NSP.

Microscopy

The normal colonic mucosa consists of epithelium

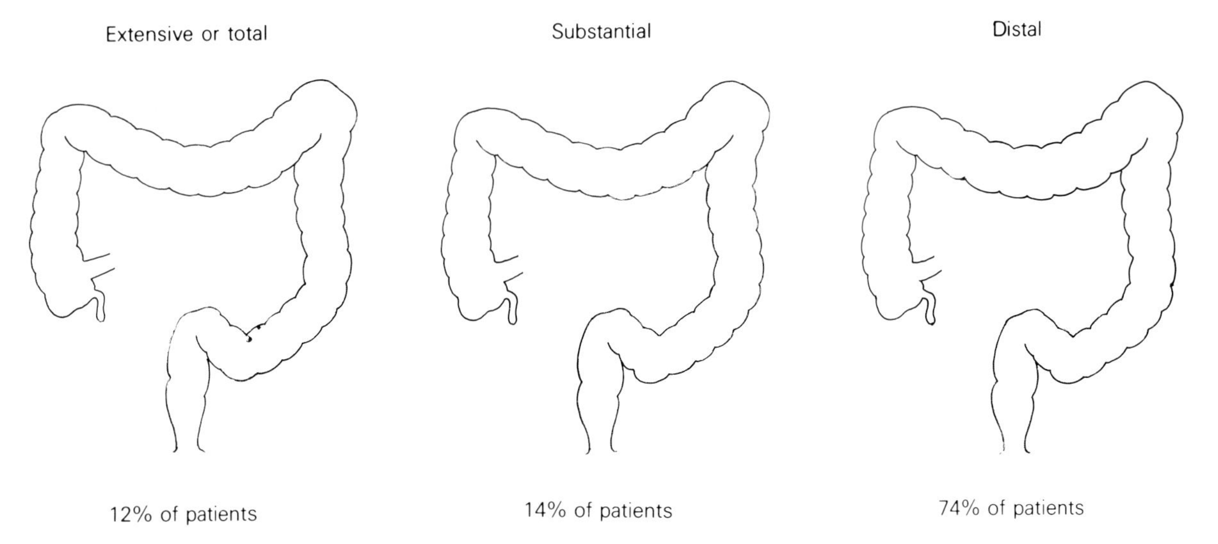

Fig. 10.3 *Extent of involvement of large bowel in NSP. (Percentages from 534 patients surveyed by barium enema in North East Scotland, 1967–75).*

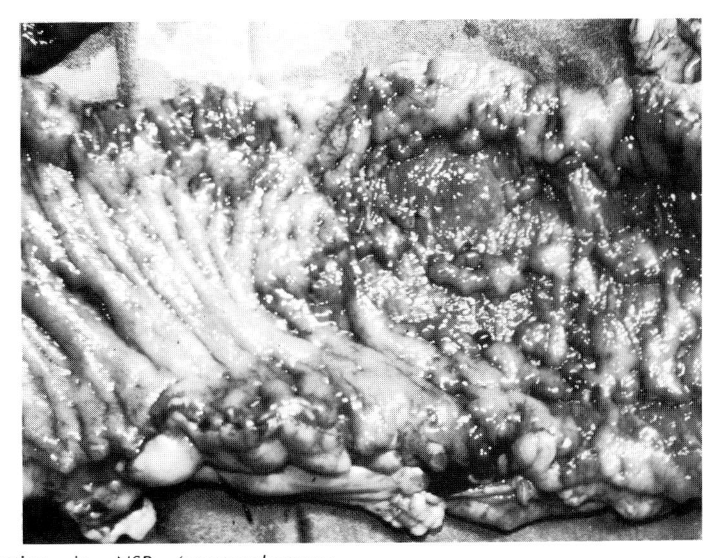

Fig. 10.4 *Severe ulceration in NSP (proctocolectomy specimen).*

characterised by regular downgrowths into the lamina propria, known as crypts. The epithelium is columnar with frequent goblet cells. Biopsies from patients with mild disease show an increased number of inflammatory cells in the lamina propria, which becomes swollen by oedema. The goblet-cell population is reduced and acute inflammatory cells, including eosinophils and neutrophils, are seen in the lamina propria. Neutrophil aggregates within crypts, producing crypt abscesses, are one of the features of NSP (Fig. 10.5).

In acute disease, adjacent crypt abscesses become confluent, with loss of the overlying

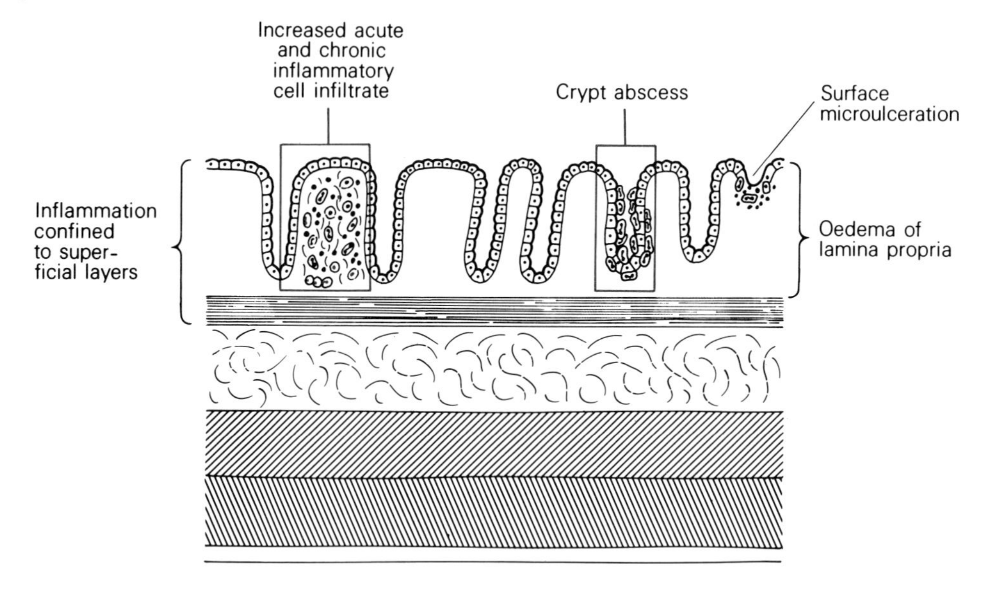

Fig. 10.5 *Diagrammatic representation of histological features of mild NSP.*

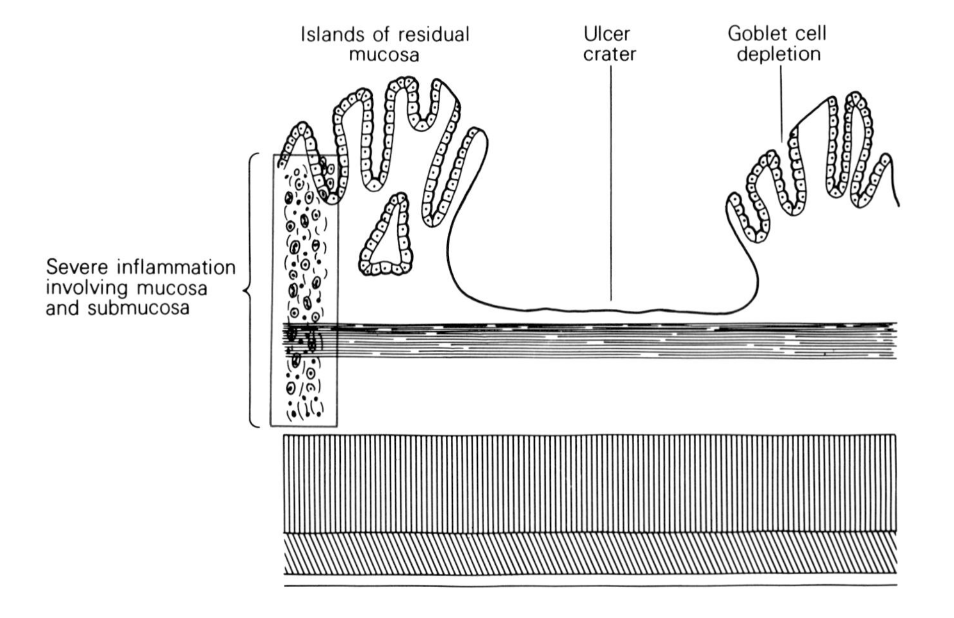

Fig. 10.6 *Diagrammatic representation of histological features of severe NSP.*

mucosa, so producing ulceration (Fig. 10.6).

As activity subsides, goblet cells reappear but the gland pattern is distorted and shortened.

In long-standing NSP, dysplasia of the mucosa may be seen. This is an important finding because, if severe, it may be a warning that cancerous change is occurring (see below).

Crohn's Disease

Crohn's Disease differs radically from NSP because it can affect any part of the alimentary tract (Fig. 10.7). The most characteristic Crohn's lesion is a severe inflammatory thickening of the terminal ileum, which becomes a rigid tube, with a great increase in mesenteric fat, and fleshy lymph node enlargement. The wall of the ileum is so thick that there may be obstruction of the lumen (Fig. 10.8), and the mucosa shows linear ulceration, producing a 'cobblestone' appearance. Fissures may penetrate the wall of the bowel, leading to fistulae forming into adjacent hollow organs. These changes may extend into the caecum.

In Crohn's colitis, the changes may be very similar to NSP, but typically there are relatively normal areas of colon between areas of ulceration (skip lesions), the rectum is often less inflamed than the colon, and perianal sepsis is a very common manifestation.

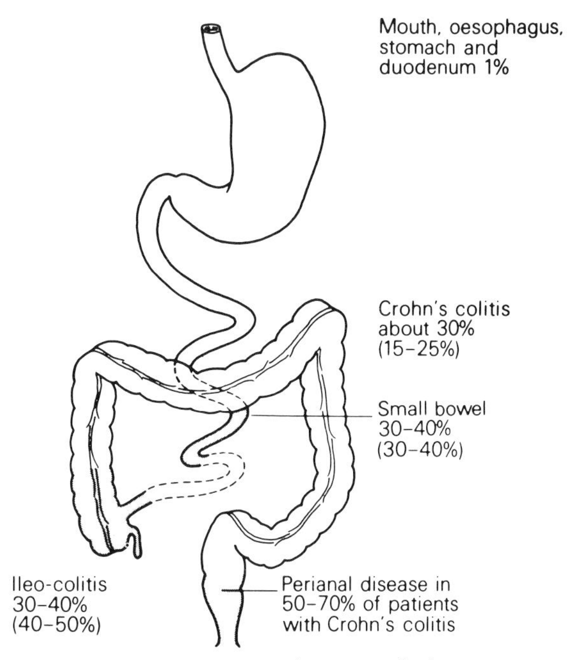

Fig. 10.7 *Diagram showing the areas of alimentary tract affected by Crohn's disease in British Isles. (Figures in brackets from survey in USA).*

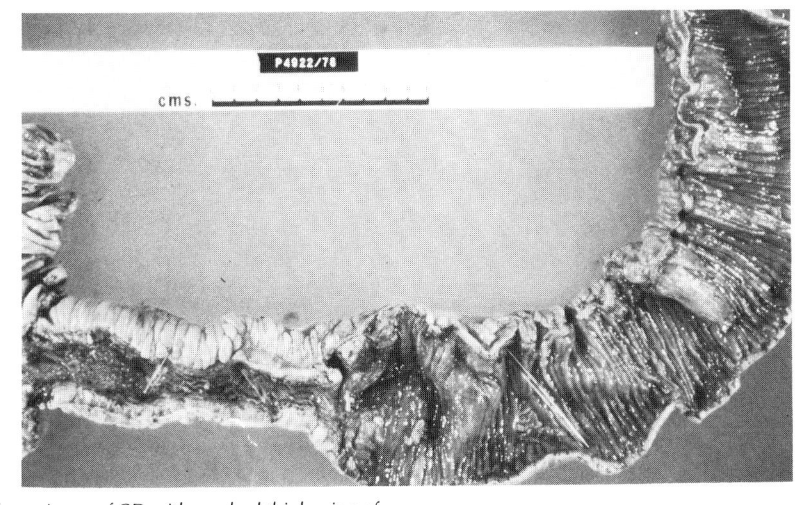

Fig. 10.8 *Resected specimen of CD with marked thickening of wall of terminal ileum and cobblestone ulceration of mucosa. The proximal bowel shows the signs of intestinal obstruction.*

Microscopy

The typical microscopic changes of CD include severe inflammation affecting all layers of the bowel (transmural inflammation: Fig. 10.9). The inflammatory cells include lymphocytes arranged as lymphoid aggregates, and plasma cells as well as neutrophils.

A histological hallmark of CD is the presence of granulomata, reminiscent of sarcoidosis. These granulomata consist of modified macrophages (epithelioid cells) and occasional giant cells. They are found in 60% of cases, usually in the submucosa (Fig. 10.10).

Crypt abscesses are not so frequently seen in CD but aphthoid ulceration, characterised by microabscesses deep in the lamina propria, is a useful diagnostic feature. Fissure formation, extending from the surface through a variable depth of the bowel wall of the intestine, is commonly seen. Despite the characteristic transmural inflammation, the incidence of free perforation and megacolon is rather less than in NSP. Although the changes affecting related lymph nodes are mostly those of reactive hyperplasia, in some cases epithelioid granulomata are seen within the lymph nodes.

SYMPTOMS

Non-specific Proctocolitis

Symptoms vary according to the extent of disease. Patients with distal disease (proctitis and proctosigmoiditis: Fig. 10.3) do not necessarily have diarrhoea and may even be constipated; passage of blood and mucus per rectum is often accompanied by lower abdominal pain, urgency and tenesmus. Patients with more extensive disease will tend to have large-volume diarrhoea, pass

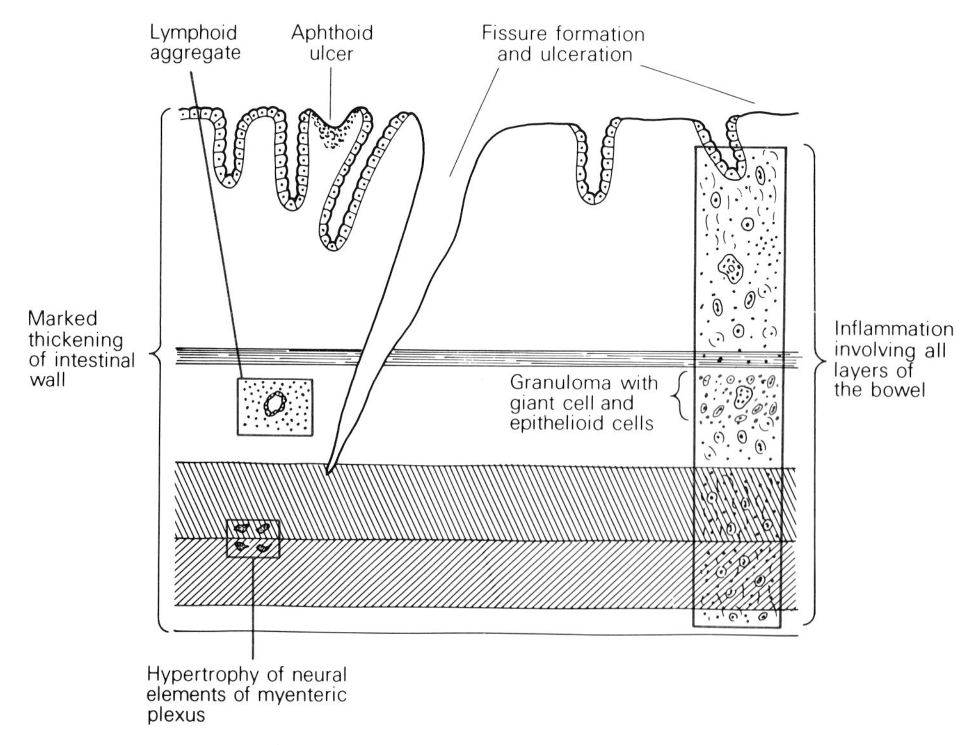

Fig. 10.9 *Diagrammatic representation of histological features of Crohn's disease.*

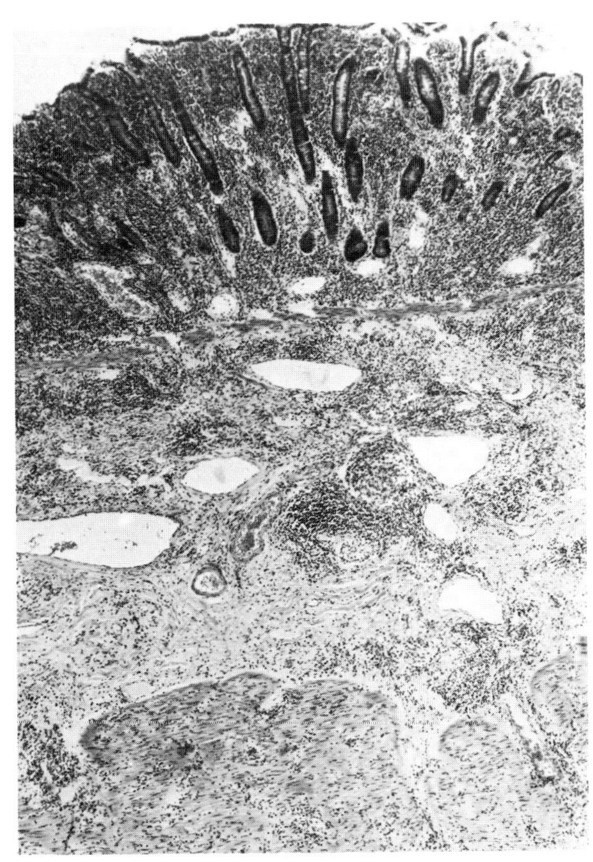

Fig. 10.10 *Photomicrograph of histological changes in Crohn's disease: inflammatory cell infiltration, and numerous granulomata in submucosa.*

blood and mucus per rectum and, in addition, are frequently systemically ill with weight loss and anorexia. Rarely, patients may become acutely ill with disease of such severity that vigorous resuscitation is required.

Occasionally, extra-intestinal manifestations such as arthritis, iritis or skin rashes are the predominant presenting complaint.

Crohn's Disease

A great variety of symptoms occur, and they vary according to the extent and site of gastrointestinal tract involvement. Patients with predominantly colonic disease may be impossible to differentiate clinically from patients with NSP. Small-bowel disease can produce diarrhoea, steatorrhoea, pain, or symptoms of obstruction if a stricture is present. Bleeding per rectum is less common than in NSP. Extra-intestinal manifestations similar to those associated with NSP are occasionally encountered. Crohn's disease is generally a more insidious disease. In childhood and adolescence, patients tend to present with retarded growth, and alimentary tract symptoms are only recognised after close questioning. At all ages, patients with CD may have pyrexia of unknown origin, recurrent abdominal pain, or anorexia and weight loss as their major complaint: in these circumstances the diagnosis can go unsuspected for some time.

In contrast to NSP a substantial number of patients with CD will present initially with perianal problems.

PHYSICAL EXAMINATION

Non-specific Proctocolitis

General

It is common to find no abnormality on physical examination. Patients with extensive and severe disease may show evidence of weight loss. The mucosal and nail changes associated with iron-deficiency anaemia may be seen. In an acute exacerbation, tachycardia and fever may be evident and, if significant amounts of blood and fluid have been lost, the patient becomes dehydrated and hypotensive.

Abdominal examination

Tenderness over the diseased colon is a common finding. Bowel sounds are usually normal. Abdominal distension may be pronounced when toxic dilatation of the colon occurs. Rectal examination is essential and may reveal a characteristic velvety feeling of the inflamed mucosa, with blood on the finger.

Crohn's Disease

General

There is frequently evidence of weight loss. Changes due to anaemia, including vitamin B_{12} and folate deficiency, should be looked for. Other features such as glossitis, clubbing, mouth ulceration, fever and tachycardia are common.

Abdominal examination

Abdominal findings depend on extent and site of bowel involvement. A tender right iliac fossa mass suggests ileal or ileocaecal disease. When a small bowel stricture is present, signs of acute or subacute obstruction may be present, including abdominal distension, visible peristalsis, and obstructive bowel sounds (Fig. 10.11). In patients with mild colonic or small-bowel disease no abnormality is usually found except tenderness in the abdomen.

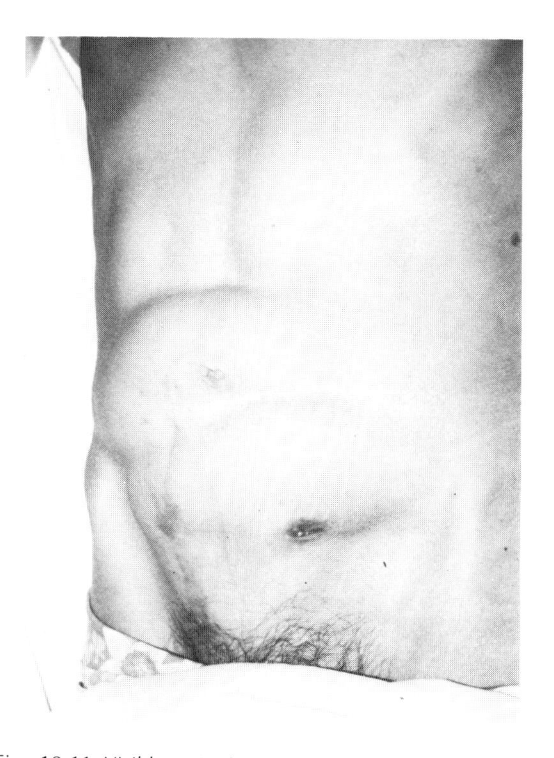

Fig. 10.11 *Visible peristalsis in obstructed small bowel above CD in terminal ileum.*

Inspection of the anus often suggests the existence of CD: oedematous skin tags and chronic relatively painless fissure formation are common. The anal canal may be indurated and narrow, with palpable rectal ulceration.

In all in-patients it is important to inspect the stool for evidence of malabsorption or blood loss.

SIGMOIDOSCOPY

Non-specific Proctocolitis

Sigmoidoscopy is essential for diagnosis of NSP since this disease almost always affects the rectum.

The mildest changes consist of oedema of the bowel wall together with hyperaemia resulting in loss of visibility of the normal submucosal blood vessels. If the disease is active, spontaneous or contact bleeding of the mucosa develops. Pus is sometimes visible and, when the disease process becomes severe, ulceration of the mucosa is encountered: this is seen more in the sigmoid colon than in the rectum. The rectum becomes rigid and will not distend in the usual way by inflation of air through the sigmoidoscope. mucosal islands, which are islands of hyperplastic mucosa left between extensive ulceration, are sometimes a feature of severe colitis. As the condition goes into remission, the epithelial layer heals over and looks relatively normal. A rectal biopsy should always be taken at initial sigmoidoscopy.

Crohn's Disease

Crohn's disease should be suspected on sigmoidoscopy when the inflammation in the rectum is patchy, or superficial aphthoid ulcers are seen. 'Cobblestone' ulceration and narrowing of the rectum due to fibrosis denotes severe disease.

If Crohn's disease is suspected, a rectal biopsy should always be taken because sarcoid-like granulomata are sometimes detectable on histological section, even when the rectum looks normal.

INVESTIGATION

Blood

Full blood count, erythrocyte sedimentation rate, urea and electrolytes, liver function tests and serum albumin are essential laboratory investigations to assess the severity of any given attack of IBD. A low serum albumin is a significant indicator of severe relapse. a falling ESR is a useful indicator of progress. Anaemia is generally either an iron deficiency (hypochromic microcytic) anaemia due to blood loss or a normochromic normocytic anaemia resulting from the chronic inflammatory process. In CD, malabsorption may result in vitamin B_{12} or folate deficiency, and occasionally produces a frank megaloblastic anaemia. Serum electrolytes are commonly normal. The total body potassium may be reduced as the result of severe diarrhoea although this is not necessarily reflected in the serum potassium. In the majority of patients, liver function tests are normal but in some 10% of patients, because of associated liver disease, they are abnormal (commonly a raised alkaline phosphatase).

Stools

Two or three stool specimens should be examined by microscopy and culture in initial attacks and relapses of IBD. There are two reasons for this policy:

- The differential diagnosis of NSP includes diseases such as amoebic dysentery, antibiotic-associated pseudomembranous colitis and campylobacter infection.
- It is now known that exacerbations of IBD can be precipitated by enteric infection.

Tests of small bowel function

Tests of small bowel function are used to assess the degree of malabsorption present in the patient with Crohn's disease (see p. 122).

Radiology of NSP (Fig. 10.12)

Plain abdominal x-ray is not only useful in detecting toxic dilatation or perforation but may also give information on the extent of disease. Diseased colon tends to be empty of faeces and

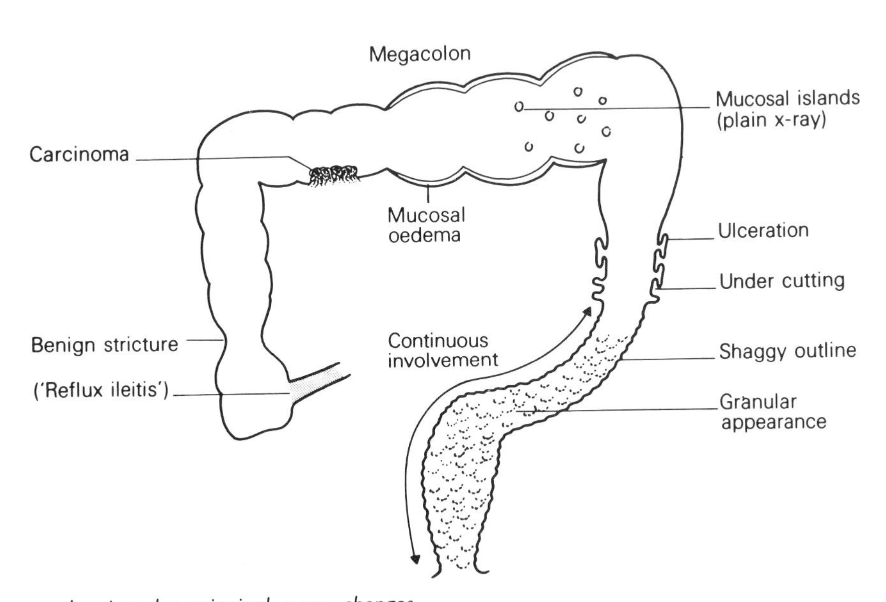

Fig. 10.12 *Diagram showing the principal x-ray changes found in NSP.*

occasionally bowel gas outlines clearly the diseased segments of bowel.

Barium enema is not advisable in a patient with severely active disease because of the risk of perforation. With moderately active disease, a barium enema can give important information about the state of the colon. In quiescent colitis a double contrast barium enema should show enough mucosal detail to give an accurate assessment of the extent of disease. The usual features are fine mucosal granularity, superficial and occasionally deep ulceration (Fig. 10.13). With long-standing disease, shortening of the colon with loss of haustral pattern will also be seen. NSP extends proximally and continuously from the rectum, unlike CD which may show patchy colonic involvement. Strictures are comparatively uncommon; especially in long-standing disease, the presence of a stricture should always raise a suspicion that malignant change has occurred.

Radiology of Crohn's disease (Fig. 10.14)

Intestinal obstruction is a fairly common complication of ileocaecal CD, and a plain abdominal x-ray

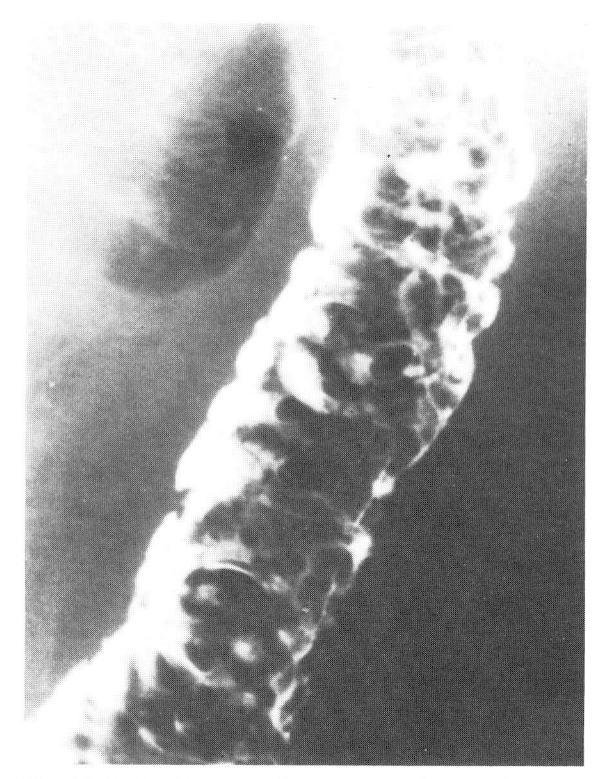

Fig. 10.13 *Double contrast barium enema showing ulceration in severe NSP.*

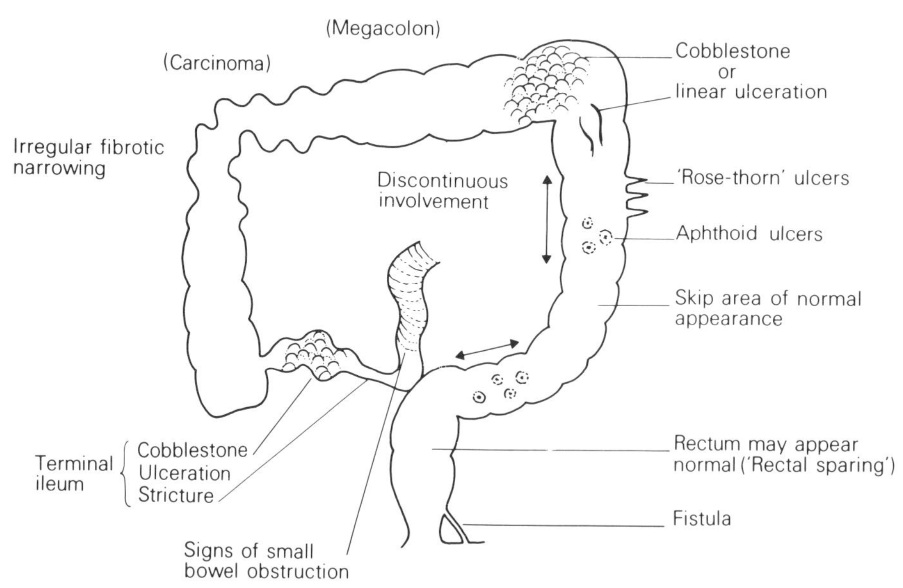

Fig. 10.14 *Diagram showing the principal x-ray changes seen in barium studies in CD.*

will show dilated loops of bowel, possibly with fluid levels. The radiological investigation of CD usually involves barium studies of both the small and large bowel. The radiological changes of Crohn's colitis differ little from those of NSP except that the lesions may be patchy and deeper with more mucosal undermining. Discrete ulcers on double contrast barium enema are seen as a small pocket of barium surrounded by a halo of radiolucency due to oedema. If the small intestine is involved, patchy changes with oedema, ulceration and/or stricture formation should be looked for on a small-bowel meal or enema (Fig. 10.15).

COMPLICATIONS OF INFLAMMATORY BOWEL DISEASE

Local Complications

Perianal disease

Perianal problems are less common in NSP than in CD, but there is still a greater incidence of perianal abscesses, fistulae and fissures among patients with NSP than in the normal population. The treatment of each complication is generally the same as for a patient without colitis (see p. 252).

In contrast, most clinicians would recommend nonoperative treatment for the perianal problems of CD, except when an acute abscess is present. Anal fistula is a particularly difficult complication to treat satisfactorily in CD.

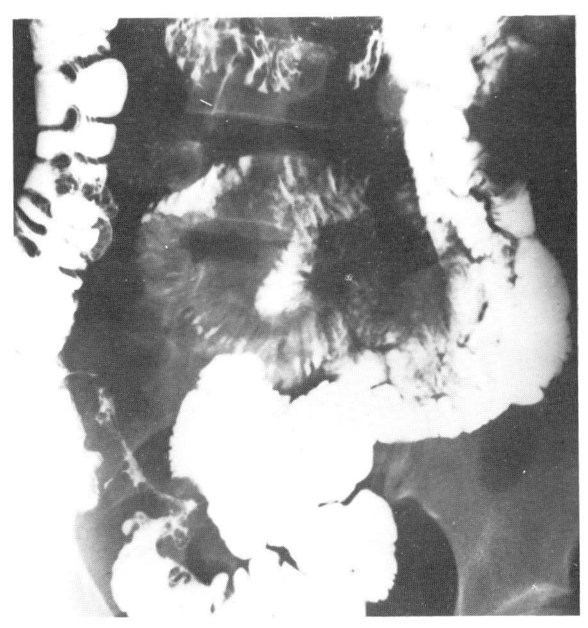

Fig. 10.15 *Small-bowel barium meal in CD. There is marked narrowing and irregular mucosal pattern in terminal ileum.*

Intestinal obstruction

The inflammation in CD is transmural so that an element of obstruction may be a problem in many cases. Stenosis of a more permanent kind is seen in patients with long-standing disease, where fibrosis as well as repeated inflammation may play a role. In most cases it is the small bowel which is the site of the obstructing lesion. Many of these episodes settle on conservative management but sometimes resection of the appropriate area is needed.

Fibrous strictures

These may be present in the small or large bowel in CD, but only involve large bowel in NSP. It is unusual for fibrous strictures to produce a significant degree of obstruction in the large bowel. The clinical importance of finding such a stricture in a patient with NSP lies in the strong possibility that it may be malignant.

Perforation of the bowel

This is an unusual complication of both CD and NSP. Almost all the perforations reported in patients with CD have been in the small bowel, whereas perforation necessarily occurs only in the large bowel of patients with NSP. Toxic megacolon is often a precursor to the development of perforation in patients with NSP.

Toxic megacolon

This rare but dangerous complication is seen in NSP more than in CD. It only affects patients with severe disease in whom ulceration of the colon involves the muscle layers. Consequent loss of tone allows expansion of the colon beyond its normal dimensions, the transverse colon being most commonly affected. Dilatation of the colon may be exacerbated by administration of certain anti-diarrhoeal agents, notably opiates (morphine, codeine phosphate). A barium enema performed during an attack of disease may be a further precipitating factor. There are usually, but not invariably, signs of toxicity, including high fever and tachycardia. There may be a paradoxical diminution in the number of stools. Abdominal distension is a feature, and abdominal tenderness is common. However, the abdominal signs may be dangerously masked by administration of corticosteroids.

The diagnosis is made on plain x-ray of the abdomen (Fig. 10.16). The transverse colon is generally the most severely distended area. If mucosal islands with intervening ulceration are seen, this is a signal for immediate surgery, because perforation is imminent (see p. 241).

The reported mortality associated with toxic megacolon has been as high as 30% but in most centres it is now nearer 10%.

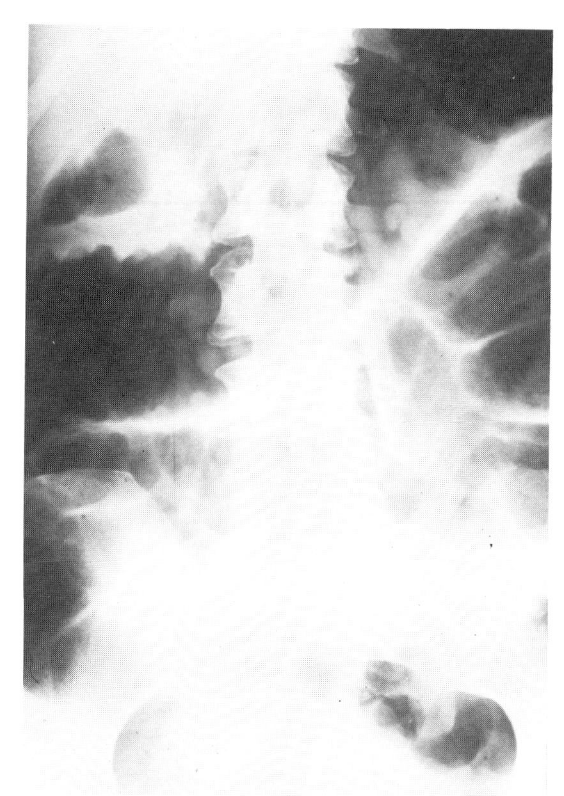

Fig. 10.16 *Plain abdominal x-ray showing toxic dilatation of transverse colon in severe NSP. Irregular thickened outline of colon, with mucosal islands visible between areas of ulceration.*

Large-Bowel Carcinoma as a Complication of Inflammatory Bowel Disease

Nonspecific proctocolitis is a premalignant condition. Although this fact has received much publicity, it is important to recognise that carcinoma only rarely develops. Over 70% of patients with NSP have distal disease (Fig. 10.3). In them the risk of colorectal cancer appears to be no greater than in the general population. The patients at risk are the 10–15% who have total or near-total colitis, and who have had their disease for 10 or more years: in this group, the risk is about 30 times that in the general population. Between 10–20 years, the risk for the individual appears to be about 1 in 200 for each year, rising to 1 in 60 after 20 years. Patients who develop NSP in childhood may be particularly at risk (Fig. 10.17). However, carcinoma developing in a colitic large bowel accounts for only about 1% of all colorectal cancers.

Cancer develops insidiously, particularly because patients are used to irregularity of the bowels and bleeding, and the patient's symptoms often change little until the tumour is no longer curable. Consequently a determined effort has been made in the last few years to try to predict the development of this complication.

Dysplasia has been found in rectal biopsies of some, but not all, patients with cancer developing elsewhere in a colitic colon. Other patients who have not already developed carcinoma have also been found to have these changes, and it is thought that dysplasia may indicate the potential for the development of carcinoma.

However, dysplastic change is far from uniform; it is difficult to assess histologically and it is still not clear how far established dysplasia foretells the development of a carcinoma. In this difficult field

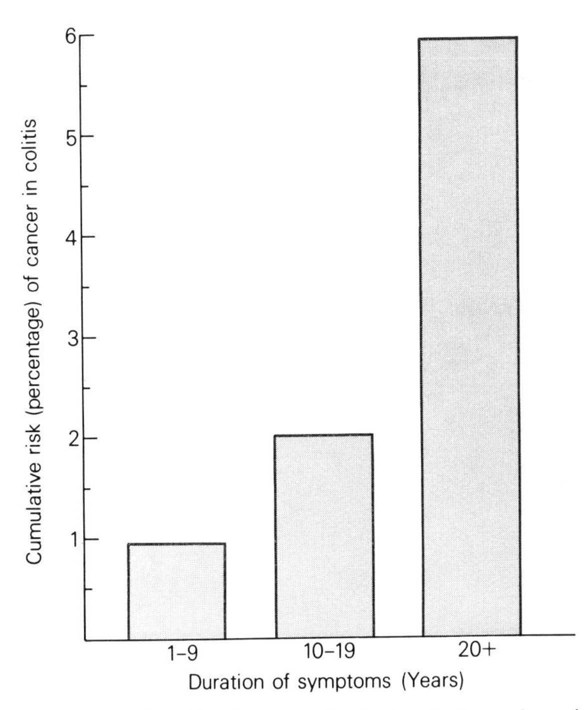

Fig. 10.17 *The risk of cancer developing in the colon of patients with extensive or total NSP.*

it is absolutely essential that patients who have had pancolitis for more than 10 years should be seen once or twice a year, even if their disease is quiescent. Sigmoidoscopy and rectal biopsy must be undertaken at each visit and, every two years, it is advisable for these patients to have a colonoscopy, with multiple biopsies of the colon. Patients who show severe dysplasia in several biopsies should be advised to undergo prophylactic proctocolectomy. In a proportion of these, a focus of carcinoma will be found, but with this close type of supervision the prognosis after radical resection appears to be good.

The risk of carcinoma developing in a patient with Crohn's colitis is very much less than the risk for a patient with NSP, and those with small bowel involvement are very unlikely to develop a carcinoma.

Extra-Intestinal Manifestations

Arthritis of large joints, uveitis, erythema nodosum, and liver disease are the commoner extra-intestinal manifestations associated with both diseases. (Fig. 10.18). Pyoderma gangrenosum, a necrotising skin disorder, is seen very rarely in patients with NSP. Patients may present with low back pain due to sacro-ileitis, though this is frequently asymptomatic and is seen simply on routine radiology.

The pathogenesis of these manifestations is unclear, although there is some evidence that circulating immune complexes are involved.

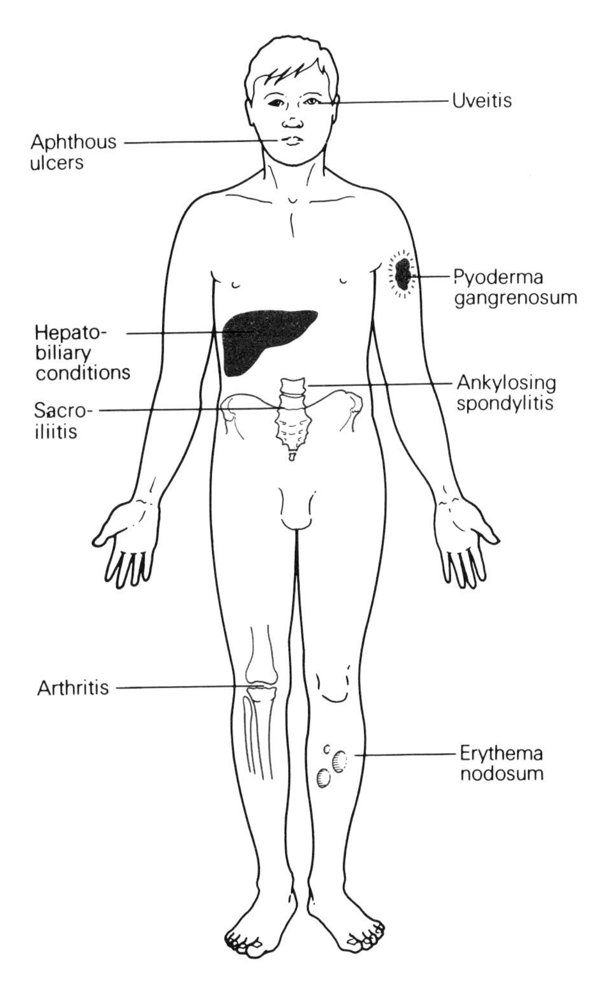

Fig. 10.18 *The extra-intestinal manifestations of inflammatory bowel disease.*

Associated liver disease can take many forms, including fatty change, chronic active hepatitis, cirrhosis, sclerosing cholangitis, pericholangitis, and carcinoma of the bile duct. In general, the severity and progression of liver disease is not influenced either by the state of the disease or by removal of the colon.

The overall frequency of extra-intestinal manifestations varies from 2–10% of patients.

MANAGEMENT OF IBD

The aim of management is to relieve symptoms, to induce remission, and to prevent relapse. Sometimes it is necessary to deal urgently with complications.

Almost every patient with IBD is going to require a long period of supervision, with many visits to hospital and, in a few cases, quite long spells of in-patient treatment. The nature of the disease demands patience and understanding on the part of both patient and doctor. This relationship may have to meet difficult situations, with major decisions to be taken, e.g. about the establishment of a permanent stoma, so it must be based on mutual respect and trust. In severe or complicated disease, surgery can produce an excellent result, although in CD this may be followed by further relapse.

The treatment of IBD employs three main methods:

Drugs,
Nutritional support,
Surgical resection.

Drug Treatment

Corticosteroids

When given by mouth or parenterally, these drugs are of great value in controlling severe attacks and relapses. Prednisone is generally preferred, although hydrocortisone or ACTH is given intravenously in severe attacks.

In less severe attacks, oral prednisone is often used, but only for limited periods, because all systemic corticosteroids have important side-effects and the aim is to use them only over a limited period, to achieve maximum effect.

In addition to the systemic and oral routes, corticosteroids can be given through the anal canal. In localised proctitis, prednisone suppositories are very useful, and in proctosigmoiditis prednisone 21-phosphate in water can be given as a retention enema, or administered as a foaming preparation. This local treatment can be used over quite long periods, and side-effects are generally slight.

Sulphasalazine (Salazopyrin)

This is a compound of sulphapyridine and 5-amino salicylic acid, which is split into its two components by bacterial action in the colon (Fig. 10.19). It is now accepted that 5-amino salicylic acid is the active component.

This drug is the mainstay of maintenance therapy (as opposed to treatment of acute attacks) in NSP because it reduces the frequency and severity of relapses, and many patients continue to take it prophylactically over years. Unfortunately it is not so helpful in preventing relapse in quiescent Crohn's disease, although it does have a useful effect in active CD.

Side-effects are common, especially nausea and vomiting, but they are lessened by using enteric-coated tablets. Other side-effects include skin rashes, headaches and, rarely, blood dyscrasia. Oligospermia occurs, but is reversed if the drug is discontinued. Some patients who are sensitive to sulphasalazine can be desensitised by gradual increase from a minute starting dose.

Azathioprine (Imuran)

There is evidence that this drug is of value in maintaining remission in chronic active CD. Some believe that it promotes the healing of fistulae. Side-effects, especially on haemopoiesis, can be severe and it should only be used when other treatments are ineffective. Regular blood counts

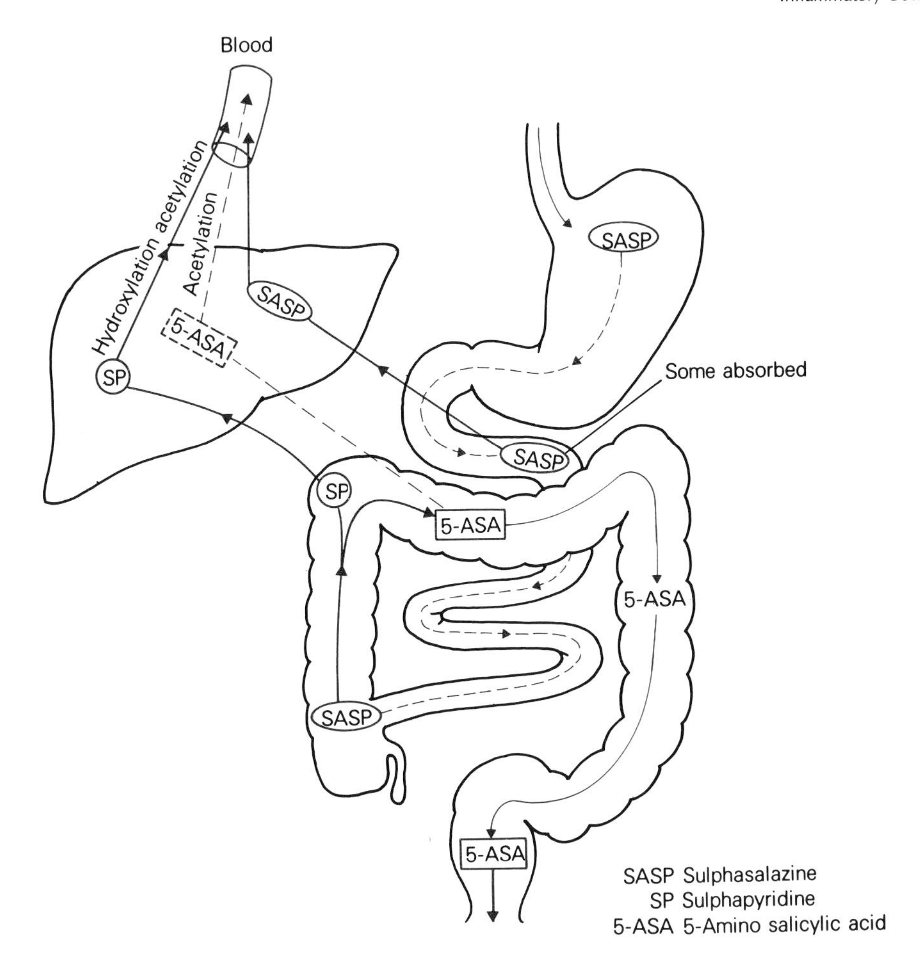

Fig. 10.19 *Diagram showing the absorption of sulphasalazine (SASP). SASP is converted to sulphapyridine (SP) and 5-aminosalicylic acid (5-ASA), probably by bacterial action in the colon.*

must be made. Azathioprine may be helpful in NSP, but is only used when other methods have failed.

Disodium cromoglycate (Nalcrom)

This drug is not of proven value.

Treatment of symptoms

If colitis is active it is a serious mistake to give constipating drugs such as codeine phosphate or loperamide: they are not very effective and there is a strong suspicion that they may precipitate toxic megacolon. However, after disease has been excised by right hemicolectomy, or colectomy and ileorectal anastomosis, these drugs are very helpful. After terminal ileal resection, cholestyramine may be useful. Sometimes lower abdominal pain is a feature of relapses and may be helped by antispasmodics such as mebeverine or propantheline.

Nutritional Support

This is an extremely important aspect of treatment of everyone with CD, and of all those with extensive NSP. Ulceration of the colon means that there will be losses of blood and protein in the exudate from the ulcerated granulating areas. Furthermore, patients who are generally unwell with IBD are likely to have a poor appetite and therefore their intake of foodstuff is below their requirements. In CD a degree of intestinal obstruction may further restrict intake, and inflammatory change in the small bowel may result in malabsorption, including reduced absorption of vitamin B_{12}.

There are therefore a number of reasons why the nutrition of patients with CD and severe NSP might be impaired.

Dietary assessment by a qualified dietitian, measurements of height and weight, and estimation of serum protein, are all useful. Sometimes the design of an attractive oral diet is enough to make good the deficiencies. Supplemental feeding via a fine nasogastric catheter during sleep can be most valuable.

Elemental diets made up of amino acids, glucose, and medium-chain triglycerides, with minerals and vitamins, have been extensively promoted but they are not very palatable and have not proved of great practical value.

Some workers believe that, in severe disease, exclusion of oral nutrition for a period of time with total parenteral nutrition (TPN) helps to induce remission. The difficulties and dangers of TPN should not be underestimated and it should only be embarked upon in units with proper experience of the technique. TPN has an important place in the management of severe fistula problems (either intra-abdominal or external) and as a temporary supportive measure prior to excisional or restorative surgery.

Iron, vitamin B_{12} and folic acid may all be poorly absorbed, especially in ileal CD, and most patients on a poor diet need vitamin supplements.

It is possible that a diet low in fibre and high in refined carbohydrate, is associated with the development of IBD. Conversely, there is no direct evidence that a high-fibre diet is helpful in the treatment of IBD, but this is being investigated. There is certainly no benefit to be gained from the traditional low-residue diet.

Nutritional problems are of exceptional importance when IBD affects children and adolescents, because limitation of growth due to illness and poor food intake is a most serious aspect of IBD at this age, and needs specific attention.

Surgical Treatment

The indications for surgery are somewhat different in the two main forms of IBD. They are summarised in Tables 10.2 and 10.3.

Proctocolectomy

This remains the standard operation for NSP. All large-bowel mucosa is removed, so that the disease cannot recur, and the patient can therefore

Table 10.2
Indications for Operation (Non-specific Proctocolitis)

Emergency operation	*Urgent operation*	*Elective operation*
Perforation	Failure of a fulminating attack to settle on full medical treatment	Repeated failure of good medical treatment
Toxic megacolon	Repeated need for blood transfusion	(Severe extra colonic complications)
(Haemorrhage)		Severe epithelial dysplasia
		Carcinoma of colon

be offered complete relief. This is at the cost of living with a permanent ileostomy. In elective surgery it is vital to discuss the implications of an ileostomy with the patient and it is often helpful for the patient to meet someone with an established ileostomy.

The whole colon is removed, from the ileocaecal valve. The rectum must be carefully removed; this involves close perimuscular dissection from the abdominal approach and, from the perineal end, an intersphincteric dissection between the internal and external sphincter (Fig. 10.20). In this way the pelvic autonomic nerves are not disturbed and there should be no interference with bladder or sexual functions – a very important matter, because most patients requiring this operation are young.

An ileostomy is fashioned in the right iliac fossa

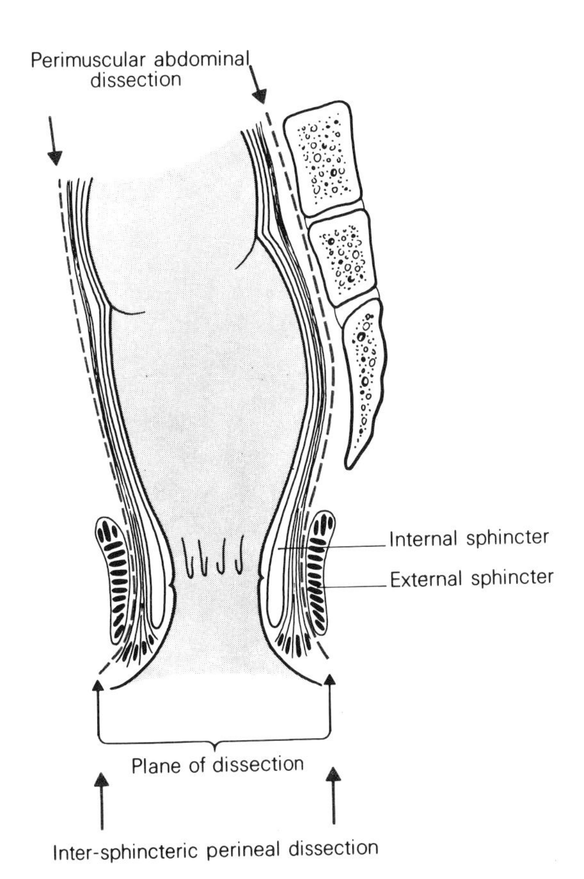

Fig. 10.20 *Rectal dissection from above and below during proctocolectomy is kept very close to the rectal wall.*

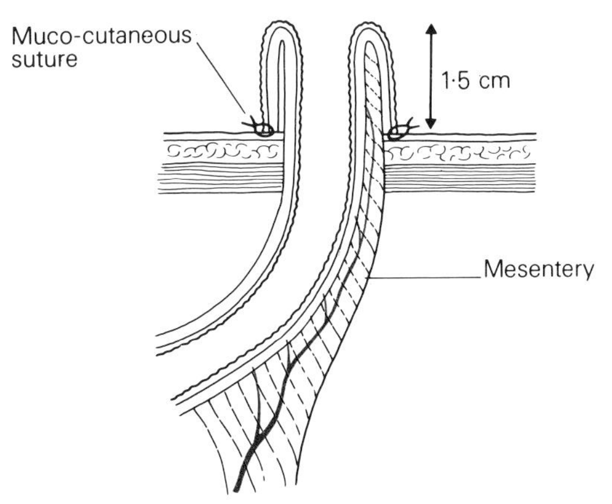

Fig. 10.21 *Diagrammatic section through a spout (Brooke) ileostomy, showing the eversion of the bowel which produces the spout.*

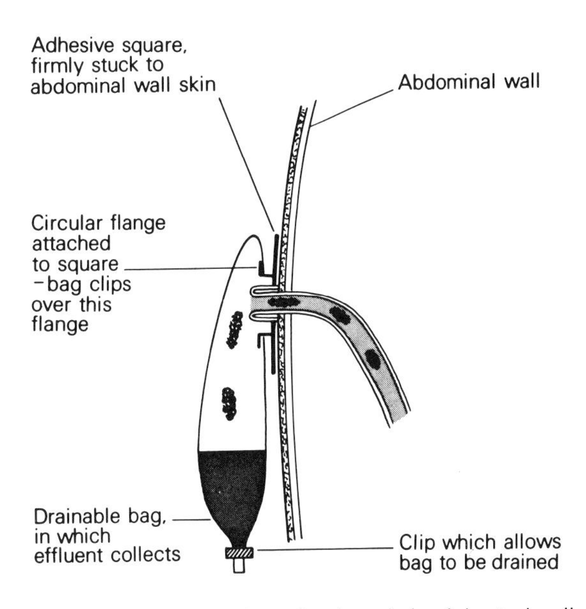

Fig. 10.22 *Diagrammatic section through the abdominal wall showing ileostomy apparatus* in situ.

by bringing the cut end of the ileum through a carefully sited circular hole cut in the abdominal wall of the right iliac fossa. The ileum is turned back to form a spout and the edge of the ileum sutured to the skin edge (Fig. 10.21). An ileostomy bag is immediately applied which fits snugly around the ileostomy and receives the ileal effluent (Fig. 10.22).

Sometimes, when a patient who is very ill has to undergo emergency colectomy, it is wise to limit the excision to the colon, and to leave the rectum *in situ*. The bowel is divided through the lower sigmoid colon and the distal end brought out as a mucous fistula at the lower end of the incision. An ileostomy is fashioned (Fig. 10.23). This avoids the rectal dissection which is the difficult and time-consuming part of the operation, and is a safe and effective alternative for the very sick patient.

Substitutes for ileostomy

Although proctocolectomy is a very successful operation in restoring patients with NSP to full health and activity, and although (with the help of modern apparatus) ileostomists adapt remarkably well to their new method of defaecation, it is not a fully satisfactory outcome to an operation which often has to be performed on teenagers and young adults. Not surprisingly, there has been much effort directed to finding an alternative.

There are three possible approaches:

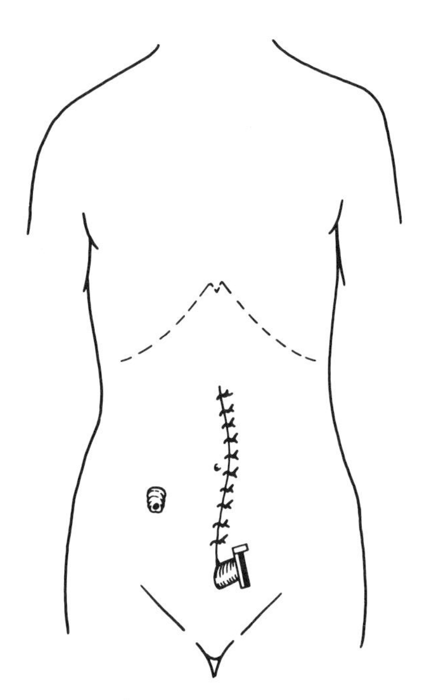

Fig. 10.23 *Total colectomy, with ileostomy and exteriorisation of sigmoid colon through lower end of incision.*

1. *Total colectomy with ileo-rectal anastomosis.* This operation has been in limited use for 40 years. Only a few patients are suitable for it, and it is usually reserved for patients under the age of 45 who have no perianal or ischiorectal sepsis, and in whom the rectum is not severely ulcerated and the rectal capacity is adequate. The procedure is usually done in a single-stage operation. The whole colon is excised and the ileum anastomised to the recto-sigmoid junction. Many patients will have fewer than three bowel movements each day after this procedure, although others will have unacceptable frequency. The other main disadvantage of the procedure is the problem of continued inflammation in the rectum and the small risk of carcinoma developing in the rectal stump: this makes it essential for patients to accept the need for an annual sigmoidoscopy. For many young people with NSP, however, the advantage of avoiding an ileostomy makes the operation acceptable, and in 50-60% of patients so treated the result is highly satisfactory.

2. *Kock's ileostomy.* This involves making an S-shaped pouch of ileum containing a valve which prevents the contents reaching the stoma at skin level. The pouch is emptied by intermittent catheterisation. Consequently, the patient wears only a small flat dressing over the stoma instead of a bag (Fig. 10.24).

Although some patients who are averse to wearing an ileostomy bag prefer this operation,

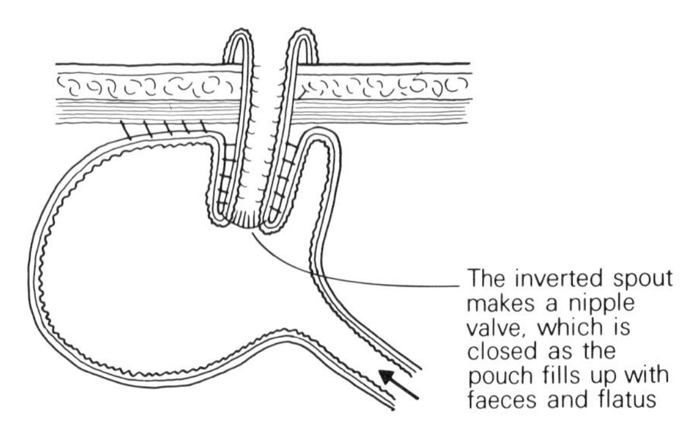

Fig. 10.24 *Kock's ileostomy, which consists of a pouch of ileum with a continent flush stoma.*

there is quite a high complication rate and it should only be done on the strong request of the patient. It is not suited to patients with CD.

3. *Perineal reservoir*. This is a recent development with considerable potential, although it is still too early to make a final assessment. The whole colon and the upper half of the rectum are removed. Then the lower rectum is denuded of mucosa down to the dentate line. An S-shaped pouch of ileum is fashioned, to act as a reservoir, and the efferent limb is brought down and sutured to the upper end of the anal canal (Fig. 10.25). By this method, all large-bowel mucosa is removed (so there can be no recurrence of NSP, or any threat of carcinomatous change) but the anal sphincter mechanism is intact, so faeces can accumulate in the reservoir and be passed through the anal canal, under voluntary control. A few patients have to empty the pouch by passing a catheter, but many achieve normal defaecation, emptying the pouch 3–4 times daily.

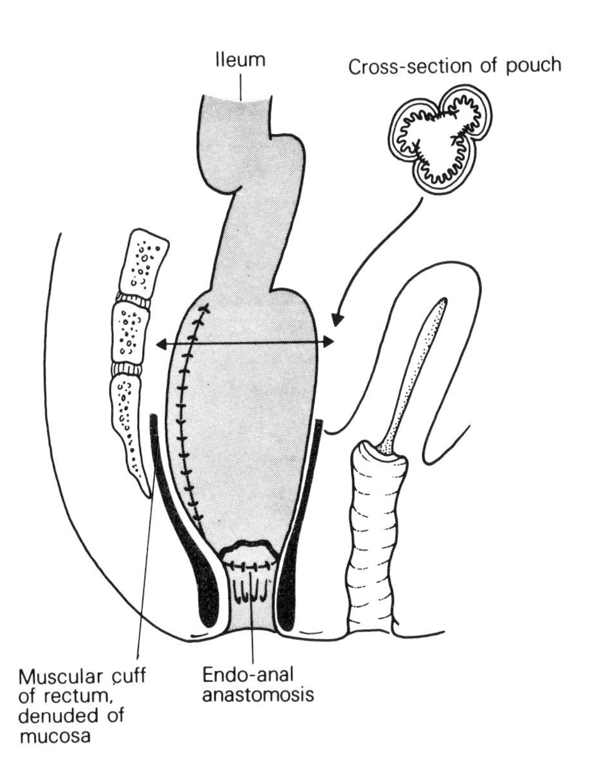

Fig. 10.25 *Construction of Parks' perineal reservoir (or S-pouch), with ileo-anal anastomosis, following excision of the whole colon and most of the rectum.*

Surgery for Crohn's disease (Table 10.3)

This falls into two broad categories:

surgery for ileocaecal disease
surgery for Crohn's colitis and peri-anal disease.

The surgery of Crohn's colitis differs very little from that of NSP. The risk of later recurrence of disease in the remaining ileum makes it unwise to fashion the complicated pouches necessary for Kock's ileostomy or the perineal pouch procedure. Consequently the two main operations are procto-colectomy and total colectomy with ileo-rectal anastomosis, the choice depending on the degree of rectal and anal involvement. Both are open to the risk of recurrence of disease in the ileum, but at least 50% of patients secure a good long-term result, and many others do well after a second operation to resect a further length of small bowel.

The risks of carcinomatous change are much smaller in long-standing Crohn's colitis than in NSP.

The majority of operations for Crohn's disease are performed for disease localised in the small bowel or the ileocaecal region.

Subacute small bowel obstruction which does

Table 10.3
Indications for Operation (Crohn's Disease)

Urgent operation	*Elective operation*
Toxic megacolon (rare)	Small bowel obstruction
Perforation	Fistula into bladder or vagina
(Haemorrhage)	Some patients with enterocutaneous or enterocolic fistula
(Intestinal obstruction)	(Systemic manifestations of disease)
	Perianal disease
	Carcinoma (rare)

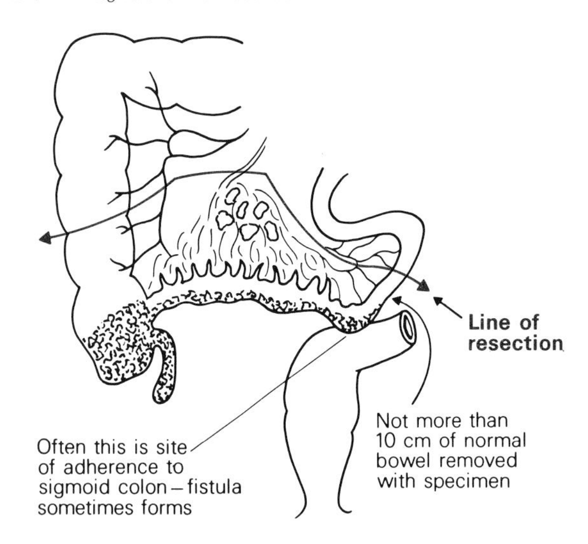

Fig. 10.26 *Right hemicolectomy for Crohn's disease.*

not respond to a period of medical treatment is a common indication for operation, which usually takes the form of a right hemicolectomy (Fig. 10.26).

Persistent pain and diarrhoea, especially when associated with a palpable mass or fistula into another viscus, is another indication for operation, especially in young people, whose growth is affected and who are losing much schooling.

There is always reluctance to operate when there is evidence of widespread disease of small bowel because resection of all the diseased bowel would not leave enough for nutritional needs.

The main surgical principle in Crohn's disease is to relieve the complications whilst removing as little normal tissue as possible. There is no evidence that removing enlarged lymph nodes or lengths of normal-looking bowel on either side of a diseased segment does anything to improve prognosis.

THE MANAGEMENT OF ATTACKS OF NSP

Proctitis and Proctosigmoiditis

This group includes 75% of all patients with NSP, and the great majority of these patients are managed throughout as out-patients. The diagnosis is made at sigmoidoscopy, at the first visit, when a rectal biopsy is taken and treatment commenced.

If the inflammation is restricted to the lower rectum, a suppository containing prednisone or sulphasalazine is inserted each evening on going to bed, and may be all the treatment required. In procto-sigmoiditis, a retention enema or foam enema containing prednisone will penetrate up to the sigmoid. These topical treatments will sometimes need to be supplemented by sulphasalazine by mouth in a dose up to 3 g daily, and this may be usefully continued to prevent relapse.

Some of these patients respond quickly to local treatment and have no further trouble; others slowly improve but need to continue with some treatment; a few have continuing symptoms, which vary in severity. Over the space of 20 years, about 20% of patients will show gradual proximal extension of the inflammation.

Active Chronic Proctocolitis

This is a very troublesome form of the disease. The patients are not severely ill and will try to lead a normal life but they are in fact generally tired and rundown, with troublesome diarrhoea and urgency of defaecation: this last symptom is a particular nuisance, forcing them to be careful about all journeys outside the home as well as over the choice of a job and the taking of holidays.

The proctitis, which causes the urgency, can be helped by using a steroid enema or foam application: these can penetrate some way up the colon. Regular oral sulphasalazine is nearly always used, and some patients benefit from azathioprine. Generally these patients should not be maintained on oral corticosteroids, because of the danger of side-effects: however, a few derive so much benefit that a small maintenance dose is given, perhaps only on alternate days.

The extent of colitis varies in these patients, although severe symptoms can occur with only the distal half of the colon affected. If symptoms are really troublesome and do not respond to medical treatment, surgery must be considered. The patients tend to soldier on, in poor health, partly from apprehension about surgery and a permanent ileostomy. It is important to remember the great improvement in health and quality of life which may follow surgery.

Acute Proctocolitis

Indicators of a severe acute attack of proctocolitis are:

more than 6 stools per day, with blood
fever over 38.5°C
pulse over 90 per minute
haemoglobin less than 10 g/l
a high ESR.

The greater the extent of the colon affected, and the deeper the ulceration, the more severe the attack. In the severest forms, the patient's life is in grave danger from bacteraemia and from the threat of perforation and peritonitis. Close consultation between physician and surgeon is essential from the outset, because the decision to undertake emergency colectomy may have to be made at any time.

On admission, complete bed rest is provided in a calm but necessarily active atmosphere. Hourly recordings of temperature, pulse and blood pressure must be made. An accurate fluid balance chart is essential, including the volume of stools passed. A full blood count, analysis of serum chemistry, and a blood culture must be done. A full physical examination, with particular attention to the abdomen, is performed, probably with a gentle, limited sigmoidoscopy. Plain abdominal x-rays play a very important part in this assessment. Free subdiaphragmatic gas is a clear sign of perforation, and is an indication for operation as soon as the patient can be prepared. Wide dilatation, especially of the transverse colon, is always a serious sign, especially in conjunction with a thick irregular outline and mucosal islands (a sign of very deep and dangerous ulceration): megacolon is generally regarded as another indication for emergency colectomy. It is dangerous to perform a barium enema in these circumstances.

Fulminant colitis can develop very rapidly, so a thorough review of the whole patient at least twice a day is essential – recordings, stool frequency, fluid balance, general condition and particularly abdominal signs, haemoglobin, urea and electrolyte levels must all be considered by the same team, so that developments can be recognised. Fresh plain abdominal x-rays and serum protein levels are needed at least every day. Any deterioration in general condition must be most carefully considered, because perforation can occur, in a patient on a high dose of corticosteroids, with little change in abdominal physical signs.

Apart from those few patients who are immediately prepared for colectomy because of perforation or severe megacolon, the majority are commenced on an intensive course of treatment, along the following lines:

1. Parenteral corticosteroids are given by continuous intravenous infusion, using either hydrocortisone 300–400 mg, or prednisolone 60 mg, over 24 hours.
2. The bowel is rested by allowing only sips of water, and fluid is administered intravenously. These patients are usually dehydrated, anaemic, hypoproteinaemic, and deficient in sodium and potassium. They therefore require electrolyte solutions, blood, and plasma in carefully calculated proportions.
3. Frequently these patients are sufficiently poorly nourished that peripheral intravenous feeding is required.
4. In a situation in which blood cultures are often positive, there is a strong case for immediately giving wide-spectrum antibiotics, e.g. gentamicin or cefotaxime and metronidazole.

There is some controversy over how long this intensive care should be continued before deciding on colectomy. The situation is a dangerous one: the particular fear is that perforation will occur in spite of the treatment but, on the other hand, experience shows that patients can recover from these severe attacks. Some authorities believe that, if there is no clear improvement in a fulminating attack after five days of intensive treatment, then surgery is indicated, whilst others would continue the regime for 7–10 days. Fever nearly always responds to corticosteroid therapy but continued high stool frequency with losses of the order of 1000 g per day, tachycardia, abdominal distension and tenderness, continued colonic dilatation on repeated x-ray, and difficulty in maintaining the haemoglobin and the serum proteins are all indications that the colon has been irreparably damaged and colectomy is needed. There are no rules for reaching this decision; experience and judgement must play the main part.

Severe Disease

There are a considerable number of patients who do not have fulminant disease but who have still suffered a severe first attack or relapse. They require hospital admission, complete rest, completion of investigations, and the establishment of a course of treatment. Treatment will usually include the use of oral corticosteroids in a dose of 40–60 mg prednisolone , or the parenteral route may have to be used. These patients may tolerate topical corticosteroid treatment in the form of a saline-based enema or a rectal foam injection. They can usually be allowed a light, high-protein, high-calorie diet. Correction of anaemia is very important. The best methods of assessing progress are by twice-daily clinical examination, temperature and pulse recordings, and daily stool volumes and weights.

Corticosteroid treatment should not be continued for more than a few weeks because there is no convincing evidence that they prevent further relapses, and side-effects are potentially dangerous. There is, however, the occasional patient who requires a longer period of such treatment to achieve control but this will require close supervision.

Some of these patients improve steadily and require no more than 2–3 g of sulphasalazine daily to keep them in remission: this should probably be continued over several years because there is good evidence that continued use does prevent relapse.

Other patients will not settle so well, and move into the group, already described, of active chronic proctocolitis (see p. 240).

Follow-up of NSP

All patients require regular follow-up, although some need only be seen infrequently.

Once the initial severe attack has been weathered, it is interesting to note that the long-term mortality of patients with NSP is not significantly greater than that for an age- and sex-matched population.

THE MANAGEMENT OF CROHN'S DISEASE

Crohn's disease is a relapsing condition, so it is never possible to say that a patient is permanently cured.

In a disease which often affects the small bowel, nutrition is particularly likely to be affected, and this has been considered (p. 235).

The care of Crohn's colitis is along lines similar to the care of patients with NSP.

Diffuse small-bowel CD, with weight loss, anaemia, diarrhoea and steatorrhoea often responds to oral or parenteral corticosteroids in large doses, for a short time. Sulphasalazine can also help in these circumstances. Azathioprine can act as a useful adjuvant to corticosteroids, and may be helpful as a substitute for them in prevention of relapse.

Secondary infection in deeply ulcerated bowel may be usefully treated with metronidazole.

There are some situations where attempts at medical treatment are inappropriate. The patient with a large, inflammatory, palpable mass which on radiology is shown to contain multiple internal fistulae and abscesses, or the patient with symptomatic small-bowel or colonic strictures, should probably be referred directly for surgery. Extensive disease is not necessarily a contra-indication to surgical treatment when mechanical defects such as fistulae or strictures are the main cause of symptoms.

Maintenance of Remission

Some patients enjoy long remissions on no specific treatment. For others, who experience many relapses of predominantly small bowel disease, azathioprine has been shown to be useful in reducing relapse frequency and severity: it may also be helpful when fistulae are present. The side-effects of azathioprine include upper gastro-intestinal symptoms, which may require withdrawal of the drug, but they usually resolve if the patient can persevere with treatment. Blood dyscrasias can be severe, with either an aplastic anaemia, leucopenia or thrombocytopenia, and patients should have regular blood counts during follow-up. In colonic or ileocaecal disease, sulphasalazine is the drug of choice. Long-term corticosteroid treatment should be avoided. If used in the treatment of an acute attack, it should be given in a large dose for a week or two and then tailed off.

Operations for Recurrent Crohn's Disease

Even if Crohn's disease recurs after surgical treatment, there is good evidence that it is worthwhile performing further surgery at a later date if there are reasonable indications. The disease may recur either at a previous anastomosis or in a new site. Revision surgery is often made difficult by dense adhesions.

Follow-up of Crohn's Disease

Because of the prolonged and relapsing nature of this disease, long-term follow-up is important. This is especially directed to detection of:

- early signs of recurrence
- development of nutritional problems
- side-effects of the drugs used for control of CD.

The overall prognosis varies greatly in this disease. Patients may have very long remissions and appear to be cured. Others, despite efficient treatment, continue to show signs of active disease. Following surgical resection, about 50% of patients do very well: the other 50% will at some time show relapse. Sometimes, when this is localised, a further resection can be followed by an excellent result. Somewhat surprisingly, the long-term mortality of CD is not significantly greater than for an age- and sex-matched population.

ANTIBIOTIC ASSOCIATED PSEUDOMEMBRANOUS COLITIS

(see also p. 335)

Although pseudomembranous colitis had been clearly described in the pre-antibiotic era, the reports of several cases of this condition occurring after administration of lincomycin or clindamycin in 1973 and 1974 suggested that the condition was a specific complication of this form of antibiotic therapy. Within a short time reports appeared in the literature of pseudomembranous colitis developing after courses of many other antibiotics, often used in combination.

The condition tends to occur in patients after operations involving postoperative antibiotic cover. Diarrhoea is usually the initial presenting symptom. Passage of mucus in the stool is common, but blood is not usually present. Abdominal pain is occasionally complained of. Nutritional impairment with low serum albumen was present in nearly 80% of one series of patients. In a few patients the severity of the fluid loss through diarrhoea, and the general toxaemia, produce a very serious illness.

The diagnosis may initially be made on sigmoidoscopic appearances, but it is important to realise that the typical sigmoidoscopic changes may take several days, or even weeks to develop; moreover the rectum may be relatively spared and the characteristic macroscopic appearances may therefore not be visible. Typically there are raised white plaques of varying size in the rectum, with oedematous intervening mucosa. Barium enema may show changes suggestive of ulcerative colitis with a varying extent of colonic involvement.

Biopsy of affected large bowel shows distension

of glands and an outpouring of mucus, pus and fibrin to form a pseudomembrane. The histological appearances of the intervening mucosa shows non-specific inflammatory changes only.

A further valuable addition to the diagnostic criteria for this condition came with the discovery in 1977 that a toxin was present in the stools of patients with antibiotic-associated pseudomembranous colitis. The test involves incubating faecal suspensions on Hela cell monolayers. The diagnosis is positive when the cells become disrupted. The effect is neutralised by incubation with *Clostridium sordelli* anti-toxin. The organism *Clostridium difficile,* now thought to be responsible for the disease, can be identified, with its toxin, in most patients with antibiotic-associated pseudomembranous colitis.

Treatment

If the patient is very ill at the time of diagnosis, supportive therapy such as administration of intravenous fluids may be necessary. Most patients were treated similarly to patients with acute nonspecific proctolitis using corticosteroids, until it was discovered that vancomycin rapidly eliminated *Clostridium difficile* and toxin from the stools of affected patients and resulted in rapid clinical improvement. This is now the treatment of choice in this condition. Metronidazole is said to be a useful alternative. Only very rarely is surgical treatment indicated, for threatened perforation or megacolon. In resistant cases the diarrhoea can sometimes be controlled by cholestryramine, which is claimed to bind the toxin.

NECROTISING ENTEROCOLITIS

Although occasional examples of this grave disease of the intestines of the newborn baby had been seen for many years, it is only in the last 15 years that it has become generally recognised. The reason for this appears to be that it almost exclusively affects premature babies (often about 1500 g), or those who had a complicated birth, with hypoxia and shock. Until 15 years ago the mortality among these babies was very high, but with the development of neonatal intensive care most now survive, and become potential subjects for necrotising enterocolitis.

About the third or fourth day (sometimes later), often whilst still on assisted ventilation, one of these small babies shows signs of abdominal distension and passes blood per rectum. Plain x-ray of the abdomen reveals a highly characteristic picture of pneumatosis intestinalis, i.e. the wall of the bowel (usually colon) is outlined by intramural gas. If this is speedily treated by nasogastric suction and broad-spectrum antibiotics, the condition can resolve, although later fibrosis can cause a stricture. If the process progresses, then gangrene of the intestinal wall, and perforation, mean that surgery is indicated. Laparotomy reveals ischaemic necrotic bowel (usually terminal ileum and the proximal half of the colon), with visible intramesenteric gas, and often several perforations, with peritonitis. Resection of ischaemic bowel and terminal ileostomy is frequently followed by slow recovery and, after some months, continuity of ileum and the remainder of the colon can be restored by anastomosis at a second operation.

It seems likely that the basic problem is that, in shock, the mesenteric vasoconstriction is so profound that pathogens in the gut are able to penetrate and multiply in the wall of the bowel, producing a combination of ischaemic and infective gangrene: no specific organism has been identified. However, outbreaks tend to occur in neonatal units and to be brought under control by very strict barrier nursing techniques. Happily, this seems to be a condition whose incidence is falling.

11

Anorectal Disorders

The major function of the anal canal is to provide a continent passage through which there can be a controlled evacuation of flatus and faeces. It is of considerable surgical importance because it is prone to a number of disorders, and is a valuable portal for the examination of the large intestine.

ANATOMY AND PHYSIOLOGY

The anal canal (Fig. 11.1) is about 3 cm long in the adult; the lower 2 cm is lined by squamous epithelium, which terminates at the pectinate line. Here a number of anal valves, or crescentic folds, mark the junction between the sensitive modified skin of the anal canal and the rectal mucosa. Above the anal valves are a number of pockets, the anal crypts, into some of which open the anal glands.

Immediately deep to the lining of the anal canal lies the vital anal sphincter mechanism. This consists of an inner smooth muscle tube (the internal sphincter), which is a condensation of the

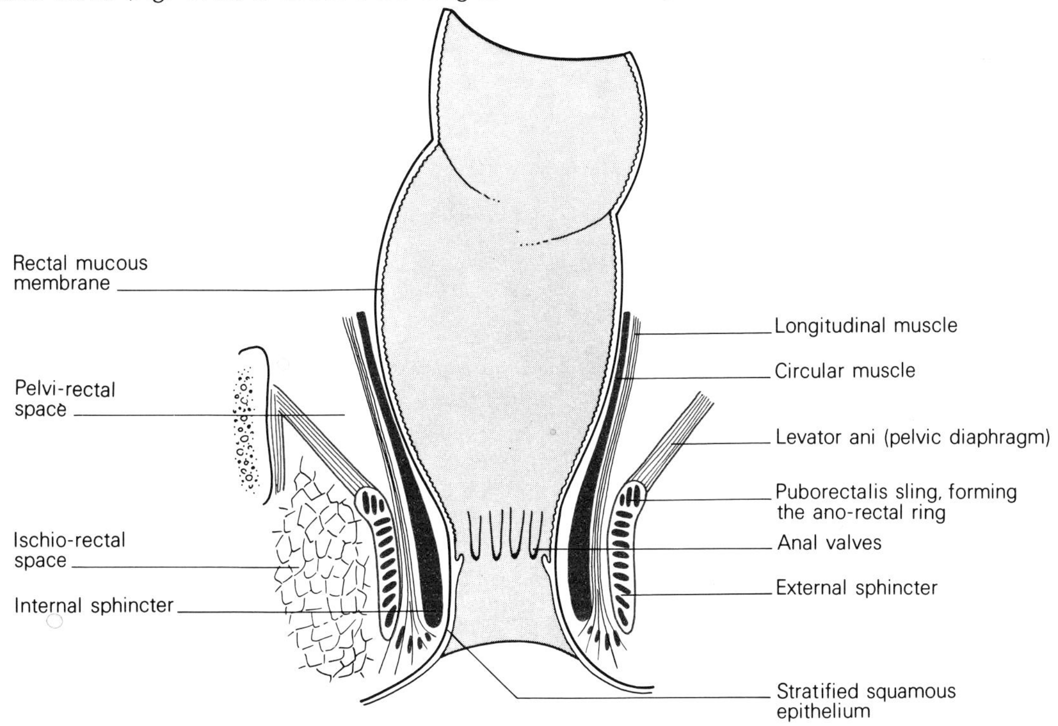

Fig. 11.1 *Anatomy of the anal canal.*

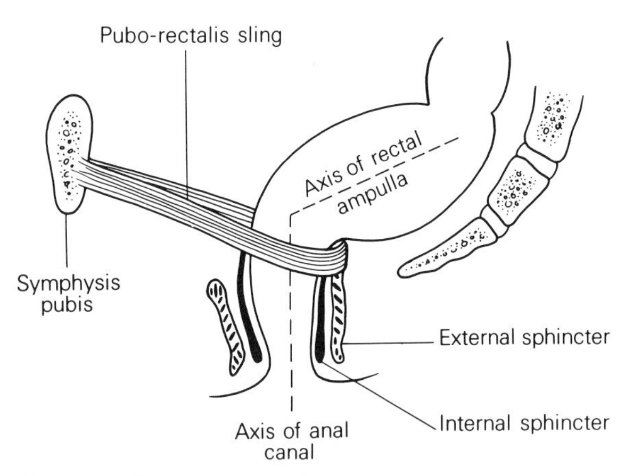

Fig. 11.2 *The puborectalis sling.*

circular muscle of the gut, and the outer striated muscle ring (the external sphincter). At its upper border the external sphincter is in continuity with the pelvic diaphragm, i.e. the levator ani muscle. An important part of this muscle is the puborectalis sling, which is attached to the back of the symphysis pubis and pulls the junction of rectum and anal canal (the anorectal ring) forwards, so creating a valvular mechanism important in maintaining continence (Fig. 11.2). On either side of the puborectalis, the levator ani muscle fans out radially as the pelvic diaphragm and is attached to the walls of the pelvis.

Anal Continence

Except when defaecation has to be postponed, and the striated muscle of the levator ani and external sphincter is voluntarily contracted, continence depends on the unconscious working of several factors:

1. Normally, the lower rectum is empty and the puborectalis sling maintains an angle of 70–80° between anal canal and rectum. Intra-abdominal pressure therefore tends to press the anterior rectal wall against the posterior wall and prevent passage of faeces and flatus (Fig. 11.2).

2. The resting tone in the internal anal sphincter maintains a pressure zone in the anal which is higher than the intrarectal pressure.

3. A vital aspect of anal continence is the sensory mechanism by which rectal filling is recognised, and discrimination between flatus and faeces achieved. The sensation of flatus or faeces entering the rectum is perceived in the stretch receptors sited in the levator ani, rather than the rectal wall itself. 'Sampling' of the contents is carried out by a relaxation of the anal sphincter mechanism which allows the rectal contents to come into contact with the sensory epithelium of the anal canal: this enables the individual to decide whether it is safe to pass flatus without fear of soiling – a process which may go awry when the stool is fluid (Fig. 11.3).

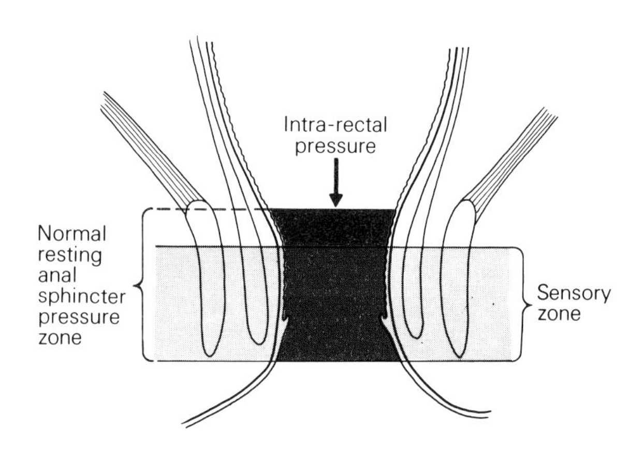

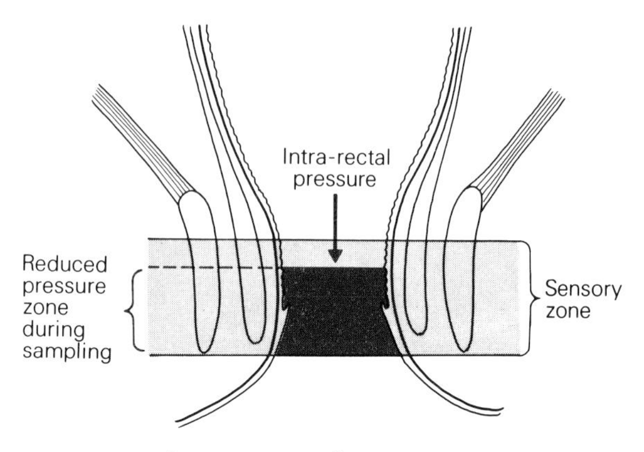

Fig. 11.3 *Anal continence – the sampling process (after Duthie, 1980).*

When stool begins to enter the rectum, as the first phase of defaecation, the rectum relaxes to accommodate it, and the receptors signal that filling is occurring. The sampling process indicates that faeces are present as well as flatus. The external sphincter can be contracted voluntarily for a minute or so but then the process of defaecation has to take place. This involves complete relaxation of the levator ani, as well as of the anal sphincter, which allows the rectal angle to straighten. Expulsion has to take place in the squatting position and is assisted by the Valsalva manoeuvre, which increases the intra-abdominal pressure.

Anal incontinence

The involuntary leakage of faeces through the anal canal has a number of causes:

1. Extreme urgency. This is likely to occur in acute gastroenteritis or severe inflammatory bowel disease, and may occur in low rectal cancer. The patient cannot control a liquid stool for long enough to reach the toilet.
2. Soiling. This is usually due (especially in the very young and in the elderly and the bedridden) to impaction of faeces in the rectum. A large faecal mass distends the rectum and, around it, liquid faeces finds its way and leaks out through the patulous anus. All too often these patients are said to have diarrhoea, but the diagnosis is immediately revealed by digital rectal examination. The treatment is to break up and evacuate the faecal mass, and then aim to keep the rectum empty: in infants this requires a long period of controlled use of laxatives and toilet training.
3. True faecal incontinence is due to an actual weakness of the sphincters.
   a. The most severe forms are seen in patients with divided sphincters. This condition sometimes dates from a third-degree tear during labour which was inadequately repaired; from a penetrating wound of the perineum; or, rarely, as a sequel to operations for anal fistulae. Many of these patients can be helped by direct repair of the sphincters.
   b. Some cases are due to neurological deficit in organic disease, such as meningomyelocoele, spinal cord injury, or diabetic neuropathy. It is very difficult in these cases to produce much improvement.
   c. There are a number of patients in whom there is no evident cause for incontinence. Among these are elderly patients whose weak sphincters seem to display an aspect of ther ageing process. Others, however, are middle-aged women who may also have rectal prolapse: they can often be helped by rectopexy (p. 256), combined with a repair of the puborectalis and pubococcygeus.

HAEMORRHOIDS

This is one of the most common conditions to afflict the citizens of Western countries, and there is considerable evidence that it is related to the refined Western diet. Certainly rural Africans, who eat a diet with high fibre content, are rarely constipated and hardly ever suffer from haemorrhoids (piles).

Haemorrhoids form either in the internal haemorrhoidal plexus (when they are known as internal piles) or in the external plexus (external haemorrhoids).

Internal haemorrhoids are much the commoner and may affect as many as 50% of those over 50 years of age living in Western countries. There is considerable controversy over aetiology, although the usual explanation is that a combination of constipation, sustained straining at stool and (in the case of women) pregnancy leads to engorgement of the veins of the internal haemorrhoidal plexus, which are radicles of the superior rectal vein.

Between the faecal mass and the muscle wall lie the mucosa and the vascular tissue. Pressure exerted between the faecal mass and the anal sphincter tends to obliterate free flow of blood and, since arterial blood continues to flow into the internal plexus, it becomes engorged. As time goes on, prolapse of the pile occurs and becomes greater if excessive straining continues, with resultant enlargement of the haemorrhoidal masses. As the haemorrhoids become larger, squamous epithelium may extend onto the surface of the haemorrhoid normally covered by columnar epithelium – usually known as squamous metaplasia.

Classification of Haemorrhoids

Haemorrhoids are normally classified as follows (Fig. 11.4):

First degree	bleeding only
Second degree	prolapsing but reduce spontaneously
Third degree	prolapse which does not undergo spontaneous reduction

Symptoms

In addition to bleeding and prolapse, other symptoms may occur. Pain is uncommon unless thrombosis is present. Itching (pruritis) is common and discharge of mucus is present if the haemorrhoids are large.

Examination

In addition to external examination of the anal region, and digital examination, it is important to examine the anal canal with a proctoscope while the patient bears down. This will give an accurate assessment of the size of the haemorrhoids and the degree of prolapse. Sigmoidoscopy should always be performed since there is a high incidence of coincidental rectal disorders which may be the true cause of the symptoms.

Treatment

The multiplicity of methods for the treatment of haemorrhoids suggest that no one method gives perfect results. For first-degree and some second-degree haemorrhoids, an outpatient method such as injection with sclerosing solution or banding of the haemorrhoids gives good results, whereas third-degree haemorrhoids are probably best dealt with by a ligation and excision method. Newer

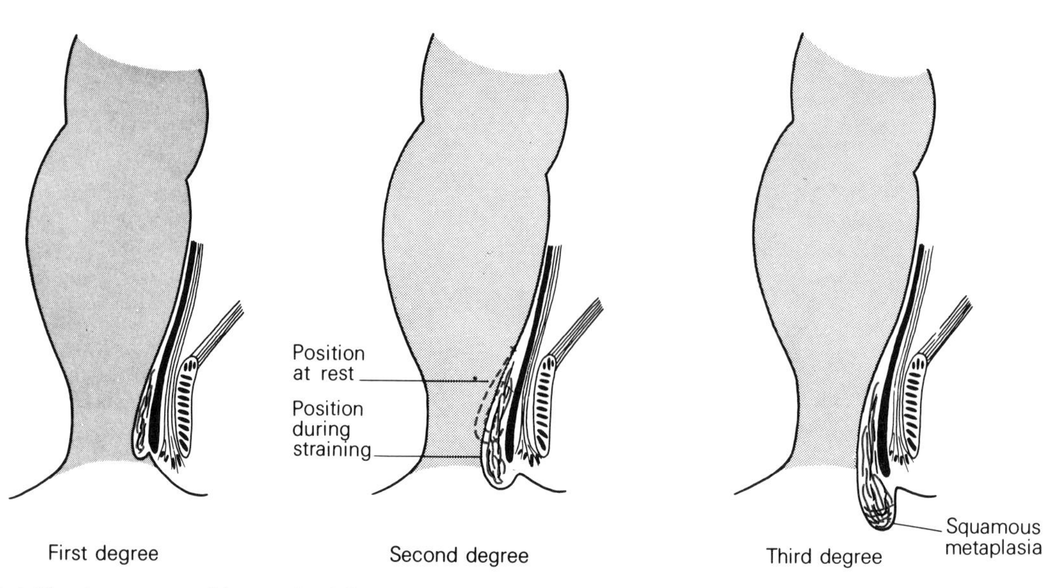

Fig. 11.4 *The three stages of haemorrhoid formation.*

treatments include cryotherapy, manual dilatation of the anus, lateral sphincterotomy and thermo-coagulation using the infra-red coagulator.

Sclerosing treatment

The solution most commonly used in the injection of haemorrhoids is 5% phenol in arachis or almond oil. A proctoscope is inserted and injections are made in nonsensitive columnar epithelium immediately above the haemorrhoid at the level of the anorectal ring (Fig. 11.5). All the three usual haemorrhoidal sites may be injected in one session. Injections are generally made into the submucosa and not into the venous plexus itself. The agent sets up an inflammatory reaction which causes obliteration of the haemorrhoids and allows the mucous membrane lining to adhere to the underlying internal sphincter apparatus.

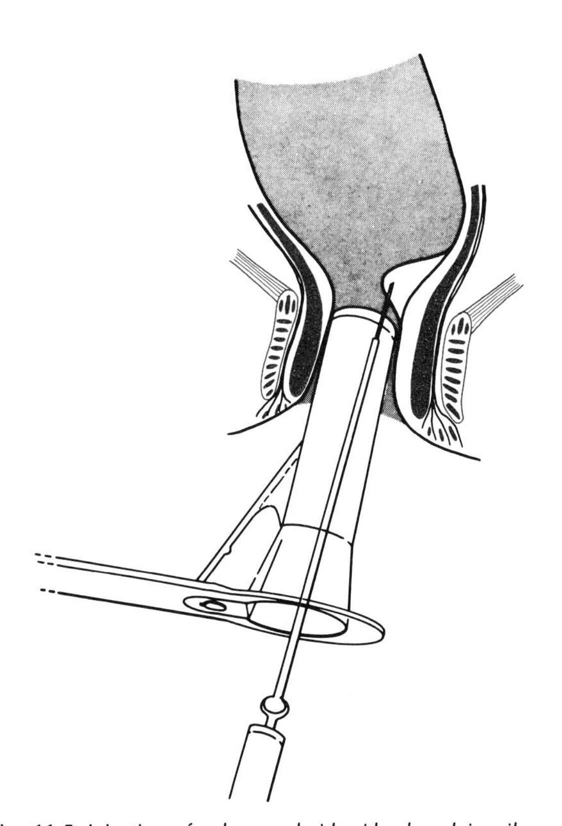

Fig. 11.5 *Injection of a haemorrhoid with phenol in oil.*

Ligation with rubber bands

These are applied through a proctoscope with a special band applicator around the base of an internal haemorrhoid. They produce ischaemia with consequent necrosis. If severe pain is to be avoided, it is important that they are not applied to innervated squamous epithelium. One or more bands can be applied in one session (Fig. 11.6).

Ligation and excision

This method is particularly recommended if there are third-degree haemorrhoids with large skin tags present. The haemorrhoid is dissected off the internal sphincter, commencing in the perineum outside the anal margin. The haemorrhoidal pedicle is transfixed and ligated well up in the anal canal and the haemorrhoid excised (Fig. 11.7).

ANAL FISSURE

Anal fissure is a very painful and common condition. The pain occurs during defaecation but may persist for a variable length of time afterwards.

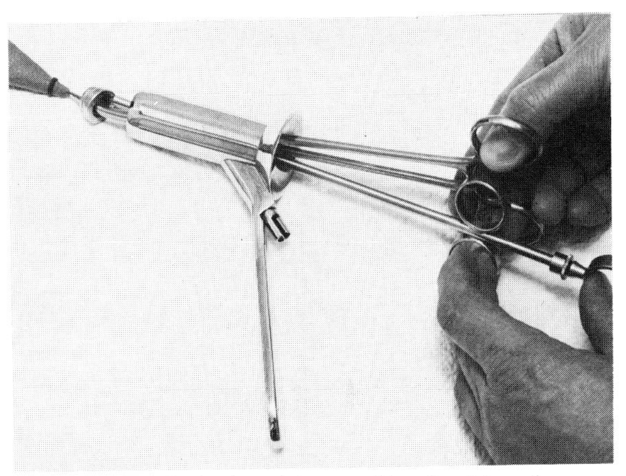

Fig. 11.6 *Method of applying a rubber band to a haemorrhoid, through a proctoscope.*

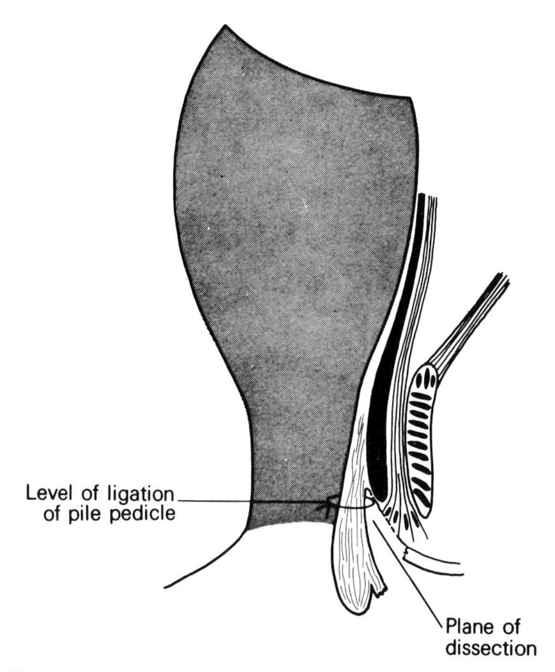

Fig. 11.7 *Haemorrhoidectomy.*

Aetiology

The precise cause is not known but constipation with abrasions of the anal canal occurring during defaecation may be a factor. It more commonly affects the posterior aspect of the anus in the midline but, in female patients, fissures are occasionally seen anteriorly, especially after childbirth. The elliptical shape of the lower end of the external sphincter leaves the anterior and posterior aspects of the anal canal in the middle relatively less well supported, and this may go some way to explain the common site for occurrence of fissures. A persistent anal fissure should raise a suspicion of Crohn's disease.

Examination

A fissure is seen at the anal margin as the buttocks are gradually parted, and involves the anal canal up to the level of the pectinate line. There is frequently a hypertrophied anal papilla at the upper end of the fissure, whereas at the lower end of the fissure a sentinel tag is commonly seen (Fig. 11.8). The base of the fissure characteristically consists of fibres of the internal sphincter, which may be interspersed with fibrous tissue in chronic fissures. It is not advisable to attempt digital examination once fissure has been diagnosed since there is intense spasm in the sphincter apparatus causing severe pain. Acute fissures do not generally have a sentinel tag and are more superficial.

Treatment

The pain of an acute fissure may resolve in a few days with the help of a laxative and application of some local anaesthetic jelly. If the condition becomes chronic, the two most popular treatments consist of either anal dilatation or lateral internal sphincterotomy. Both treatments are designed to

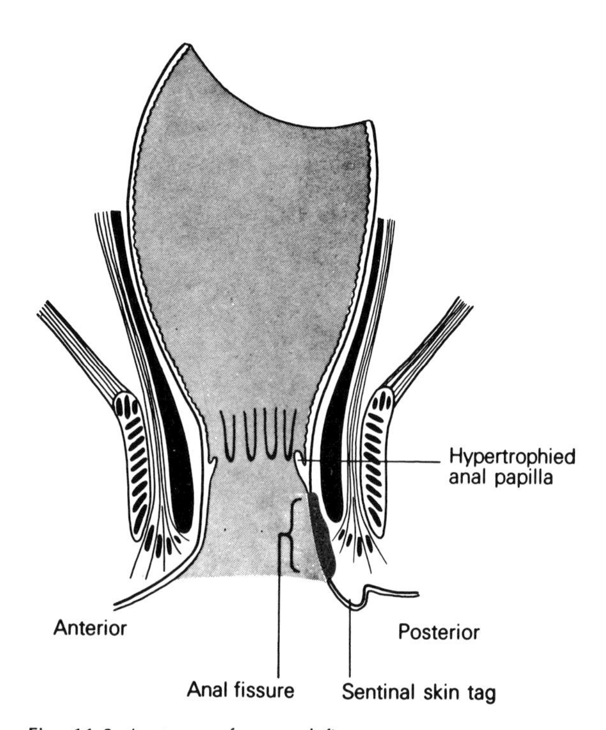

Fig. 11.8 *Anatomy of an anal fissure.*

produce relaxation of the sphincter spasm which in turn allows the fissure to heal. Stretching of the sphincter is done under general anaesthetic with the patient well relaxed. The results are generally satisfactory, although in some patients disturbance of anal continence may occur.

Division of the internal sphincter is best done by cutting the internal sphincter in the left lateral position below the level of the pectinate line. The two commonly used methods consist of (a) closed subcutaneous sphincterotomy using a tenotomy knife and (b) open sphincterotomy through a small incision at the anal margin. Both are easy to perform and have a high success rate. Disturbance of anal continence is less common than after anal stretching. Pain relief is usually dramatic. The sentinel tag and the hypertrophied anal papilla should both be removed at the time of operation.

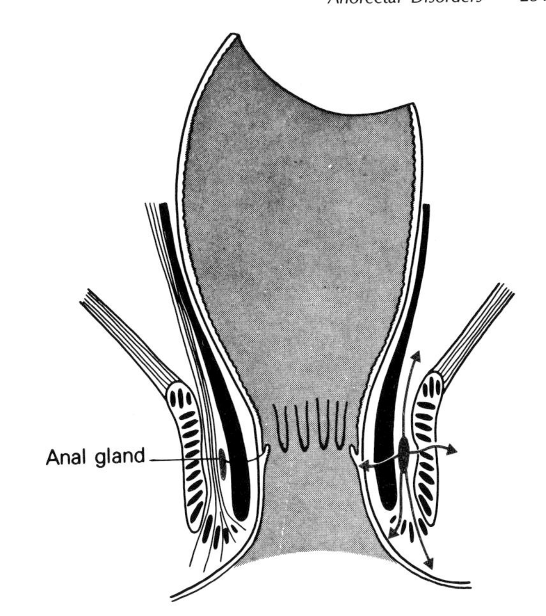

Fig. 11.9 *Diagram to show the direction of spread of infection in the anal region, originating in an anal gland.*

ANORECTAL SEPSIS

An abscess in the anorectal region is a fairly common event although, in view of the heavy bacterial population of the area, it is perhaps remarkable that sepsis is not seen more often, and that, when it does occur, it is usually due to staphylococcal infection.

There is no certainty about the origin of anorectal abscesses, but the favoured theory is that infection arises in an anal gland (Fig. 11.9) and then tracks superficially or deeply along one of the planes in the area to initiate an abscess. Abscesses which point on the skin beside the anus, having spread along the intersphincteric plane, are the commonest and are known as perianal abscesses (Fig. 11.10). When sepsis spreads through the external sphincter to the ischiorectal space, then the resulting abscess is termed an ischiorectal abscess. In both these sites of sepsis, the original anal gland abscess may drain through the internal sphincter into the anal canal and it is easy to see how, in those circumstances, a fistula may arise, once the abscess is drained on to the skin outside the anus. Rarely, sepsis spreads through the leva-

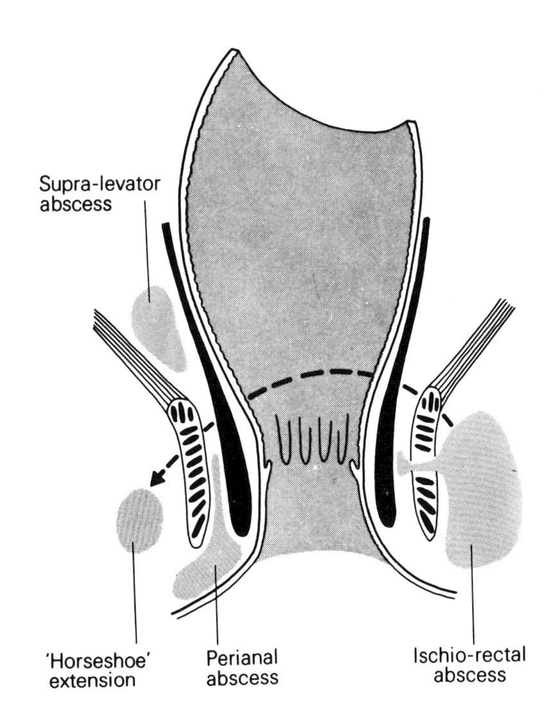

Fig. 11.10 *The sites of the commoner abscesses of the anus and rectum.*

tor ani (or along the intermuscular plane) to form a supralevator abscess.

Perianal abscess presents as a very painful and acutely tender swelling beside the anus. An ischiorectal abscess develops slowly, the patient becoming aware first of a throbbing and then of acute pain to one side of the anal canal, with the pain being much accentuated on defaecation. The skin over the affected fossa is swollen and very tender, and the induration can be felt on digital rectal examination. It is a much larger abscess than a perianal one, and has a tendency to spread around the anal canal to the opposite ischiorectal fossa ('horseshoe' extension). These patients are usually ill and feverish.

The aim of treatment is to provide good drainage as soon as possible so that the abscess cavity can collapse, granulate and heal. Most can be drained by direct incision over the swelling: often some skin is excised and a Milton gauze pack tucked into the cavity so that it heals from the bottom.

ANAL FISTULA

It is essential to recognise that virtually all fistulae arise at the time of occurrence of an abscess: for one reason or another, early and complete decompression and drainage is not achieved and a track persists between the anal canal (rarely, the rectum) and the perianal skin. This results in intermittent discharge of pus and faeces beside the anus, and in itching and discomfort in the perineum.

Much the commonest type of fistula is the low-level type which probably originates from an intersphincteric abscess bursting both medially, through the internal sphincter, and downwards to the perianal skin (Fig. 11.11). Much less common is a trans-sphincteric fistula, originating from an ischiorectal abscess.

There is usually one, but sometimes two or more external openings, which discharge pus, and the internal opening is usually felt at the level of the

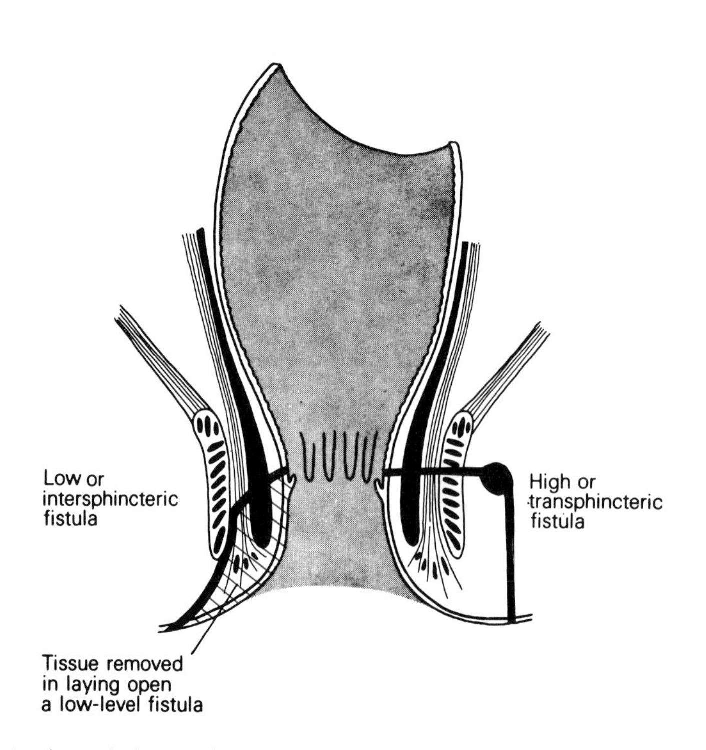

Fig. 11.11 *Diagram showing the track of inter-sphincteric and trans-sphincteric anal fistulae.*

pectinate line. With care, a probe can usually be passed along the fistula into the anal canal, and this helps in deciding on its anatomy.

In treating low-level, and some high-level fistulae, the fistulous track is laid open, with removal of surrounding skin (Figs 11.11 and 11.12). It is essential to know, before doing this, that the anorectal ring will be left intact, otherwise incontinence could result. These racquet-shaped wounds, left open to granulate, heal surprisingly quickly and soundly and rarely leave any residual disability.

The relatively uncommon fistulae which have

(b)

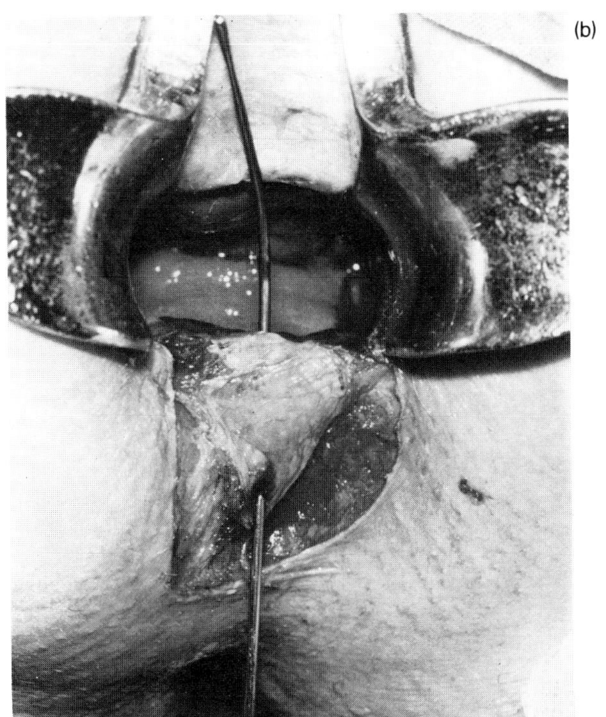

(a)

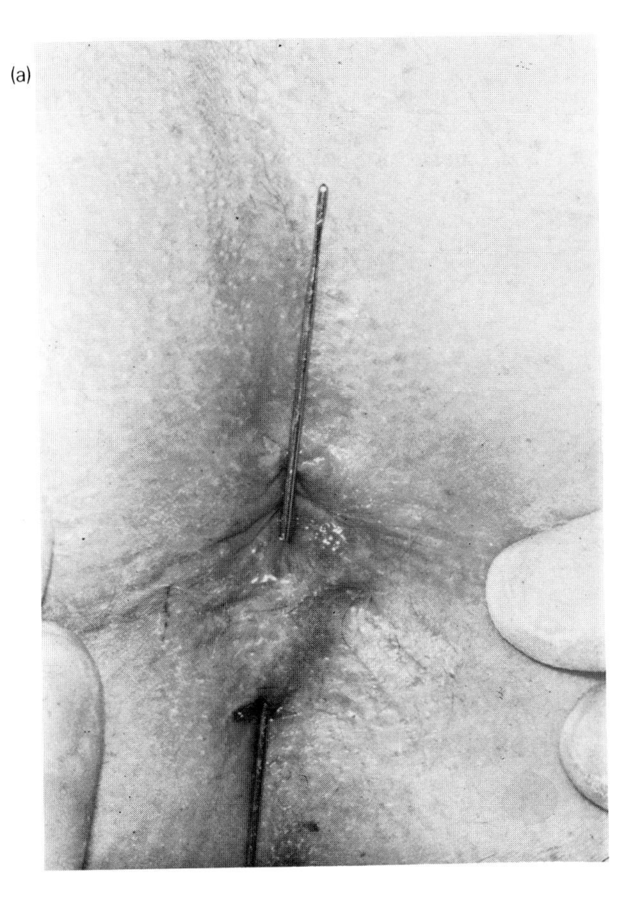

(c)

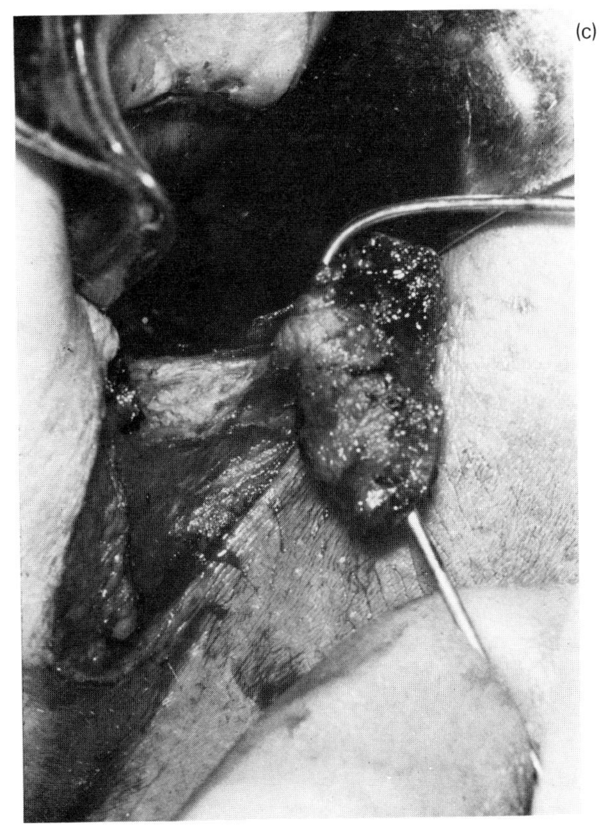

Fig. 11.12 *Excision of a low-level inter-sphincteric anal fistula. (a) A probe has been passed along the track of the fistula, and emerges through the internal opening, in the anal canal. (b) The fistula is being excised, along with surrounding skin and connective tissues. (c) Final stage of dissection, looking up anal canal: the whole length of the fistula is being excised, along with any superficial fibres of the external sphincter which may be involved (Fig. 11.11).*

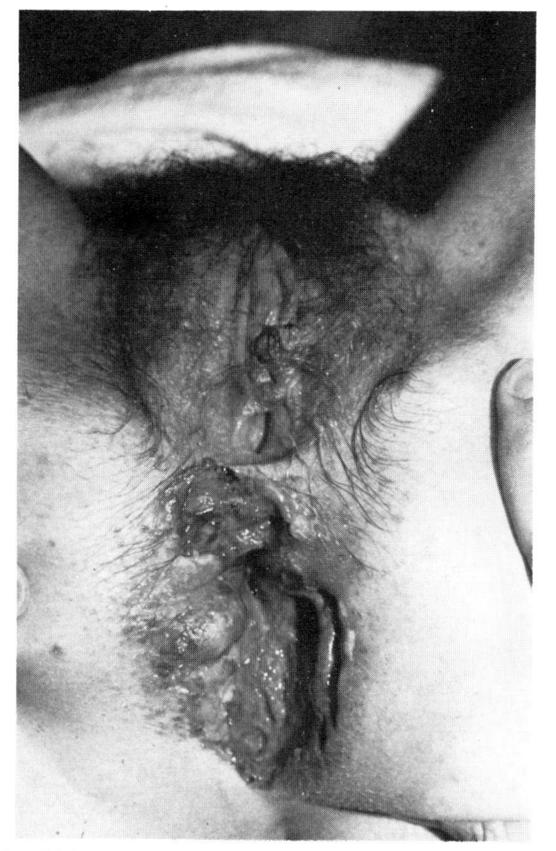

Fig. 11.13 *Perianal region of a girl of 15 who complained of three weeks' discharge: she proved to have severe Crohn's colitis.*

an internal opening into the rectum, above the anorectal ring, cannot be treated by complete laying-open, and a temporary colostomy may have to be established to stop the faecal leak along the fistulous track: then the opening into the rectum can be sutured and the fistulous track allowed to close by granulation.

Perianal sepsis and anal fissure are common complications of Crohn's disease, and may be the presenting feature (p. 228, and Fig. 11.13).

RECTAL PROLAPSE

Definition

Rectal prolapse occurs when the whole circumference of the rectum descends through the anus. The term mucosal prolapse is used when only the mucous membrane and submucosa protrudes, and complete prolapse denotes descent of the full thickness of the rectal wall (Fig. 11.14).

Presentation

The problem usually presents in childhood or in the middle-aged and elderly. During childhood, most cases occur in the first two years of life. About 80% of cases among adults are female and the maximum incidence in this group occurs in patients over 40–50. In affected males there is no such tendency towards developing the problem in older age, the cases being evenly distributed throughout adult life. It has been shown that the adult problem is more commonly seen in nulliparous women than in those who have children. The reason for this is not understood.

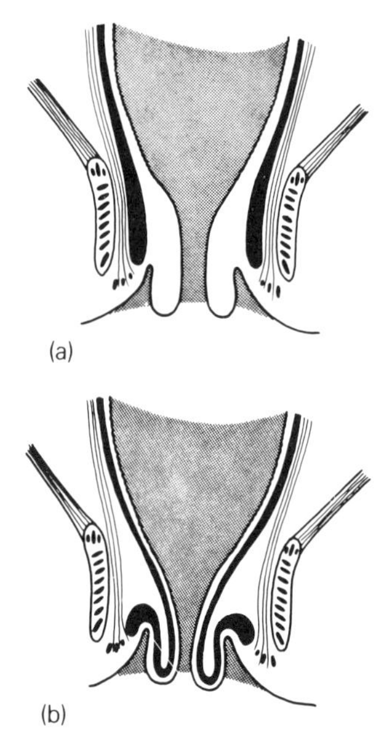

Fig. 11.14 *(a) Mucosal and (b) complete rectal prolapse.*

Aetiology

It has been suggested that a common precursor to rectal prolapse in childhood is straining at stool due to diarrhoea or constipation. A further aetiological factor is the absence of the sacral curve in childhood so that the rectum lies in the same vertical line as the anal canal, instead of the substantial angle which exists between rectum and anal canal in the adult. Rectal prolapse may complicate cystic fibrosis (see p. 109).

The aetiology of adult rectal prolapse is unknown, but several important observations have been made on these patients. Many of them tend to have a deep rectovaginal pouch (Fig. 11.15) and it used to be thought that many patients initially developed a hernia of the pouch of Douglas which eventually progressed and brought down the full circumference of the bowel wall with it. More recent work using cineradiography has demonstrated that, in many patients with prolapse, the descent of the prolapse commences as an intussusception of the mid rectum. The reason for this is not clear. However, it is important to recognise that complete rectal prolapse is a form of abdominal hernia.

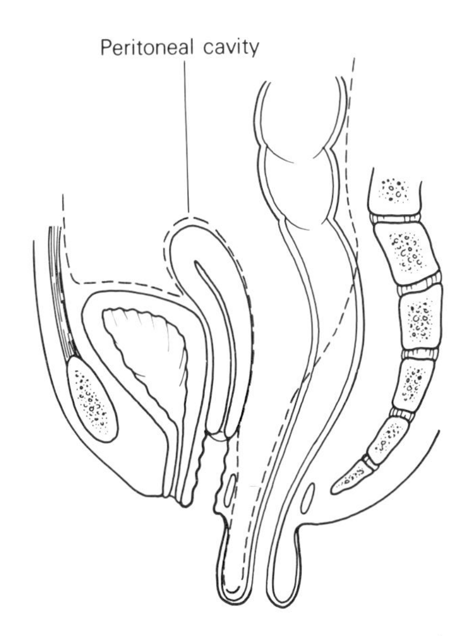

Fig. 11.15 *Section of pelvis to show the anatomy of complete prolapse.*

Although rectal prolapse may rarely occur in patients with cauda equina lesions, the weakness of the sphincter mechanism found in many patients with rectal prolapse is though to be secondary to the prolapse rather than being important in the aetiology of the condition.

Clinical Features

In most children the prolapse can be felt on digital examination to be of the mucosal prolapse variety, but occasionally it may be a complete prolapse. The rectum may prolapse several inches outside the anus.

Adults complain of prolapse initially during defaecation only, with either spontaneous reduction or requiring manual replacement. As the condition becomes more severe, prolapse occurs when standing and during ambulation. It is often associated with a bearing-down sensation, discharge of mucus, and incontinence of faeces due to sphincter weakness.

Careful examination is important to assess whether the problem is mucosal or complete prolapse. This may be decided on such criteria as the extent of prolapse, digital assessment of the thickness of the prolapsed bowel wall, and the tone of the sphincters.

Treatment

Children

In small children it is well known that the condition is generally a self-limiting one which responds to simple measures such as treatment of constipation and strapping the buttocks together. Rarely, injection of the lower rectal mucosa with sclerosing solution will be necessary. If abdominal operation is necessary, rectosigmoidectomy with anastomosis of the two ends of bowel is preferable to operations where implants are used.

Adults

Mucosal prolapse is best treated using local

methods to the anal canal. Injection sclerotherapy is of value in patients who have minor problems and haemorrhoidectomy has been found to benefit patients with more extensive mucosal prolapse. In addition to removing a good part of the prolapsed mucosa, the operation works by creating a large raw area which heals by secondary intention thus producing some narrowing and rigidity of the lower rectum and the anal canal.

Complete prolapse: The simplest operation advocated for this problem is insertion of a Thiersch wire around the anal canal. Most surgeons who use this method now use a monofilament suture such as nylon or polypropylene, but the results are not very satisfactory because it is difficult to obtain the correct degree of tightness.

The most popular method of treating complete rectal prolapse is ivalon sponge rectopexy. After dissection of the rectum, completely separating it from the sacrum and from the vagina, with its blood supply intact, a sheet of polyvinyl alcohol sponge is wrapped around the rectum, apart from a small anterior strip. The sheet is sutured to the reduced rectum and to the presacral fascia, and in the weeks after the operation the sheet stimulates fibrosis which fixes the rectum and prevents prolapse.

Although this operation is good for arresting prolapse, a number of patients continue to have some trouble with incontinence, and the wrap operation is often combined with suture of the weakened levator ani.

SQUAMOUS CARCINOMA OF ANAL REGION

Compared to carcinoma of rectum, squamous carcinoma of the anal region is a rare problem. It is equally common in men and women. Squamous carcinoma of the anal canal is more common in females, whereas squamous carcinoma of the anal margin area is more common in males. Lesions of the anal margin and perianal region are commonly well differentiated whereas those in the anal canal tend to be poorly differentiated.

Presentation

The complaints include anal pain, bleeding at defaecation, feeling a lump or rectal discharge. If the lesion is more advanced there may be tenesmus or even incontinence.

Examination

The lesion is frequently misdiagnosed, and it is important to biopsy any lesion in the anal region which is remotely suspicious since the appearance of an early lesion may closely resemble a chronic anal fissure or a thrombosed haemorrhoid. The appearances may vary from a superficial ulcer to a warty growth, and advanced lesions cause anal stenosis and distortion of the anal canal. The inguinal lymph nodes should be examined carefully for evidence of metastatic spread.

Treatment

Localised squamous carcinomas in the perianal region and around the anal margin may be adequately treated by wide local excision or by radiotherapy. It is important to follow up these patients closely to look for evidence of recurrence of tumour. If tumours within the anal canal extend above the pectinate line, the risk of development of metastases to the nodes around the rectum is high so that the most commonly recommended treatment consists of abdominoperineal excision of the rectum with formation of a colostomy (p. 211). The patients are closely followed up and, if inguinal lymph node metastases develop later, a block dissection of the inguinal region is performed. The overall results of treatment of carcinoma of anus and anal canal are poorer than for carcinoma of rectum. Some workers have claimed 5-year survival rates of up to 50% of those patients subjected to operation.

PRURITUS ANI

Itching in the perianal area is a fairly common

symptom and one which, in a severe case, is extremely distressing to the patient. A useful approach is to regard pruritus as a symptom of anorectal disease, and first to carry out a complete examination of the area. Any condition which allows faecal or mucous leakage will tend to aggravate pruritus, so it is important to identify and treat prolapsing haemorrhoids, an anal fistula, proctitis, or occasionally a low rectal carcinoma or villous papilloma. Threadworms are an important and readily-treated cause, and can be easily seen in active movement on proctoscopy. Scabies and pediculosis pubis can affect the perianal area, and perianal warts can make anal cleansing very difficult. Weakness of the anal sphincter sufficient to allow some leakage of faecal material can be difficult to assess unless it follows accidental injury or surgery for major fistula: it is more often seen in the elderly, when treatment can be difficult.

Lack of cleanliness can be an important cause, because, once scratching begins, this in itself can cause minor abrasions of the soft moist perianal skin, which in turn invite secondary infection with pyogenic bacteria, fungi or yeasts. A mycotic infection typically has a well-defined reddened edge, and microscopic examination of a scraping from the edge will show the agent, and then specific treatment can begin. It should be remembered that corticosteroid and antibiotic ointments, though often used, may themselves perpetuate pruritus through causing a sensitivity reaction.

When the possible primary causes of pruritus have been treated, the main aim must be to help the patient not to continue scratching. Good local hygiene, light clothing, avoidance of antibiotic ointments, use of a dusting powder or simple calamine and phenol lotion may help. In cases of long standing, with thickening and pallor of the perianal skin, it can be very difficult to produce a lasting relief.

Proctalgia Fugax (see p. 10)

PERIANAL CONDYLOMATA ACUMINATA

Viral warts in the perianal region (perianal condylomata acuminata) are being seen with increasing frequency (Fig. 11.16). The lesion affects the perianal skin and the epithelium of the lower end of the anal canal. Varying numbers of warts are seen in different patients, and warts may also be seen on the penis and genital area in the same patient. It is thought that the infection is frequently transmitted by sexual activity. There is little doubt that these lesions are caused by a transmissible virus, the human papilloma virus, one of the papova viruses.

Treatment

If there are only a few small lesions present the best method of treatment is to use 25% podophyllin in tincture benzoin compound. If the lesions are large or do not respond to this method of treatment then operative treatment should be undertaken.

Diathermy excision

Diathermy excision of these lesions is a popular

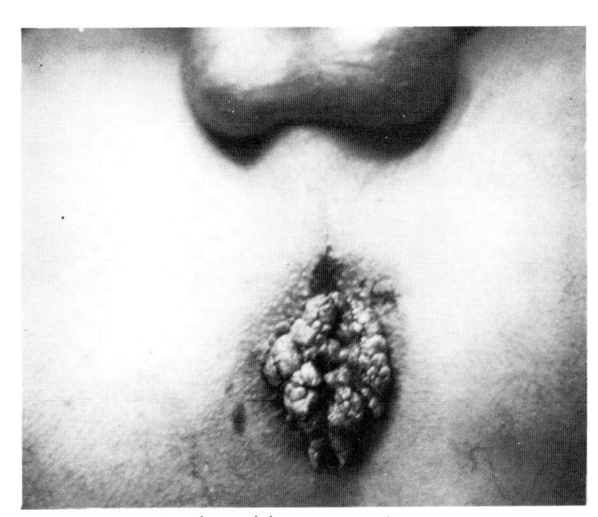

Fig. 11.16 *Perianal condylomata acuminata.*

method, but it is difficult to determine how much tissue damage is produced.

Scissor dissection

This has recently been described, and appears to give good results without much scarring. The perianal area is infiltrated with saline with 1/300 000 adrenaline so that the warts are separated from each other. They can then be removed individually, leaving healthy skin between each excised area. Bleeding is minimal and healing is rapid.

SEXUALLY TRANSMITTED DISEASES

One aspect of the remarkable change which has come over the presentation of the so-called venereal diseases is that some 70% of patients now diagnosed as having infectious *syphilis* are homosexual males. A primary chancre may be seen at the anal verge or in the anal canal and an important additional sign is marked inguinal adenitis. In the secondary stage the perianal area may show condylomata lata – scattered grey or pink papules – again with marked inguinal adenitis.

Venereal proctitis is usually due to *gonorrhoea*. In women this is likely to be due to spread from a vaginal discharge but in men it will generally be due to anal coitus. The signs are of a localised acute granular proctitis with an unusually profuse purulent exudate.

Herpes simplex can occur in passive homosexual males and is extremely painful, with much anal spasm and consequent constipation. Scattered areas of erythema or vesication around the anus are usually seen.

Perianal warts (condylomata acuminata, p. 257) are unusually common in homosexual males.

12

Congenital Deformities

All parts of the alimentary tract, from the mouth to the anus, can be the site of a malformation which has arisen *in utero*. The effects of these anomalies vary in severity. Thus, a baby born with a cleft palate can be difficult to feed but generally develops normally and the effect of the cleft on speech will create social rather than medical difficulties. On the other hand, most of the malformations of the gut have immediate and far-reaching effects and survival is rarely possible without major surgery during the first days of life.

Most deformities arise within a few weeks of conception, whilst the vital early stages of organ formation are taking place. The mechanism is not clear, although the frequent association with other major developmental defects (for example, duodenal atresia with Down's syndrome, rectal abnormalities with genito-urinary deformities) suggests some general harmful influence operating during the first three months of fetal life: this may be viral or, in most cases, an unknown agent. The most striking example of a genetic influence occurs in cystic fibrosis of the pancreas, which is caused by a recessive gene, with a one in four chance that siblings will be similarly affected. Hirschsprung's disease and hypertrophic pyloric stenosis occur predominantly in male babies.

The incidence of malformations varies considerably within and between countries and races, but congenital abnormalities of the alimentary tract have an incidence of about 1 in every 1000 births (a frequency similar to Down's syndrome), and produce about one-third of all admissions to a neonatal surgical unit.

The need for these units has become generally recognised over the last 30 years. The sick newborn needs highly specialised care and equipment. Almost all these babies are nursed in individual incubators, using miniaturised equipment. The nursing care of these babies is highly specialised and the paediatricians, surgeons and anaesthetists who care for them all need considerable special experience. Best results are therefore obtained in units where experience can be concentrated. The aim in western Europe and North America is to produce a neonatal surgical unit for every 3 million people. In practice in Great Britain this means that each Area Health Board supports one unit. With rapid medically-supervised transport in a portable incubator, these babies can be safely transferred considerable distances.

CLEFTS OF THE LIP AND PALATE

These are due to a failure of the maxillary and nasal growth centres to fuse in a normal manner (Fig. 12.1). All forms of failed fusion may be seen:

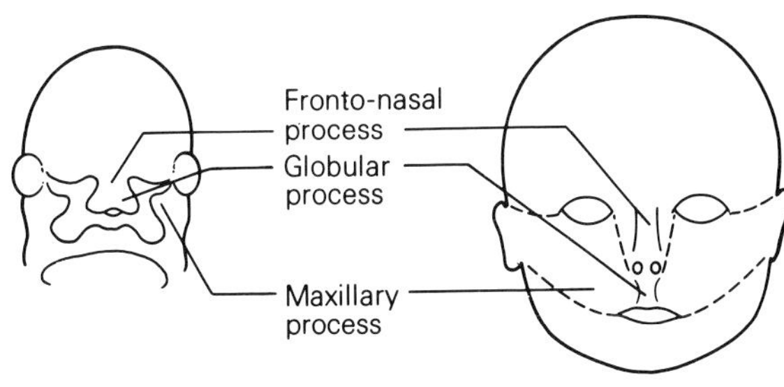

Fig. 12.1 *Embryology of the face, showing the formation of the upper lip by fusion of the maxillary and fronto-nasal processes.*

there may be a small notch in the red margin of the lip, or a bifid soft palate, or there may be complete failure of both maxillary growth centres to meet the median nasal growth centre, resulting in complete bilateral clefts of the lip and total cleft palate (Figs 12.2, 12.3).

These deformities cause little actual medical disability, but if a palate is not skilfully repaired the social disadvantage of cleft palate type of speech are severe, and the appearance of an uncorrected cleft lip is very unpleasant. With timely and expert plastic surgery during the first two years, these disabilities are nowadays almost completely overcome.

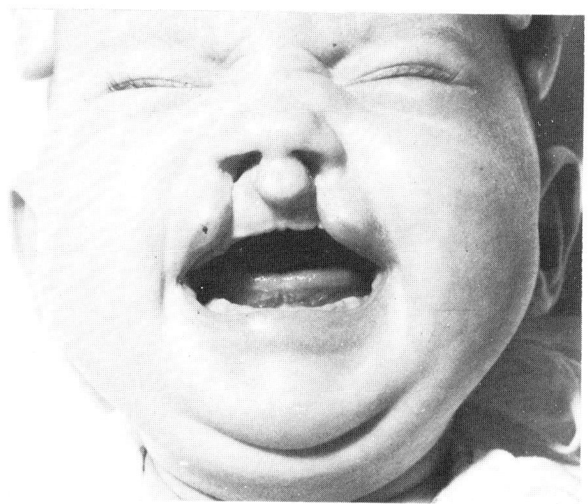

Fig. 12.2 *Double cleft lip. The part of the lip formed by the frontonasal process is clearly seen.*

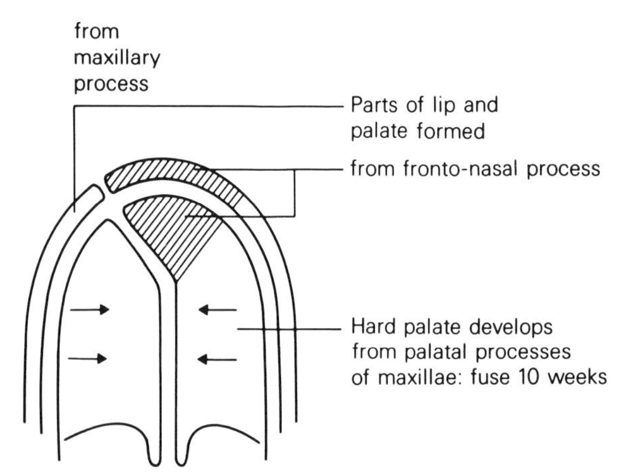

Fig. 12.3 *Complete cleft of lip and palate, viewed from below. The cleft of the lip and anterior palate is due to failure of fusion of the fronto-nasal process and the right maxillary process: the cleft of remaining palate is due to non-union between the palatal processes.*

OESOPHAGEAL ATRESIA

This anomaly occurs about once in every 3000 births, so it is one of the commoner major deformities of the alimentary tract. In the normal course of events the trachea and larynx split off from the foregut about the fourth to sixth week of fetal life, so this must be the stage at which oesophageal anomalies develop, but there is no understanding of why this should happen: associated anomalies in the heart and renal tracts and in

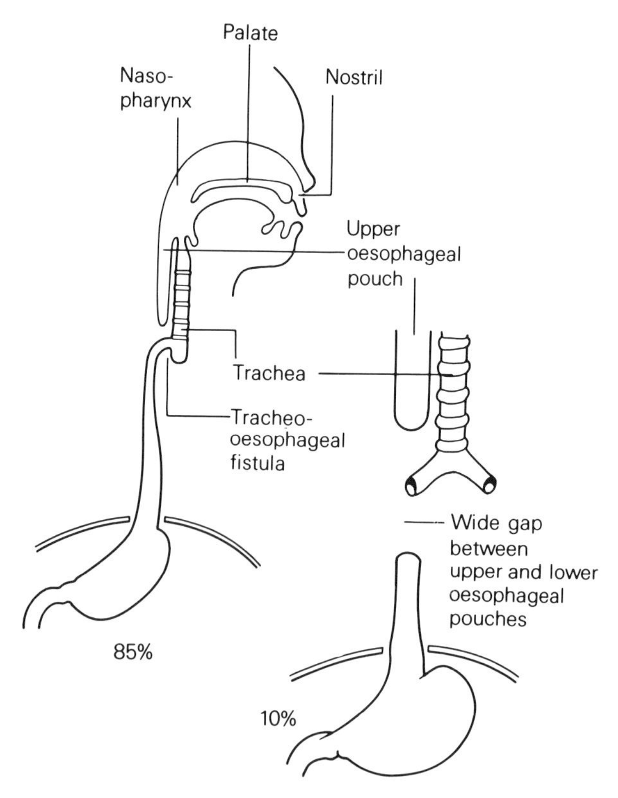

Fig. 12.4 *Sagittal sections showing the two major forms of oesophageal atresia.*

the rectum occur in about half the babies with oesophageal atresia, so some general influence appears to be affecting development at this very early stage after conception.

Much the commonest deformity (85%) is a complete atresia of the upper oesophagus with a fistula between the tracheal bifurcation and the lower oesophagus. A few (10%) babies have a long gap between the two oesophageal pouches and no fistula (Fig. 12.4).

Clearly, these newborns cannot swallow and at a very early stage are 'frothy' and 'bubbly', and cough and splutter. Whenever this is noted, a stiff catheter should be passed through the mouth; it will be found to arrest about 10 cm below the incisor teeth.

Since the first successful repair of an oesophageal atresia in a neonate in 1941, this has become a regular operation for paediatric surgeons. The right chest is entered extrapleurally, the tracheo-oesophageal fistula is divided and oversewn, and the two blind ends of oesophagus mobilised and joined together. In good risk babies, over 2 kg weight, mortality is now negligible, which is a remarkable tribute to refined anaesthetic techniques and delicate surgery.

NEONATAL INTESTINAL OBSTRUCTION

Obstruction can occur at any level from the duodenum to the anus. The higher deformities in the duodenum and small bowel tend to present quickly, during the first 24–48 hours, with characteristic bright green vomiting, quite different from the yellow vomit which many babies produce: this must always be regarded as evidence of organic obstruction. Inspection of the abdomen will often show visible peristalsis in stomach, or generalised distension, and plain radiography provides some very characteristic pictures.

Duodenal Obstruction

There are two major causes, one intrinsic and one extrinsic.

Intrinsic obstruction

In this case, there is a blockage of the lumen due either to a membrane, or to actual discontinuity of the lumen (atresia, Fig. 12.5). All have the same effect: complete or nearly complete obstruction. Occurring so high in the alimentary tract, they produce very early vomiting which is characteristically grass-green in colour, and the distended stomach may be visible. The plain abdominal x-ray shows a characteristic 'double bubble' (Fig. 12.6). Sometimes the obstruction can be relieved by excision of the membrane. In atresia the usual treatment is to anastomose jejunum to the distended duodenum above the obstruction (Fig. 12.7). There is a strong but unexplained association of the these anomalies with mongolism, which occurs in 25%, and the further association with cardiac abnormalities suggests a general

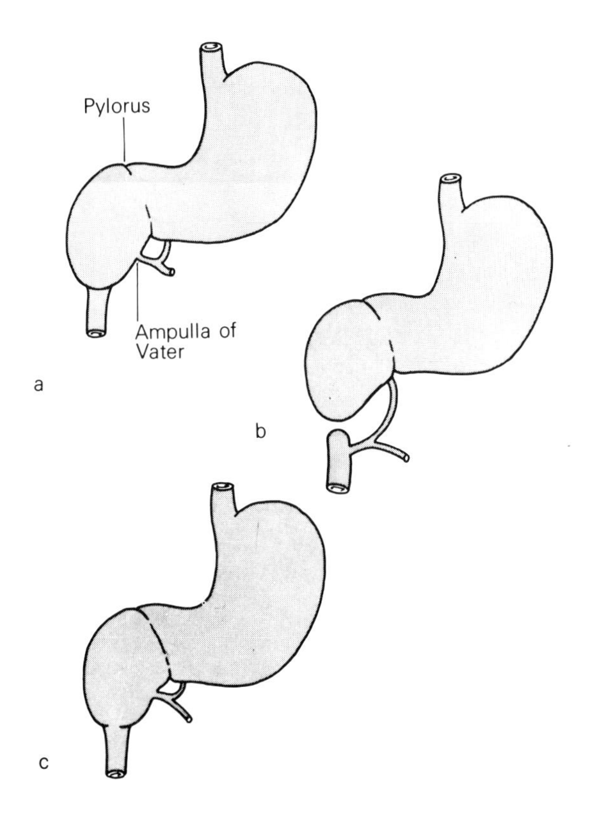

Fig. 12.5 *Types of intrinsic duodenal obstruction: (a) complete membrane, (b) atresia, also rarer type with the ampulla of Vater below the obstruction, (c) membrane with small central opening. In types (a) and (c) the vomit will be bile-stained.*

harmful influence operating around 8–12 weeks of fetal life.

Extrinsic obstruction

Here, the rotation of the midgut has gone awry.

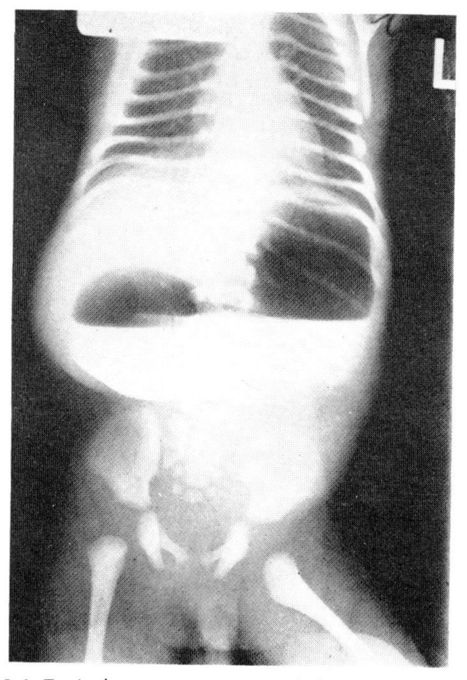

Fig. 12.6 *Typical x-ray appearance of duodenal atresia.*

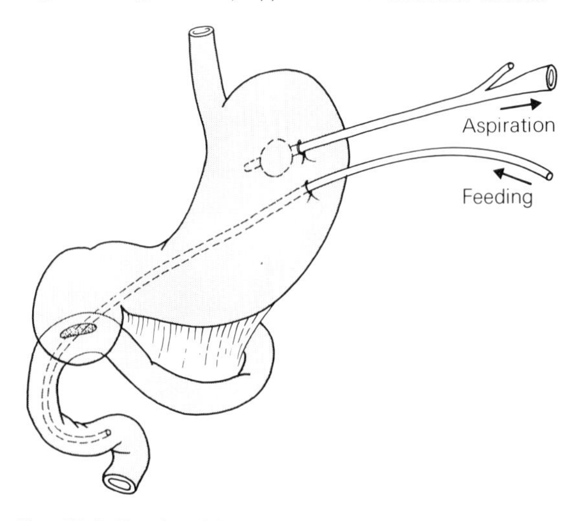

Fig. 12.7 *Duodenojejunostomy. Gastrostomy allows aspiration of the dilated stomach, and the transanastomotic tube allows early feeding, whilst the dilated stomach and duodenum are regaining tone and normal function.*

Normally the duodenal loop becomes applied to the posterior abdominal wall and is crossed by the mid-gut artery, with the colon then coming to lie around the periphery of the abdomen (Fig 12.8). If the anticlockwise rotation of the colon becomes arrested over the duodenal loop, bands (named after Ladd, a paediatric surgeon in Boston, USA) are formed which can obstruct the duodenum (Fig. 12.9). Furthermore, the base of the small bowel mesentery is very short, so it is easy for volvulus to occur (i.e. rotation of a loop of bowel around the axis of its mesentery, causing obstruction). Sometimes complete non-rotation of the midgut occurs, and this also creates the conditions for volvulus. (Fig. 12.10). If volvulus occurs, the duodeno-jejunal flexure is necessarily obstructed.

These babies tend to feed normally for a few days after birth, and then volvulus occurs, followed by green vomiting: this can, however, occur later in life. Treatment entails division of Ladd's band, untwisting the volvulus, and placing the small bowel on the right, and colon to the left side of the abdomen. The caecum then lies in mid-abdomen, so the appendix should be removed.

Small Bowel Obstruction

Small bowel obstruction in the newborn is most often due to atresia or stenosis. It seems likely that these babies have had a normal bowel and then, at some stage of development, there has been an accident to the mesenteric circulation of part of the small bowel (perhaps due to volvulus or strangulation round a band): sterile ischaemic necrosis of a segment of bowel occurs, followed either by its total disappearance (atresia) (Fig. 12.11), or

Fig. 12.8 *Normal rotation of the midgut. (a) During the sixth to tenth week of fetal life the midgut herniates out into the umbilical cord. The vitello-intestinal duct extends to the placenta. (b) Midgut rotation, which occurs anticlockwise, has commenced. (c) The left colon has returned to the abdomen and occupies its normal position. The proximal colon is in process of taking up its normal position (arrow) and will settle and become attached in the right iliac fossa. The duodenal loop is now partly retroperitoneal and the third part is crossed by the superior mesenteric artery.*

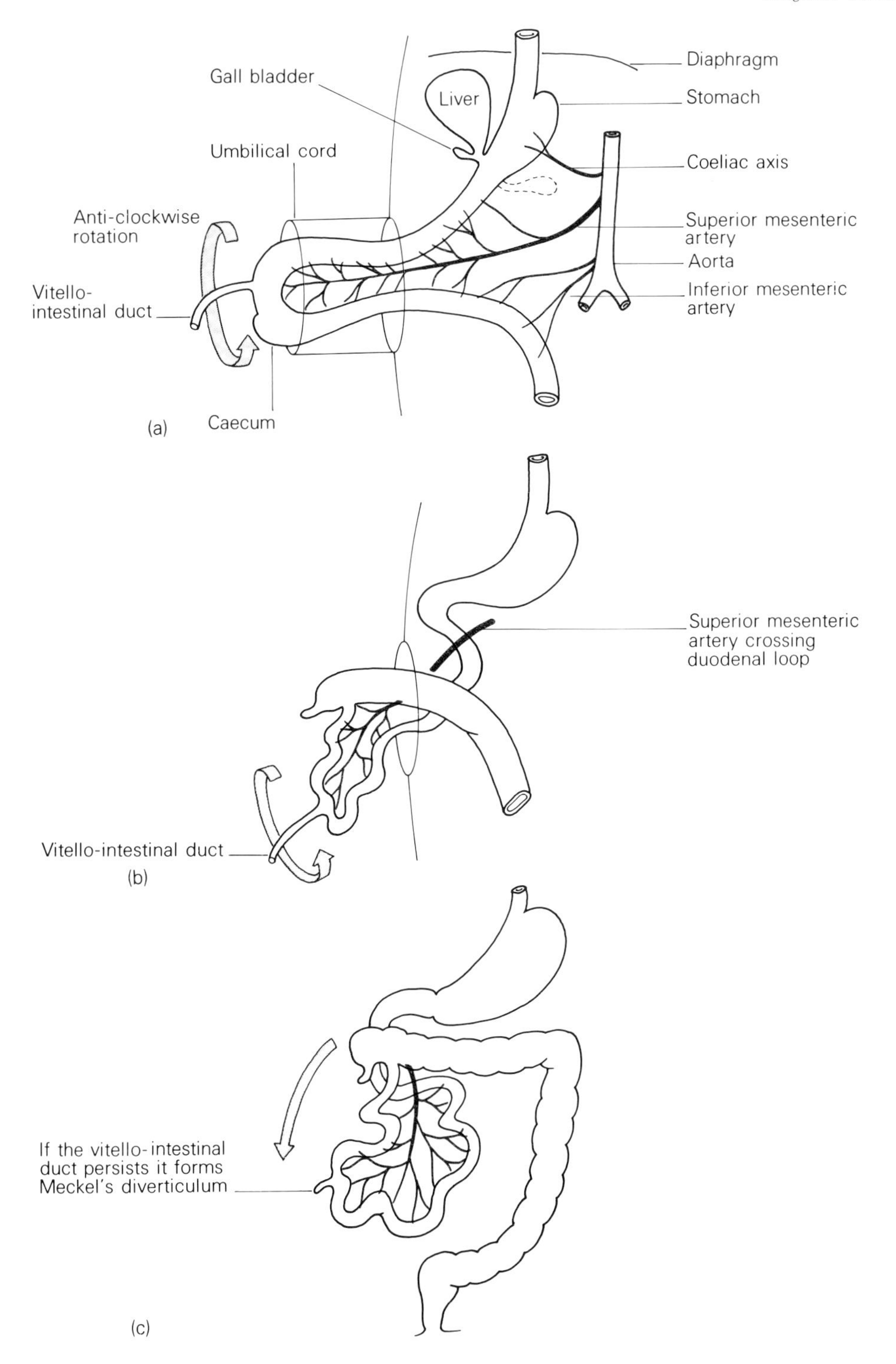
Diaphragm
Gall bladder
Liver
Stomach
Umbilical cord
Coeliac axis
Anti-clockwise rotation
Superior mesenteric artery
Aorta
Vitello-intestinal duct
Inferior mesenteric artery
(a)
Caecum
Superior mesenteric artery crossing duodenal loop
Vitello-intestinal duct
(b)
If the vitello-intestinal duct persists it forms Meckel's diverticulum
(c)

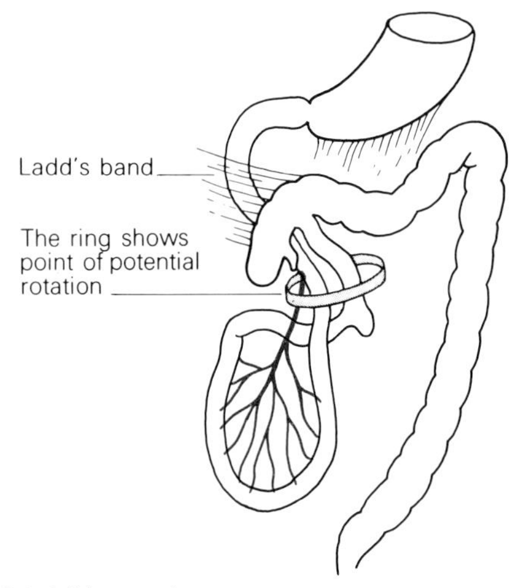

Fig. 12.9 *Midgut malrotation.*

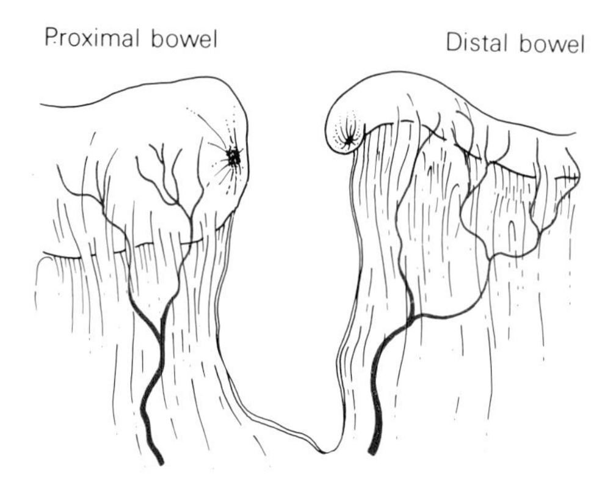

Fig. 12.11 *The anatomical defect in atresia of jejunum or ileum. Note the disproportion between the two ends, the retraction and fibrosis induced by the ischaemic process in the distal stump, and the gap in the mesentery.*

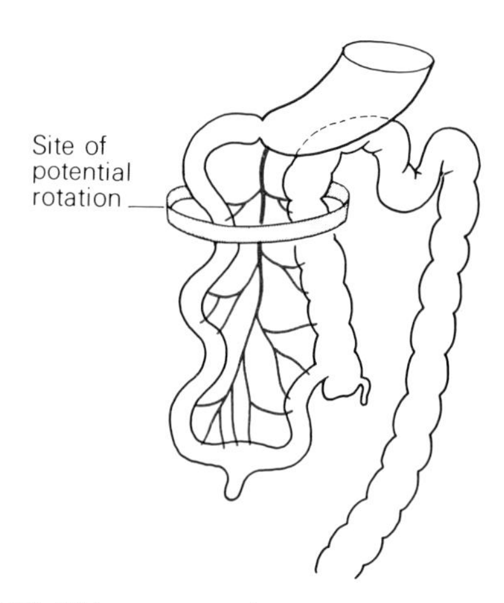

Fig. 12.10 *Midgut non-rotation.*

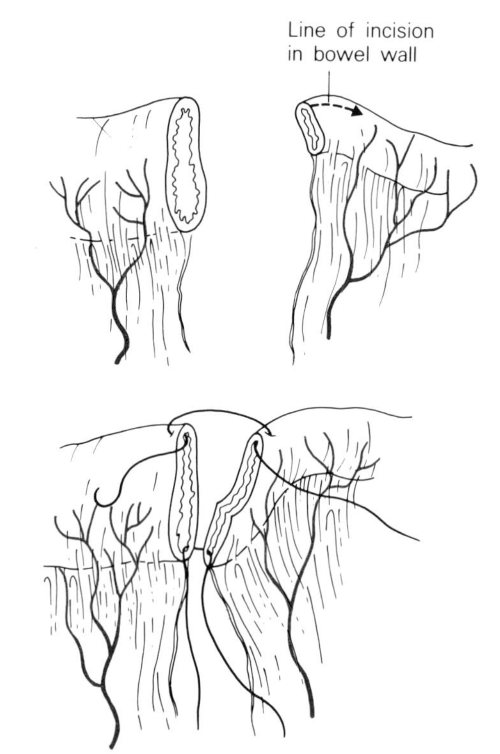

Fig. 12.12 *'End-to-back' anastomosis. A single layer of interrupted inverting sutures is inserted.*

ischaemic fibrosis leading to severe stenosis. Very few of these babies have other congenital deformities so a local accident seems more probable than a general factor influencing development.

These babies also present within 24–48 hours of birth with green vomiting and very marked abdominal distension. A plain film shows an extraordinary degree of dilatation of small bowel, due to the fact that obstruction has been building up over several months during which the baby has been nourished through the umbilical cord. Resection and end-to-back anastomosis produces excellent results (Fig. 12.12).

Intraluminal Obstruction

This is an unusual cause of bowel obstruction at any age. It is well illustrated by meconium ileus,

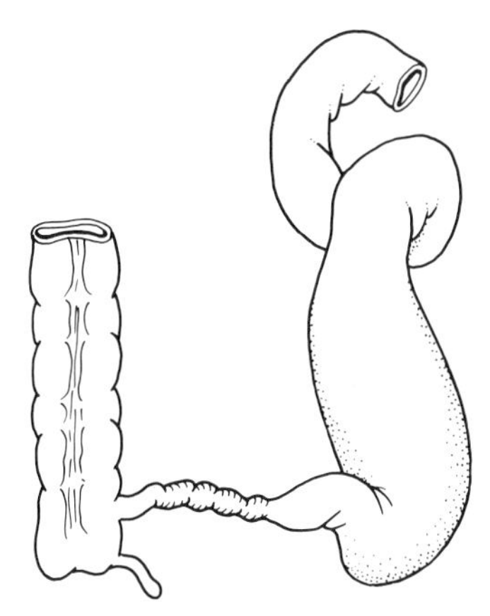

Fig. 12.13 *Typical appearances of the distal ileum in meconium ileus. Hard pellets of meconium cause obstruction to the viscous, putty-like meconium distending the ileum above them.*

which affects a few children with cystic fibrosis of the pancreas (see p. 109). Secretion of pancreatic enzymes is so deficient that meconium (which consists of swallowed amniotic fluid, bile and other secretions, lanugo, and squamous epithelium, and is normally of creamy consistency) is so viscous that it has the qualities of masticated chewing gum. The viscosity of this material is so high that it cannot be propelled through the small bowel, and intestinal obstruction results (Fig. 12.13). Presentation is very similar to small bowel atresia. Treatment usually entails resection of terminal ileum, which contains the most immovable material, and manual clearance of the viscous meconium from the rest of the bowel. Some babies are successfully treated by administration of a hypertonic enema of gastrografin; this stimulates hypersecretion of intestinal juice and the obstructing meconium is washed out of the ileum into the wider colon, whence it is then evacuated naturally.

These and all other babies with cystic fibrosis are very liable to respiratory infection and will require lifelong ingestion of pancreatic extract to make good the deficient pancreatic secretion (see p. 110).

Megacolon

Megacolon describes a condition in which the colon is grossly dilated and distended. This can be an acquired disorder (see p. 220), but most patients with megacolon suffer from a congenital malformation generally known as Hirschsprung's disease.

Hirschsprung's Disease

Hirschsprung was a physician in Copenhagen and in 1886 he described two children who had never had a normal bowel action and who showed enormous abdominal distension due to dilatation of the colon above an apparently normal rectum. Until 1948, when Swenson and Bill showed that the distension disappeared when a colostomy was formed in the dilated colon, it was thought that the colon became so large because it was mysteriously lacking in contractility. It was then recognised that the apparently normal rectum contained no ganglia in the submucosal and myenteric nerve plexuses, and therefore was totally inactive and unable to expel faeces. It is now known that the intestinal autonomic innervation migrates down the gut from above: occasionally (about once in every 5000 neonates) this migration stops short of the anal canal, leaving a length of colon devoid of ganglia. This deformity may affect only a few centimetres of rectum or, more commonly, the whole rectum and part of the sigmoid colon (Fig.

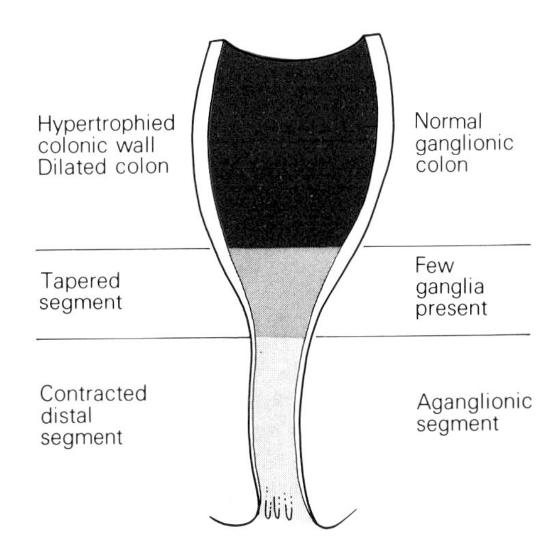

Fig. 12.14 *Pathology of Hirschsprung's disease.*

12.14). More rarely, most of, or the whole of, the colon is aganglionic.

Clinical presentation in the neonate

The majority of cases present in the neonatal period. Boys outnumber girls by 5 to 1. A family history of Hirschsprung's disease is present in 7% of all cases. There is delay in passage of meconium. Abdominal distension is common and feeding is slow. Rectal examination demonstrates an area of rectum which is tight around the examining finger and if the segment involved is short there is often release of flatus and meconium as the finger is withdrawn. Plain x-rays show many gas-distended loops of bowel.

Valuable confirmation of the diagnosis can be obtained from a limited barium enema (Fig. 12.15) which shows the narrow rectum and dilated colon above the zone of transition from ganglionic to aganglionic bowel.

In some infants the presentation is more insidious, with failure to thrive being the major problem. Abdominal distension and constipation is intermittent in these children and the diagnosis may only be arrived at after several admissions to hospital. Diarrhoea due to enterocolitis is a presenting feature of Hirschsprung's disease in a small percentage of babies, and this complication carries a high mortality.

Occasionally, children who survive infancy will present with chronic constipation in later childhood or even as adults. Usually these patients have relatively short segments of the colon involved.

Management

It is most important that all infants with Hirschsprung's diease should have either a colostomy fashioned, or definitive surgery completed, before leaving hospital because of the danger of enterocolitis developing.

Biopsy

Biopsy of the rectum should be performed to

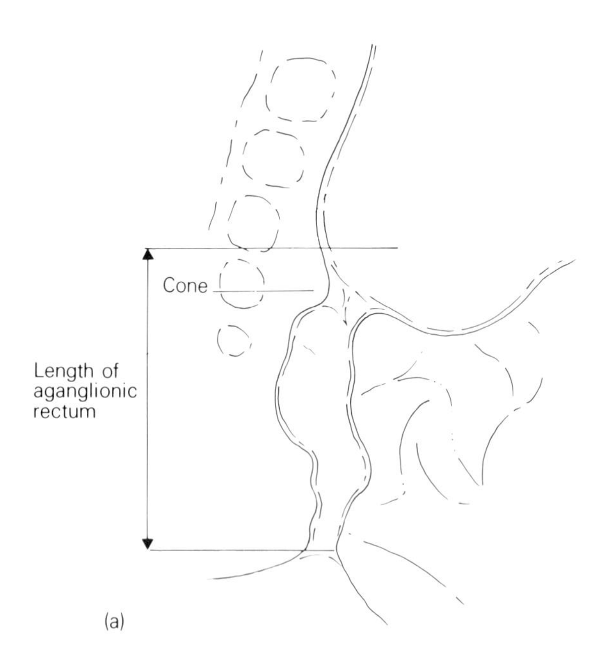

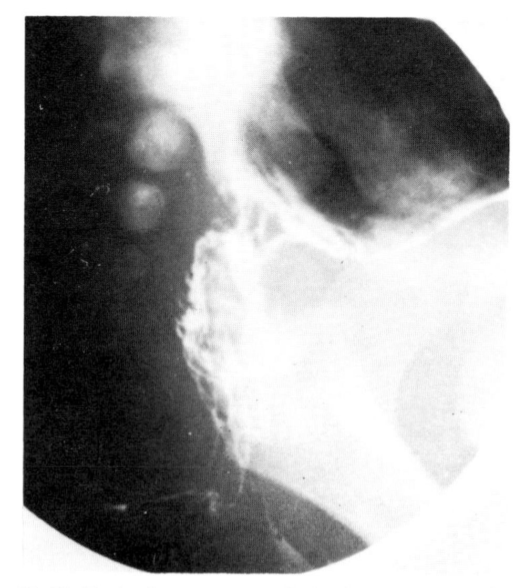

Fig. 12.15 *Typical appearance of a barium enema carried out on a newborn with Hirschsprung's disease.*

confirm the diagnosis. The most widely used method was to take a full-thickness biopsy of the rectal wall posteriorly under general anaesthetic, to include the muscle layers. The defect was sutured. The alternative approach, taking mucosal and submucosal biopsies with a suction biopsy instrument, is now increasingly used. Histological confirmation is obtained when ganglia are absent from the submucosal and myenteric plexus. In addition, there is an increase in the number of nerve fibres seen in the interface between the circular and longitudinal muscles. A further refinement in histological technique utilises a method designed to stain sections for acetylcholinesterase to identify cholingergic fibres, and identification of adrenergic fibres using a catecholamine fluorescent technique.

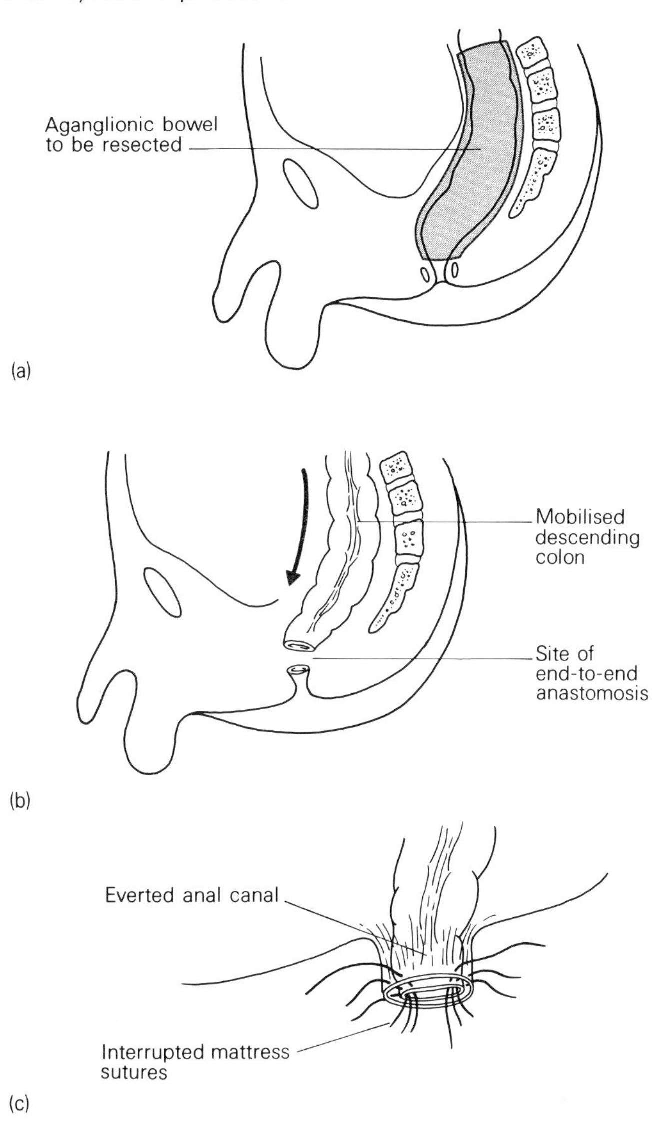

Fig. 12.16 *Swenson's operation. (a) The segment of bowel to be resected. (b) The restoration of continuity. (c) Detail of performing anastomosis on everted anal canal; once completed the everted anus is restored to its normal situation, as in (b).*

Surgery

Preliminary colostomy. Surgery ought to be undertaken as soon as the diagnosis is made. If the obstruction is complete and the child is ill, then it is best to operate before definitive histology is obtained. The initial step in the neonate should always be formation of a colostomy. This must be made in ganglionic bowel; ideally the presence of ganglia ought to be confirmed using frozen-section histology. If this facility is not available then it may be best to make the colostomy in the transverse colon rather than immediately above the transitional zone in the sigmoid colon. An opportunity is available at the time of operation to take biopsies above and below the transitional zone so that, when the later definitive operation is performed, the length of aganglionic bowel is definitely known.

Definitive surgery. The definitive operation is usually delayed until, with the bowel decompressed and evacuating normally via the colostomy, the baby has grown and is an otherwise normal 9–12-month-old child.

Two operations are commonly used, and both involve excision of aganglionic bowel, followed by anastomosis of normal colon to the anal canal.

In Swenson's operation (Fig. 12.16), all aganglionic bowel is excised and the mobilised ganglionic colon is anastomosed end-to-end to the anal canal by a pull-through operation.

In Duhamel's operation the rectum is retained, the ganglionic colon is joined to the posterior half of the anorectal ring, and then the common wall between rectum and colon is destroyed (Fig. 12.17), so forming a capacious new rectum.

Both operations require considerable care and expertise for their performance, but yield excellent long-term results.

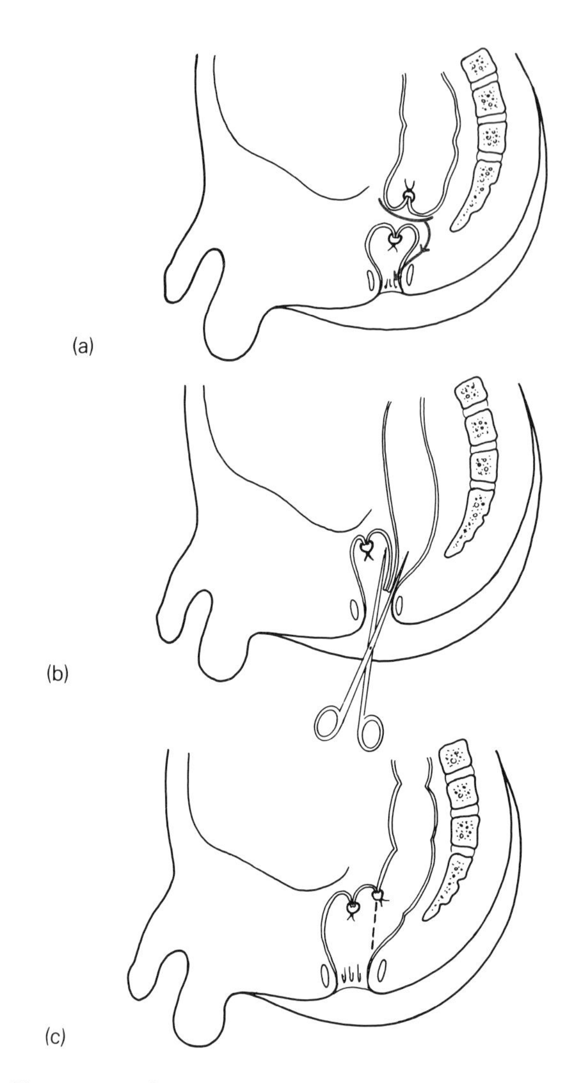

Fig. 12.17 *Duhamel's operation. (a) Aganglionic sigmoid and upper rectum has been resected but the lower half of rectum retained and closed by suture. (b) Ganglionic colon brought through the posterior half of anorectal ring and the common wall crushed. (c) End result.*

Anorectal Anomalies

In the four-week-old fetus the hindgut ends in the cloaca. In the following weeks, the cloaca is split vertically into an anterior urogenital sinus and a posterior rectum. Anomalies are divided into high and low deformities. High deformities – those lying above the levator ani – are associated with disordered division of the cloaca by incomplete descent of the urogenital fold. Low deformities, which only affect the rectum and anus below the levator ani and pelvic diaphragm, are associated with abnormalities in the disappearance of the cloacal membrane. (Fig. 12.18).

There should be little delay in suspecting an anorectal anomaly because one look at the

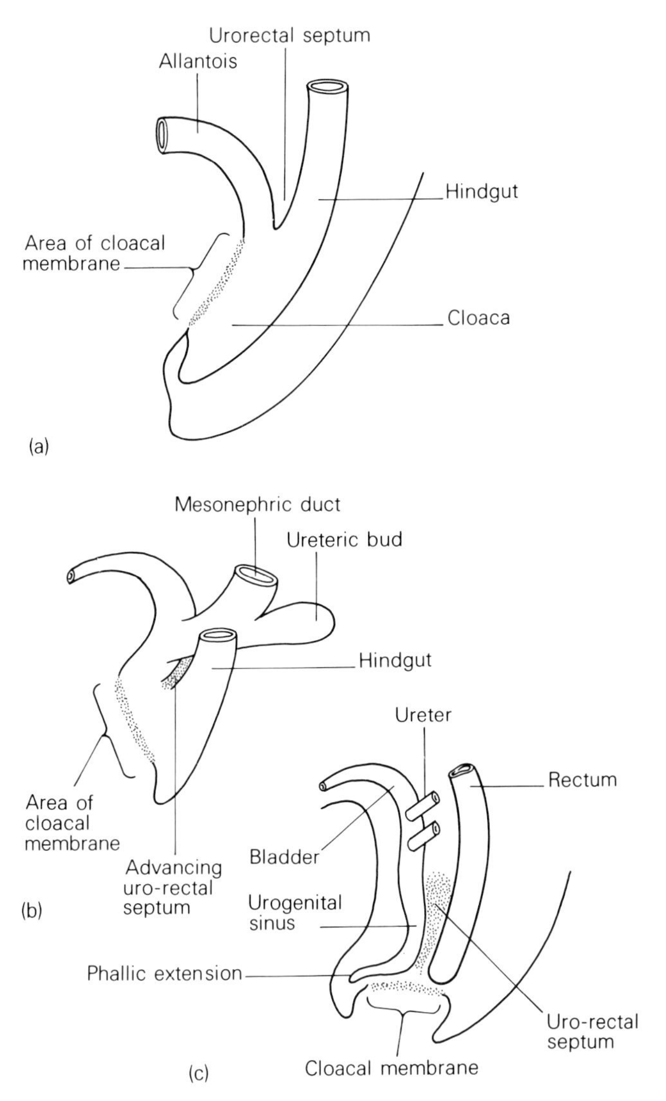

Fig. 12.18 *Normal development of the hindgut. (a) About 4 weeks of fetal life. (b) At 5–6 weeks. (c) At 8–10 weeks. It can be seen how incomplete advance of the urorectal septum will leave the rectum in communication with the urogenital sinus (posterior urethra). On the other hand, a failure of disappearance of the cloacal membrane will leave a normal rectum but no exit through the anal canal.*

perineum will show that something is amiss. Accurate analysis is important because half these lesions can be relieved by minor surgery. The incidence of these anomalies is about 1 in 5000 births.

Low anomalies

In males, *covered anus* (Fig. 12.19a) is the usual form of the low anomaly. There appears to be no anus, but usually a ridge can be seen running forwards to a tiny punctum on the back of the scrotum. If a probe is passed, and the skin ridge cut back, a normal anus is revealed. In girls this type of anomaly results in either a 'shotgun' perineum, with the anus alongside the fourchette, or a vestibular ectopic anus (Fig 12.19b), the opening lying between the fourchette and the hymen: these

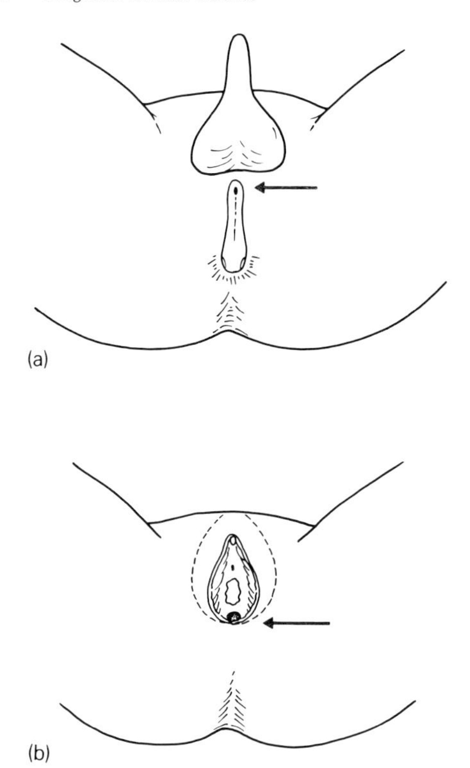

Fig. 12.19 *Low anorectal anomalies. (a) Covered anus in a boy. (b) Vestibular ectopic anus in a girl. (The arrows indicate point of opening of hindgut.)*

can be corrected by a relatively simple perineal operation which transplants the anal orifice posteriorly. Although a common term for all forms of anorectal anomaly is 'imperforate anus', such a deformity is in fact very unusual. The vital point in all low anomalies is that the puborectalis sling is intact and these children are continent.

High anomalies

These are much more serious because no part of the rectum exists at or below the level of levator ani. In boys the rectum opens into the back of the posterior urethra, i.e. there is a recto-urethral fistula (Fig. 12.20). In girls, the rectum may end blindly or communicate with the top of the vagina. Four out of five babies with a high anomaly are boys, and the diagnosis is often revealed by meconium appearing at the tip of the penis. There is fairly general agreement that these babies are

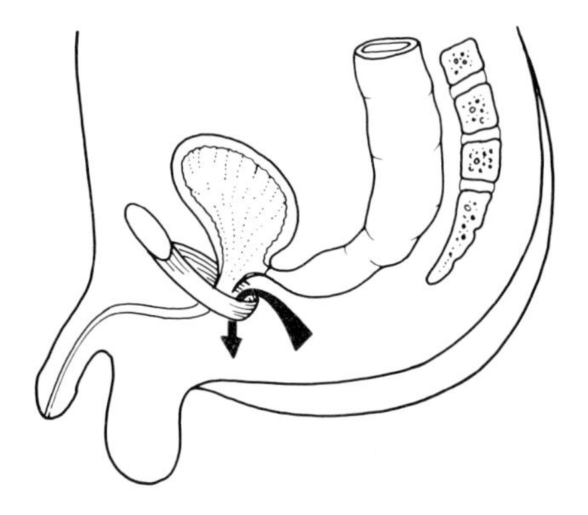

Fig. 12.20 *High anorectal anomaly; rectourethral fistula in a boy. (Arrow indicates the puborectalis sling, and level of levator ani.)*

best treated by a colostomy at birth, with construction of a rectum and anus at 9–12 months of age. The total absence of an external sphincter apparatus makes it very difficult to produce a satisfactory degree of continence.

EXOMPHALOS AND GASTROSCHISIS

There are two striking deficiencies in the development of the anterior abdominal wall.

In *exomphalos* (Fig. 12.21), all or most of the epigastric abdominal wall fails to develop and there is a major herniation of liver and gut through a wide defect which is covered only by a glistening transparent avascular membrane composed of amnion and peritoneum. This begins to disintegrate as it dries out and loses the nourishment derived *in utero* from amniotic fluid, and so repair is an urgent matter. The hernia is often too big to allow a full-scale repair of the abdominal wall. Sometimes a temporary repair can be effected by excising the sac and dissecting up the skin of the abdomen and using this as a cover for the abdominal contents. This creates a skin-covered hernia, and the muscle layers can be repaired when the child has grown and is fit, around one year of age.

A *gastroschisis* (Fig. 12.22), is an open defect of the abdominal wall, beside the umbilicus, which has allowed intestine to spill out of the abdomen *in utero:* this appears to happen days or weeks before delivery. At birth there is a striking prolapse of

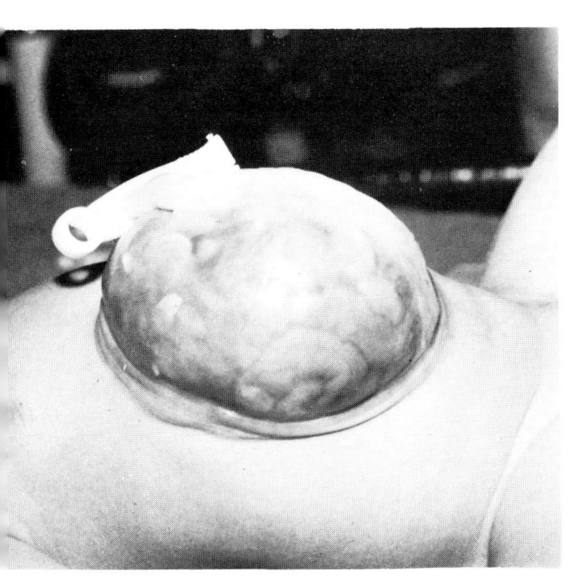

Fig. 12.21 *Exomphalos, showing the glistening transparent membrane.*

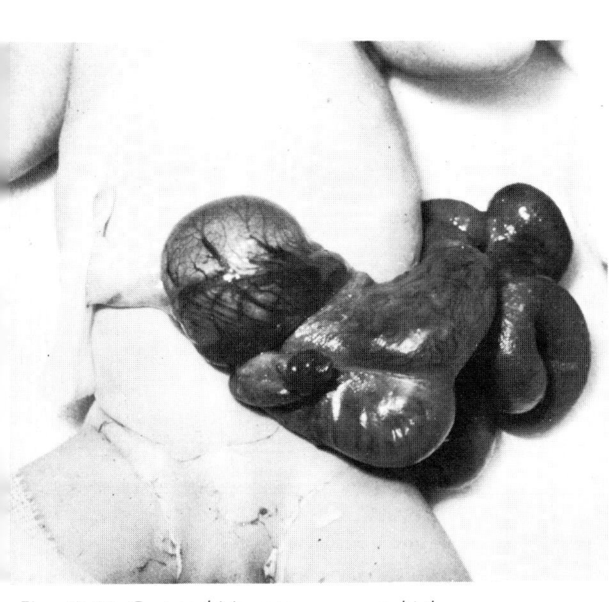

Fig. 12.22 *Gastroschisis; appearance at birth.*

small bowel through the deficiency, and urgent repair is needed. If the bowel is cleansed and replaced in the abdomen, and the defect repaired, most of these babies do remarkably well.

HYPERTROPHIC PYLORIC STENOSIS OF INFANCY

Although this is generally considered to be a congenital abnormality, there is usually no hint of the existence of this condition until the baby begins to vomit in the third or fourth week of life. In the established case, the pathological anatomy is most striking – a dilated thickened stomach with huge hypertrophy of the pyloric circular muscle sufficient to produce severe obstruction to the gastric outlet. The pylorus is an ovoid mass 1.5–2.0 cm long and about 1 cm in diameter which, when contracted, is hard and readily palpable through the abdominal wall.

What causes this striking development of the pyloric sphincter is unknown. It is certainly commoner in some families, and it particularly affects firstborn boys of high birth weight. It is a fairly common condition and occurs at the rate of about 3 per 1000 births.

In a typical case, a well-built baby boy, who has fed normally for about 3 weeks, begins to vomit, and over the space of days this becomes progressively more frequent and forceful. The child is always hungry but no sooner is a full meal readily taken than it is rejected. On inspection of the abdomen, gastric peristalsis is usually visible and careful palpation under the edge of the right lobe of the liver reveals an intermittently palpable lump like a large hard garden pea: it is usually easier to feel this lump during a feed. Nowadays few babies reach the stage of serious dehydration and malnourishment which used to make this a dangerous and lethal condition. As soon as the diagnosis is confirmed the child will be operated on: the circular muscle ring is divided longitudinally in Ramstedt's operation (Pyloromyotomy, Fig. 12.23). This is now a very safe and successful operation although, as recently as 1940, it carried a 25% mortality: this was almost entirely due to cross-infection and subsequent gastroenteritis.

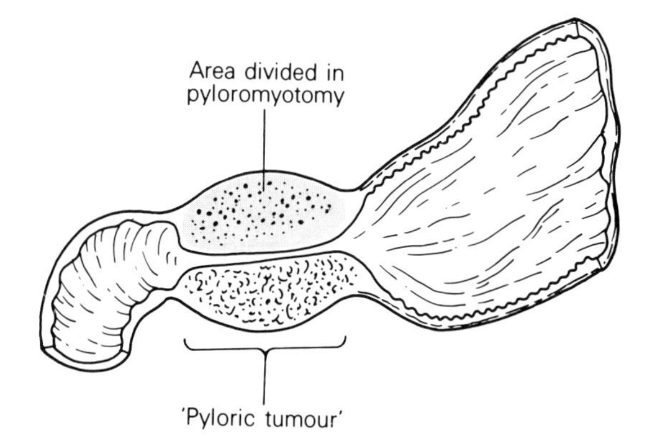

Fig. 12.23 *Sketch of the pyloric tumour of hypertrophic pyloric stenosis, showing the area of the muscular ring which is divided by pyloromyotomy.*

MECKEL'S DIVERTICULUM

This small remnant of the vitello-intestinal duct (see Fig. 12.8) is the commonest congenital deformity of the alimentary tract, being present in 2–3% of the population: only about one-third of diverticula, however, prove to be pathogenic.

The majority exist as an unattached diverticulum projecting from the antimesenteric surface of the ileum, sited some 60 cm above the ileocaecal valve (in the adult), and averaging 5 cm in length. There is a characteristic blood supply via the omphalomesenteric artery (Fig. 12.24). A few diverticula are attached to the back of the umbilicus, and of these a minority are patent, so intestinal juices are discharged through the navel. Between 50–60% of diverticula contain ectopic gastric mucosa, secreting acid and pepsin.

Most diverticula remain silent, and they may be found incidentally at a laparotomy. Of the one-third which produce symptoms, 80% will present during childhood, and of these 5 out of 6 exist in boys. There are a number of ways in which a Meckel's diverticulum can prove pathogenic:

1. The gastric secretions may cause a peptic ulcer to form in the adjacent ileum; this may erode a vessel, causing *rectal bleeding* (see p. 309), or penetrate the wall of the ileum, causing *perforation* and *peritonitis* (see p. 286).

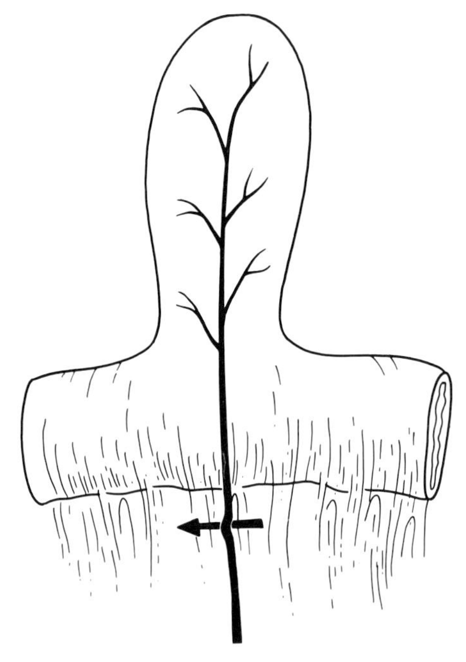

Fig. 12.24 *A Meckel's diverticulum, showing the omphalomesenteric artery. The arrow shows a foramen beneath the artery under which a piece of bowel could be caught and strangulated.*

2. Acute inflammation of a diverticulum can occur. Both pathologically and clinically this is very similar to acute appendicitis.
3. Small intestinal obstruction can occur for two separate reasons. An unattached diverticulum can form the leading point of an intussusception (see p. 298). An attached diverticulum can also act as a peritoneal band (see p. 290), or be the point of rotation of a volvulus.

In all these situations, treatment involves excision of the diverticulum with closure of the defect in the wall of the ileum.

BILIARY ATRESIA AND CHOLEDOCHAL CYST

These are fairly rare abnormalities (an incidence of about 1 in 15 000 births), but the sight of an otherwise healthy newborn, gradually becoming more deeply jaundiced and finally dying, after some months, with advanced biliary cirrhosis, has presented surgeons with a major challenge.

The defect in these babies is that they have either no detectable extrahepatic bile ducts, or they are only threads, and there is little or no flow of bile possible from liver to duodenum (Fig. 12.25a).

A great deal of speculation has gone into explaining this anomaly and, whereas this was thought to be a congenital malformation, it is now believed that these babies are suffering from a progressive obstructive cholangiopathy which may well be viral in origin, and could be related to the virus of hepatitis B.

The fact that these babies only become jaundiced days or weeks after birth suggests that there is a developing situation, not a static duct atresia, and much pathological evidence has now been accumulated favouring the concept of a progressive cholangitis.

Physiological jaundice of the newborn is very common but when it fails to fade, or a baby becomes progressively more icteric, with a palpable liver, then no time must be lost in undertaking investigation. Some of these babies have a neonatal hepatitis with normal bile ducts; these tend slowly to improve, with a slowly falling serum bilirubin. Babies with abnormal ducts show a rising bilirubin, acholic stools, and failure of injected ^{131}I-rose bengal to be excreted from liver to duodenum. It is vital to make a precise diagnosis before too much liver damage occurs, and this is best done before the tenth week of life, by performing operative cholangiography under local anaesthesia. If no extrahepatic ducts are outlined, the prognosis is very serious, but remarkable success has been obtained by exploration of the porta hepatis (Fig. 12.25b), identification of the junction of the right and left hepatic ducts, and anastomosis to an isolated loop of jejunum (Fig. 12.25c). Occasionally, hepatic transplantation has to be considered.

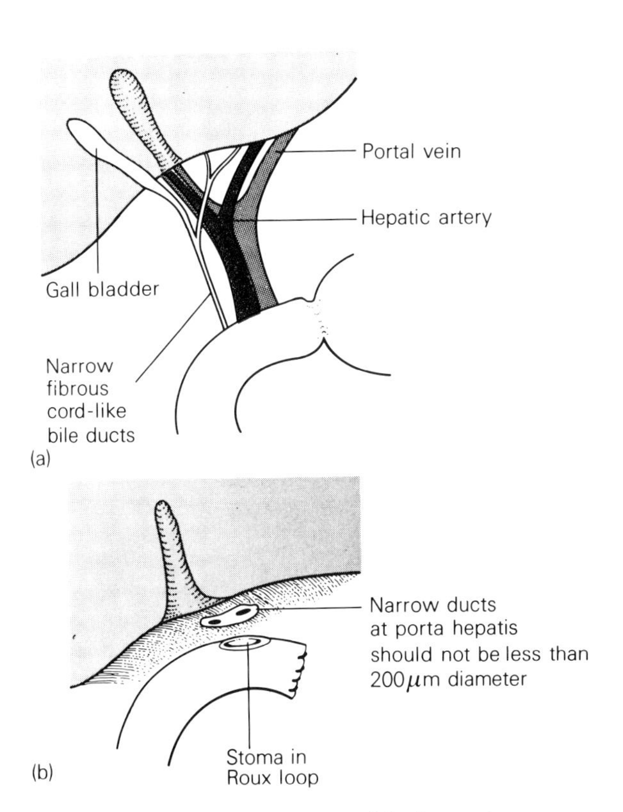

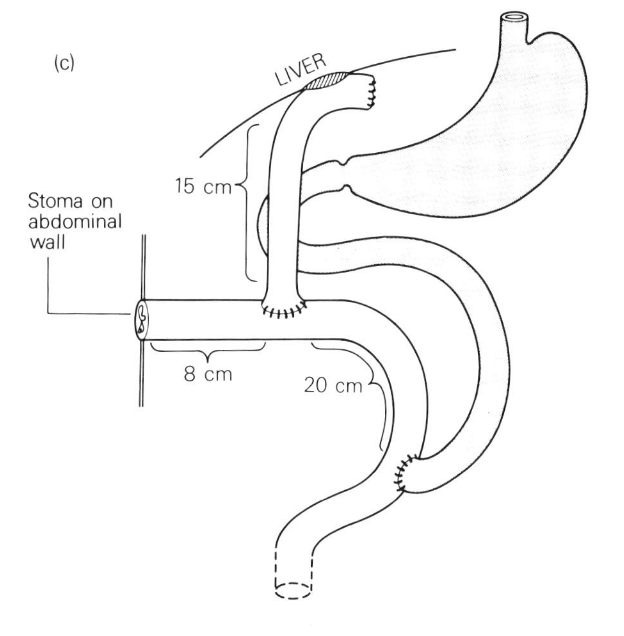

Fig. 12.25 *Biliary atresia. (a) Typical findings at laparotomy. (b) The porta hepatis has been explored and the fibrosed ducts followed into the liver – ready for anastomosis between the ducts and a jejunal loop. (c) Completed anastomosis.*

Choledochal Cyst

This is a rare anomaly (Fig. 12.26) which may present early in life with progressive jaundice and a mass in the right upper quadrant. In other patients there is a history over months or years of recurring pain and jaundice, and the cyst is found after investigation. Sometimes excision of the cyst is possible, but more often it is drained through a Roux jejunal loop.

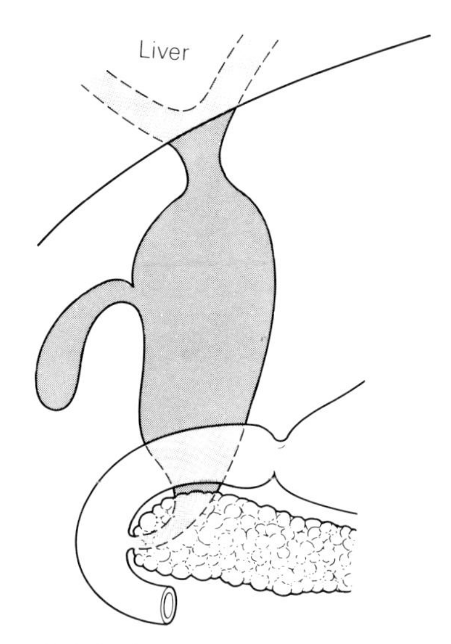

Fig. 12.26 *Choledochal cyst.*

13

The Acute Abdomen

This is one of the most interesting, demanding and rewarding areas of medical work: it is now almost unique in medicine in so far as most patients are managed by decisions made at the bedside, without recourse to complex investigations. Many of these decisions have to be made for patients whose illnesses offer potential (and not infrequently real) threats to life, so the practice of emergency abdominal surgery makes serious demands on clinical skills, and the surgery required can be technically difficult and occasionally distinctly dramatic. Surgeons are no more skilful now than their forbears of fifty years ago, but the major recent advances in anaesthesia, resuscitation and antibiotic therapy mean that the great majority of patients with serious abdominal emergencies can now be returned to normal health: this includes both the aged and newborn infants.

The major part played by bedside assessment of the patient makes this sphere an important training

Table 13.1
Admissions to Surgical Wards with Acute Abdominal Pain

552 Patients, Adult Surgical Wards, Leeds, 1972	*Percent of total*	*363 Patients up to 13 years old, Royal Aberdeen Children's Hospital 1974*	*Percent of total*
Acute appendicitis	26.3	NSAP	30.0
Cholecystitis	7.6	Acute appendicitis	28.0
Small-bowel obstruction	3.6	Constipation	11.0
Perforated peptic ulcer	3.1	Upper respiratory tract infection	8.0
Pancreatitis	2.9	Urinary tract infection	6.9
Diverticular disease	2.0	Gastroenteritis	3.6
Miscellaneous	4.0	Bronchopneumonia	2.2
NSAP	50.5	Small-bowel obstruction (inc. intussusception)	2.2
		Mesenteric adenitis (operated)	2.2
		Abdominal injuries	1.0
		Infective hepatitis	1.0
		Torsion of the testicle	less than 1%
		Acute pancreatitis	less than 1%
		Otitis media	less than 1%
		Acute glomerulonephritis	less than 1%
		Diabetic acidosis	less than 1%

NSAP = non-specific acute abdominal pain: see p. 281.

ground in clinical skills, and experience is rapidly built up, with the accuracy of diagnosis being quickly tested at emergency laparotomy. However, by no means all patients who are referred to surgical wards have a surgical cause for their acute abdominal symptoms, so the emergency surgeon needs also to be a good physician. This need is well illustrated in Table 13.1, which shows the final diagnoses made in patients admitted to paediatric and adult surgical wards with acute abdominal pain. Among the children, only one-third actually required an operation; another one-third had a specific medical illness requiring diagnosis and treatment, whilst the remaining patients recovered spontaneously. Among the adults, nearly half those admitted did not need surgery. It is therefore a prime requirement in abdominal surgeons that they should be skilful bedside diagnosticians, discriminating in their choice of surgery but quick to operate on the real emergency.

Diagnosis

These patients are usually anxious and in pain, upset at having to leave home and family unexpectedly. A quiet and understanding approach is vital. Sit rather than stand, so that the patient feels you are speaking to him on the same level, and have time to listen to his story (Fig. 13.1). In emergency surgery, the history is every bit as important as the physical examination and should build up a reasonably complete picture of the present complaint and past medical history. A record sheet (Fig. 13.2) is very useful in prompting the memory at 3 am, and shows the important features which should be explored in taking the history. Let the patient say what he or she wants to say but do not hesitate to expand that story with necessary questions – e.g. the history of a missed period may be an essential clue in diagnosis, but few women will volunteer this information.

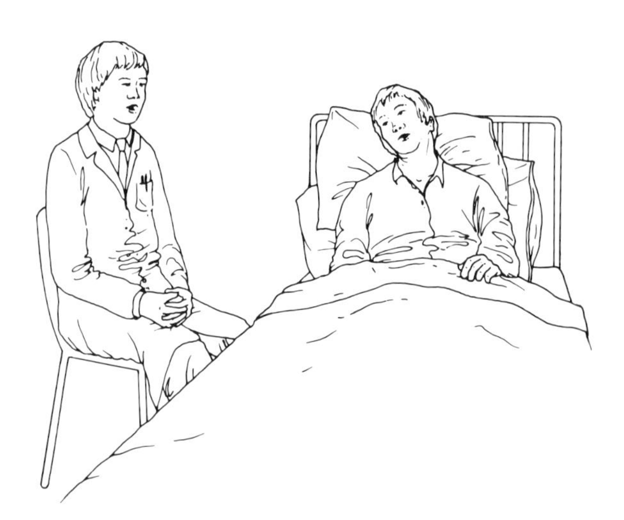

Fig. 13.1 *Listening to the history.*

It is essential to be clear about the site and character of abdominal pain, vomiting, diarrhoea and constipation, and these topics have already been considered in detail (pp. 32–36).

The physical examination of the patient commences as soon as the doctor sits down at the bedside. The appearance of the patient, the general behaviour, the readiness or reluctance to move, occurrence of spasmodic pain and distress, are all vital signs which will become apparent during the taking of the history.

Aggravation of pain by movement is characteristic of any condition causing peritoneal irritation, so all these patients move only slowly and cautiously. Patients with intestinal, biliary or ureteric colic, on the other hand, move restlessly around, seeking a more comfortable position.

It is a matter of choice and opportunity in what order the examination proceeds. In a few pale, shocked and hypotensive patients the first priority may be to start resuscitation and only then, when intravenous fluids are expanding the depleted blood volume, to return to the physical examination.

It may be wise to start with abdominal examination; this will seem logical to the patient, and it is especially important in children to grasp a time when they are quiet and the abdomen can be quickly examined (Fig. 13.3). Observe the respiratory movement of the abdomen, and any swelling (local or generalised), and take the first opportunity to inspect and palpate the hernial orifices and the scrotal contents because they must never be

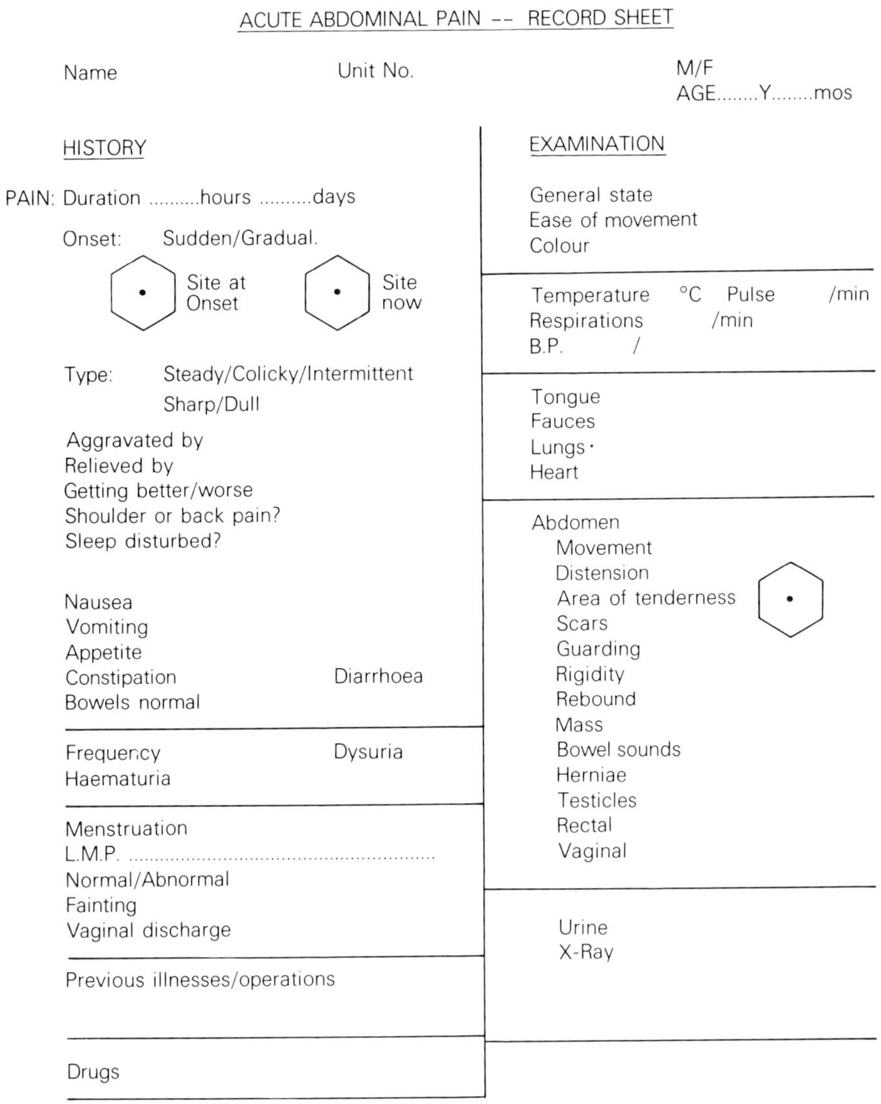

ACUTE ABDOMINAL PAIN -- RECORD SHEET

Name Unit No. M/F
AGE........Y........mos

HISTORY

PAIN: Duration ....hours ....days
Onset: Sudden/Gradual.
Site at Onset
Site now

Type: Steady/Colicky/Intermittent
Sharp/Dull

Aggravated by
Relieved by
Getting better/worse
Shoulder or back pain?
Sleep disturbed?

Nausea
Vomiting
Appetite
Constipation Diarrhoea
Bowels normal

Frequency Dysuria
Haematuria

Menstruation
L.M.P. ....
Normal/Abnormal
Fainting
Vaginal discharge

Previous illnesses/operations

Drugs

EXAMINATION

General state
Ease of movement
Colour

Temperature °C Pulse /min
Respirations /min
B.P. /

Tongue
Fauces
Lungs
Heart

Abdomen
Movement
Distension
Area of tenderness
Scars
Guarding
Rigidity
Rebound
Mass
Bowel sounds
Herniae
Testicles
Rectal
Vaginal

Urine
X-Ray

Fig. 13.2 *Record sheet for the patient with acute abdominal pain.*

forgotten (Fig. 13.4). Abdominal palpation should be done with the examiner seated, the flat warm hand being placed gently on the part of the abdomen least likely to be tender (Fig. 13.5). The area of tenderness is gently defined and then, most important, the area of muscle guarding. Peritoneal irritation, due to the presence of inflamed tissue, alimentary juices or blood in contact with the peritoneum of the anterior abdominal wall, will set up reflex tightening of the overlying abdominal muscles and this can be appreciated by the hand. In a typical case of acute appendicitis it is easy to palpate deeply in the left iliac fossa but the reflex contraction of the muscles overlying the inflamed appendix will produce a tightening of the muscles covering the right iliac fossa so the hand is not able to depress the abdominal wall so far – the more pressure is applied the more the protective muscle

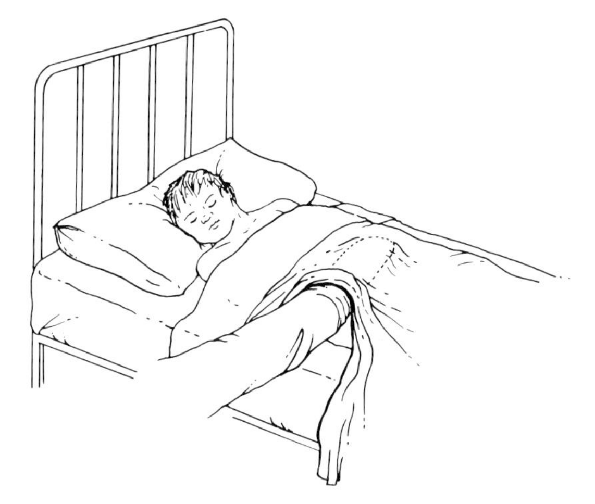

Fig. 13.3 *Examining the sleeping child.*

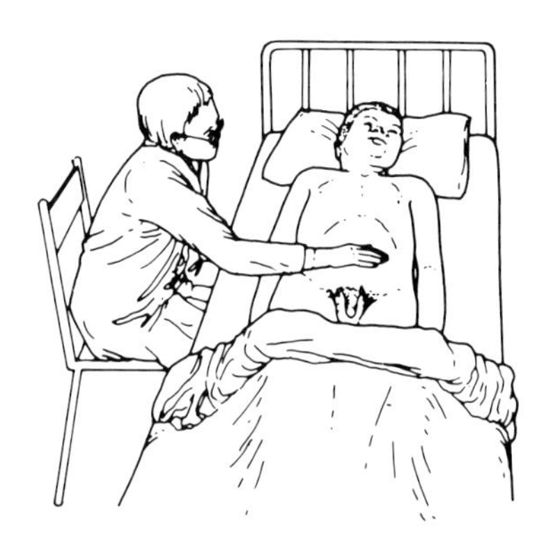

Fig. 13.4 *No abdominal examination is complete without a search for an external hernia or, in males, palpation of the testicles.*

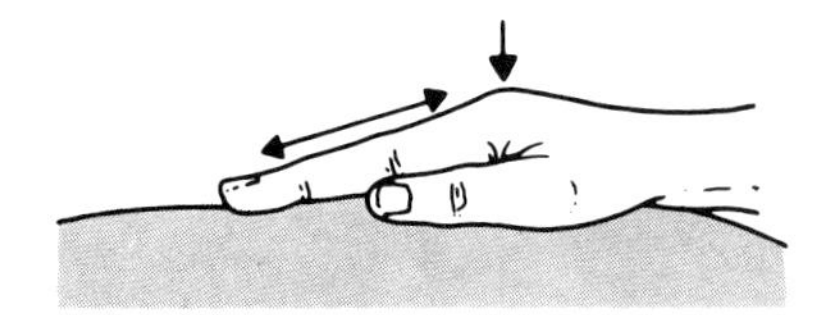

Fig. 13.5 *Abdominal palpation. It is easier to palpate gently when sitting down, with the flat hand. To detect tenderness and guarding, dip lightly by flexing the staight fingers at the metacarpophalangeal joints.*

contraction increases in strength. When the underlying focus of irritation is very marked, the overlying muscle will actually be rigid: thus, when a perforation of a peptic ulcer occurs, the considerable chemical peritonitis set up by spillage of acid gastric juice causes intense generalised parietal peritoneal irritation and the whole abdominal wall may be found to be rigid.

The signs of tenderness and guarding are essentially related to parietal peritoneal irritation. Tenderness in acute appendicitis or cholecystitis is not appreciated in the organ, which is basically insensitive to compression, but in the overlying peritoneum. This is most important and is the reason why, for instance, acute inflammation of an appendix situated in the pelvis or behind the terminal ileum will not show much tenderness on abdominal palpation (see p. 283). This is a reminder that there are two other vital ways of eliciting abdominal tenderness – by vaginal and rectal examination. Fortunately the pelvic peritoneum, in the rectovaginal and rectovesical pouches, is accessible to the examining finger and so inflammation in the pelvis, remote from the anterior abdominal wall, can be detected by a finger which compresses the inflamed tender parietal pelvic peritoneum. It is quite essential to remember that no patient with acute abdominal pain has been completely examined until such a pelvic examination has been made (see p. 43).

Tenderness and muscle guarding are by far the most important signs, but others are useful. Much is talked of rebound or release tenderness. This means that, when the palpating hand is lifted off the abdomen, the patient feels pain, which is due to sudden movement of the inflamed parietal peritoneum – a sign similar to the reluctance with which patients with peritonitis sit up or turn over in bed because these movements involve movement of the abdominal wall, which is painful. These signs of parietal peritoneal inflammation are useful in differentiating intra- from extraperitoneal disease.

Auscultation of the abdomen can be of great value, especially when the high-pitched splashing sounds of small bowel obstruction are heard. However, both the presence of normal sounds and complete silence should be interpreted with care:

normal folk, especially when digestion of a meal is complete, have periods of silence, whilst normal sounds can be heard in the early stages of peritonitis.

Other signs are of great importance. The temperature, pulse and respiration rate should always be measured and the tongue and fauces inspected. Not all patients with an acute abdomen have a dirty tongue, especially children. A raw throat and palpable cervical nodes may suggest acute upper respiratory tract infection, which may be associated with mesenteric adenitis. It is vital to examine the chest – an early bronchopneumonia with pleurisy can easily cause referred pain along a thoracic root, which is felt in the abdomen (Fig. 13.6).

Urine examination is an integral part of abdominal examination. Everyone must have a test for albumin and sugar – diabetic ketosis can, for instance, give a good imitation of acute appendicitis. It is essential to examine the urine microscopically: a right-sided pyelitis can cause appreciable tenderness in the right iliac fossa, so the finding of many pus cells in the urine could be an important diagnostic clue (Fig. 13.7).

Plain films of the abdomen are not needed in most patients but, when doubt exists, they can be of crucial importance. Perforation of a hollow viscus means that some gas will escape; this finds its way through the peritoneum and may be seen in an erect film as a gas bubble trapped under the dome of the diaphragm (Fig. 13.8). When intestinal obstruction occurs, the swallowed air in the bowel cannot pass the obstruction and will outline the distended loops in a very characteristic manner, helping to establish both the existence of obstruction and its level in the bowel (Fig. 13.8). The finding of radio-opaque calculi in the urinary or biliary tracts may greatly help in establishing a diagnosis.

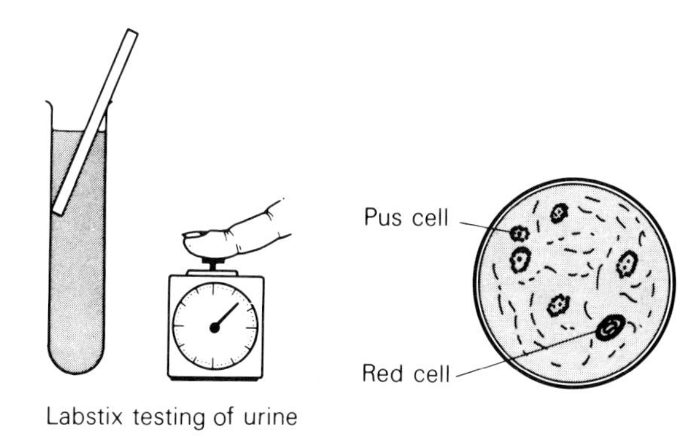

Fig. 13.7 *Examination of the urine. Chemical examination of the urine for glucose and albumin, and a microscopic search of the shaken deposit for pus and red cells, are integral parts of abdominal examination.*

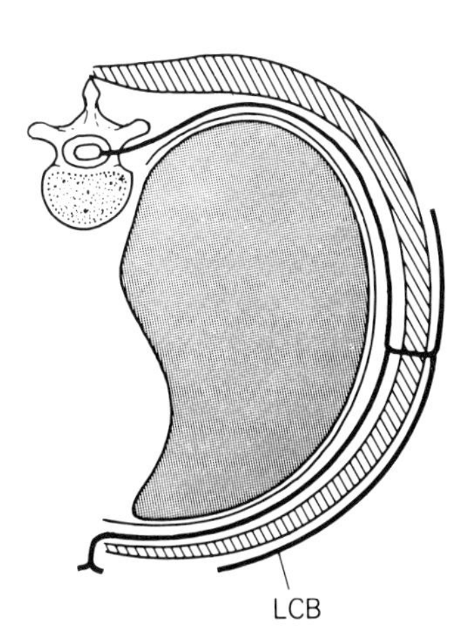

Fig. 13.6 *Innervation of abdominal wall. The lower thoracic nerves innervate not only the parietal pleura (which may be affected by an adjacent area of pleurisy), but also the anterior abdominal wall, via the lateral cutaneous branch.*

Babies and infants with acute abdominal pain present the surgeon with special problems. They are too young to understand why the doctor should come and prod their sore tummy and make the pain worse, so they are very likely to protest by crying. This means a tense abdomen and the end of useful abdominal examination. Some children are easy-going and will respond to distracting conversation, or a toy to play with, whilst a warm gentle hand is slipped under the sheets and the abdomen examined. Other infants are not taken in by any of these stratagems and shout defiance from the start: sometimes this defence suddenly collapses but in others no persuasion is of any avail and these children must be sedated. A good method is to instil diazepam into the rectum in a dose of 5 mg up to 3 years and 10 mg above this age; this quickly soothes the child without the pain of an injection and allows a peaceful examination

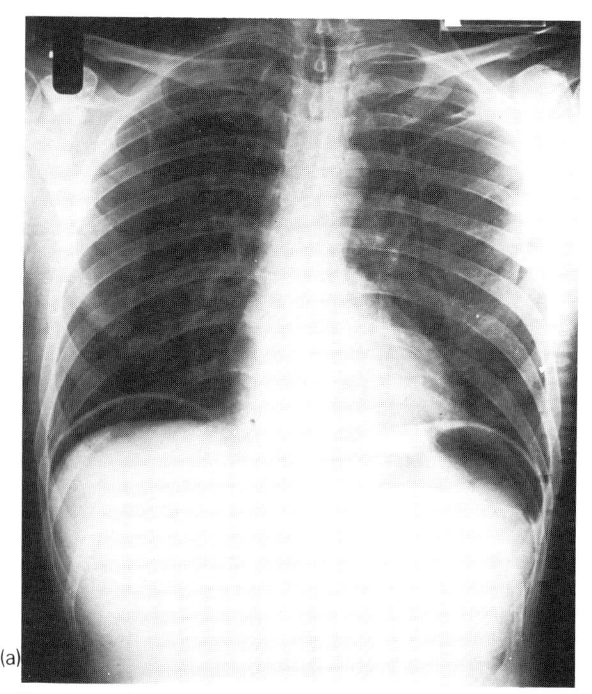

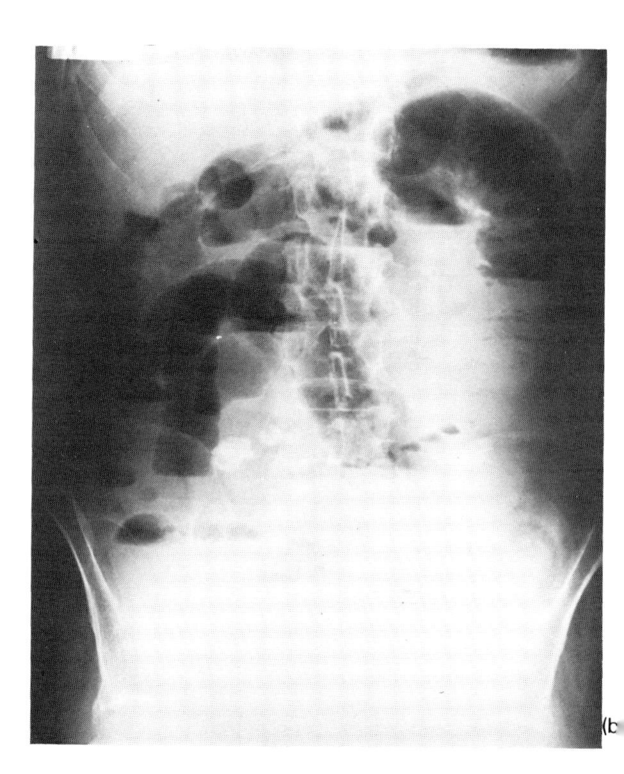

Fig. 13.8 *Plain erect abdominal x-rays showing: (a) free sub-diaphragmatic gas, (b) distended small bowel loops containing fluid levels, (c) supine film showing characteristic pattern of obstructed small bowel.*

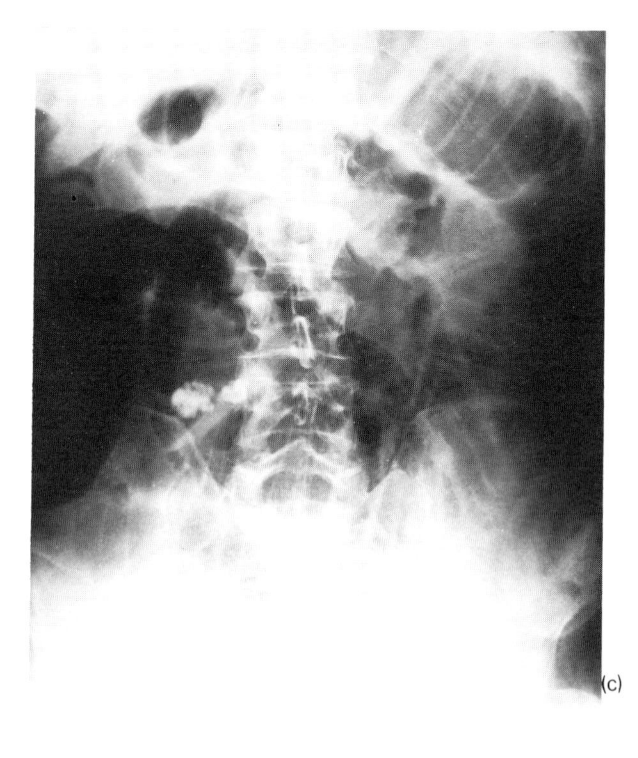

in which areas of tenderness and guarding can be picked up, or a mass felt. The absence of a history direct from young children is usually compensated by the shrewd and experienced observations of parents.

One of the most important implications of the fact that only one-third of surgical admissions for acute abdominal pain need a surgical operation is that many patients will need careful medical evaluation, a process known as 'active observation' (Fig. 13.9). When patients are first admitted and thoroughly examined, it will be clear that a number of them require prompt operation. Most of these patients will have acute appendicitis; in some there will be intestinal obstruction; and others will have a perforated viscus. However, in the majority there will be either a suspicion of a medical condition (e.g. a stone stuck in the biliary or urinary tracts, or pneumonia, or a urinary tract infection) or there will be doubt whether any identifiable disease is present. 'Active observation' means that all these patients remain under

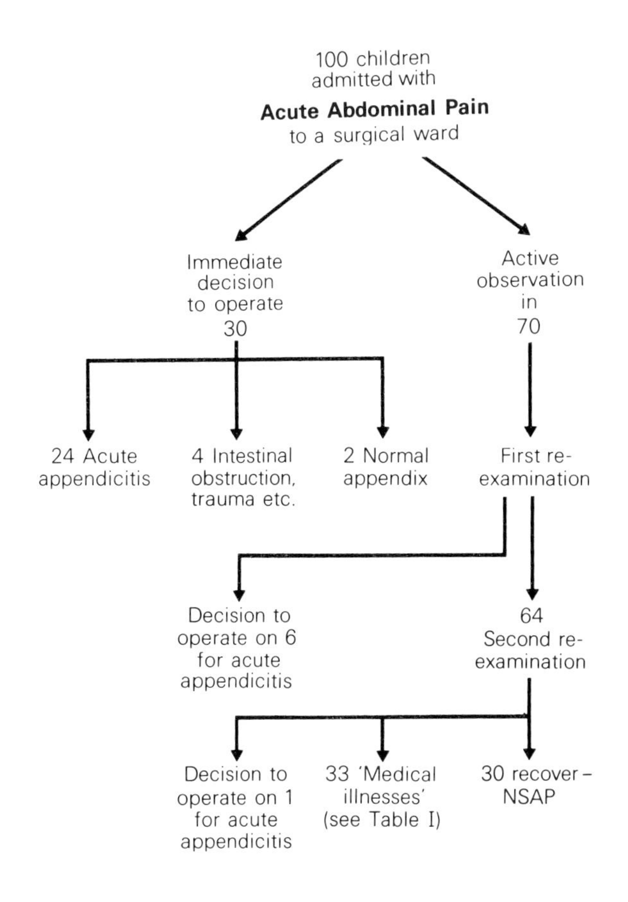

Fig. 13.9 *Flow chart showing the outcome when 100 children, admitted to a surgical ward with acute abdominal pain, are managed by 'active observation'.*

close scrutiny, the nursing staff record temperature and pulse every hour, nothing is given by mouth (in case a general anaesthetic is required), and special radiographic and chemical tests are made. After 2–3 hours, the surgeon who originally saw the patient returns to make a careful re-examination. In some cases this examination, taken with the results of investigations now to hand, will confirm a medical diagnosis, and appropriate treatment can be started. In others, signs that were unconvincing on admission may have become clearer and it will be evident that, on arrival, the patient was in the early stages of a surgical disease such as acute appendicitis and now needs operation.

In others the pain will be easing and the signs becoming less marked, so these patients can be given a drink and observation continued. If a third examination a few hours later shows continued improvement, it can be concluded that no serious condition exists and they can be allowed home. Then, and only then, they join the large number of patients to whom the term 'non-specific acute abdominal pain' (NSAP) is applied. This is a very common condition (perhaps related to the irritable bowel syndrome) which, in its early stages, gives a good imitation of acute appendicitis, but which resolves in 12–24 hours.

It may reasonably be asked why the family doctor cannot pick out these patients and avoid sending them to hospital. There are several important reasons for this. Individual general practitioners see comparatively few patients with serious acute abdominal disease – perhaps 3 or 4 patients per year with acute appendicitis – but they see many more patients with acute abdominal complaints, and successfully diagnose some as having, for instance, acute tonsillitis with associated abdominal pain, whilst others have no convincing signs and settle with 24 hours starvation and rest. The patients that the general practitioner refers to hospital are those whose clinical picture make him or her suspect serious disease, and always at the back of his mind is the knowledge that, although many cases of acute surgical abdominal disease are easy to diagnose, others are much more difficult. It is these which are the dangerous ones, because delay tends to occur, and therefore early reference to hospital, where the patient can be seen by experienced surgeons and subjected to investigation, is a reasonable course. The practitioner is trying to steer a course between unnecessary admission and harmful delay: experience helps in this situation but even the most experienced surgeon, seeing patients with acute abdominal complaints every few days, knows how difficult precise diagnosis can be, so considerations of safety rightly mean that the genuinely doubtful patient is sent in.

It must not be forgotten that the first necessity is for the patient (or parents or friends) to react to the onset of acute abdominal symptoms. It should be a part of health education that anyone in whom acute abdominal pain continues unabated for 6 hours needs medical examination.

ACUTE APPENDICITIS

Acute inflammation of the vermiform appendix is a disease of the 20th century and of Western-style civilisations (see p. 25). At present, in Great Britain, the chance of a newly-born baby developing acute appendicitis during his or her life is about one in five, falling to one in ten by the age of 20. Some 70 000 new cases are seen each year, making acute appendicitis the commonest surgical emergency in both adults and children (see Table 13.1, p. 275). Now that acute appendicitis is so widely recognised, it is generally treated promptly and the mortality rate of all cases in Britain is less than 1 in 200. However, too many patients still come to operation with peritonitis due to perforation, and 88% of deaths occur in this group. It is a grave mistake to think that acute appendicitis is always readily diagnosed and treated: this is true for four patients out of five but, in the minority, the presentation can be misleading and the delay causes these patients to suffer a very serious illness. Modern surgery and anaesthesia and the use of antibiotics mean that almost all – except the very young and the very old – survive, but the threat to life from undiagnosed acute appendicitis is still a real one and means that every patient with acute abdominal pain needs very careful examination and observation. Two-thirds of patients arrive in hospital within 24 hours of the onset of appendicitis but, even so, 28% have already perforated. Among children under 5 years, three out of four have perforated by the time they come to operation, a reminder that special care is needed in examining every child with acute abdominal pain (p. 279). No matter how young the baby is, acute appendicitis is still a possibility and must be actively considered.

Pathology

The most important form of acute appendicitis

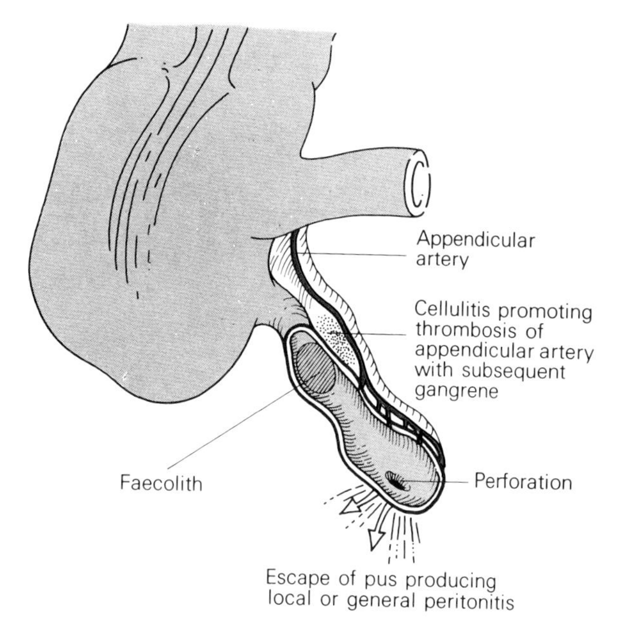

Fig. 13.10 *Acute obstructive appendicitis.*

occurs when the lumen becomes obstructed by a faecolith or calculus and an abscess forms beyond the obstruction. This can quite quickly lead to a stinking necrotic bag of pus which perforates either spontaneously or whilst the fragile appendix is being removed (Fig. 13.10). The black purulent contents are highly infective and dangerous and teeming with anaerobes as well as faecal aerobic bacteria. In many cases of acute appendicitis, however, there is no obstruction but a generalised acute inflammation, the cause of which is unknown: perforation can also occur in these appendices, although the process is slower. The pathological lesson for the public and for the medical profession is clear: recognise and treat acute appendicitis before perforation occurs.

Symptoms

All patients complain of abdominal pain and this is almost always the first symptom. In about 60% of patients this is at first an ache around the umbilicus, which may progress to severe colic if the appendix is obstructed. After a variable time the progression of inflammation causes local parietal peritonitis and pain shifts to the right iliac fossa. This is a steady pain, aggravated by coughing and movement. In some 40% of patients, pain starts and remains in the right lower quadrant, especially if the appendix is not obstructed.

Vomiting usually follows a few hours after the start of pain; this is particularly marked in obstructive appendicitis, but is absent in one patient in five. Diarrhoea occurs in about 20% and is a very important symptom because, when combined with vomiting, it may suggest the commoner condition of gastroenteritis (p. 333). However, when diarrhoea and vomiting occur with abdominal pain, the first thought must be to suspect appendicitis: diarrhoea is particularly characteristic of pelvic and retro-ileal appendicitis – both difficult forms of acute appendicitis to diagnose.

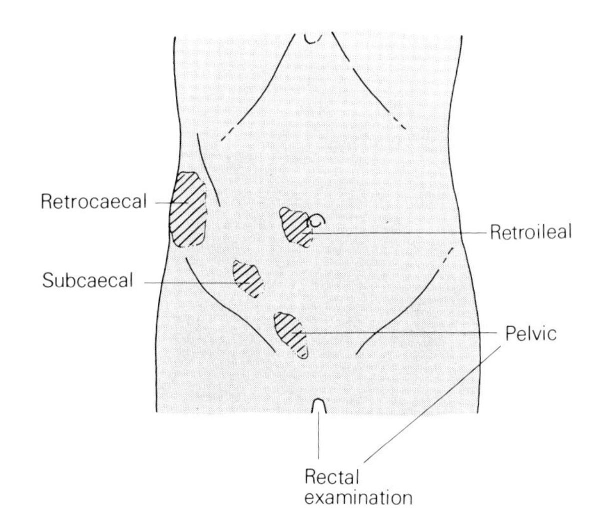

Fig. 13.11 *The sites of tenderness in acute appendicitis, which depend on the position of the appendix.*

Signs

Patients with acute appendicitis may walk into the surgery or ward and do not necessarily look ill at first, so that this can be misleading. In two-thirds of patients the temperature is not above 37° C, and the pulse rate is barely raised in early appendicitis. However, tachycardia is a very important sign of local peritonitis and must never be overlooked in a difficult case. Furring of the tongue and foetor of the breath are nonspecific signs which are quite often absent. Patients tend to lie still and move only with care.

Local tenderness over the appendix is the one sign present in every patient and must be sought carefully and accurately. Unfortunately, there is a widespread belief that patients with acute appendicitis show maximal tenderness over McBurney's point – many do, but the site of maximal tenderness depends on the position of the appendix. Retrocaecal appendicitis will show most tenderness above and lateral to the anterior superior iliac spine, retro-ileal appendicitis will produce rather diffuse deep tenderness near the umbilicus: a pelvic appendicitis may only be positively diagnosed when a tender bulge of the rectovesical pouch is found on rectal examination (Fig. 13.11). Guarding of the overlying abdominal muscles, the other vital sign of acute appendicitis, has already been considered (p. 277). When the appendix has perforated and there is a spreading peritonitis, the overlying abdominal wall is likely to be rigid and this is a most important warning sign of a serious situation requiring speedy treatment.

Rebound tenderness is a useful sign when examining a patient in the early stages of acute appendicitis – it is often present in these patients but generally absent in those who prove to have NSAP (p. 281).

Sometimes a tender mass can be felt in the right lower quadrant. This is because, in some patients, protective adhesions quickly form around the inflamed appendix, the omentum covers the area, and adheres to adjacent loops of bowel. Consequently, when the appendix perforates, the pus cannot spread and a localised appendicular abscess forms.

Investigations are of very little help in the diagnosis of acute appendicitis. Quite often there is no leucocytosis and, although a radio-opaque faecolith is a valuable sign, it is rarely seen, and it is not necessary to x-ray every patient with a suspect appendix.

Differential diagnosis has already been considered (p. 280). The most difficult group are young women, in whom salpingitis, rupture of an ovarian follicle, or ectopic pregnancy can produce signs very like those of acute appendicitis. Active observation will usually allow patients with NSAP to be identified and spared laparotomy. Microscopy of the urine is important because an acute right-sided pyelonephritis can produce a surprising amount of tenderness and even guarding, so the finding of pus cells on microscopy is very important.

The incidence of appendicitis rises to its peak at 15 years of age, and many cases are therefore seen throughout childhood. Irrespective of age, the first thought when a child complains of abdominal pain for more than 6 hours must be to suspect acute appendicitis: in infancy the necessary examination and observation can call for much care and patience (p. 279).

Treatment of Acute Appendicitis

Once the decision to operate has been taken, all patients benefit from an analgesic and some intravenous fluid. The majority, who have an acutely inflamed but unruptured appendix, can go to theatre as soon as is convenient. The operation to remove the acutely inflamed appendix is often fairly simple (though it can occasionally be technically demanding) and these patients generally recover quickly and return home in a few days.

There is, however, a most important group who require quite a different scale of care – those with a gangrenous perforated appendix, with local or general peritonitis. In three out of four infants, and a majority of elderly patients, the appendix has perforated by the time of admission, so at the two extremes of life, when risks are necessarily higher, (and in many young and middle-aged patients as well), a carefully planned regime is essential for a safe outcome.

Anybody with acute appendicitis is likely to have drunk less than usual, and to have vomited several times, and therefore will be dehydrated. This will be much more marked in patients with peritonitis because they have usually been ill for longer, have vomited more often, will have alimentary secretions lying in dilated bowel, and will have been forming peritoneal exudate. Patients with severe peritonitis can have their blood volume reduced by 20–30%. These patients tend to maintain blood pressure by vasoconstriction in the mesenteric and peripheral vascular tree but, when they are anaesthetised for laparotomy, this vasoconstriction is relaxed: if no preoperative restoration of blood volume has been made, then a disastrous fall of blood pressure can occur as a depleted blood volume is distributed through an expanded vascular bed.

A dehydrated adult with peritonitis is likely to have an extracellular fluid deficit of many litres: most adults normally ingest about 2.5 l of water daily so, if the patient has been starving for 48 hours and has also been vomiting, a deficit of 5–6 l can soon be built up. The infusion is usually commenced with Hartmann's solution (Table 13.2): any hypotension due to oligaemia should be corrected with a colloid solution such as dextran 70. At least 3–4 hours must be spent on this rehydration, but care must be taken over giving large intravenous infusions quickly, especially in the elderly, and central venous pressure measurement is a valuable guide. Careful calculations must, of course, be made in infancy and childhood.

While rehydration is proceeding, it is equally important to be treating any possible bacteraemia with well-chosen intravenous antibiotics. There is now a very wide range of choice, but a regime which has stood the test of time is: gentamicin (5–6 mg/kg/day in three divided doses), ampicillin (500 mg 4–6-hourly, half dose in children), and metronidazole (500 mg thrice daily, 7.5 mg/kg thrice daily in children).

Safe removal of the gangrenous appendix requires a skilful operation through a generous incision. It is important to remove any faecolith shed from the necrotic appendix, which could lead to continued suppuration. It is now clear that the operation should conclude with thorough peritoneal debridement, in which all contamination is aspirated, fibrinous plaques are removed, and all quarters of the peritoneum and intestines thoroughly lavaged with an antibiotic solution, e.g.

Table 13.2
Electrolyte Concentrations in Common Intravenous Fluids, Compared with Normal Plasma Values (millimoles per litre)

	Na^+	K^+	HCO_3^-	Cl^-	Ca^+
Normal plasma	142	4.5	26	103	2.5
Sodium chloride 0.9%	150	—	—	150	
Sodium chloride 0.18% and dextrose 4%	30	—	—	30	
Hartmann's solution	131	5	29 as lactate	111	2.0

tetracycline 0.1% in warm normal saline. This has been shown to substantially reduce the chances of residual abscesses in the peritoneum or incision.

A high level of postoperative care is as important for these patients as an expert operation, and some are going to require a spell in the intensive therapy unit. Gram-negative bacterial infection aggravates the effects of dehydration by producing vasodilatation by activation of the kinin system, and causing loss of circulatory volume by vascular endothelial damage. If these have caused a period of severe hypotension then some acute renal tubular damage may be reflected in a period of reduced renal function, which will require expert supervision of fluid and biochemical balance and will occasionally call for treatment by renal dialysis. Loss of fluid into lung tissue causes loss of compliance and impaired lung efficiency (shock lung), so periods of mechanical respiratory assistance may be essential. It is these grave possible sequelae of advanced acute appendicitis (in common with all severe endogenous infections from the alimentary tract, p. 327) which cause some deaths, generally among the elderly. These infections continue to cause very serious illness at all ages and expert management is needed, along the lines just outlined.

Happily, most patients with a perforated appendix make a slow but straightforward recovery. After operation the reaction of the gut to trauma – whether it be the handling of bowel at operation, or the effects of peritonitis – is for peristalsis effectively to cease. This period of reparative inactivity is usually followed by return of peristalsis, signalled by the passage of flatus per rectum and deflation of any distension of the abdomen. This cannot be hurried in any way and it is essential to keep the bowel at rest during this process by giving fluids intravenously and keeping the stomach empty of swallowed air and secretions by aspiration through a nasogastric tube. If general peritonitis resolves naturally, it will be 3–4 days before flatus passes and bowel sounds return. If this process is delayed, it is usually due to a residual abscess, which may be under the diaphragm (subphrenic), amongst adherent coils of bowel (interloop abscess), or in the pelvis. This continued failure of return to normal peristalsis is called 'paralytic ileus'. At first the only thing to do is to maintain fluid and electrolyte balance by carefully controlled intravenous fluid administration but, if ileus continues for more than 5–6 days, parenteral feeding through a caval catheter will have to be commenced so that the patient's metabolic state does not become harmfully depleted (p. 4). Once a paralytic ileus has continued for more than one week it becomes a difficult problem for the surgeon to know whether there is also an adhesive kink providing a mechanical block (which may need freeing) or whether a residual abscess is also causing a hold-up (good ultrasonic scanning is a great help in this situation). If a residual abscess is suspected, because the patient looks unwell, has a high swinging fever and a tachycardia, perhaps with objective evidence of an abscess, then it will usually require surgical drainage (Figs 13.12, 13.13).

It is these serious complications which cause

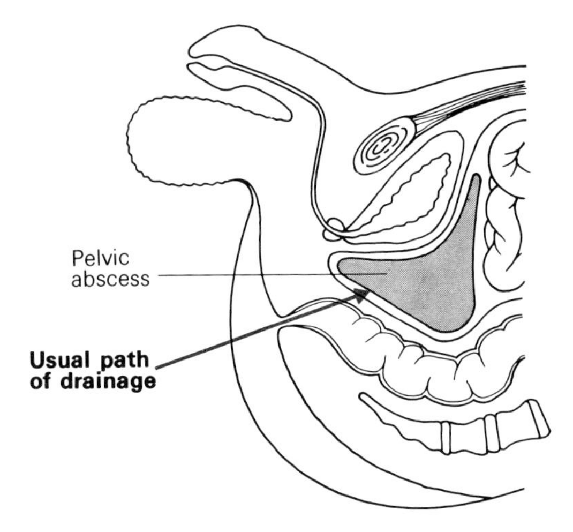

Fig. 13.12 *Sagittal section of male pelvis, showing the relation of a pelvic abscess to the rectum. Some pelvic abscesses will point and drain spontaneously through the anterior rectal wall, or in females into the posterior fornix: others require surgical drainage.*

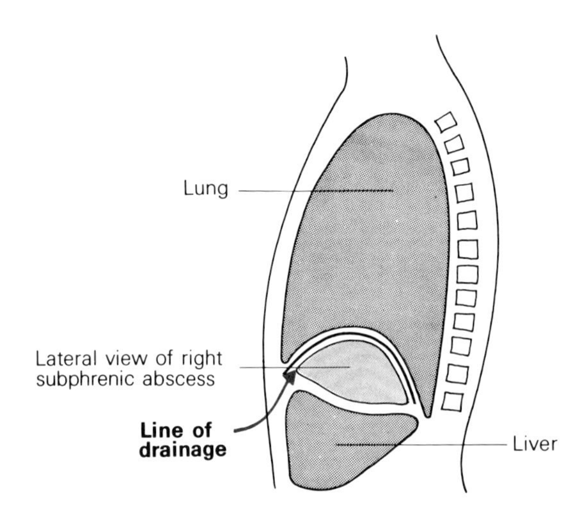

Fig. 13.13 *Sagittal section of upper abdomen showing a right subphrenic abscess. This is usually drained through a short incision under the costal margin.*

deaths from appendicitis and are likely to be seen in infancy (where the perforation rate is around 80%) and, especially, in the elderly, who tend to present late with a high perforation rate.

There is general agreement among surgeons that the correct treatment for acute appendicitis is emergency appendicectomy. The only exception to this would be in isolated conditions, such as a ship far from land, when it would generally be safer to stop fluids by mouth, to maintain an intravenous infusion, and to give suitable antibiotics. Most patients with acute appendicitis will recover on this regime although it is much more hazardous than immediate appendicectomy in a properly equipped hospital.

The treatment of appendicular abscess is a little more controversial. There is no doubt that many well-localised abscesses will resolve with rest in bed and a fluid diet. Most surgeons would recommend that these patients should have a planned appendicectomy three months later because a recurrent attack of appendicitis quite often occurs. If conservative management is adopted, the patient needs careful observation because some of these abscesses become larger and more tender and require surgical drainage before they will resolve.

The fact that death from acute appendicitis is now so rare (approximately one patient in 200) does not mean that vigilance can be relaxed, because this is still a very difficult condition to diagnose in some patients and peritonitis is still a dangerous condition. Infants are especially at risk because of their high perforation rate and the difficulty of examining them, and so are the elderly, who tend to tolerate abdominal pain for longer and therefore present later than younger patients.

GENERAL PERITONITIS

Although modern anaesthesia and antibiotics have robbed general peritonitis of most of its terrors, it is still a very serious abdominal condition. In patients with acute uncomplicated appendicitis the mortality rate is now down to 1 in 1500 but, when peritonitis is present, one patient in 50 succumbs. What produces this 40-fold increase in mortality and, among the survivors, many patients who only recover after a serious and often gruelling illness?

Peritonitis produces four distinct effects:

1. A fibrinous inflammatory exudate forms throughout the peritoneal cavity, which is

followed by paralysis and dilatation of the intestines. This causes sequestration of alimentary juices in the bowel and is followed by repeated vomiting.

2. With these changes, intake of fluids by mouth stops, so there is progressive dehydration.
3. Bacterial growth occurs rapidly in the exudate and is very likely to lead to bacteraemia. Children are liable to hyperpyrexia. Most patients have a mixed aerobic and anaerobic infection, and *E. coli* and *Bacteroides fragilis* are the commonest organisms: this has an important bearing on the choice of an antibiotic in treatment.
4. The adhesions caused by the sticky exudate often result in encysted collections of pus, especially under the diaphragm (subphrenic), in the pelvis or between adherent loops of bowel (interloop abscesses).

As a late effect, these adhesions may cause intestinal obstruction or, in females, occlusion of the Fallopian tubes.

The major cause of generalised peritonitis is perforation of a hollow abdominal vicus. This may be caused by blunt or penetrating injury of the abdomen, or a variety of diseases. In Western countries the commonest of these are:

acute appendicitis
perforated peptic ulcer
acute colonic diverticulitis
perforation of colonic carcinoma
    or, rarely, a small bowel neoplasm
fulminating inflammatory bowel disease
gangrene of bowel, e.g. mesenteric arterial
    obstruction or strangulation of bowel
acute obstructive cholecystitis
perforated typhoid ulcer (wherever typhoid
    fever is endemic)
leakage from an intestinal or gastric anastomosis.

Irrespective of cause, all patients with generalised peritonitis share a common clinical picture. They look drawn and ill and take care to lie still, and only move with caution. They give a history of continuing abdominal pain and vomiting, are toxic and dehydrated, and have a fever and a fast, thin pulse. In late cases, the abdomen is likely to be diffusely distended and tender, showing the signs of paralytic ileus: this contrasts with the rigid flat abdomen of a patient with a recent perforation of a peptic ulcer. By far the most serious group are those with a faecal peritonitis due to a colonic perforation: these patients rapidly show the signs of gram-negative bacteraemia and, though they may be flushed, soon become hypotensive.

Treatment is a matter of great urgency, but there is no question of these patients being rushed to theatre because they need careful preoperative preparation along the lines already suggested on p. 284. When the patient becomes fit for surgery, the essentials are to remove the source of peritoneal contamination, and carry out a thorough peritoneal debridement. In any case of colonic perforation, excision of the affected colon and the establishment of a temporary colostomy is almost always essential (p. 217). Good postoperative care, with all the facilities of an intensive therapy unit, plays as important a part in the recovery of some of these patients as the operation itself (p. 285).

INTESTINAL OBSTRUCTION

When, about 100 years ago, surgeons began to open the abdomen, intestinal obstruction was still regarded as too dangerous a condition to operate on. Although this attitude changed by the beginning of the century, a comprehensive review in 1932 showed a mortality of 40% in adhesive and neoplastic obstructions, and of 14% for strangulated external hernia. These figures are a measure of the seriousness of the subject and a consideration of the pathology of intestinal obstruction will show why this is so.

Obstruction of the intestine produces four effects:

1. *Loss of alimentary secretions*

The normal adult produces some 7–9 litres of

alimentary secretions each day, but only about 100 ml of this is lost in normal faeces (Fig. 13.14). In small-bowel obstruction, much of these secretions are lost, both by vomiting and by sequestration in widely dilated loops of small intestine. Distended bowel also secretes more juice than normal bowel. In a number of ways, therefore, the patient loses water and electrolytes, and it is an important part of treatment to replace these by intravenous infusion before operation.

2. *Intestinal distension*

This will always occur, although in high small-bowel obstruction the jejunum can be decompressed by regurgitation into the stomach. Some patients with colonic obstruction show an extreme degree of distension: pressures over 25 cm of water can occur, impeding the circulation in the bowel wall and eventually causing necrosis.

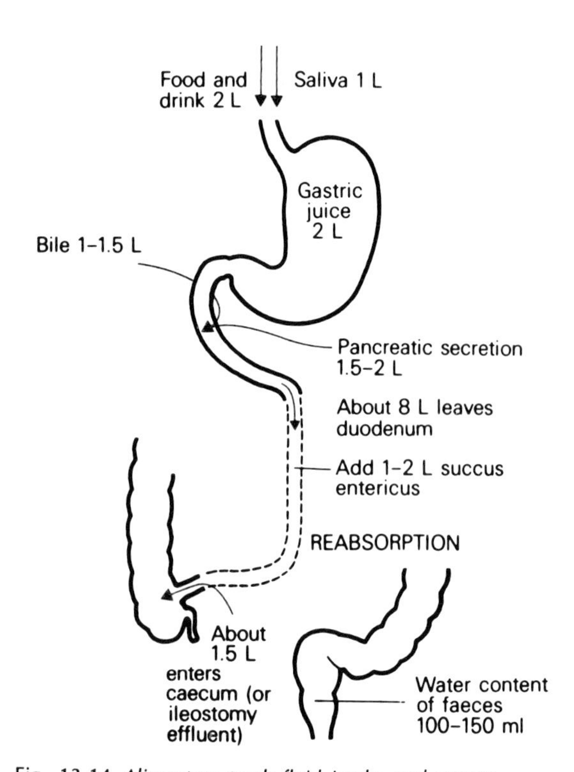

Fig. 13.14 *Alimentary track fluid intake and output.*

3. *Bacterial growth*

The normally clean small intestine is, when obstructed, rapidly populated by intestinal bacteria, hence the offensive faeculent vomitus seen in late small-bowel obstruction. This highly infected fluid is very dangerous if spilt into the peritoneum or accidentally aspirated into the respiratory tract.

In some cases a further serious pathological change occurs:

4. *Strangulation*

This means interruption to the mesenteric blood flow. Most of these patients have a loop of bowel caught under a band or impacted in a hernial orifice. This usually arrests venous return which, if continued long enough, leads on to venous gangrene. Coincidentally there is very severe bacterial overgrowth in the ischaemic loop, which plays an important part in hastening proteolysis and disruption of the ischaemic bowel wall, and this in turn will result in perforation and peritonitis (Fig. 13.15).

The great majority of bowel obstructions are due to a mechanical block – a demonstrable and usually removable cause. A small number of patients have a functional obstruction, due to cessation of peristalsis, known as paralytic ileus (see p. 285).

The mechanical causes can be classified (Fig. 13.16) as being due to:

Pressure upon the bowel, e.g. a strangulated hernia or a band obstruction.

Disease in the wall of the bowel, e.g. a carcinoma grows to encircle and narrow the colon so much that faeces cannot pass the stricture. Fibrotic strictures due to Crohn's disease and diverticulitis are other examples.

An object impacted in the lumen. An example of this occurs when a large stone ulcerates through the wall of the gall bladder into the duodenum and passes down the small bowel, finally impacting in the terminal ileum. Dried fruit, poorly chewed and quickly swallowed, can swell in the intestine and impact.

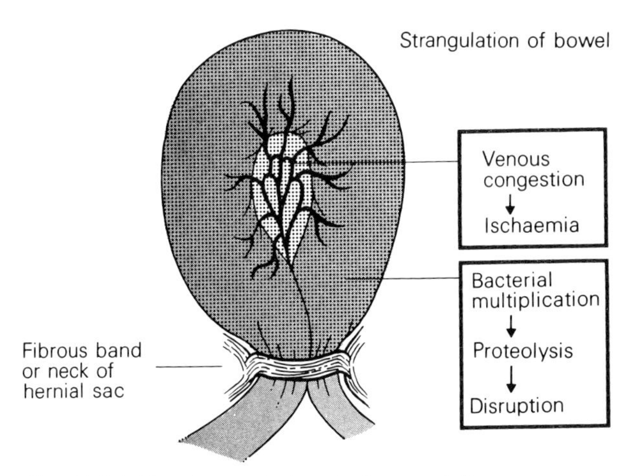

Fig. 13.15 *The changes in intestinal strangulation.*

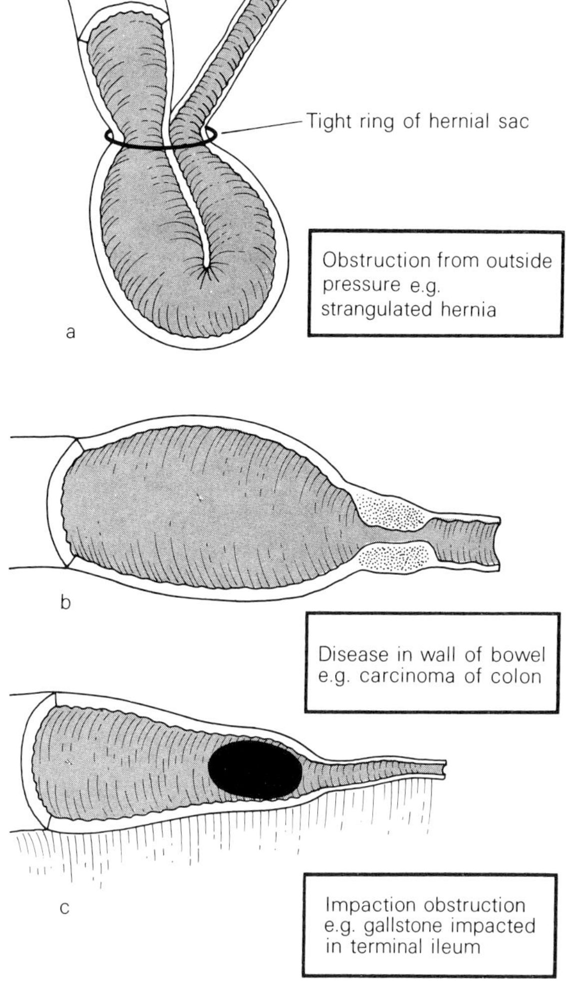

Fig. 13.16 *The mechanical causes of intestinal obstruction; (a) pressure from outside, (b) disease in the wall, (c) impaction in the lumen.*

Although they operate in different ways, all these causes produce the same effect – blockage of the lumen of the bowel. The patient complains of the classical triad: colicky abdominal pain, vomiting, and constipation, but the emphasis varies according to the level of obstruction.

In small-bowel obstruction the copious secretions above an obstruction produce frequent vomiting accompanied by severe small-bowel colic. Inspection of the abdomen often shows central distension provided there is a fair amount of distended small bowel above the obstruction, and loud splashing bowel sounds can be heard. This is an acute distressing picture which nearly always leads to an early call for medical advice.

The picture in large-bowel obstruction is generally quite different. Recurrent lower abdominal discomfort has often been felt for days or even weeks, with increasing difficulty in moving the bowel. Some patients notice that the abdomen has become swollen, but the whole picture is slower and less demanding. Nevertheless, the most impressive degrees of tympanitic abdominal distension can be seen, and sometimes the distended caecum can be seen and felt. This is a very important sign because perforation of a tensely distended caecum is a distinct possibility.

Any patient with a mechanical obstruction of the bowel will have hyperperistalsis and this can be heard through a stethoscope as frequent high-pitched splashy sounds – these are quite characteristic and can be an important clue to the presence of an obstruction. Rectal examination and a search for irreducible herniae must never be forgotten. Plain abdominal x-rays may be of great value. Gas distension of loops of bowel shows up very clearly in a supine abdominal film, and an erect film will show the presence of fluid levels in the bowel. In low colonic obstructions the distended colon shows a very characteristic gas pattern on x-rays.

Adhesive and Band Obstructions

It is one of the natural functions of the peritoneum, when injured in any way, to form a fibrinous exudate: this is how the beneficent adhesions which limit the spread of appendicitis are formed. Handling of the bowel at operation, resecting parts of it, forming anastomoses, all leave many injured areas and lumps of ischaemic tissue where ligatures have been applied, so adhesions form after all abdominal operations. In some people, reabsorption by fibrinolysis is almost complete, in others massive adhesions persist. In some patients, a few strands of fibrin become organised to form strong fibrous bands: these are dangerous because they can form the axis around which a volvulus may occur or a small strong ring through which a loop of small bowel can pass and become strangulated.

Four out of five adhesive obstructions arise after laparotomy and may occur either early (in the immediate postoperative period) or late.

Those which occur during the phase of recovery from a laparotomy are difficult to distinguish from a slow return of peristaltic activity or paralytic ileus. This distinction requires considerable vigilance and diagnostic skill and largely hinges on signs that the obstruction is progressive and confined to the small intestine.

The great majority of adhesive obstructions occur months or years after a laparotomy, and are due to a loop of small bowel being trapped under a tight strong band (Fig. 13.15). This leads to immediate hyperperistalsis above the obstruction, colicky central epigastric pain, vomiting, and cessation of the passage of flatus per rectum. If such a patient has an abdominal scar, a slightly tumid tender abdomen, and audible obstructive bowel sounds, then a band obstruction must be suspected. This is a serious diagnosis because the entrapping band may be short and strong and lead to obstruction of venous return, i.e. the patient will have not only intestinal obstruction but also strangulation: this bowel needs urgent release if it is not to die and then have to be resected.

The operation may be a simple one of dividing a band and releasing a trapped kinked loop of intestine or it can be a very difficult one of painstakingly dividing innumerable adhesions and bands until the obstructing adhesion is found. The most difficult part of these operations is deciding whether a loop of bowel which has been strangulated under a band is viable – in doubtful or definite cases of gangrene a resection and anastomosis is required.

It is a serious mistake to exclude a band obstruction because there is no scar on the abdominal wall. Some patients form spontaneous bands, others have a Meckel's diverticulum with a band connecting to the umbilicus. The obstruction which occurs can be just as severe as those due to postoperative adhesions.

Adhesions and bands account for about one-third of all bowel obstructions in Western countries. They are the legacy of an increasing number of abdominal operations, which have in turn been done because of the frequency in Western societies of diseases such as acute appendicitis, malignant disease of the colon and rectum, and peptic ulceration. In every adhesive obstruction there is a strong possibility of strangulation and this must make the surgeon very vigilant. The mortality rate is still 8–10%: this is partly a consequence of an ageing population, but is also due to the difficulties of positively diagnosing strangulating obstructions.

Strangulated External Hernia

At the start of the 20th century this was everywhere the commonest cause of intestinal obstruction, and it still is much the most usual cause in the Third World, where few patients have abdominal surgery, and where colorectal cancer is rare. In all these herniae a loop of intestine is forced through the narrow neck of a hernial sac and thus kinked and trapped: with progressing venous engorgement, the trapped loop becomes larger and less likely to reduce spontaneously.

Although inguinal hernia is much commoner than femoral, strangulation occurs in one-third of femoral herniae but in only one inguinal herniae in 20. As a consequence, roughly equal numbers of strangulated inguinal and femoral herniae are seen. Strangulated femoral hernia is three times commoner in women than in men, whilst strangulated inguinal hernia is seen ten times more often in men than in women.

Strangulated umbilical, incisional, and obturator hernias are rare but important.

Strangulated inguinal hernia

Few patients with a strangulated inguinal hernia will be missed because, in addition to severe central abdominal pain and vomiting, the patient will complain of a lump in the groin that became tense and painful when the abdominal symptoms started (Fig. 13.17). Ninety-seven per cent of these herniae are oblique and 80% will contain small bowel, so these patients will have the signs of a small-bowel obstruction and a tender lump above the inguinal ligament, frequently extending into the scrotum. In 5%, large intestine will be strangulated; although these patients may not have pressing abdominal symptoms, the hernia will be obviously tense and tender: these cases are important because the infective complications are serious.

A number of elderly men have an irreducible inguinal hernia, but these are not tender and there are no abdominal complaints. The surgeon who always examines the testicle as well as the hernial sites will not be misled by the occasional torsion of an inguinal ectopic testicle.

Strangulated femoral hernia

This can, in contrast, be very easily missed. A typical patient is a fat middle-aged woman who complains of the onset of colicky abdominal pain, vomiting and constipation, but who is unaware of any pain or lump in the groin. Only one patient in four complains of a painful lump (Fig. 13.18). Without symptoms directing attention to the groin it is very easy to overlook a small tense lump hidden in the fat of the groin and upper thigh, and the difficulty is compounded by the fact that, in half of these patients, the lump is not tender. This is so different from the tenderness of strangulated inguinal hernia that it can make the examiner question the diagnosis, but it should not do so. It will now be seen why one of the essential aphorisms of emergency medicine is: 'in any case of acute abdominal pain always examine the hernial orifices'.

Diagnosis is made no easier by the fact that so many patients are obese, which makes abdominal examination difficult: auscultation over several minutes may be rewarded by hearing a rush of obstructive bowel sounds.

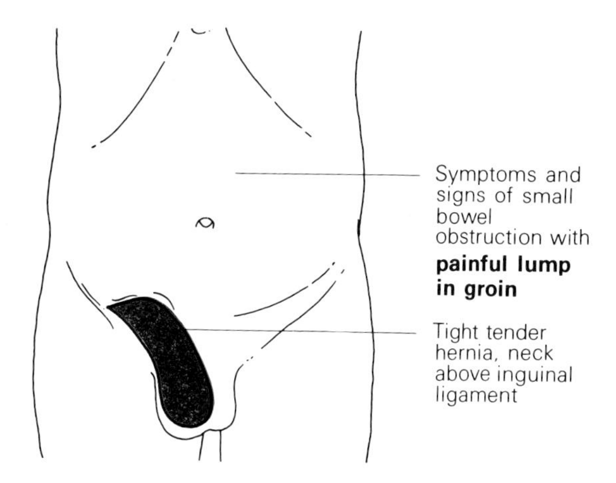

Fig. 13.17 *Strangulated inguinal hernia.*

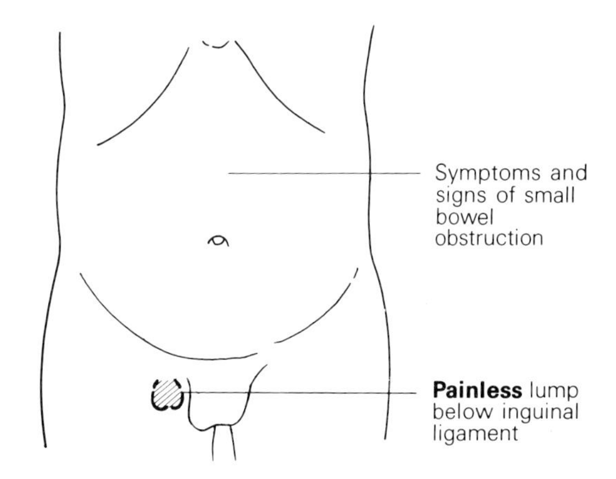

Fig. 13.18 *Strangulated femoral hernia.*

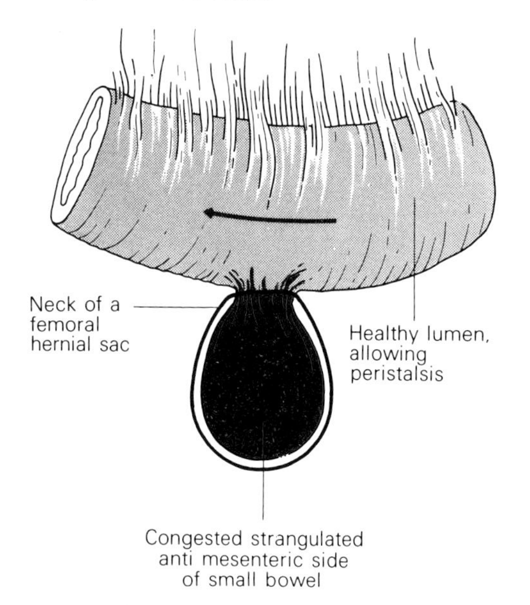

Fig. 13.19 *Richter's hernia.*

Most difficult of all these patients are those who have strangulated a portion of great omentum. They have vague abdominal pain and a lump over the saphenous opening. These must be explored because a Richter's hernia (Fig. 13.19) gives similar signs, i.e. a strangulated hernia which affects only the antimesenteric portion of the intestinal wall, so reducing but not obliterating the lumen of the intestine, and there will *not* be signs of intestinal obstruction.

Strangulation of a para-umbilical hernia (Fig. 13.20)

This only accounts for about one in ten strangulated herniae, but the mortality rate is treble that of inguinal and femoral herniae. The reasons for this include the facts that most patients are elderly and fat, have had the hernia for a long time, and do not notice or bother about some abdominal pain and hardening of the hernia. The contents of the hernia are typically omentum and transverse colon, so vomiting is a late feature. Even when a doctor is summoned, it can be difficult to decide whether a hernia which has for long been irreducible has become strangulated – this usually depends on the general signs of intestinal obstruction and tenderness of the sac. If a loop of small bowel has slipped into the sac and become strangulated, then the fairly acute onset of pain and vomiting makes diagnosis much easier. These patients are often poor operative risks.

Incisional hernia

The same difficulties arise when strangulation occurs in an incisional hernia. During the past 10

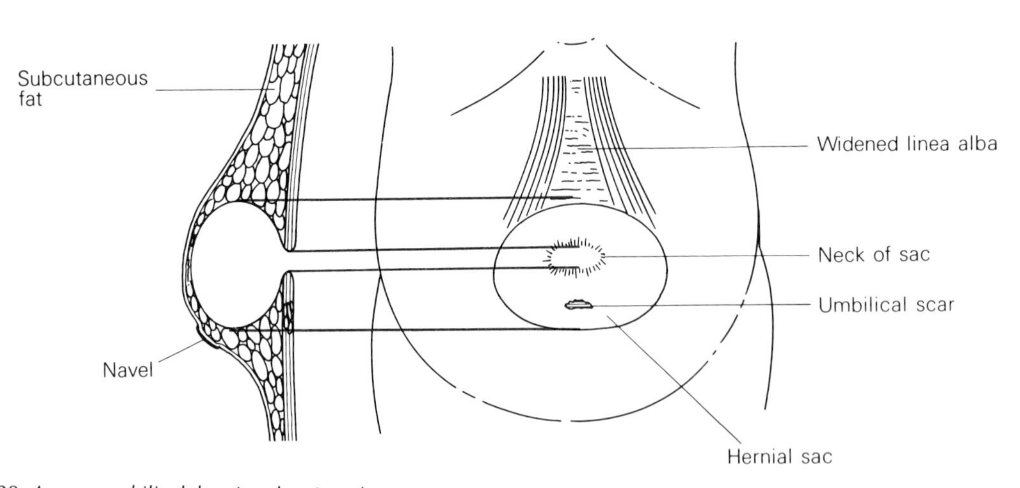

Fig. 13.20 *A para-umbilical hernia, showing sharp narrow neck, compared to capacious sac. These patients are generally obese, so it is difficult to appreciate the full size of the sac.*

years, surgeons have taken increasing interest in the secure closure of abdominal incisions, so fewer herniae are seen: this is largely due to the abandonment of catgut, which is absorbed before the wound is soundly healed, and the adoption of monofilament nylon or polypropylene suture material. A majority of these herniae occur through lower midline incisions made for gynaecological procedures, and again these patients are often fat and have had a lump for some time. Diagnosis follows the same lines as for para umbilical hernia, with a strong bias towards exploration owing to the difficulty of being sure whether strangulation has occurred.

Strangulated obturator hernia

This is an interesting rarity. The herniation occurs where the obturator artery and nerve leave the pelvis by perforating the obturator membrane (Fig. 13.21). The obturator canal has tough edges so when, rarely, a herniation of peritoneum occurs alongside the nerve and artery, strangulation of bowel easily arises if a loop of intestine slips into the hernial sac. This hernia causes no external swelling and is very difficult to palpate but, in addition to abdominal pain and vomiting, the pressure of the impacted loop of bowel on the nerve produces characteristic pain in its area of distribution, i.e. over the anteromedial aspect of the thigh from the perineum to the knee.

This is clearly a difficult but satisfying diagnosis to make; fortunately most patients clearly have an acute small bowel obstruction and the cause is revealed at laparotomy.

The treatment for all these herniae is a short period of preoperative rehydration and preparation followed by operative relief of the obstruction and repair of the hernia. In inguinal and femoral hernia, the important step is to remove the hernial sac and to repair the widened inguinal or femoral canals, usually with a fascial flap. Umbilical and incisional herniae can be large and often occur in obese patients, presenting the surgeon with a difficult repair – again the preparation and suture of rectus sheath flaps is usually the method of repair.

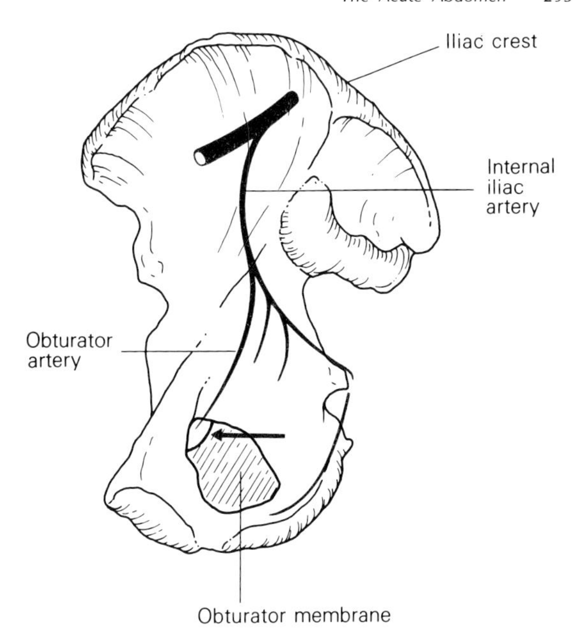

Fig. 13.21 *View of inside of right pelvis, showing path of exit (arrow) of obturator hernia.*

The results of operative treatment are mostly quick and satisfactory, but the occurrence of strangulation and the need for resection adds a material risk and most large series of strangulated herniae carry a mortality of about 5%.

Internal Abdominal Herniae

Intestinal obstruction due to bowel being trapped in one of the internal hernial sites is a rarity. Most cases present with signs of small-bowel obstruction, but there is no abdominal scar to make the surgeon suspect adhesions, and no external herniae. The true cause of the obstruction is only revealed at laparotomy. Most occur in the peritoneal folds at the extremes of the small bowel, which can be deep enough to trap a knuckle of bowel or, occasionally, to accommodate many loops of small bowel (Fig. 13.22).

Strangulation of bowel or stomach in a diaphragmatic hernia is by far the most important of this group because this is a relatively common event and constitutes a real threat to life. The

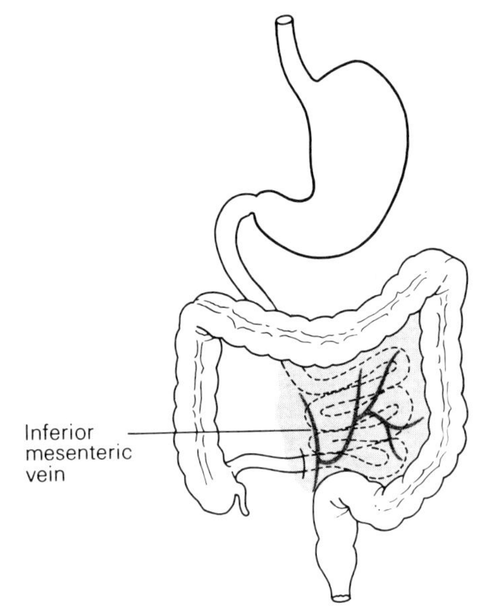

Fig. 13.22 *A left paraduodenal hernia. During rotation of the midgut, the duodenum is formed normally but, instead of the jejuno-iluem lying in front of the mesocolon, it becomes covered by mesocolon, so only the terminal ileum is intraperitoneal. Obstruction occurs when a loop of bowel prolapses and is trapped at the hiatus of the hernia, which lies behind the inferior mesenteric vein.*

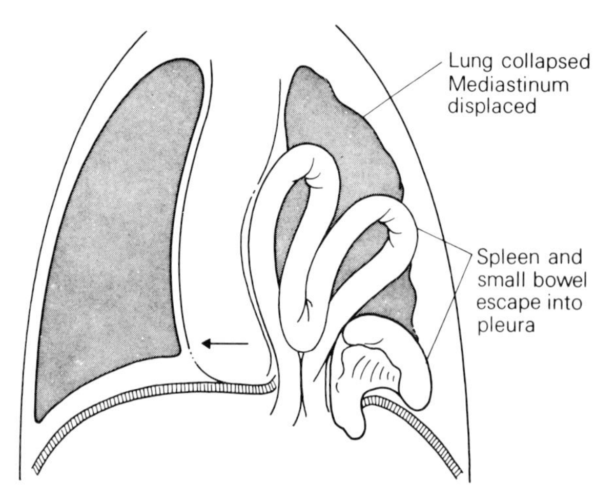

Fig. 13.23 *Traumatic rupture of the left dome of the diaphragm: spleen, stomach and small bowel are likely to be found in the pleural cavity.*

hernia may be a congenital defect, a traumatic rupture, or an acquired paraoesophageal hernia. These have all, usually, been quite silent until the patient complains of upper abdominal pain and vomiting. The essential key to suspicion of a complication of diaphragmatic hernia is that the patient is short of breath, and careful clinical examination may show poor movement and air entry into the affected chest. An urgent chest x-ray will nearly always reveal a tell-tale shadow of the herniated stomach or small bowel, with mediastinal shift (Fig. 13.23). Operation to reduce the strangulated bowel is an urgent necessity.

Obstruction of the Large Intestine

The differences between large and small bowel obstructions are numerous. Small-bowel obstruction is about three times commoner, is due to many causes, and is often complicated by strangulation, but in Western countries there is only one common cause of obstruction of the large bowel – i.e. carcinoma – and strangulation is rare. Small-bowel obstructions produce acute symptoms with a short history, colonic obstructions are generally much slower to develop.

Neoplastic obstruction

It is a characteristic of colonic neoplasms that they extend circumferentially around the bowel wall, so narrowing it (Fig. 13.16). When this reaches a certain stage, the semisolid material in the distal colon can no longer pass through the stenosis. This explains why 70% of obstructing neoplasms lie at or beyond the splenic flexure.

The initial reaction of a hollow viscus to obstruction is to increase the propulsive power of peristalsis by hypertrophy of smooth muscle proximal to the obstruction: when this can no longer force faeces through the stenosis, a build-up of faecal material occurs, with gradual dilatation. In the colon, this process tends to go unnoticed by patients because they often have a period of frequent passage of small liquid stools. Only when obstruction becomes complete does gas begin to build up and it is this which causes increasing abdominal distension.

Pain is rarely severe, but 'windy pains' across the lower abdomen are a nuisance and the patient realises the constipation is becoming complete. Vomiting is unusual.

Examination shows a patient who is not notably distressed or acutely ill, though there may be signs of anaemia and weight loss. The abdomen is very noticeably and generally distended, and hyper-resonant. It is rare to find tenderness or a mass, but in a thin patient it is often possible to see and feel the distended caecum. In the 25% of patients who have an obstruction in the caecum or ascending colon, the signs will be those of gradual small-bowel obstruction, and visible peristalsis is often seen. Rectal examination usually reveals a dilated empty rectum.

Plain radiology of the abdomen can be invaluable. Distal obstructions result in a characteristic accumulation of gas throughout the colon, which is maximal in the caecum: in the erect film a very wide fluid level is often seen in the caecum (Fig. 13.24). The wide transverse colon often shows characteristic haustration, and the width and anatomical distribution of the distended bowel leaves little doubt that the obstructed bowel is large and not small bowel (Fig. 13.25). Often the high pressure in the caecum causes compression of the lips of the ileocaecal valve so that small bowel does not share in the distension: the

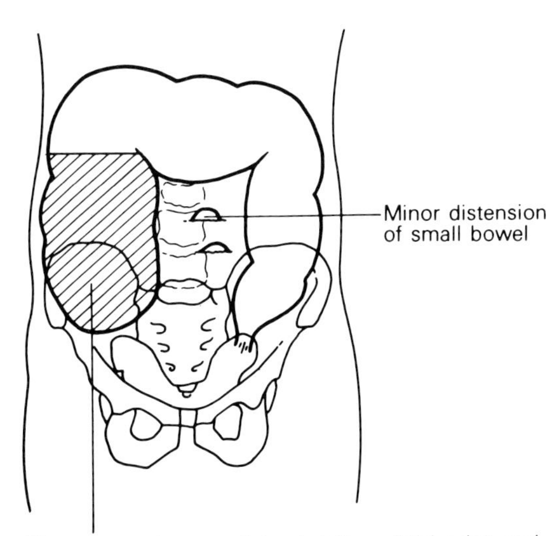

Fig. 13.24 *Typical plain x-ray appearance of obstruction of distal colon by carcinoma of the sigmoid.*

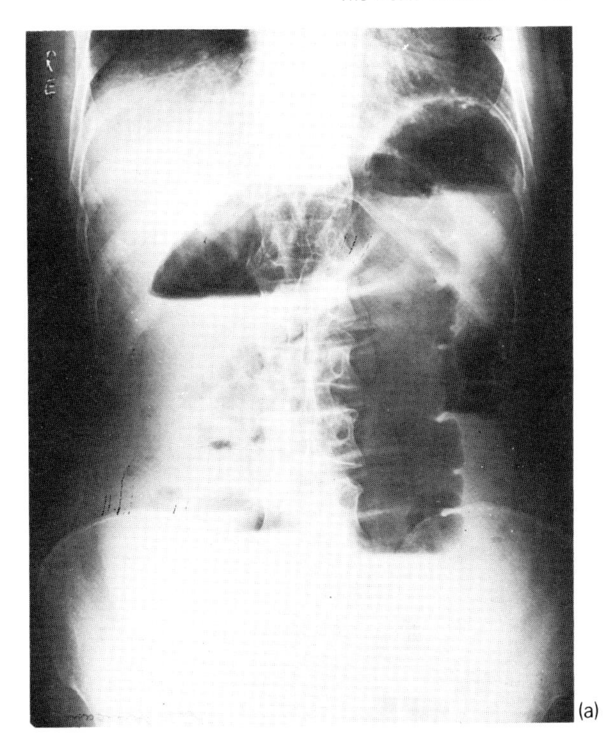

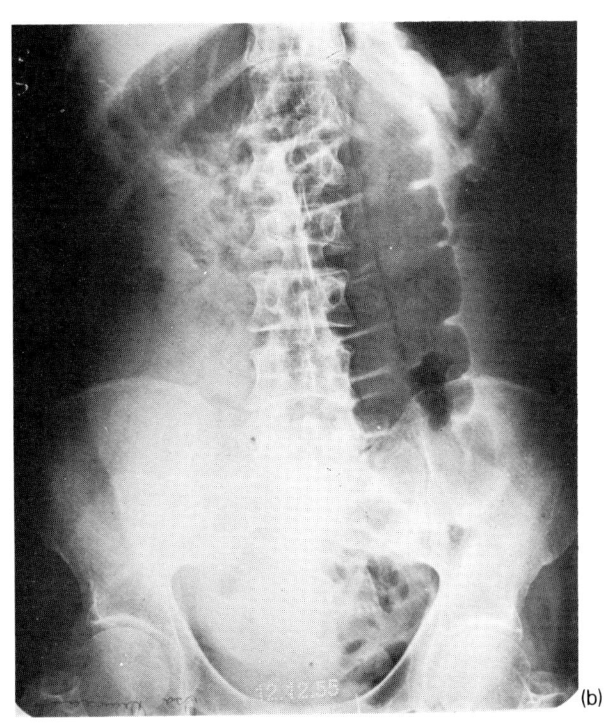

Fig. 13.25 *Erect (a) and supine (b) x-rays, obstructed carcinoma of sigmoid colon.*

closed loop so created produces a dangerous rise of pressure and caecal rupture is a real threat in these circumstances.

There is often doubt about the level of a colonic obstruction and then an emergency barium enema can be a great help in localising the obstruction and excluding pseudo-obstruction.

Treatment is still controversial, but most surgeons would recommend immediate resection of obstructing proximal neoplasms, with anastomosis of terminal ileum to colon: this gives excellent results (Fig. 13.26).

When the obstruction lies beyond the splenic flexure there are two main methods available. One school of surgeons prefers to make an emergency decompression by establishing a transverse colostomy, leaving the patient to recover for 2–3 weeks before carrying out an elective resection and anastomosis (Fig. 13.27). Even this relatively simple treatment carries a mortality of 10–15%. The other school believes it better to carry out an immediate resection often followed by anastomosis: alternatively a Hartmann's operation may be done (Fig. 13.28), with later reconnection of colon to rectum. The great majority of patients with an obstructed colon are elderly and so not all are fit for immediate resection, but in the hands of an experienced surgeon the mortality is below 10%

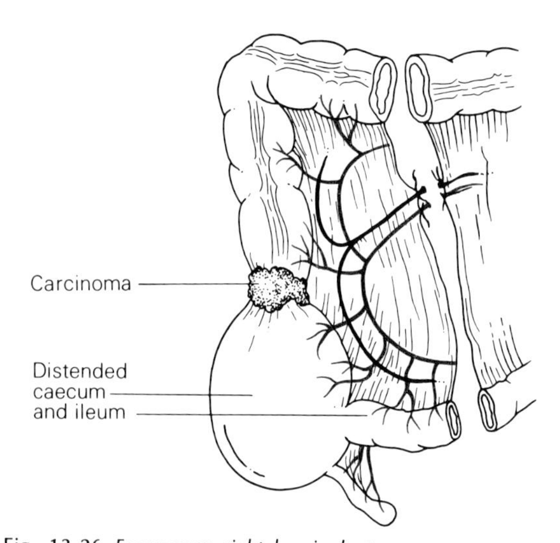

Fig. 13.26 *Emergency right hemicolectomy.*

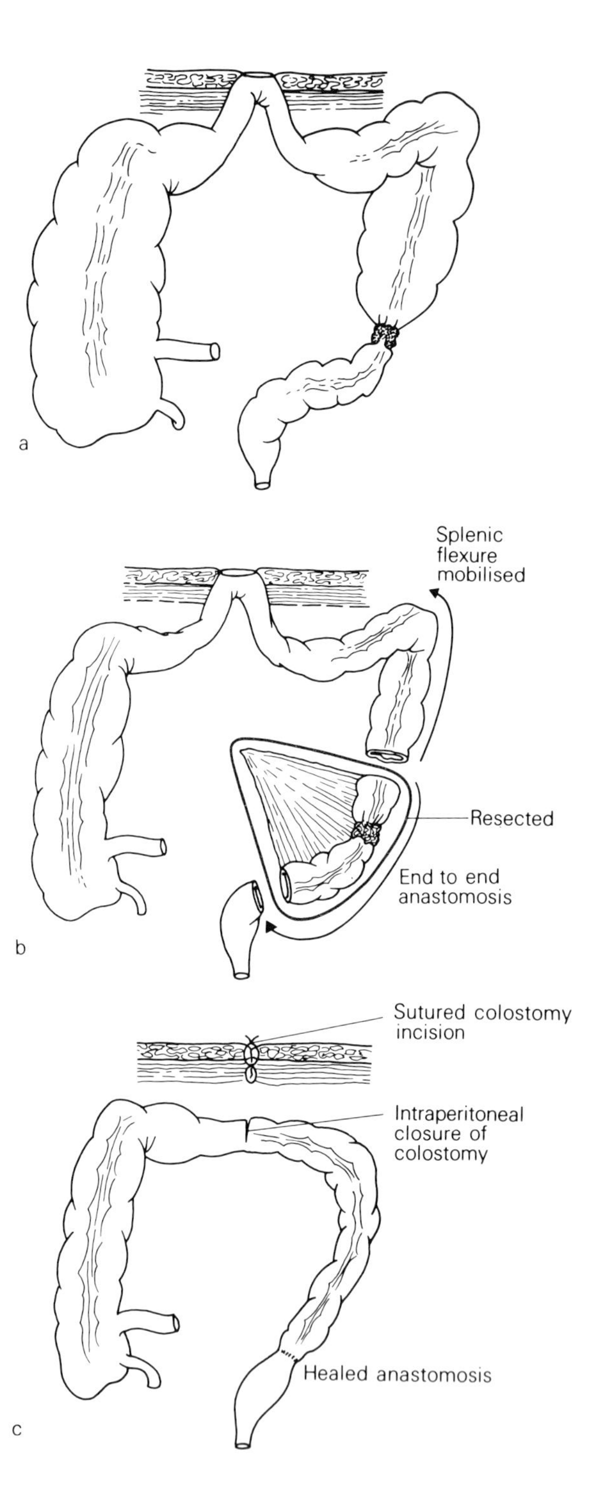

Fig. 13.27 *Three-stage treatment of obstructed distal carcinoma of colon. (a) Emergency colostomy. (b) Resection and anastomosis. (c) Closure of colostomy.*

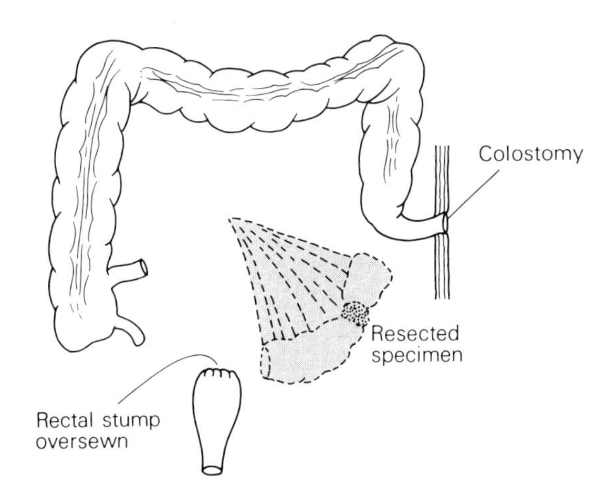

Fig. 13.28 *Hartmann's resection. At the emergency operation a radical resection of the carcinoma is performed and a terminal colostomy formed.*

and the patient has a potentially curative operation in one stage. There is a strong suggestion – but as yet no proof – that immediate resection carries a better long-term prognosis than staged resection.

Volvulus of the colon

The sigmoid colon is anatomically liable to volvulus, having a long mesentery with a narrow base. In Western countries this is fairly unusual (about 5% of all obstructions) but in Eastern Europe, the Middle East and Africa, sigmoid volvulus is the cause of about one-third of all obstructions. It appears to be much more common among those who eat a bulky natural vegetable diet. There is an unexplained high incidence among inmates of mental hospitals.

Volvulus is the only common cause of ischaemic necrosis of the colon, but it may take 3–4 days to reach the stage of perforation so there should be time for treatment to forestall this.

Onset of an attack is acute, with cessation of passage of flatus, lower abdominal colic, and rapidly progressive abdominal distension. Tight gaseous distension is the striking abdominal finding even shortly after onset, and obstructive sounds may be heard. Tenderness should raise a strong suspicion of gangrene.

The plain abdominal film is very helpful, showing a huge sigmoid loop occupying most of the abdomen with a characteristic curved stripe running down the centre of the abdomen where the two loops are pressed together. Big fluid levels may be present (Fig. 13.29).

Most patients who are seen with sigmoid volvulus have a past history of similar attacks and, once one or two patients have been seen, this condition is fairly easily recognised.

For a long time the treatment of volvulus of the sigmoid was detorsion, either by laparotomy or, for the past 50 years, by passing a sigmoidoscope and using it to thread a rectal tube through the twist: this releases large quantities of gas under pressure, and liquid faeces.

More recently, resection of the sigmoid has been favoured because of the strong tendency to recurrence after untwisting. Most of these are done a few days after sigmoidoscopic deflation. However, a very careful watch must be kept for the minority of patients with gangrene – these must be treated by immediate resection of all ischaemic bowel and establishment of a terminal colostomy: the rectal stump is oversewn and, in fit patients, reconnection of the colon to the rectum can be considered after recovery is complete (Fig. 13.28).

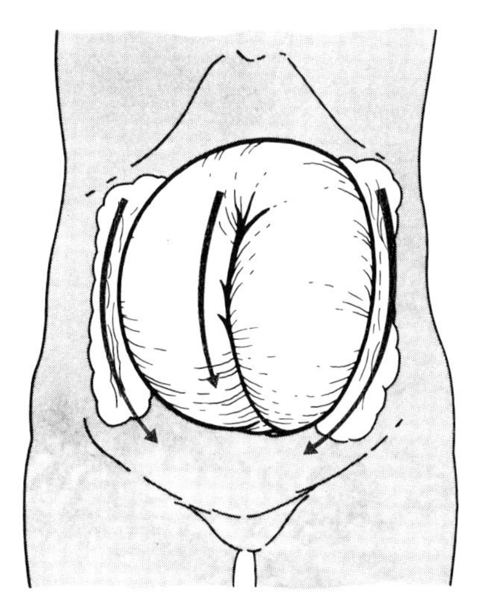

Fig. 13.29 *Typical appearance of plain x-ray in sigmoid volvulus; note the three converging lines.*

Torsion of the caecum is rare, but it is serious because of the threat of gangrene. The symptoms are those of acute small-bowel obstruction and the diagnosis is likely to be made at laparotomy. However, the x-ray may show the tensely distended viscus lying above and to the left of the usual position of the caecum. Recurrence is likely, so emergency right hemicolectomy seems a reasonable treatment.

Torsion of the transverse colon is very rare.

Pseudo-obstruction of the colon

Although not common, this is seen often enough to be an important differential diagnosis in patients with a large-bowel obstruction. It appears to be comparable to 'paralytic ileus' and is sometimes called 'ileus of the colon' because, though the whole colon may be tightly distended, there is no mechanical obstruction.

Sometimes a cause can be identified, such as a severe systemic infection, the puerperium (especially with Caesarean section), episodes of hypoxia, or hypotension.

These patients show the signs of a large-bowel obstruction, but close scrutiny of the plain abdominal film almost always shows some gas in the rectum. A close watch should be kept for this condition because it is most undesirable to undertake an unnecessary laparotomy on patients already seriously ill. An emergency barium enema is a valuable and relatively harmless way of confirming this diagnosis. However, there is a small risk of caecal rupture and this must not be forgotten when awaiting recovery.

Intussusception

This is a form of intestinal obstruction which is most often seen, in a unique way, in infancy, but which can occur in older patients. The word is derived from the Latin *intus* meaning 'within' and *susceptum*, 'caught up.'

The mechanism by which intussusception occurs is that a solid lesion, e.g. an adenoma, arises in the mucosa of the intestine. As it develops, the peristaltic waves passing the tumour pull on it, and as it grows in size it is pulled upon the more strongly. This often results in formation of a polyp, with a stalk of normal, stretched mucosa. If the pull exerted by peristalsis should actually invert the wall of the bowel then an intussusception has been initiated and the polyp at the apex may travel some distance, so inverting a length of bowel behind (Fig. 13.30). Not only does this narrow the lumen of the intestine, but it also means that the mesentery is drawn in with the intussuscepting bowel and, necessarily, subjected to considerable compression. The veins are occluded first, producing engorgement of the intussuscepted bowel (hence the passage of altered blood per rectum which is typical of intussusception) and, later, gangrene. Intussusception is, therefore, a form of strangulating bowel obstruction and so requires early diagnosis.

In infancy, typically, a child of 6–18 months of age is suddenly seized with abdominal colic and may vomit. Attacks of colic recur, with screaming and drawing-up of the legs, and some dark red

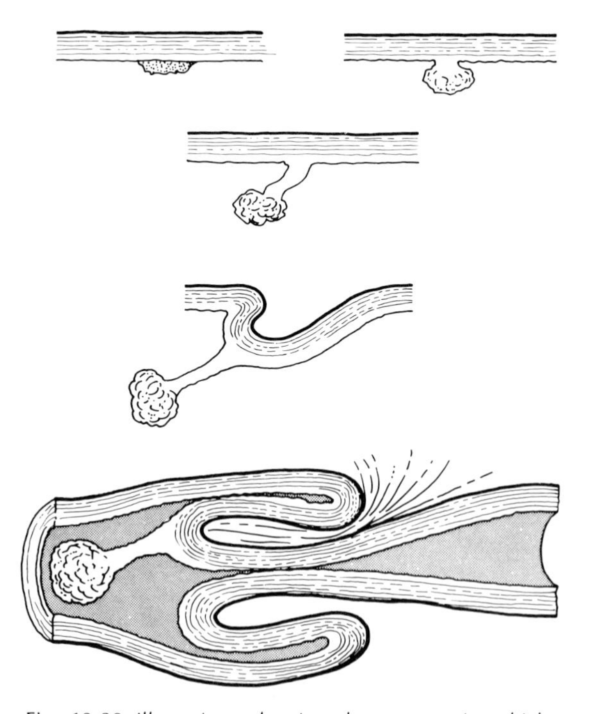

Fig. 13.30 *Illustrations showing the manner in which an intestinal adenoma grows to become a polyp which can, in turn, initiate an intussusception.*

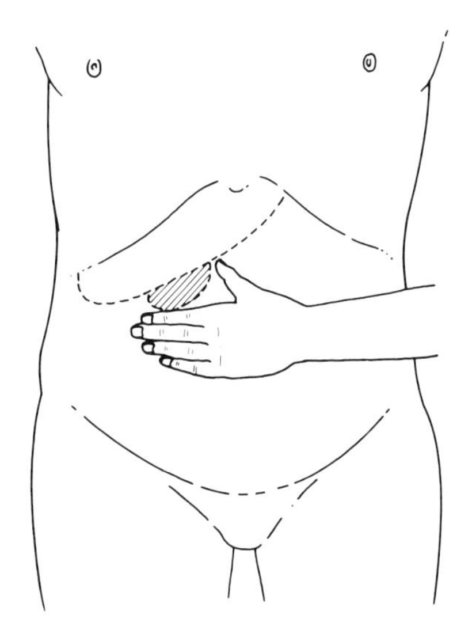

Fig. 13.31 *The best way to palpate the mass of an intussusception in infancy is to use the flat hand – most often the mass is felt under the liver edge.*

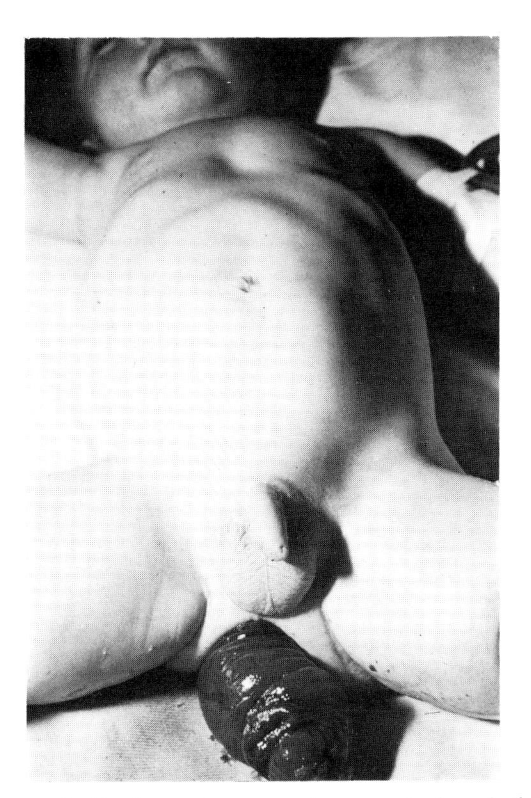

Fig. 13.32 *Rarely, an insussusception presents through the anal canal.*

blood is often passed per rectum. Abdominal examination reveals a sausage-shaped mass in the upper abdomen, and obstructive bowel sounds (Fig. 13.31). Rectal examination shows mucus stained with dark red blood (Fig. 13.32). At operation, the distended ileum is seen to enter a mass consisting of the colon enclosing the intussuscepted iluem and proximal colon. In most cases, pressure on the apex of the intussusception results in reduction and when the whole intussusception has been unravelled it will be seen that the apex is an indurated area in the wall of the terminal iluem: this is, in fact, a greatly hypertrophied Peyer's patch of lymphoid tissue (Fig. 13.33). Viral studies make it almost certain that this is due to an adenovirus infection which probably enters via the nasopharynx and spreads to the abdominal lymphoid tissue. As the baby gets older, immunity to these viruses builds up and it is rare to see this specific form of intussusception after the age of 2 years.

However, older children may suffer intussusception of a Meckel's diverticulum and, in adults, an intussusception of the colon is seen from time to time, with an adenomatous polyp or a carcinoma at the apex.

Small bowel neoplasms

These are fairly unusual but, because of the relatively small calibre of the small intestine, they may present early with intestinal obstruction. Roughly equal numbers of benign and malignant neoplasms occur, the benign tumours (adenoma, lipoma) being likely to form the apex of an intussusception in an adult. (Sometimes several adenomas are associated with melanin deposits in the mucosa of the lips and cheeks – the Peutz–Jeghers syndrome: these patients are also liable to intussusception.)

For every malignant small-bowel neoplasm, the surgeon in Great Britain is likely to see about 50 colorectal and 30 gastric carcinomas. Roughly one-third are carcinomas, one-third are lymphomas (there is an association with coeliac disease) and one-third are carcinoids. All tend to produce gradual narrowing of the bowel lumen and so the

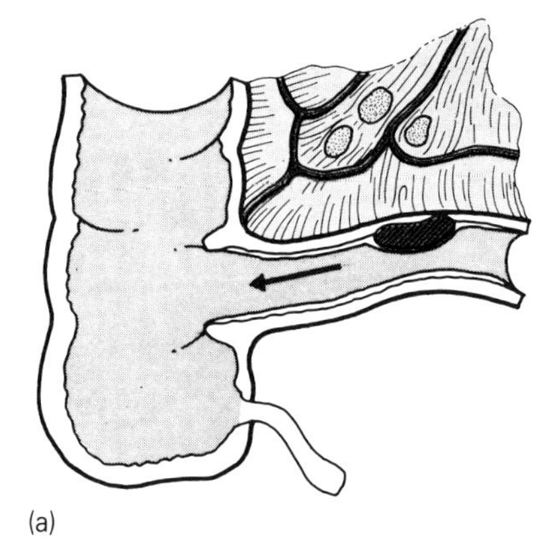

(a)

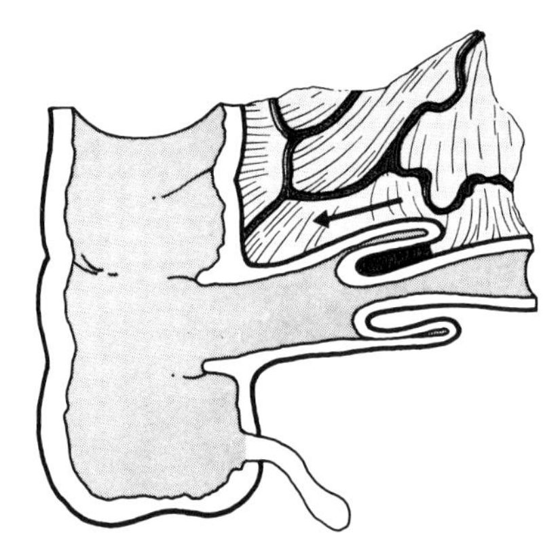

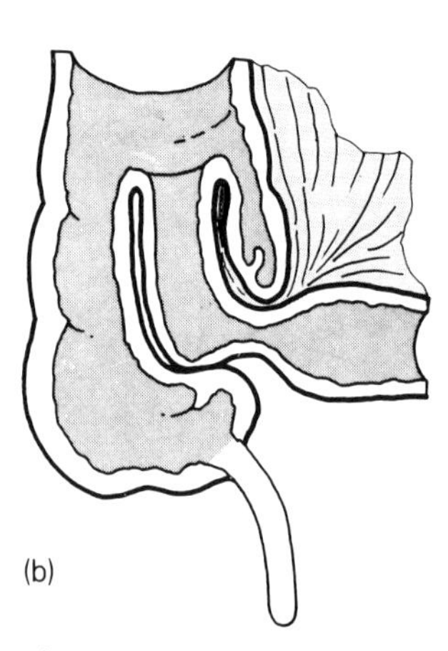

(b)

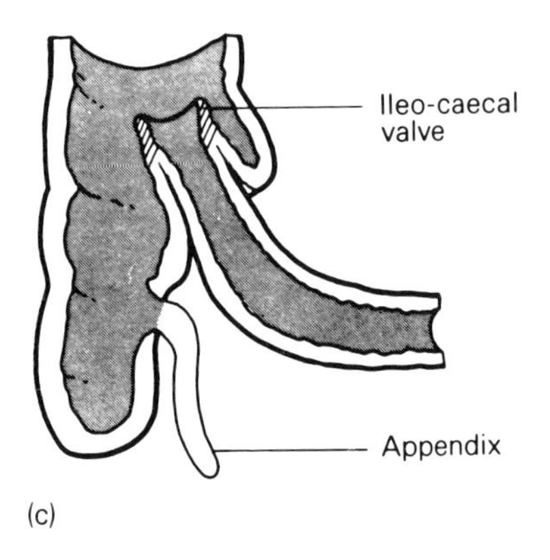

(c)

Fig. 13.33 *The aetiology of intussusception in infancy. (a) The enlarged Peyer's patch. (b) Development of intussusception, initiated by the enlarged Peyer's patch. At first an ileo-ileal intussusception, this becomes ileo-colic in character. (c) Ileo-caecal intussusception, i.e. the ileo-caecal valve is the leading point of intussusception.*

patient experiences increasing small-bowel spasm and colic (especially after meals) and gradually the signs of intestinal obstruction develop.

The carcinoid tumour (or argentaffinoma, or Kulchitzky cell carcinoma), is an unusual neoplasm which occurs most often as a yellowish lump in the tip of the appendix of young people, where its behaviour is usually benign. In the ileum of older people, carcinoids arise deep in the mucosal layer, producing a characteristic yellow nodule in one wall and, as they grow, are likely to produce intestinal obstruction. Although carcinoids are to be regarded as carcinomas of low-grade malignancy, once they have spread to adjacent lymph nodes the outlook becomes more serious because spread to the liver often follows.

It is characteristic of carcinoid tumours to secrete 5-hydroxy-tryptamine (5 H-T or serotonin) and other humoral substances, which are metabolised by monoamine oxidase in the liver to 5-hydroxyindoleacetic acid (5-HIAA), which is excreted in the urine. When the volume of 5-HT produced by hepatic and other extra-intestinal metastases exceeds the capability of the liver to inactivate it, then the circulating 5-HT and other secretions, e.g. histamine, are likely to produce symptoms of the carcinoid syndrome, i.e. intestinal hurry going on to diarrhoea, and flushing of the face. Attacks tend to be precipitated by exercise and taking alcohol. The diagnosis is confirmed by finding more than 25 mg of 5-HIAA in a 24-hour collection of urine.

Early resection before metastasis is the treatment

of choice for intestinal carcinoids. In the appendix, appendicectomy is usually sufficient (The occurrence of carcinoids is an important reason for invariably sending the excised appendix, however inflamed, for histological examination). The progression of metastases is usually slow, with a mean survival time of some three years: symptoms of the carcinoid syndrome can be relieved by drugs which inhibit 5-HT production, e.g. methysergide, cyproheptadine.

PERFORATED PEPTIC ULCER

This is one of the classical abdominal emergencies, perhaps because it is a dire event for the patient and presents striking signs to the surgeon. Like acute appendicitis, it appears to have been unknown until the middle of the nineteenth century, when reports of perforations of gastric ulcers in young single anaemic women began to appear: these were rapidly fatal. The first successful suture was performed (by candlelight!) in the home of a man of 41 in 1892, in North Germany. With the coming of the twentieth century, duodenal ulcer in men became increasingly common, and the curious syndrome in young women disappeared. By the time of the Second World War, perforated duodenal ulcer in men was one of the commonest surgical emergencies. After 1950 there was a steady fall for fifteen years, but the incidence seems now to have stabilised. There are still interesting regional and national differences. There are more perforations in Scotland and the North of England (about 20 per 100 000 population per annum) than in the South (about 10 per 100 000). More duodenal than gastric ulcers are seen in the North: during 1944–53 in Glasgow the ratio was 17:1, but is now half that figure. Similarly the male to female ratio was 6:1 and is now 4:1. Perforations occur fairly evenly throughout adult life.

Clinically, the striking feature is the instantaneous onset of severe upper abdominal pain which rapidly spreads to involve the whole abdomen. Phrenic reference of pain to one or other supraclavicular nerve distribution is classical. Movement is intensely painful and patients tend to lie where they have been struck by the pain. Vomiting often occurs. Only two-thirds of patients give a history of recurrent dyspepsia, a reminder that perforation of an acute ulcer is quite often seen after only a day or two of upper abdominal pain.

When a peptic ulcer causes sufficient penetration of the gastric or duodenal wall to breach it, there is a point at which the ulcer base gives way and the gastric content is suddenly released. The appearance of such a perforation is striking – a neat circular hole appears to have been drilled out, with smooth vertical sides. Peritoneal contamination can be very severe if a meal has recently been taken, and food can be recovered from all quadrants of the abdomen. If the stomach is empty, gastroduodenal juices still cause severe peritoneal irritation but the signs tend to be rather less severe.

The appearance of a patient with a perforated peptic ulcer is highly characteristic – in obvious pain, pale and sweaty, lying absolutely still, taking short quick respirations. However, the pulse is rarely much quickened or blood pressure lowered during the first 6–8 hours after perforation. When the abdomen is inspected, the tight recti stand out and there is no trace of respiratory movement; the rigidity of the abdominal muscles is board-like. For this reason tenderness may seem to be slight because no impression can be made on the tense muscles. Bowel sounds are often absent, but may be heard in the first few hours after perforation. When a rectal examination is made, the pelvic peritoneum is often tender.

In 60% of patients, sufficient swallowed air escapes through the perforation for it to be visible in an erect x-ray film of the diaphragmatic area – this is a highly charcteristic and useful confirmatory sign (Fig. 13.8). When it is absent, acute pancreatitis is another condition which produces severe sudden upper abdominal pain, but it rarely causes such marked abdominal signs (Fig. 6.8).

Sometimes a small perforation seems to cause only a slow leak and the signs are localised to the upper abdomen. These perforations tend to produce so marked an inflammatory exudate in adjacent omentum, liver, and colon that the spillage is localised and in some cases the perforation is in fact sealed off by fibrous adhesions.

This is the practical basis of one of three possible methods of treating a perforation, i.e. the non-operative regime, in which the stomach is kept empty by effective nasogastric suction, nothing is taken by mouth, and fluids are supplied intravenously. If this regime is effective, the patient rapidly improves and the abdominal signs regress. It is not much used but can be valuable in selected patients who are already improving when admitted, or who have such severe cardiorespiratory disease as to be unacceptable for surgery.

The classical treatment for a perforated peptic ulcer is simply to close the perforation by deep under-running sutures of catgut, often incorporating a patch of omentum (Fig. 13.34). This is speedy and effective treatment, but it has its limitations. Some perforations are so large as to be technically uncloseable and these usually require partial gastrectomy as do those perforations complicated by severe haemorrhage: some perforated gastric ulcers are actually carcinomas, which may go unrecognised unless a generous biopsy is taken: patients who have only simple suture of a chronic peptic ulcer tend to have further trouble and often need elective surgery.

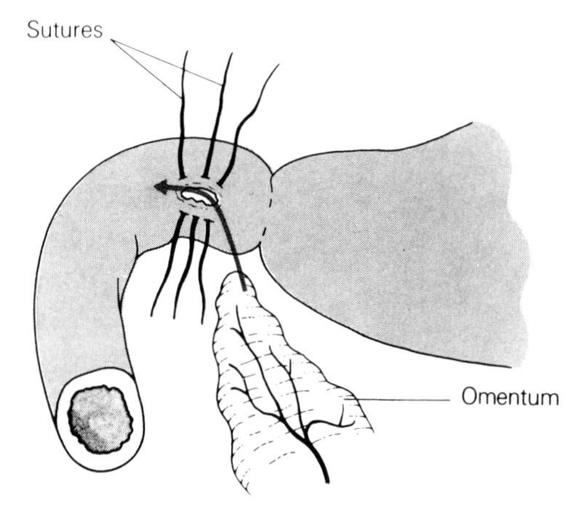

Fig. 13.34 *Suture of a perforated duodenal ulcer.*

This has led many surgeons to look at the possibility of carrying out definitive ulcer surgery at the time of perforation. Most patients who come speedily to hospital are quite fit for such an operation and then the major requirement is a surgeon sufficiently experienced to make a wise choice of operation and perform it skilfully. There are good reasons to advise partial gastrectomy (Fig. 5.30), for most perforated gastric ulcers because many are large and are prone to leak after simple closure, whilst roughly one in every ten will in fact be a perforated carcinoma: these are not easily recognised as neoplastic nor is wedge biopsy of the ulcer edge by any means always positive.

There is a good case, also, for emergency definitive surgery for the perforated chronic duodenal ulcer, because two-thirds of these patients, if treated by simple closure of the perforation, require later elective surgery. The popular operation for this group at present is truncal vagotomy and a pyloroplasty (Fig. 5.27), but some duodenums are so scarred when they perforate that these patients require closure of the perforation and a gastrojejunostomy and vagotomy. A few experts in highly selective vagotomy have done this, after having closed the perforation.

Whatever operation is adopted, it is important to remember that there is widespread contamination of the peritoneal cavity. Sometimes food fragments have to be picked out manually and every patient should have the peritoneal cavity thoroughly washed out with several litres of warm saline, containing 0.1% tetracycline, paying special attention to removal of debris from the subphrenic space, where a residual abscess is especially likely to occur.

The mortality of perforated duodenal ulcer is now very low (2–4%, except in the elderly) but for gastric perforations the mortality rate is 10–15%. The reasons for this are that gastric perforations are larger, patients are more severely ill with peritonitis when admitted, and are more prone to postoperative complications than patients with duodenal perforations.

ACUTE INTESTINAL ISCHAEMIA

When acute obstruction of the superior mesenteric artery occurs, the flow of blood to the midgut is more or less completely interrupted. Emboli from the left ventricle of a patient with auricular fibrillation or a recent myocardial infarction are the classic cause of the occlusion, but these are now rarely seen, and most cases are due to thrombosis of an atheromatous vessel. Occasionally mesenteric venous thrombosis occurs and this can also cause circulatory arrest in the midgut. In the elderly, cardiac failure or arrhythmias may reduce circulation through the gut to a critical level.

In a typical example of acute intestinal failure, a middle-aged or elderly person with a history of cardiac disease complains of the sudden onset of severe general abdominal pain, usually followed by vomiting. At first, there is little abdominal tenderness, and so delay in diagnosis may occur. Some bloody diarrhoea may give a warning, but there is only about 6 hours from the onset of the obstruction during which, if the circulation is restored, the bowel may recover its viability. To achieve this, both family doctor and surgeon must react quickly to the picture of an ill anxious patient with severe pain but few signs: a white cell count over 20 000/mm^3 is nearly always found.

Ideally, superior mesenteric embolectomy or thrombectomy is performed, with restoration of circulation to still-viable bowel. More often, extensive ischaemic necrosis necessitates resection of much of the small bowel and proximal colon, and only a minority of patients survive this: if they do, the problems of maintaining adequate nutrition with only a short length of small bowel are considerable (p. 135).

Inferior mesenteric artery occlusion is considered on p. 218.

ABDOMINAL INJURIES

Throughout the history of warfare and fighting, it has been recognised that penetrating wounds of the abdomen, whether made with spear, arrow, dagger, or bullet, were frequently lethal. Peritonitis due to wounds of the gut, or haemorrhage from fragmentation of solid organs, were generally irremediable until very recent times. Until the advent of fast road traffic made serious street accidents a commonplace, it was not generally realised that blunt (non-penetrating) abdominal injuries can be equally dangerous and fatal.

During wars, experience in the management of abdominal injuries advances rapidly, and this has been seen throughout the years since 1914. There are marked cultural differences in the incidence of peacetime abdominal injuries. Where fighting among communities or gangs is common, penetrating injuries may outnumber blunt injuries. In Western Europe, road accidents are the common cause of abdominal injuries, which affect both pedestrians knocked down, and occupants of cars thrown about in collisions. Some 40–50% of deaths among European children between 5 and 14 years of age are due to accidents: most of these fatalities are from head injuries, but abdominal injuries are the cause of about 8% of deaths. Most of them are due to children crossing a road and being knocked down by a passing vehicle, but a number are due to falls whilst at play.

A blunt injury of the abdomen may be due to a direct blow on the abdomen which, though leaving no external mark beyond a little bruising, directly ruptures an underlying organ. Alternatively, an organ such as the spleen or liver may be torn by sudden acceleration or deceleration. The important rule is always to suspect that closed abdominal injury may have occurred in anyone who has met with a violent accident, whether it was a knock-down car injury, a fall from a height, or a violent street fight.

In the conscious patient, there will be a history of an accident, a complaint of abdominal pain and tenderness and, often, signs of blood-loss. The severity of bleeding varies greatly, from a small leakage to an overwhelming and irreparable loss. The organs most often fractured are the solid ones – kidney, spleen and liver. Most renal injuries tend to resolve with time and tears of the liver which have ceased to bleed are best left alone. Splenic injuries usually require splenectomy because suture is difficult and unreliable. Major tears of the liver cause very copious haemorrhage and can be very difficult, and sometimes impossible, to repair. Blunt rupture of the bladder and intestines occur and can be difficult to recognise, there being a latent period after injury when there are very few signs. It is vital to examine the abdomen very carefully in anyone who complains of any abdominal pain after injury and to practise 'active observation' (p. 280) over some hours, because the signs of tenderness and guarding may only develop slowly.

Special care is needed in patients who have not recovered full consciousness after a head injury. They cannot draw attention to abdominal discomfort. Anyone with a head injury who shows hypovolaemic shock should be suspected of internal haemorrhage – either in the abdomen, chest or a large limb fracture – because head injuries themselves rarely produce hypotension. Very careful examination is then needed, including x-rays of the chest and pelvis, and diagnostic peritoneal lavage can be a valuable help in detecting intra-abdominal bleeding.

In penetrating injuries, whether with knife or bullet, there is little doubt that an injury has occurred. The problem is to identify all the structures which have been injured and repair them. High-velocity gunshot wounds are especially serious in producing widespread damage: particular care has to be taken over injured large bowel, with a preference for resection and temporary colostomy rather than any sutured repair.

Much diagnostic skill and good operative judgement are needed in this branch of surgery.

SPLENECTOMY

Apart from accidental rupture, and the need to remove the spleen to achieve radical resection of a carcinoma of the stomach or splenic flexure, almost all the indications for splenectomy are haematological. Some of them are integral elements of treatment, e.g. thrombocytopenic purpura or hereditary spherocytosis, whilst others are diagnostic, e.g. the staging of lymphomas. In Gaucher's disease the spleen may require removal on account of its great size, sometimes associated with hypersplenism.

The operation of splenectomy is generally a straightforward anatomical exercise. First, the spleen is mobilised by dividing the lienorenal ligament, allowing the spleen to be brought up to the surface (Fig. 13.35), and then the gastrosplenic ligament is divided to allow a good view down

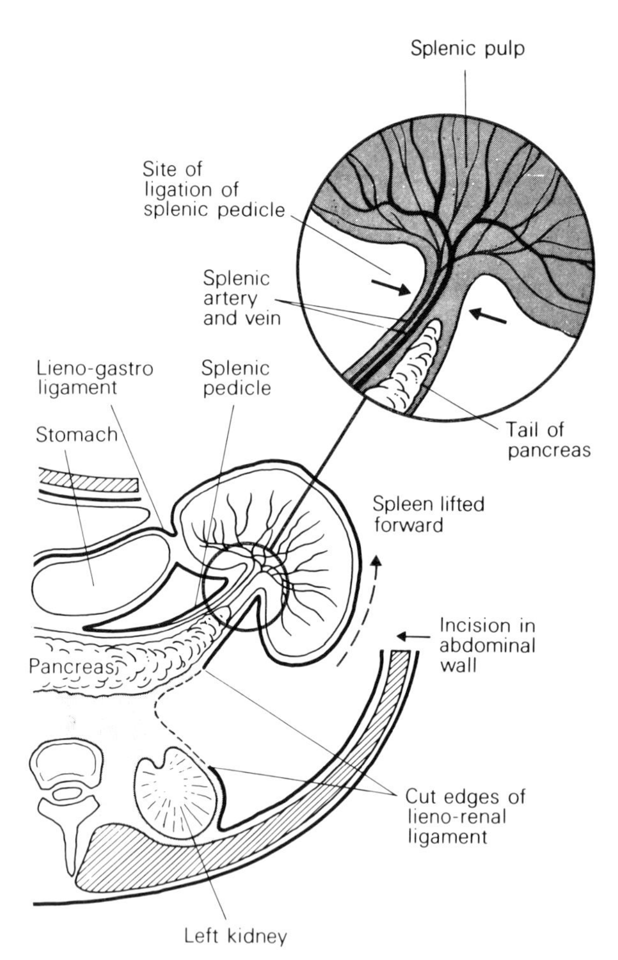

Fig. 13.35 *Cross-section of left upper quadrant of abdomen. The lienorenal ligament has been divided and the spleen brought up into the wound. The next step will be to open up the space between stomach and spleen and ligate the short gastric vessels, to permit a good view down onto the splenic pedicle. The splenic pedicle has been isolated and the tail of the pancreas can be clearly seen. The splenic artery and vein will be defined, ligated and divided, and then the spleen removed.*

onto the splenic pedicle. Taking great care to see and avoid the tail of the pancreas, the splenic artery and then the vein are tied and divided (Fig. 13.35), or the branches may have to divided within the hilum: the spleen is then removed.

Because many of these patients have disordered haemostasis, it is especially important to leave a dry field and incision, and patients with thrombocytopenia often have to be operated on under cover of a platelet transfusion.

There is a particular liability to postoperative pulmonary complications at the left lung base, where a watch must be kept for signs of consolidation or fluid: physiotherapy is used from the time of operation to try to forestall such an event.

There is good evidence that, if splenectomy is carried out on a child under the age of five years, the immune resonse to infection is reduced, and considerable effort is taken to avoid splenectomy in early life. If it proves to be essential, then long-term prophylactic antibiotic treatment is used.

OTHER CAUSES OF ACUTE ABDOMINAL PAIN

It is an observed fact that more normal appendices are removed as an emergency from young women than from men of the same age group. This is due to the pelvic positioning of the female genitalia, and their response to the monthly hormonal cycle.

Rupture of the graafian follicle some 14 days after the onset of menstruation can sometimes be acutely painful (mittelschmerz), probably associated with the effect of blood from the torn surface irritating the local peritoneum. This can give short-lived but marked signs, and an accurate menstrual history is vital (p. 276). The precision of the history, if needed by direct questioning, is equally vital in picking up the missed or abnormally brief menstrual vaginal loss which can be the essential signal of the presence of an ectopic pregnancy. Implantation of a fertilised ovum in the fallopian tube means that trophoblastic invasion occurs in a thin-walled viscus not designed for this intense vascularity: rupture will at some stage occur and can cause very severe intraperitoneal haemorrhage about the 6–8th week of pregnancy. This can be both a difficult and a dangerous emergency calling for skilful diagnosis and management.

In acute salpingitis due to an ascending infection from the vagina, the symptoms and signs are, not surprisingly, similar to those of the peritonitis set up by pelvic appendicitis. However, the illness is more influenza-like, with headache and high fever, and speculum examination of the cervix shows a purulent discharge. If the diagnosis can be firmly made, the condition responds well to bed rest, fluids, and a broad-spectrum antibiotic.

Torsion of an ovarian cyst causes sudden very acute lower abdominal pain, usually with an easily palpable, rounded tender mass.

Acute abdominal emergencies occasionally arise during the course of a normal pregnancy and can cause considerable difficulties in diagnosis, because the pain tends to be explained in terms of the pregnancy, and abdominal signs can be significantly more difficult both to detect and interpret during pregnancy and the puerperium. This is a situation calling for great care from both obstetrician and surgeon because although, with modern anaesthesia and intensive care, the risks to the mother are low, a surgical emergency arising during pregnancy can present a very significant threat to the continuation of the pregnancy.

Other important abdominal surgical emergencies such as acute cholecystitis (p. 187), acute colitis (p. 231) and acute diverticular disease of the colon (p. 216) are considered elsewhere. It is also vital to remember that there are some important medical causes of acute abdominal pain (p. 280).

Many patients are admitted to surgical wards with acute retention of urine, and with acute ureteric obstruction, which are both very painful complaints. However, a careful history and examination will usually reveal the correct diagnosis: in the case of acute ureteric pain, an emergency intravenous pyelogram can be of great assistance.

The symptoms of threatened or commencing rupture of an abdominal aortic aneurysm are being increasingly recognised. An elderly person, nearly always a man, suddenly collapses with very severe gripping abdominal pain, which may be maximal in the left loin. In about two-thirds of patients, the pulsation of the aneurysm can be felt, and the patient is hypotensive: emergency ultrasound can be very helpful in confirming the diagnosis. Success depends very much on speedy diagnosis and transfer to theatre for operation by an expert vascular team.

RECURRENT ACUTE ABDOMINAL PAIN

This is a common problem which is particularly associated with childhood. Boys and girls are equally affected and are usually between 8–12 years of age. It is an observed fact that in most of these children no organic cause for the pain can be found, but two important facts follow from this. First, it is important to detect the minority who have a correctable cause for the pain. Second, although no organic cause may be found, a great deal of anxiety is aroused by these attacks (mostly centred around the possibility of a 'grumbling appendix') and they can lead to considerable loss of schooling. The whole family is affected by these attacks.

The most important step is to give time to the taking of a careful history. A precise description of the attacks is needed. The site of the pain must be accurately localised, and its timing, duration and character noted. Disturbance of sleep, appetite, and bowel action must be enquired for. In a typical case of the syndrome, the child rubs a hand around the umbilical area when describing the site, occurrence is confined to the waking hours, appetite remains healthy, and bowels are undisturbed, although in almost every case the child is described as going pale and having to lie down during an attack. There are no abnormal findings on examination, the blood count and ESR are normal, and urine microscopy and culture (which must never be omitted) are negative.

Sometimes these attacks seem to occur in the morning before school, and not during the holidays, but reluctance to attend school is by no means the only problem: further enquiry often reveals tensions of one kind or another in the family, and there can be little doubt that most of these children are reacting to stress of some sort.

It is helpful to remember that, whenever pain is localised to one side of the abdomen, an organic cause is more probable, and in particular an IVP should be done. Congenital abnormalities of the urinary tract – especially hydronephrosis due to pelvi-ureteric junction obstruction – are easily overlooked because symptoms are intermittent and, between attacks, the patient is well. It is also important to remember the minority who have major but rare conditions such as duodenal ulcer, Crohn's disease, or gallstones. With an accurate history, these rarities may be suspected and radiological investigation should as far as possible be limited to these patients.

The 'grumbling appendix' is a concept which has no basis in pathology. True recurrent attacks of acute appendicitis certainly occur, but these are accompanied by anorexia, fever, and localised tenderness and guarding over the appendix – quite a different picture from typical recurrent pain. It is abundantly clear that elective appendicectomy for recurrent pain, without objective evidence of previous appendicitis, is a useless operation.

It is intriguing to speculate on the possible connection between these childhood attacks and the pain of the irritable colon.

14

Alimentary Tract Haemorrhage

INTRODUCTION

There are as many patients admitted annually to hospital with alimentary bleeding as with pneumonia or cardiac failure. Despite advances in medical and surgical care, this common clinical problem continues to carry unacceptably high mortality and morbidity. This often results from the failure to recognise that the normal pathophysiological responses to alimentary bleeding may be considerably modified by increasing age and the presence of coincidental disease, especially cardiorespiratory. Moreover, it is important to realise that there are many unpredictables. For example, a fairly similar-looking duodenal ulcer may present disconcertingly as life-threatening haemorrhage in one patient, and as trivial blood loss in another. Although the urgency will depend on the severity and rapidity of the bleed, all patients with gastrointestinal bleeding should be investigated.

The management of the rapidly bleeding patient is an emergency, posing a major diagnostic and therapeutic challenge that is best dealt with by an experienced team including physician, surgeon and radiologist, ideally in specially designed hospital premises. An energetic diagnostic and therapeutic approach is essential if mortality is to be reduced to a minimum. The team should examine the patient at frequent intervals during the early hours of management and closely monitor progress. In this way, rational judgements can be made on the timing of investigative procedures and surgical intervention.

Patients whose blood loss is initially assessed to be minor or chronic require early rather than emergency investigation and treatment. The severity or chronicity of the initial bleed gives little clue to the causative lesion.

Blood loss can present in a number of ways which may suggest at an early stage whether bleeding is arising from the upper (principally oesophagus, stomach and duodenum) or lower (principally colon) gastrointestinal tract.

Haematemesis

This means the vomiting of fresh blood, blood with clots, or blood which has been subject to digestion by gastric juices (with reduction of haem to haematin), which produces a brown fluid with brown granules—so-called 'coffee-ground vomit'. The presence of fresh blood in the vomitus implies recent haemorrhage, often of moderately large volume, from the upper alimentary tract, whereas the presence of 'coffee-ground' vomit suggests upper gastrointestinal bleeding, sometimes of smaller volume, over a more prolonged period.

Melaena

This means the passage of tarry black shiny stools, the discolouration again being produced by the reduction of haemoglobin, principally by the action of acid from the stomach. The presence of melaena implies bleeding from the upper gastrointestinal tract. If blood loss has been slow, the stool is formed; if, however, blood loss has been severe, bowel peristalsis is vigorously stimulated and the rapid transit of the intestinal contents produces a loose copious motion which varies in colour from shiny black to dusky red and which has an instantly recognisable offensive odour.

Fresh rectal bleeding

This may take the form of bright red blood on the surface of the stool, admixed with the stool, present on the underclothes, noted on toilet paper, or staining the water in the lavatory pan. It usually implies bleeding from the lower alimentary tract. Although many patients with painless rectal bleeding will be found to have haemorrhoids, this diagnosis must never be assumed because some patients will have rectal or colonic polyps or carcinoma. The occurrence of painful fresh rectal bleeding suggests an anal fissure. Profuse fresh bleeding suggests a more proximal colonic source, such as diverticular disease (see p. 218). When fresh rectal bleeding is associated with mucus and very little faecal material, the diagnosis is usually inflammatory bowel disease.

Occult blood loss

Occult blood loss is usually found in a patient who has presented with a hypochromic microcytic anaemia and who may have few gastrointestinal symptoms. Occult blood loss may result from lesions in the upper alimentary tract, e.g. carcinoma of the stomach, or classically from lesions of the lower alimentary tract such as carcinoma of the caecum or ascending colon. The detection of occult blood depends on the fact that certain substances such as benzidine, orthotoluidine and guaiac are oxidised in the presence of blood to form a blue compound. Because of possible carcinogenic properties, benzidine and orthotoluidine have been withdrawn. Occult blood is now detected by the less sensitive guaiac test, which is claimed to be able to detect intestinal blood loss of the order of 10 ml per day. The specimen of stool is spread on guaiac-impregnated filter paper and if a blue colour develops on addition of 2 drops of a solution of hydrogen peroxide the text is positive.

EPIDEMIOLOGY

A yearly admission rate of around 120 per 100 000 population may be expected and 25% of these patients will have bled sufficiently to drop their haemoglobin below 7.0 g/dl. There is surprisingly little seasonal variation, but in Scotland the highest referral rate is January, and Monday is the busiest day. Approximately 70% of patients will settle on conservative measures after the first bleed, and 30% will proceed to emergency or early surgery because of continuing bleeding. The main challenge is to identify these patients at an early stage and refer them for surgery.

Despite improved blood transfusion facilities, anaesthetic, surgical and medical expertise, there has been little improvement in the overall prognosis for major alimentary bleeding in the past 30 years. Reported mortality from massive gastrointestinal haemorrhage varies considerably from 5–50%, with most representative series quoting 8–15%. Blood loss from 'stress' ulceration associated with extensive burns or infection carries a high mortality. In the past decade, however, the appreciation of the need for an energetic team approach to the clinical problem has led to reports from one or two centres of strikingly reduced mortality (around 2%).

CAUSES OF PROFUSE BLEEDING

Upper Alimentary Tract

Considerable differences in the pattern of pathologies responsible for gastrointestinal bleeding occur throughout the world. Although portal hypertension with variceal bleeding is a relatively rare cause in the United Kingdom, up to 15% of patients will have this condition in Australia, USA and some parts of Europe. Duodenal ulcer (Fig. 14.1) is, however, the most common pathology, particularly in the young, with gastric ulcer becoming increasingly important in the 6th decade and later. Sometimes coincidental pathologies make it difficult to ascertain which is the source of bleeding. For example, up to 30% of patients with portal hypertension will be bleeding from lesions other than their varices. The importance of gastric irritants (aspirin, phenylbutazone, indomethacin and other nonsteroidal anti-inflammatory drugs, corticosteroids, and alcohol) is accepted through clinical experience but is difficult to prove. There is some evidence that the effects of some of these (e.g. alcohol and aspirin) may be cumulative. The

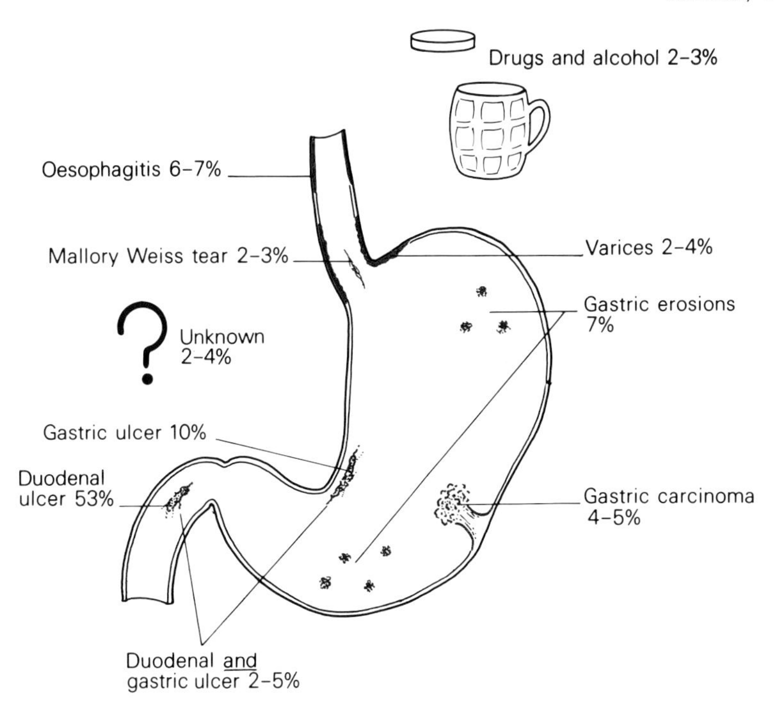

Fig. 14.1 *Common causes of upper gastrointestinal bleeding.*

widespread introduction of fibre-optic endoscopy has shown that the frequency of bleeding from oesophagitis and Mallory–Weiss tear (see p. 320) is much greater than was formerly appreciated, perhaps accounting for 10% of all cases.

Rarer causes of upper alimentary bleeding include aorto-duodenal fistulae associated with aortic aneurysms or aortic grafts, Meckel's diverticulum, pseudoxanthoma elasticum, hereditary haemorrhagic telangiectasia and haemobilia secondary to liver trauma. Systemic disorders, including renal failure, myelomatosis, or diffuse intravascular coagulation (DIC) may occasionally present as gastrointestinal bleeding from gastric erosions and are usually easily recognised by their associated signs.

Lower Alimentary Tract

In the absence of haemorrhoids, massive haemorrhage from the large bowel, especially in elderly patients, is likely to be due to diverticular disease (Fig. 14.2), bleeding being due to the rupture of an arteriosclerotic vessel in the neck of the diverticulum. The increasing use of angiographic techniques has shown that up to 20% of patients, especially

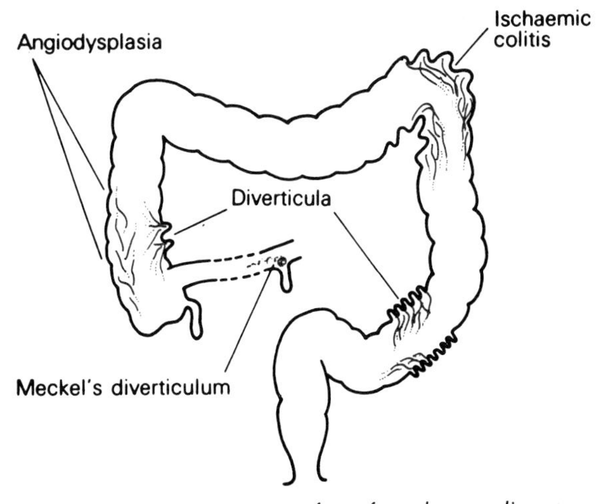

Fig. 14.2 *Common causes of profuse lower alimentary haemorrhage.*

from the 7th decade onwards, may be expected to bleed from vascular ectasia (angiodysplasia), usually found in the ascending colon. These lesions may be missed on resected specimens unless special pathological techniques involving silicone arterial injection are used. The earliest lesions consist of dilated submucosal veins; later lesions consist of dilated thin-walled ectatic veins, venules and capillaries replacing the normal mucosa and extending over an area of 1–10 mm^2. Often these lesions are multiple. Ischaemic colitis (see p. 218) usually affects the elderly, and the ischaemic lesions are commonly found in the region of the splenic flexure, where they can give rise to profuse haemorrhage. Rare causes of profuse bleeding from the lower alimentary tract include carcinoma of the colon, inflammatory bowel disease, dysentery, other infective diarrhoeas, and radiation proctitis. Potential causes of severe rectal bleeding will vary according to the age of the patient (Table 14.1).

Even after extensive investigation there remains a small group of patients (3–4%) who bleed profusely and repeatedly and in whom the source of bleeding cannot be identified even at autopsy.

Table 14.1
Causes of Severe Rectal Haemorrhage in Different Age Groups

Infancy and childhood	Meckel's diverticulum Juvenile polyps Haemangioma
Youth and middle age	Inflammatory bowel disease Endometriosis Typhoid Small bowel neoplasm (Peptic ulcer) (Haemorrhoids)
Older patients	Diverticular disease Angiodysplasia Ischaemic colitis Aorto-intestinal fistula (Carcinoma) (Coagulation disorder) (Drugs, e.g. chemotherapy)

Brackets indicate unusual causes.

CLINICAL PRESENTATION

The patient's response to blood loss depends largely on the rate and volume of loss. Other important considerations are fluid and electrolyte depletion, age and coincidental cardiovascular disease.

Acute Severe Blood Loss

This is usually defined as the loss of 1500 ml of blood, or 25% of the circulating blood volume, within a period of several minutes to several hours.

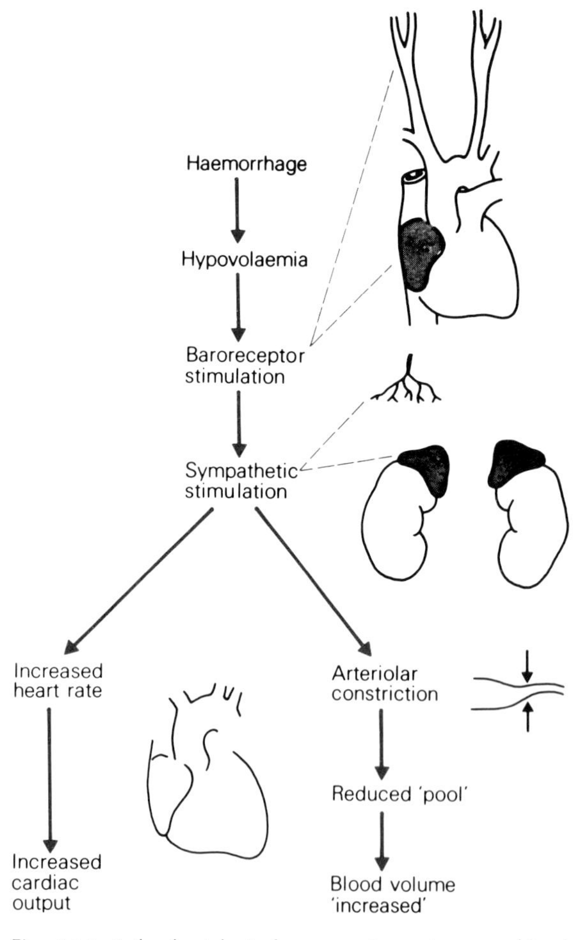

Fig. 14.3 *Pathophysiological response to acute severe blood loss – early.*

This mode of presentation is the one least likely to be missed because bleeding will manifest as profuse haematemesis or melaena, or both, and induces sufficient anxiety in the patient and relatives to ensure early referral to medical services. Prompt admission to hospital is essential.

Pathophysiological response to acute severe blood loss

Serious blood loss leads to a series of nonspecific cardiovascular responses (assuming this ability is not impaired by the presence of cardiovascular disease or of drugs such as anticholinergics and β-blockers likely to modify normal cardiac responses). As central blood volume falls, baroreceptors (Fig. 14.3) and volume-receptors are stimulated, resulting in an increase in output of catecholamines from the adrenal medulla and from the sympathetic nerve endings. This produces splanchnic and peripheral vasoconstriction with maintenance of systemic blood pressure and preservation of blood supply to vital centres in the brain and myocardium, and initially to the renal circulation. The spasm induced in the wall of the bleeding artery may be sufficient to reduce or even stop gastrointestinal haemorrhage. If this occurs, the second wave of compensatory mechanisms, which are hormonally mediated, come into play (Fig. 14.4). These include the release of antidiuretic hormone and aldosterone, acting to restore blood volume by withdrawal of extravascular fluid and reduced urine flow. The resultant expansion of circulating blood volume leads to a reduction in

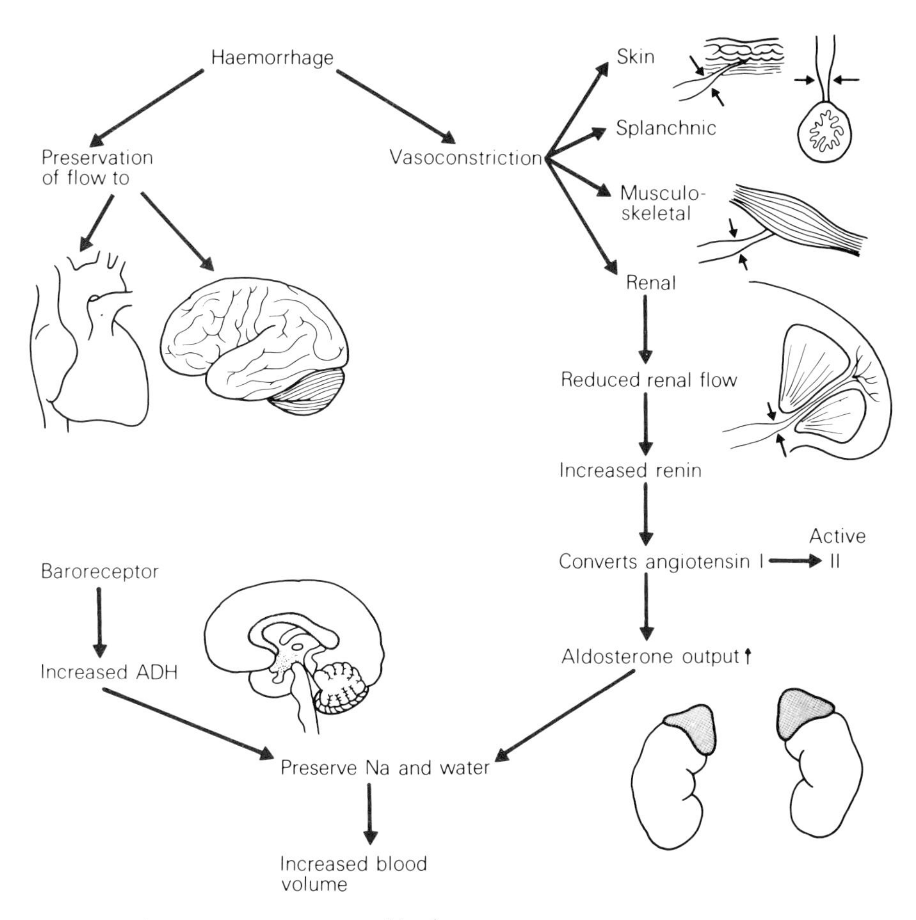

Fig. 14.4 *Pathophysiological response to acute severe blood loss – secondary mechanisms.*

haemoglobin concentration, with a fall in haematocrit and reduced oxygen carrying capacity. The patient then experiences quite marked thirst. In response to the stress of bleeding, the haemopoietic system reacts with an abrupt rise in white-cell count, and frequently with a rise in the circulating platelet count. (The marrow increases red-cell production only relatively slowly over the ensuing weeks, with peripheral reticulocytosis and gradual restoration of haemoglobin concentration.)

With continuing or severe blood loss the above compensatory mechanisms intensify and the patient enters a stage of haemorrhagic shock. Because of continuing output of catecholamines, heart rate is increased and peripheral vasoconstriction continues. The skin becomes cold and clammy and initially pale because there is minimal arterial blood flow. Because of the loss of blood volume, and the consequent reduction in venous return (Fig. 14.5), cardiac output and blood pressure both fall, thereby compounding the effects of peripheral vasoconstriction and further compromising tissue perfusion. It is therefore important to recognise that fall in mean and diastolic blood pressure is a late sign of haemorrhagic shock. The cerebral and coronary circulations are relatively well preserved, but the initial protection of the renal circulation is lost and, because of this, renal perfusion is reduced and urine output falls. The patient's initial anxiety increases as part of the shock process and, to increase oxygen supply, the respiratory rate rises. As peripheral perfusion and oxygen supply fall, tissues convert from aerobic to anaerobic metabolism and a metabolic acidosis results. This stimulates the respiratory centre to produce a further rise in respiratory rate. In the normal control of the micro-circulation, arterioles supply blood to a capillary bed. As the cells in one part of the capillary bed require oxygen for metabolism, this part of the bed opens by vasodilatation whilst other areas, whose oxygen needs have been satisfied, close down (Fig. 14.6). This results in a fluctuation of supply to various parts of the capillary bed, although the arteriolar supply remains relatively constant. In haemorrhagic shock (Fig. 14.7), arteriolar vasoconstriction results in

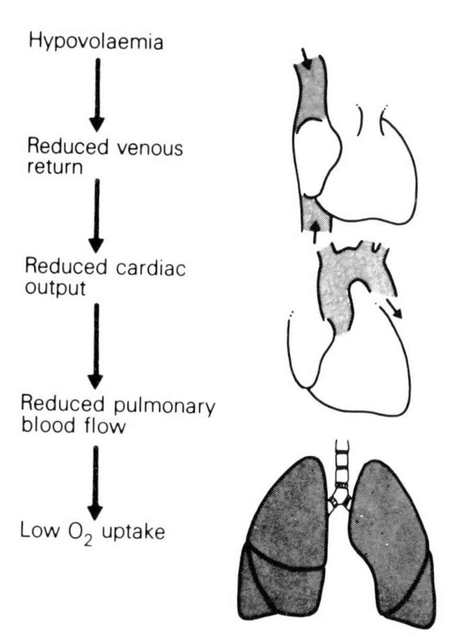

Fig. 14.5 *Pathophysiological response to acute severe blood loss – haemorrhagic shock.*

reduction of blood supply to the capillaries but, as more and more parts of the capillary bed become hypoxic, more areas vasodilate in an attempt to supply the oxygen needs of the cells, and a state of stagnant hypoxia of the capillary bed eventually results. At this stage the previous peripheral pallor becomes peripheral cyanosis as more capillary beds become filled with reduced haemoglobin. Finally, in response to haemorrhagic shock, the oxyhaemoglobin dissociation curve shows a net shift to the left. This reflects an effective mechanism of ensuring the supply of oxygen to tissues despite varying concentrations of haemoglobin and varying oxygen tensions. The affinity of the haemoglobin molecule for oxygen therefore increases, and the supply of oxygen to peripheral tissue is further reduced Resuscitation at this stage is still possible and low mortality should be the rule.

Unless the changes described are rapidly reversed by adequate resuscitation, there is breakdown of cellular and subcellular membranes (in response to hypoxia and acidosis) with the release of multiple damaging toxins. The patient is now at serious risk of developing refractory shock, which carries a mortality of between 50–95% irrespec-

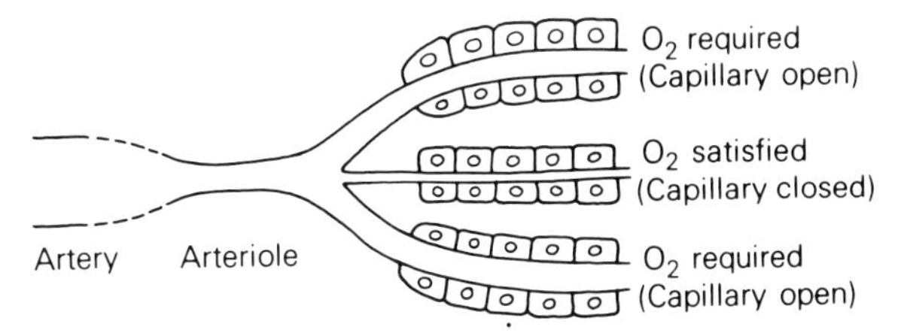

Fig. 14.6 *Normal capillary bed.*

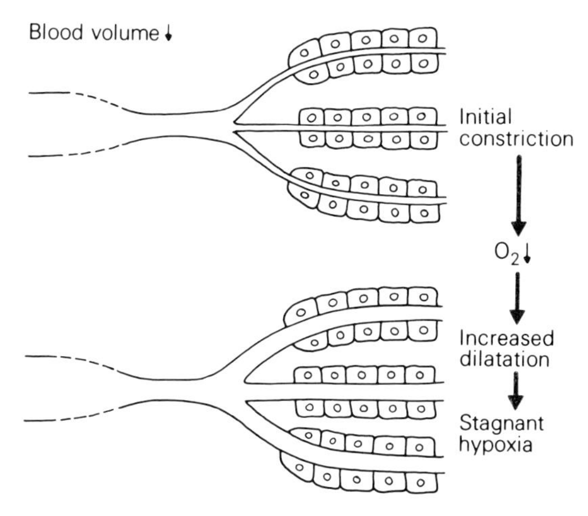

Fig. 14.7 *Capillary changes in haemorrhagic shock.*

tive of further treatment. The elderly patient, especially, now becomes extremely vulnerable to the cumulative effects of coexisting arteriosclerosis, liver, heart and renal disease.

Chronic Blood Loss from the Alimentary Tract

This is the group of patients presenting the greatest diagnostic difficulty and only by maintaining the highest index of suspicion of chronic alimentary blood loss will it be possible to avoid overlooking gastrointestinal pathology (Fig. 14.8).

Most commonly these patients present with vague signs and symptoms due to insidiously developing anaemia, and they often have no alimentary symptoms. Haemorrhage is insufficient to cause the dramatic physiological compensatory signs seen in more acute blood loss or in haemorrhagic shock. It is slowly replaced by a shift of fluid from the extravascular into the vascular space, resulting in an insidious reduction of haemoglobin level and haematocrit. The marrow responds by producing immature red cells and reticulocytes, which are found in increasing quantities in the blood, but this compensatory mechanism gradually fails to maintain the haemoglobin level.

These patients may have melaena, but this valuable clinical sign is often masked by the prescription of iron supplements before the nature of the anaemia or its cause have been defined. The patient often incorrectly attributes his black stool to his iron therapy. Iron therapy does not, however, produce a positive test for occult blood. It may be necessary for many stool samples to be examined to record a positive test, because of the relative insensitivity of the guaiac test.

Iron deficiency due to chronic blood loss may produce clinically recognisable anaemia, glossitis, koilonychia (spoon-shaped deformity of the nails) and, very occasionally, dysphagia associated with a pharyngeal web (so-called Patterson–Kelly–Brown syndrome or Plummer – Vinson syndrome). When the haemoglobin falls below 8–10 g/dl, elderly patients may develop myocardial ischaemic chest pain or signs or cardiac failure because of the combined effects of anaemia and arteriosclerosis of the coronary arteries. The combined effects of anaemia and arteriosclerosis may result in poor supply of oxygen to the brain, producing episodes of unsteadiness or syncope.

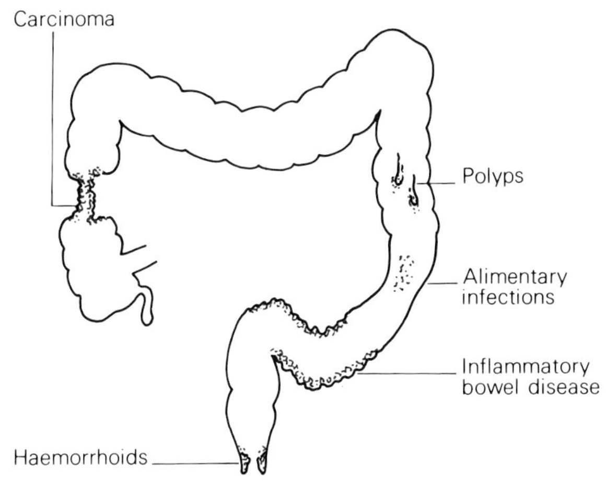

Fig. 14.8 *Common causes of chronic lower alimentary haemorrhage (see also Fig. 3.15).*

Minimal Gastrointestinal Blood Loss

This may occur from the upper or lower gastrointestinal tract.

Upper alimentary tract

Many patients are correctly admitted to hospital following reputed vomiting of 'coffee-ground' material, or a very small quantity of fresh blood. Provided there is no evidence of further bleeding the majority of these patients do not require immediate investigation or treatment. Some will be shown to have drug-induced gastric erosions or a Mallory–Weiss tear. It is important to identify these patients so that avoidance of alcohol or the precipitating medication can be advised.

Lower alimentary tract

Whilst the majority of patients with minimal bleeding from the lower alimentary tract will have haemorrhoids, or fissures, the diagnosis must never rest on the history alone (See Chapter 3). Rectal examination, proctoscopy and sigmoidoscopy must be carried out if an early rectal carcinoma is to be diagnosed.

MANAGEMENT OF ALIMENTARY BLEEDING

All but those patients with trivial blood loss should be admitted to hospital, where their care is best undertaken, ideally in specially-designed premises, by the team of general physician/gastroenterologist, surgeon and radiologist. Because of the diversity of presentation it is inevitable that the processes of clinical assessment and resuscitation will run in parallel with investigation and definitive treatment. Under no circumstances should investigative procedures (other than emergency lifesaving laparotomy) be allowed to take precedence over effective resuscitation.

Value of Clinical History

Whilst obviously important, the value of the history taken from the patient, his general practitioner, relatives or friends is limited because it gives little guidance as to the precise source of blood loss. Some judgement can, however, be made as to whether bleeding is arising from the upper or lower alimentary tract. A previous history of peptic ulcer-type symptoms along with a positive family history in a young man suggests duodenal ulceration as the likely cause. The presence of (or a previous history of) jaundice raises the possibility of portal hypertension with bleeding varices. A careful drug and alcohol intake history may suggest the possibility of varices or gastric erosions. The main value of the history, however, is to help assess the duration and severity of the bleed, and to establish the severity of symptoms related to anaemia and coexistent pathology which may require early treatment, such as cardiac failure or coagulation difficulties resulting from prescription of anticoagulants.

Immediate General Management of Major Bleedng

The urgent need is to stabilise the patient's clinical state and to decide at an early stage if and when surgical intervention is required. This decision may be reached logically and rapidly through a series of interrelated steps (Fig. 14.9)

1. assessment of the severity of the bleeding episode
2. decision on the need for transfusion
3. judgement of when the patient's condition is stable (see Chapter 3).
4. detection of the source of bleeding.

Occasionally blood loss is so catastrophic that all efforts must be directed immediately to resuscitation and urgent laparotomy.

Assessment of severity of bleeding episode

When bleeding is profuse, the clinical history is of limited value in assessing volumes of haematemeses and/or melaena.

Physical examination is much more rewarding. If signs of shock (as described above) are present, it

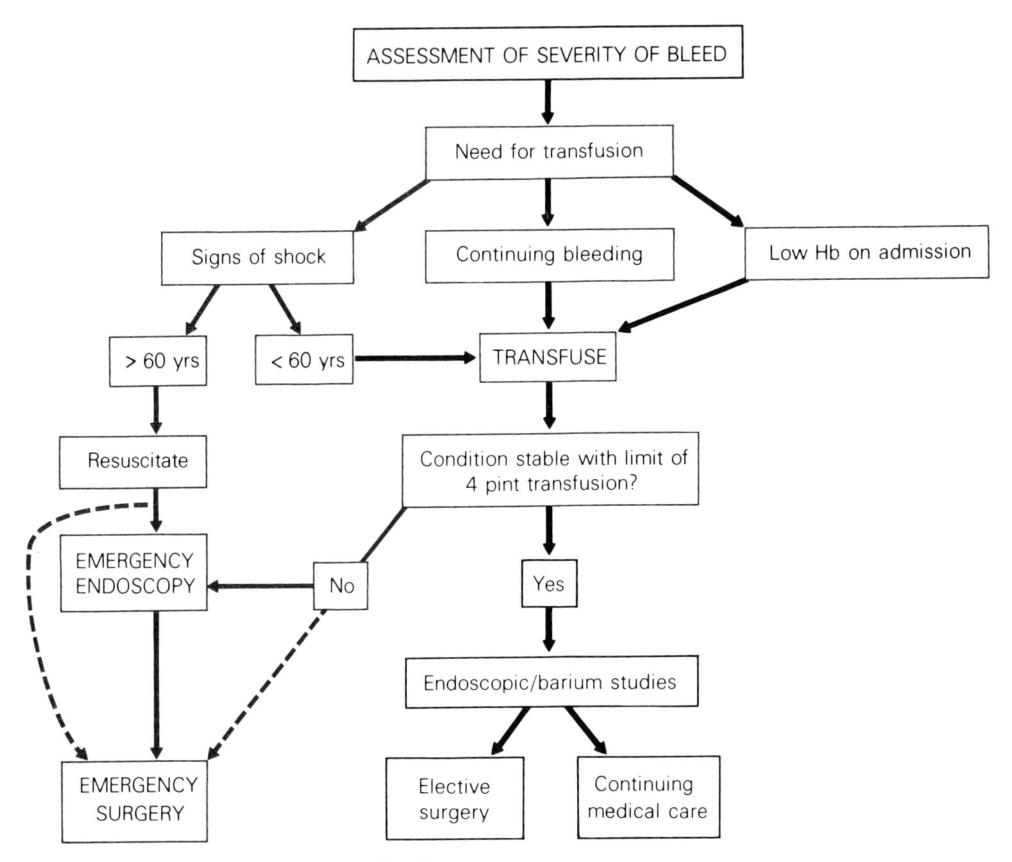

Fig. 14.9 *Management of upper alimentary bleed.*

can be assumed that the patient has lost at least 25% of his or her blood volume. In the absence of shock, continuing tachycardia and active bowel sounds suggest continuing bleeding. For reasons previously explained (p. 312), the measurement of blood pressure in this regard is less helpful. Continuing fresh rectal bleeding suggests major haemorrhage. Hepatomegaly, splenomegly, ascites, spider naevi and other signs of chronic liver disease suggest portal hypertension with varices and the likelihood of a major bleed. At this stage rarer signs, e.g. the lip and tongue lesions of hereditary haemorrhagic telangiectasia and the skin changes and angioid streaks on the retina of the patient with pseudoxanthoma elasticum, may be noted. Evidence of bleeding elsewhere may suggest coagulation disorders, especially in children, or alert the clinician to the possibility of warfarin overdosage; in either situation, once started, bleeding is likely to be major. Haemodilution is not likely to be complete at this stage and the haemoglobin estimation may be misleading: if it is already low, the episode of bleeding has been major and has occurred over a longer period than perhaps initially appeared.

Indication for transfusion

Signs of haemorrhagic shock indicate the urgent need to reestablish an adequate circulation to vital organs (Fig. 14.10). This must take precedence over all investigations. Whilst quickly establishing fast-running intravenous infusions (see p. 316), blood is taken for cross-matching and sent urgently to the blood transfusion service. (It will be of later value in the management of the patient if some of the original sample is also used for haematological analysis and estimation of the blood urea and

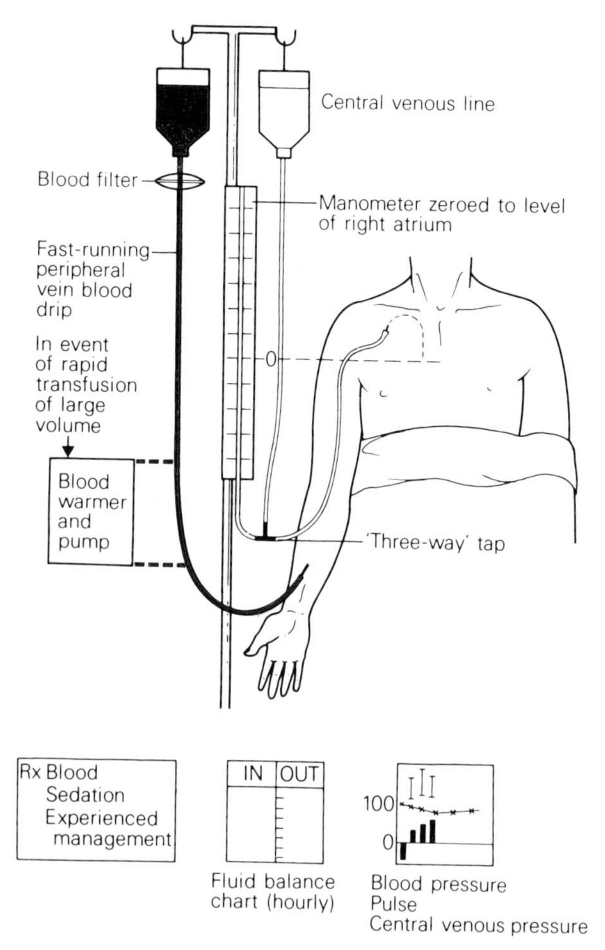

Fig. 14.10 *Immediate management of profuse alimentary haemorrhage.*

electrolytes.) An efficiently working central venous line, inserted via the right subclavian or basilic vein and x-ray-screened into the right atrium, gives useful information on central venous pressure (CVP) and is especially valuable in the frail, the elderly, and those with massive gastrointestinal bleeding. Transfusion should be sufficient to maintain a CVP of at least 5–10 cm of water above the midaxillary line (to coincide with the level of the right atrium) with the patient lying flat. *In extremis,* the central venous line may afford a valuable additional route of infusion. For the reasons previously mentioned it is important to ensure an adequate urinary output by adequate transfusion and this is best monitored by inserting a urinary catheter and charting hourly urine volumes. An hourly urine output of 40 ml or more is acceptable. In the elderly patient, or in the patient with cardiac disease, there is a real danger of enthusiastic overtransfusion in response to a brisk gastrointestinal bleed. This should be avoidable if the patient's response to transfusion is carefully monitored; the CVP line is especially valuable in this regard. Sedation is nearly always necessary to help allay the patient's anxiety. Pulse should be recorded at half-hourly intervals, CVP at hourly intervals, and BP at 2-hourly intervals.

Continuing bleeding, as evidenced by continuing haematemes or melaena, persisting tachycardia, and active bowel sounds, is also an indication for blood transfusion. This clinical situation is less dire but it must be appreciated that the patient's condition remains unpredictable and precarious. Early and adequate transfusion is mandatory if mortality rates are to be reduced. In the case of upper gastrointestinal bleeding, the advent of fibre-optic endoscopy has proved useful in indicating whether or not bleeding has stopped but it must be remembered that this is a dynamc clinical situation and bleeding may begin again rapidly and unpredictably. Fibre-optic endoscopy has shown that absence of blood in nasogastric aspirate does not mean that upper gastrointestinal bleeding has ceased. Moreover, the standard nasogastric tube is of quite insufficient calibre for efficient aspiration of blood clot from the stomach. Fibre-optic endoscopy has therefore largely superseded the nasogastric tube in detecting continuing blood loss.

A low haemoglobin level (< 8 g/dl) on admission to hospital (when haemodilution will probably be incomplete) suggests that blood loss has been more chronic and severe than perhaps first judged. Early blood transfusion is again indicated.

Infusion Fluids

Ideally, carefully cross-matched whole blood should be transfused to replace the estimated loss.

This inevitably introduces a delay of the order of an hour, and in this intervening period it may be necessary to take urgent measures to reestablish an adequate circulation. In dire necessity it may be essential to transfuse 'universal donor' Group O Rhesus negative blood. In the slightly less urgent situation the circulation may be temporarily maintained by infusions of mixtures of crystalloid and colloid (e.g. dextran or plasma protein substiute).

In patients with cardiorespiratory disease it may be necessary to transfuse concentrated or 'packed' red-cell infusions and to prevent fluid overload by simultaneous administration of intravenous diuretic (e.g. frusemide).

Water and electrolyte replacement is achieved by infusing 5% dextrose and 0.9% saline or Hartmann's solution. When a large volume of blood has been transfused (4 units or more) there is a theoretical risk of circulating calcium becoming unavailable because of its reaction with citrate in the transfused blood. It is then recommended that 10 ml of 10% calcium gluconate be administered slowly into a separate vein (not into the infusion fluid, to avoid blood clotting in the intravenous cannula).

There is no compelling evidence that transfusion of concentrates of clotting factors normally elaborated in the liver (factors II, V, VII, IX, and X) will stop or reduce bleeding in patients with liver disease. Transfusion of fresh blood or fresh frozen plasma (which also contain these clotting factors) should theoretically be advantageous but again this is not proven.

Transfusion of platelet concentrates may be of temporary help in helping to stop haemorrhage, by initiating clot formation in those clinical states associated with low platelet counts and/or deficient platelet function (e.g. in patients with cirrhosis of liver or blood dyscrasias).

When is the patient's condition stable?

When the patient's pulse rate begins to slow, when urinary output is maintained, and when the patient's BP and CVP remain in the normal range, it can be assumed that the circulatory effects of the bleeding episode have been controlled. Coexisting or associated pathologies such as cardiac failure should by this time be controlled with appropriate therapy. If circulatory stability, as indicated by the above parameters, has not been achieved after transfusion of 4 pints of blood, there is good evidence that early surgery will reduce mortality.

When and what investigations?

With the exception of the few patients who require immediate surgery, investigation into the precise cause of the bleeding should be delayed until the patient's condition is stable. The effect of blood loss on cardiac and renal function in particular can be assessed before the source of bleeding is known.

Blood estimations include measurement of haemoglobin. The value and limitations of this have already been discussed. A platelet count and, when indicated, a differential white-cell count, will disclose important disorders likely to be associated with deficient clotting. In the absence of clinical signs, abnormal 'liver function' tests will indicate underlying liver disease and may give some idea of its severity. If the blood urea is raised soon after the onset of bleeding this may indicate poor renal function. A later estimation following major gastrointestinal bleeding will, even with normal renal function, show a rising urea because of the digestion of blood in the gut.

An electrocardiograph and, when the patient has been resuscitated, a chest x-ray, are essential in the elderly or when cardiorespiratory disease is suspected from the initial general examination.

The choice of investigations to be employed in the search for the source of bleeding will depend on local expertise. With upper alimentary bleeding, good barium meal examination may give a high diagnostic yield; it is now generally accepted that upper gastrointestinal fibre-optic endoscopy, if performed within 24 hours of the bleeding episode, will diagnose the source of haemorrhage in approximately 90% of individuals. To prove that the knowledge so obtained reduces mortality or morbidity is difficult. There is however little doubt that the demonstration of oesophageal or fundal varices, erosive gastritis or gastric ulcer will influence the future management of the patient. Moreover, there is now some evidence to suggest that ulcer craters which are seen at endoscopy to be deep with blood-clot or visible vessels in their base are likely to rebleed with high mortality. This especially applies to deep gastric ulcers in the elderly. Such patients, it is argued, should proceed to early surgery.

Bleeding from the large bowel is a major diagnostic and therapeutic challenge. The source may be felt or seen at rectal examination, proctoscopy and sigmoidoscopy (in the case of haemorrhoids, inflammatory bowel disease, rectal polyps or carcinoma). Barium enema examination is not likely to be helpful in massive colonic bleeding, frequently indicating only diverticula whose relevance is often difficult to decide. Furthermore, in the event of rapid colonic bleeding, the presence of barium in the colon delays other investigations. When blood loss is not severe, polyps, inflammatory bowel disease, carcinoma and ischaemic segments may be diagnosed by barium enema.

Colonoscopy has been disappointing in helping to elucidate the cause of brisk bleeding and, until the recent introduction of instruments with wide suction channels, did not offer significant advantage over good double contrast barium enema examination. Occasionally the lesions of angiodysplasia may be seen and can be fulgarised but, as with diverticular disease, unless they are actively bleeding their significance may not be

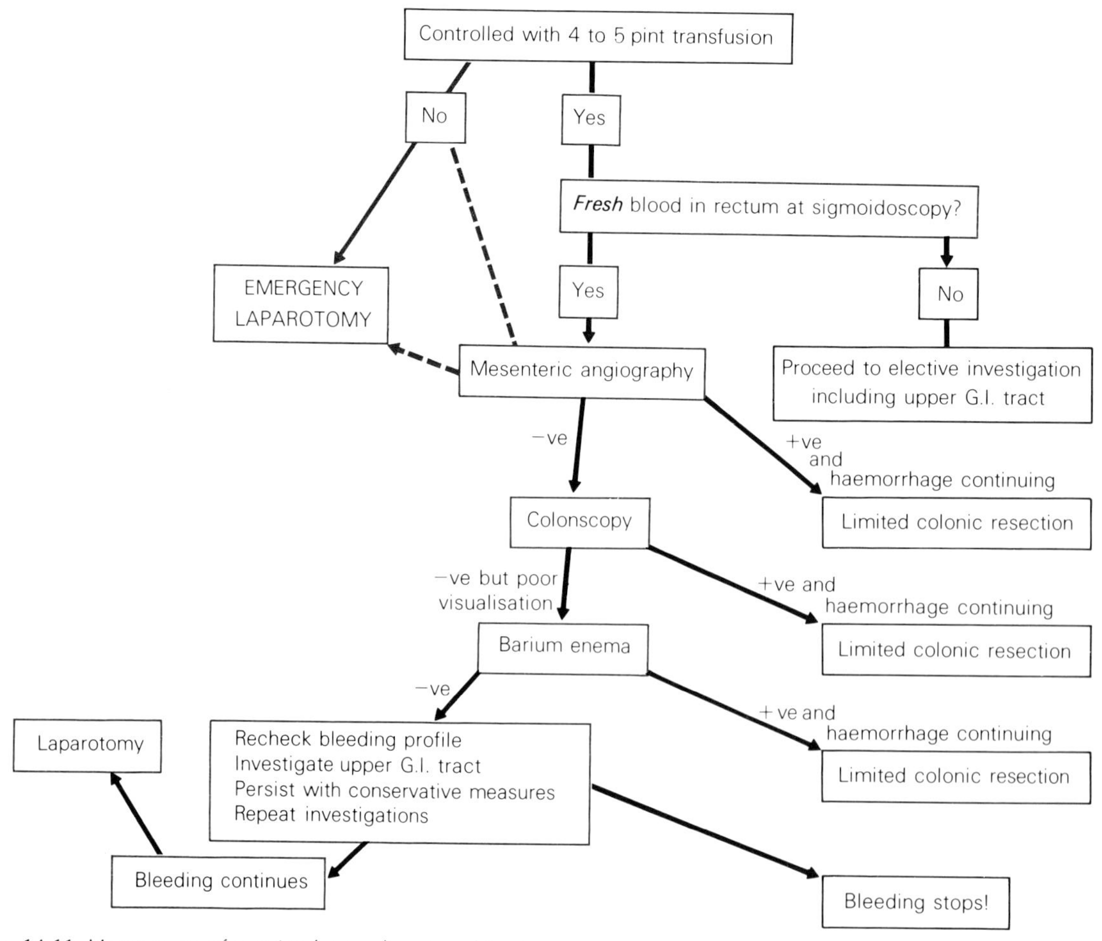

Fig. 14.11 *Management of massive lower alimentary bleed.*

clear. Polyps may be removed by diathermy via the colonoscope. Occasionally colonoscopy will detect mild but extensive inflammatory bowel disease not demonstrable on barium enema. A plan for the investigation of large-bowel haemorrhage is outlined in Fig. 14.11.

Radio-isotopic scanning techniques using technetium- or chromium-labelled red cells may help in diagnosing obscure gastrointestinal blood loss – e.g. bleeding from a Meckel's diverticulum which, after intravenous injection of technetium, may show up as a 'hot' spot under the gamma camera if the diverticulum contains functioning gastric mucosa. Chromium-labelled red cells may be reinjected into the patient and, if blood loss into the bowel is sufficiently rapid, the general area of bleeding will be indicated by a 'hot' spot under the gamma camera.

Perhaps the most significant advance in the detection of the source of gastrointestinal bleeding, and especially in the large bowel, has been the development of selective arteriography (Fig. 14.12). It is now possible to catheterise selectively the coeliac axis and the superior and inferior mesenteric arteries. This requires practice and skill as well as the appropriate radiographic apparatus. Under these circumstances it is possible to detect most sources of blood loss, provided the rate of blood loss is of the order of 2.5 ml per minute or more. In addition, it is possible to use this technique to stop bleeding by local injection of gel foam or fibrin particles and thus allow adequate resuscitation of the patient before definitive surgical treatment.

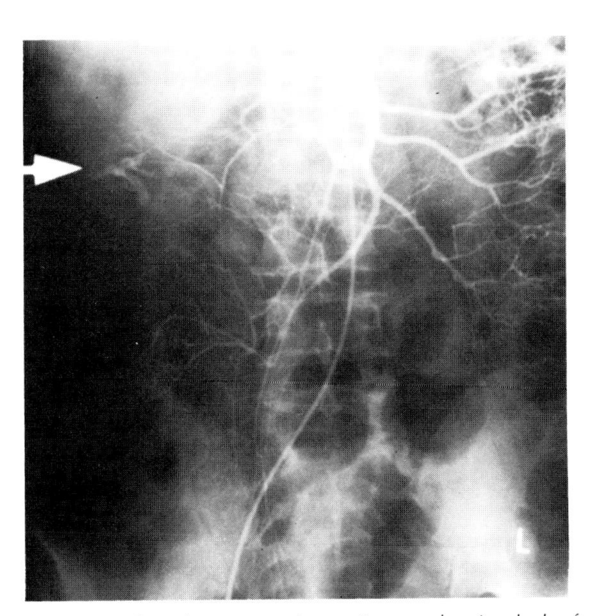

Fig. 14.12 *Superior mesenteric arteriogram showing leak of medium into hepatic flexure of colon (arrow) from a bleeding diverticulum. Confirmed at emergency right colectomy.*

Decision time

Having controlled the major problems posed by gastrointestinal haemorrhage, and having attempted to establish the source of bleeding, it is then possible to decide whether emergency surgery, elective surgery, or continued 'medical' management is appropriate.

Emergency surgery. This is indicated when there is life-threatening haemorrhage as described above, and especially in the elderly (over 60 years), and may have to be undertaken before the source of blood loss has been established. Such a decision is difficult, requires considerable experience and skill, and should be reached after early consultation between senior medical and surgical staff. Likely sources of blood loss are duodenal and gastric ulceration, varices (see p. 321), severe erosive gastritis, angiodysplasia, and diverticular disease of the colon. To find the source of bleeding in the latter two cases may be exceedingly difficult, and emergency total colectomy may be the only life-saving measure. With blood loss from a duodenal ulcer, the usual procedure is to oversew the bleeding vessel and perform a vagotomy and pyloroplasty. When bleeding occurs from a gastric ulcer, the choice of surgery will depend on the experience of the surgeon, the site of the ulcer, and the fitness of the patient (who is often old) for operation. The treatment of choice is still partial gastrectomy but sometimes circumstances dictate oversewing of the ulcer combined with a vagotomy and pyloroplasty. When bleeding is from severe erosive gastritis which has not responded to medical treatment (see p. 320), the surgeon may be forced into performing a partial or total gastrectomy to save the patient's life.

When in the large bowel the primary pathology is readily identified and is considered unlikely to respond to conservative treatment (e.g. carcinoma or solitary rectal ulcer), early surgical treatment is indicated.

Elective surgery. When a patient has bled from a gastric or duodenal ulcer on more than one occasion, there is good evidence to indicate that he or she should proceed to elective surgery. This should be carried out 4 or 5 weeks after the second bleed since operating within a week to 10 days of a gastrointestinal bleed significantly increases the risk of pulmonary thromboembolism. When bleeding has stopped, these patients should be allowed home, encouraged to be physically active, and come to elective surgery at a later date. Except for the exclusions mentioned above, the same procedure applies to colonic pathologies.

Continuing medical management. There is at present no acceptable evidence to suggest that drugs have a major part to play in stopping gastrointestinal haemorrhage. The only exception to this is the treatment with cimetidine of gastric erosions in patients with liver failure. However, once the effects of blood loss have been corrected and bleeding has stopped, the standard 'medical' treatment for peptic ulceration (see Chapter 5), diverticular disease of the colon, ischaemic colitis, and inflammatory bowel disease (see Chapters 9 and 10) is instituted.

When to feed? The pioneering work of Meulengracht and Sir Francis Avery Jones showed that early feeding reduced the mortality associated with upper gastrointestinal bleeding. It is now accepted practice for patients to be started on a bland diet as soon as it is clear that surgical treatment is not required (usually within 24 hours) and returned to a normal nutritious diet as soon as possible thereafter.

It is sound policy to tell all patients in whom aspirin or other nonsteroidal anti-inflammatory drugs have been implicated to avoid all such drugs in future.

The role of alcohol and cigarette smoking in upper gastrointestinal bleeding remains debatable, and therefore advice on moderation can only be given in general terms (see Chapter 5).

It is usually possible for all patients who do not require surgical treatment to be fully mobilised and return home within a week to 10 days. They will require a period of convalescence of approximately 3–4 weeks, during which treatment with oral iron supplements should be given.

LESS COMMON CAUSES OF GASTROINTESTINAL HAEMORRHAGE

Gastric and Duodenal Erosions

Gastric erosions are usually associated with the ingestion of gastric irritants, e.g. aspirin and the other nonsteroidal anti-inflammatory drugs and alcohol. The diagnosis is readily made at early endoscopy and the lesions usually rapidly regress with avoidance of the precipitant and the regular prescription of antacids. The 'H_2-blockers' are said to be effective in the erosive gastritis associated with liver failure. Perfusion of the stomach with ice-cold water is sometimes effective in stopping bleeding. Occasionally, surgery is necessary when haemorrhage continues (see p. 319).

Meckel's Diverticulum

This developmental abnormality, situated about 2 feet from the ileocaecal valve (see Chapter 12), occasionally contains ectopic gastric mucosa and may be the site of peptic ulceration. Difficult to diagnose before laparotomy (see above), it usually presents with profuse melaena. The treatment is surgical removal of the diverticulum.

Mallory–Weiss Tear of the Oesophagus

Recognised more frequently since the advent of fibre-optic endoscopy, this usually follows a benign course. A small tear occurs, usually after over indulgence in food or alcohol, at the junction of oesophagus and stomach. Occasionally it may occur spontaneously. Usually the patient retches repeatedly, then vomits food or alcohol followed shortly thereafter by a small quantity of fresh blood. The lesion usually heals spontaneously but occasionally surgical treatment with oversewing is necessary.

Aorto-duodenal Fistula

This fistula between aorta and duodenum is a rare cause of life-threatening gastrointestinal bleeding. Rarely it can occur spontaneously and it can bleed intermittently. Usually it occurs because of expansion of an abdominal aortic aneurysm with eventual leakage into the duodenum, or as leakage from a graft repair of an abdominal aortic aneurysm. Treatment is the repair of the aneurysm or replacement of the graft.

Henoch–Schönlein Purpura (anaphylactoid purpura)

This allergic phenomenon, sometimes following streptococcal throat infection or gastroenteritis, may (especially in children) present as abdominal pain with gastrointestinal bleeding and/or intussusception of the small bowel. The syndrome may be recognised by the purpuric rash occurring predominantly on the buttocks, the lower back, and the extensor aspects of the arms and legs. A horizontal limit to the rash just above the buttocks is usually obvious. The knees and ankles are painful and slightly swollen due to periarticular oedema, and microscopic haematuria will result from the characteristic focal nephritis.

Surgical resection may be necessary for the alimentary lesions. Bed rest usually alleviates the joint pains, and antihistamines may help the skin rash. Steroids are occasionally indicated.

Varices

Bleeding is the main clinical presentation of portal hypertension, and results from blood loss from oesophageal or gastric varices. The causes of portal hypertension include cirrhosis of the liver, hepatic fibrosis (as in schistosomiasis and congenital hepatic fibrosis) and infiltration (such as sarcoidosis and reticulosis), portal vein thrombosis, hepatic vein thrombosis (Budd–Chiari syndrome), and lesions associated with increased hepatic blood flow (e.g. tropical splenomegaly and myelosclerosis). The mechanisms involved are described in Chapter 8, and the patterns of portal venous hypertension in intra- and extra- and post-hepatic obstruction are depicted on Figs 14.13, 14.14 and 14.15. Distortion of intrahepatic portal and hepatic venous channels, and the development of shunts between hepatic artery and the portal vein, both contribute to the development of portal hypertension. The spleen enlarges and its capsule thickens. Collateral circulations develop with spontaneous anastomosis of portal and systemic circulation (see Chapter 8), and these include veins at the lower end of the oesophagus and gastric fundus which form the gastric and oesophageal varices which may bleed; anastomosis between the inferior mesenteric veins and the haemorrhoidal veins may produce haemorrhoids which can bleed profusely. It should be remem-

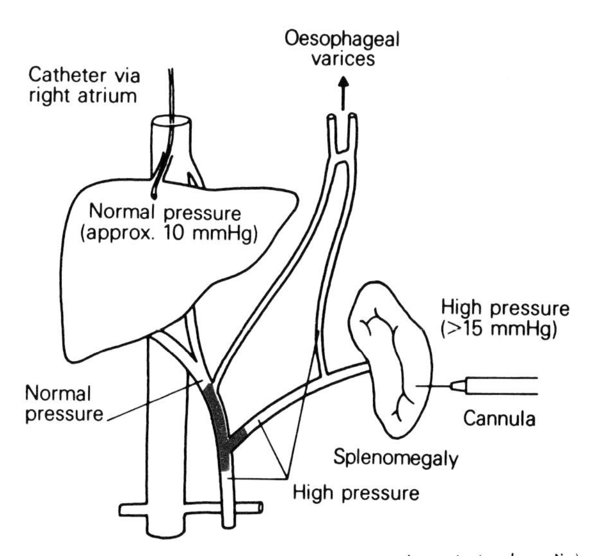

Fig. 14.13 *Portal venous pressure in extrahepatic (prehepatic) block – thrombosed portal vein.*

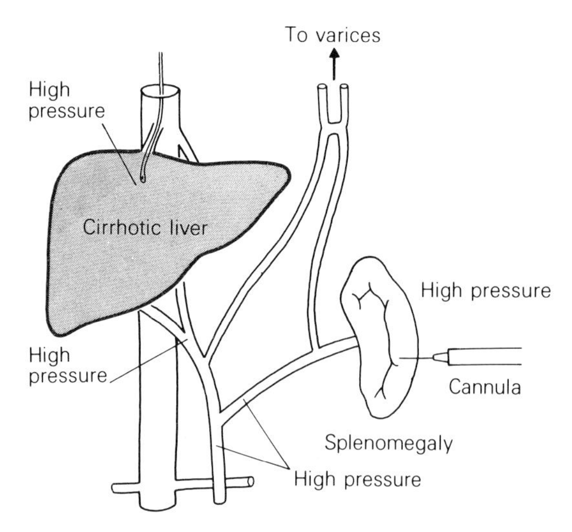

Fig. 14.14 *Portal venous pressure in intrahepatic (hepatic) block – cirrhosis of liver.*

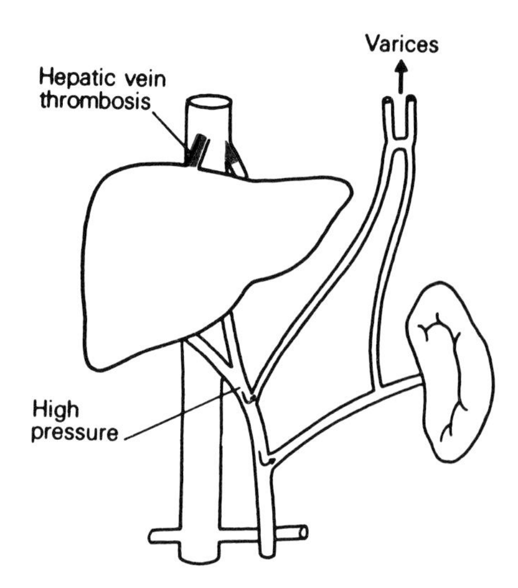

Fig. 14.15 *Portal venous pressure in posthepatic block, e.g. hepatic vein thrombosis (Budd–chiari), long-standing congestive cardiac failure, constrictive pericarditis.*

bered that portal hypertension is relatively rare and haemorrhoids, which are common in adults, rarely have this as their basis.

Clinical presentation of varices

Usually bleeding is profuse, but occasionally it can be relatively trivial and prolonged. As well as the signs of blood loss described above, the patient may well be jaundiced and have the clinical stigmata of chronic liver disease (Chapter 8), and may give a history of jaundice or alcohol abuse. The liver and spleen are often palpable and the patient may exhibit foetor hepaticus.

The diagnosis may be made on barium swallow and meal examination, but is best verified by careful fibre-optic endoscopy. Because up to 30% of patients with portal hypertension may be bleeding from coincidental pathology (e.g. duodenal ulceration or gastric erosions), it is most important to be certain of the source of bleeding. A full blood count will reveal not only anaemia due to haemorrhage but will show leucopenia and thrombocytopenia due to hypersplenism.

Management of bleeding varices

The general management is as defined in the treatment of haemorrhagic shock (p. 315) except that sedation, particularly with opiates, must be avoided. The reasons for this are explained in Chapter 8. Specific measures aimed at controlling variceal haemorrhage are as follows:

It has been shown that posterior pituitary extract (vasopressin), by virtue of its constrictive effect on the smooth muscle of arterioles, reduces both portal and systemic venous pressure. It may be given as a 20-unit infusion in 100 ml of 5% dextrose over a period of 20 minutes, or, more physiologically, as a constant infusion at a rate of about 40 units per hour. Side-effects, especially after bolus infusion in the elderly, are common and include myocardial ischaemic pain, and abdominal colic. It should not therefore be used in the elderly or in those with a history of cardiac disease. A synthetic analogue, glypressin, may be at least equally effective and is said to be free of important side-effects. Unfortunately it is not yet freely available.

Gastric cooling has been shown to be effective in some studies but it needs specialised and rather cumbersome equipment and is not routinely used.

Unless arrest of variceal haemorrhage is rapid, liver function quickly deteriorates and the prognosis is poor. If the above measures are not rapidly effective and the patient is not in irreversible liver failure, it is justifiable to attempt to arrest haemorrhage by using the Sengstaken tube, or one of its variants (Figs 14.16, 14.17). Usually this consists of a quadruple-lumen tube with connections to a gastric and an oesophageal balloon as well as suction openings in the portions of the tube in stomach and oesophagus. The tube is disposable. The balloons should always be checked in water for leaks before the tube is passed via the mouth. A little sedation may be necessary, and it helps if the oropharynx is anaesthetised with a 2% lignocaine spray before beginning. The tube may be passed with the patient sitting up, but it is much safer to do so with the patient in the left lateral position. There is a real danger of aspiration of blood and clots, and so powerful suction should always be to hand. After passing the tube, the balloons are inflated (as in Fig. 14.17) and gentle traction is applied to the tube to maintain its position; the top end of the tube is fixed to the face or head (sometimes with a special helmet). Correct siting of the tube is checked by x-ray. When the tube is in place, a nurse must remain with the patient at all times as there is a risk of the gastric balloon deflating and the tube riding up into the pharynx where, by its bulk, it will cause laryngeal obstruction; in that case, the Sengstaken tube should immediately be transected with a scissors and removed.

Regular recordings of pulse, CVP, BP and urinary output should be made, as in other situations associated with severe haemorrhage. Because of the risk of aspiration, regular chest physiotherapy and broad-spectrum antibiotics are

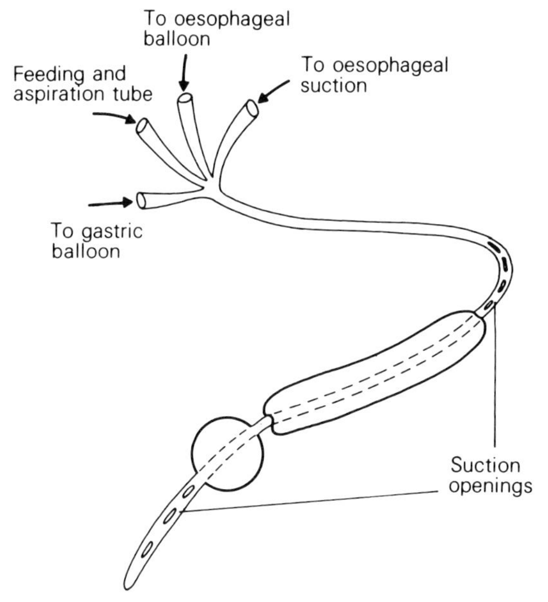

Fig. 14.16 *Modified Sengstaken tube.*

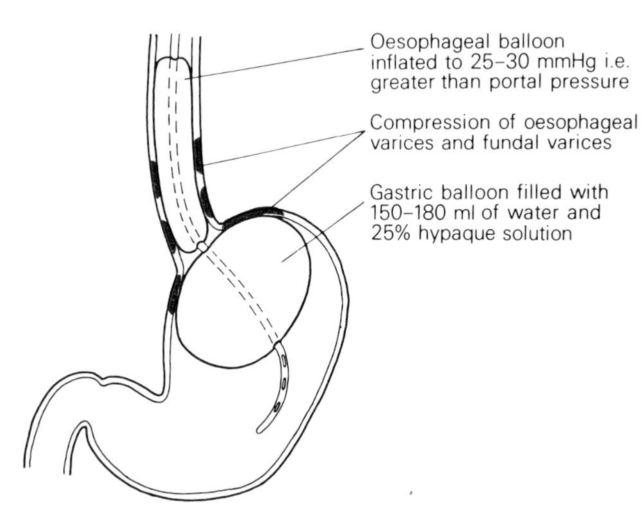

Fig. 14.17 *Inflated Sengstaken tube* in situ *with traction applied.*

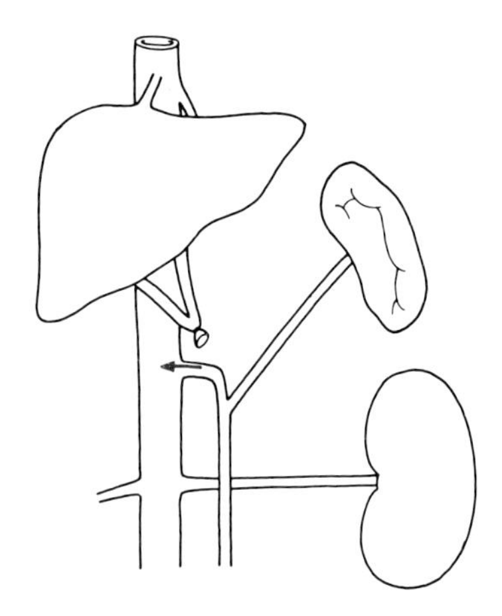

Fig. 14.18 *Portocaval anastomosis (end-to-side).*

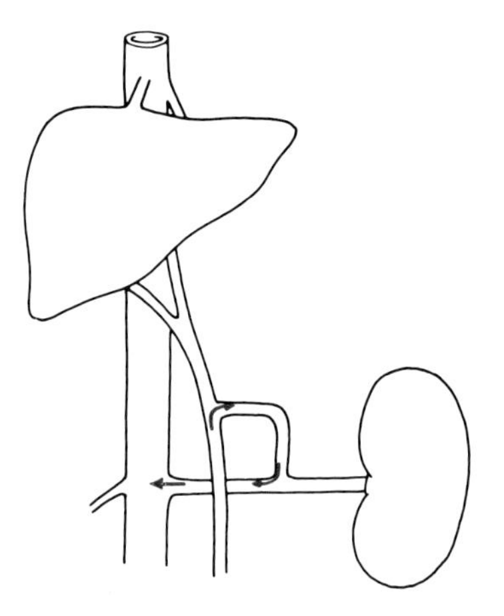

Fig. 14.19 *Splenorenal anastomosis – results are disappointing because of tendency for shunt to clot. Sometimes it is also necessary to remove the left kidney as well as spleen.*

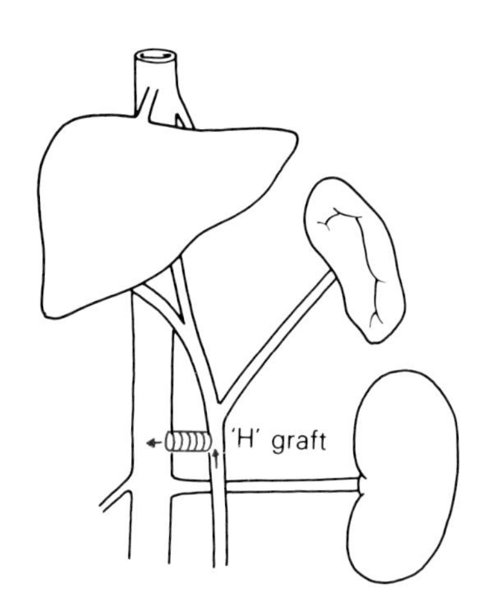

Fig. 14.20 *Mesocaval shunt – results disappointing of tendency for clotting to occur in graft. Has the advantage of being relatively easy to perform.*

necessary. The balloons are kept inflated for up to 24 hours. The oesophageal balloon is then gently deflated, followed by the gastric balloon. The tube is left in place for a further 24 hours and is removed if no further bleeding occurs.

Definitive treatment of the varices is now possible. Several approaches are available but none can claim predictable success.

The two main lines of treatment are decompression of the portal venous system and obliteration of the varices. Decompression operations to reduce portal venous pressure during an episode of acute haemorrhage remain controversial. It is, however, certain that there is no place for prophylactic shunt operations. The various common shunting precedures used are depicted in Figs 14.18 to 14.21. None can claim long-term success, and all have the disadvantage that they increase the amount of naturally-occurring shunting between portal and systemic circulation (see Chapter 8), and increase significantly the risks of hepatic encephalopathy. For a successful shunt operation there must be a patent portal vein, liver function must be adequate with no jaundice, and the serum albumin should be greater than 3 g/l; there should also be no clinical evidence of ascites or encephalopathy. A transcutaneous splenoporto-

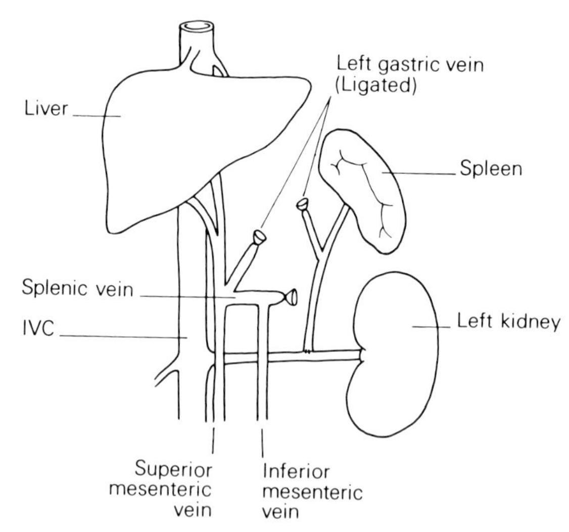

Fig. 14.21 *Distal lienorenal shunt (Warren shunt) for selective decompression of the portal venous system.*

gram will be necessary to decide whether bleeding is due to intra- or extrahepatic obstruction of the portal vein. If the spleen has been removed it will be necessary to perform coeliac axis angiography to visualise, during the venous phase, contrast returning via the splenic and portal vein (see Figs 14.13 and 14.14).

An alternative is umbilico-portography, but this can be difficult and always requires surgical help. Patients selected for such procedures should preferrably be young (under 50 years) to reduce the chance of neuropsychiatric disturbances (see p. 196). A successful shunt operation should prevent recurrence of haemorrhage, allow collateral circulations, including varices, to disappear, and reduce the problems of hypersplenism. These aims are infrequently attained and in many patients liver function deteriorates further; a high proportion develop encephalopathy and some develop secondary haemochromatosis. For these reasons shunting procedures are being used less often in the treatment of variceal haemorrhage. Their major failing is that, although they will control recurrent haemorrhage in the short term (at the expense of the above complications), shunting procedures do not increase life expectancy.

Emergency surgical treatment of varices usually consists of a direct attack on the dilated veins by gastric or oesophageal transection. The latter may take the form of complete oesophageal transection, or be more simply a trans-oesophageal ligation of varices without transection of the oesophagus. These operations carry a significant mortality (approximately 10%) but are usually successful in arresting continuing haemorrhage. Recently, the introduction of a stapling device inserted through a gastrotomy has made it possible to produce an effect similar to oesophageal transection. A ring of staples is rapidly inserted around the internal circumference of the oesophagus (Fig. 14.22). The procedure is easily carried out, with little mortality, and initial reports of success are encouraging.

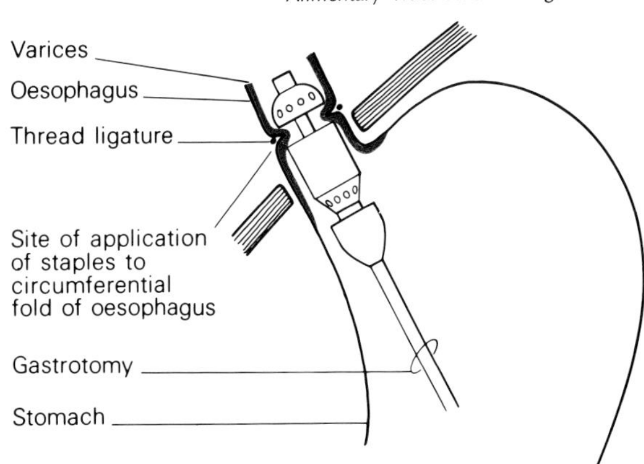

Fig. 14.22 *Oesophageal 'transection' by stapling gun.*

Because all the above procedures are palliative and do nothing to alter the incurable underlying process, considerable attention has recently been focused on the simple procedure of endoscopic sclerotherapy, which was first introduced as early as 1939. Sometimes the injection procedure is combined with the insertion of a Sengstaken tube, to prevent bleeding after injection. Injection is carried out through a long flexible needle introduced through the biopsy channel of a forward-viewing fibre-optic endoscope. A total of 10–15 ml is injected, in increments of 1–2 ml, into the submucosa adjacent to, or into, the varices from the lower end of the oesophagus upwards (Fig. 14.23). This generally requires two to four endoscopic procedures, spaced about 1 week apart. The sclerosant fluids most often used are ethanolamine or polydocanol. The aim is to produce an inflammatory response around the varices with eventual fibrous tissue formation, forcing the varices away from the luminal surface. The varices will remain as blood-carrying vessels but, enclosed in fibrous tissue, they are no longer liable to rupture and bleed.

In addition to the paravascular injection technique described above, many now employ direct intravenous injection of the sclerosant. The removal of the sclerosant from the site of the injection is prevented by compression with the tip of the endoscope and a special injection technique (Fig. 14.24). The perivascular tissue is also infiltrated during the procedure by advancing the needle a little more deeply and injecting the sclerosant whilst slowly withdrawing the needle. It is also possible to use, in conjunction with the above, a specially-designed flexible plastic sheath (the William's tube) which has a slot through which the varix bulges into the lumen. Injection then proceeds in a fashion similar to that used for haemorrhoids. The tube may be rotated to com-

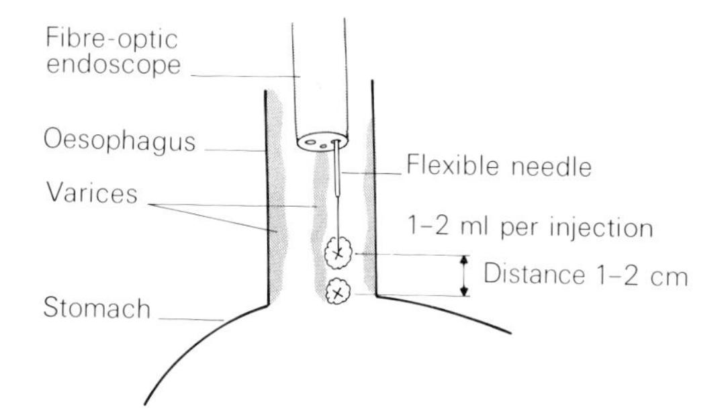

Fig. 14.23 *Oesophageal paravariceal sclerotherapy.*

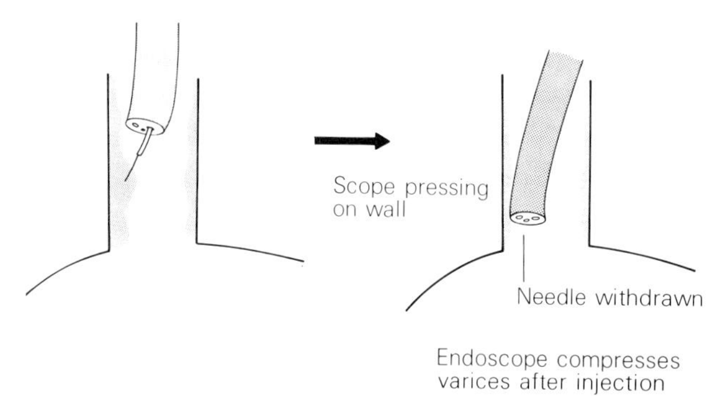

Fig. 14.24 *Intravascular sclerotherapy.*

press the varix after injection.

Present evidence suggests that sclerotherapy of oesophageal varices is now the therapy of choice for variceal bleeding that does not respond to conservative measures. In terms of stopping bleeding it appears to be equal or superior to all other surgical procedures. It is relatively easy and safe and does not increase the risk of encephalopathy. It is, however, often necessary for repeat sclerotherapy to be carried out first at three-monthly and then at six-monthly intervals. Repeated injection, especially into tissue already fibrotic, carries the risk of oesophageal ulceration, which is slow to heal and may eventually lead to oesophageal stricture.

NEW DEVELOPMENTS

Recent interest in the application of laser photocoagulation in medicine has lead to trials of lasers in the control of gastrointestinal haemorrhage. The principle of photo-coagulation with laser beams is the absorption and conversion of light energy into heat, with the resulting increase in temperature leading to coagulation. Two types of laser are currently available (differing from each other in their wavelengths) for use with flexible fibre-optic instruments. These are the argon laser and the neodymium-YAG laser. Both are currently undergoing clinical trials. Comparative studies indicate that the Nd-YAG laser produces a greater haemostatic effect but that it penetrates more deeply and is thus associated with a potentially greater risk of perforation than the argon laser. Lasers are expensive and, until the results of randomised trials are fully evaluated, their place in the management of gastrointestinal haemorrhage is uncertain. Preliminary reports suggest that a place will be found in the treatment of circumscribed bleeding such as erosions of stomach, oozing peptic ulcers, and the treatment of angiomas.

Electrocoagulation via fibre-optic endoscopes has been tried but again there are no randomised trials to prove its efficacy. At present it cannot therefore be recommended as a form of therapy.

Therapeutic angiography is increasing in importance and finds its application in the treatment of patients who are unfit for standard surgical treatment. The technique involves selective angiography and injection of vasoconstrictive drugs (e.g. vasopressin) or embolisation of the bleeding vessel with gelatin sponge, polyvinyl alcohol sponge, isobutyl-2-cyanoacrylate beads, and wire coils. Complications, which are relatively rare, include mesenteric infarction.

Transhepatic variceal obliteration is used only in some highly specialised centres. The coronary and short gastric veins are catherised and selectively embolised. Control of haemorrhage is immediate, but rebleeding frequently occurs from recanalised or newly-formed varices. Its more serious complications are intraperitoneal haemorrhage and biliary leak; in a few patients, splenic and portal vein thrombosis have occurred.

15

Alimentary Infections and Infestations

INTRODUCTION

In normal individuals the intestines, especially the colon, are a remarkable incubator and storehouse for a very large bacterial population which, after playing an important role in the enterohepatic circulation of bile salts and in vitamin B elaboration, passes harmlessly to the rectum.

Infections originating in the alimentary tract may be:

a. *endogenous*, where they are due to the normal gut commensals escaping into the body, e.g. in perforated appendicitis with peritonitis.
b. *exogenous*, where the gut is the portal of entry to the body for pathogens, which have usually been ingested in contaminated water or food.

The response to any of these infections will depend on many factors, including the general health and nutrition of the patient, the integrity of the immune defences, and the virulence and dose of the infecting organism (see Chapter 2).

Endogenous Infections

The acid medium of the normal stomach inhibits bacterial growth, and many ingested pathogens are killed in the stomach. In health, the duodenum and jejunum contain low concentrations of aerobes (10^1-10^4 per ml), mainly streptococci, staphylococci and lactobacilli: coliforms and anaerobes are unusual. In the ileum, the bacterial counts are higher (10^3-10^8 per ml) and coliforms become progressively commoner. The ileocaecal valve separates the flora of the distal gut into two main types (Fig. 15.1): on the ileal side, both gram-positive and coliform aerobes predominate; beyond the ileocaecal valve, anaerobes greatly outnumber aerobes (10^8-10^{12} organisms per ml) – largely bacteroides, coliforms and lactobacilli and clostridia. This huge bacterial population constitutes one-third of the solid bulk of faèces, with anaerobes outnumbering aerobes by at least 90 to 1.

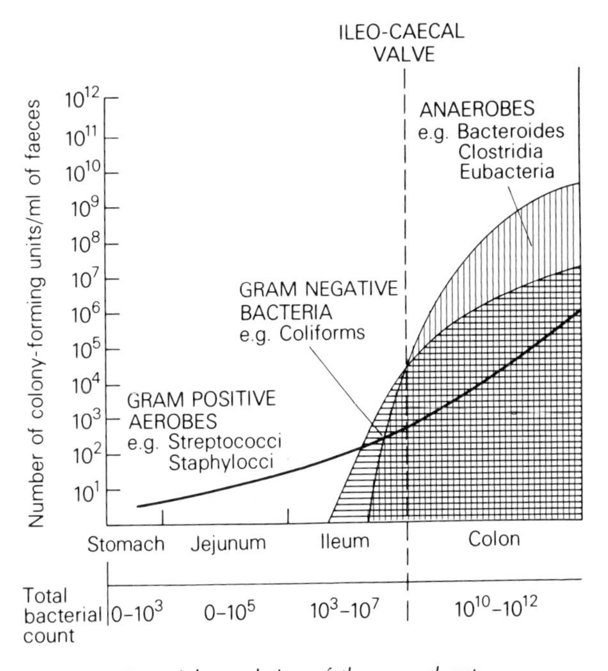

Fig. 15.1 *Bacterial population of the normal gut.*

The normal harmless progression of these bacterial, many of which are serious potential pathogens, to the rectum and anal canal may be interrupted in three different ways to produce an endogenous alimentary infection (Fig. 15.2).

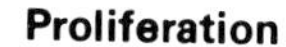

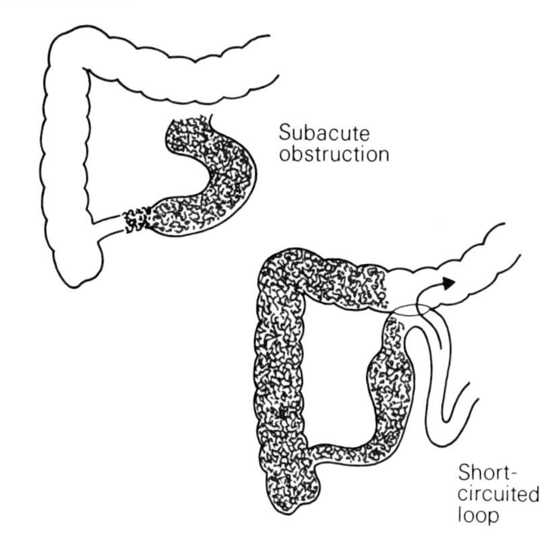

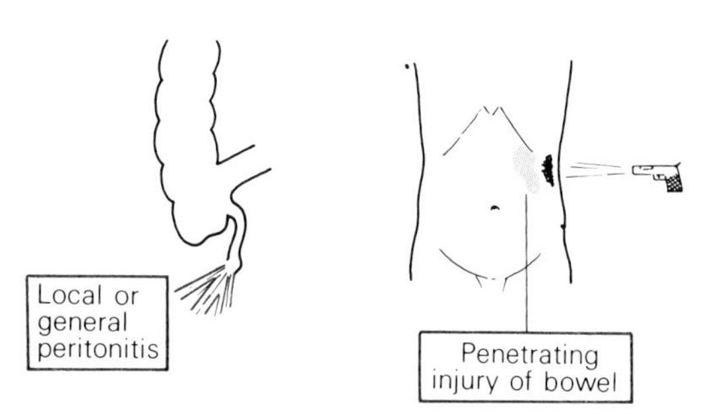

Permeation

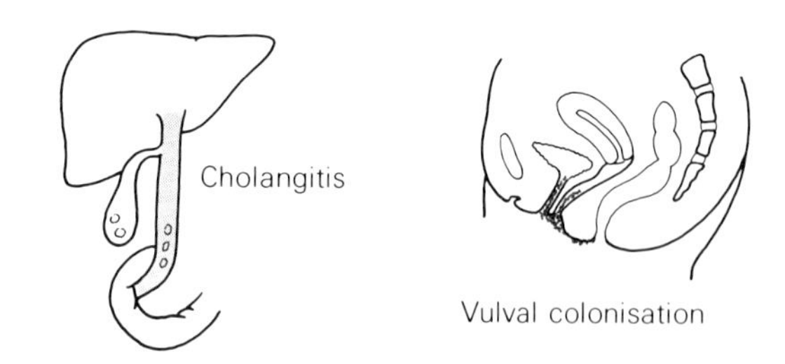

Fig. 15.2 *Endogenous alimentary infection.*

Proliferation

The numbers of organisms normally present in the small bowel will reach abnormally high levels whenever any form of obstruction to normal peristaltic flow occurs. This has already been referred to as a serious consequence of acute intestinal obstruction (p. 288) and will also occur in any gradually increasing obstruction: the resulting malabsorption, and other metabolic disturbances occurring in these 'contaminated bowel syndromes', are fully described in Chapter 7.

Perforation

Perforation of the gut, with release of aerobic and anaerobic pathogens into the peritoneum, may occur as a result of internal disease (e.g. gangrenous appendicitis) or external trauma (e.g. penetrating wound of the colon). Peritonitis will develop, which may be limited by the defences of the peritoneum, or may spread to cause a generalised peritonitis, often complicated by bacteraemia (p. 286).

Permeation

Because of anatomical proximity, gut commensals may contaminate neighbouring structures, with resulting illness. A classical example is recurrent urinary tract infection, to which many females are prone, due to ascending colonisation with faecal organisms (notably coliforms) of the introitus, then the urethra, and finally the bladder. Alimentary organisms (coliforms, *Strep. faecalis*) may also invade the biliary tree, especially in the presence of calculi, causing ascending cholangitis: subsequent invasion of the bloodstream may lead to life-threatening bacteraemia.

All these forms of endogenous infection are potentially serious and can be lethal. Treatment has three major simultaneous components:

Removal of the cause e.g. appendicectomy, resection of a stagnant loop of bowel

Appropriate antibiotic treatment

Treatment of the effects of bacterial invasion, which may entail vigorous resuscitation and often the use of all the facilities of an intensive therapy unit for several days.

The care of all patients with a major endogenous alimentary infection follows a similar pattern and has been considered in detail in the treatment of appendicitis with peritonitis (p. 284–287).

Exogenous Infections

These are of very great importance, both because of the large number of individuals involved worldwide, and because of the severity of many of these infections (Table 15.1). Diarrhoeal illnesses due to the ingestion of contaminated food or water cause the death of some 20 million children around the world each year, and yet the knowledge to prevent most of these deaths is available. Effective control of these infections and infestations demands, and will continue to demand, the concerted efforts of a remarkable range of disciplines and interests in clinical medicine, microbiology, public health, therapeutics, preventive medicine, sociology, anthropology and, not least, politics.

Only 140 years ago cholera was a regular visitor to Britain, killing 50 000 people in a year, and it was in 1856, before anyone knew the cause of cholera, that Dr John Snow demonstrated how, by removing the handle of the Broad Street pump in Central London, a cholera epidemic was terminated; subsequent excavation showed that a cesspool drained into this supposedly clean-water well. With this convincing demonstration of the role of water in the spread of alimentary disease, public opinion and politicians were convinced that major engineering was required to make certain that pure water reached homes and places of work and that sewage was safely disposed of. The remarkable sewerage system of London, still in use, was engineered by Bazalgette between 1860–75. The cholera vibrio itself was not demonstrated until 1883 – by Robert Koch – but by then epidemics in London had disappeared because of action taken on the basis of Snow's demonstration.

Table 15.1
Important Gut Pathogens and Associated Clinical Disorders

Salmonella	Enteric fever (typhoid) Gastroenteritis
Campylobacters	Abdominal pains and diarrhoea
Escherichia coli (certain subtypes)	Diarrhoea in young children Travellers diarrhoea
Clostridium difficile	Pseudomembraneous colitis
Shigella	Bacillary dysentery
Entamoeba histolytica	Amoebic dysentery
Giardia lamblia	Diarrhoea and malabsorption
Vibrio cholerae	Cholera
Staph. aureus	Enteritis (rare)
Candida albicans	Enteritis
Rota viruses	Diarrhoea

The importance of a pure water supply, efficient sewerage, and high standards of hygiene in the making and selling of foods is now taken for granted in developed countries, so when a score of Britons holidaying on a Greek island contract typhoid in a hotel employing a carrier, the news media treat the small outbreak as a major event. It is forgotten that, for at least two-thirds of the population of the World, enteric fevers, along with amoebiasis and cholera and the intestinal infestations, are a daily, often lethal, reality. It is calculated that some 200 million individuals suffer from schistosomiasis, 400 million from hook worm and no less than 1000 million from roundworm infestation. The annual death rate from cholera in India still runs into many thousands, and is likely to continue as long as social and religious customs encourage bathing in highly contaminated water.

It is therefore evident that, although the knowledge is available to allow these dangerous and unpleasant exogenous alimentary tract diseases to be largely abolished, the achievement of this state of affairs is going to demand a revolution in social and political thinking, with planning, education and engineering of enormous proportions.

In the meantime, a great range of preventive measures are practical. Every water well drilled in a Third World village is a small contribution, which is well illustrated in Calcutta, where there has been a striking fall in fatal cases of cholera following improvements in the water supply. A whole range of measures are everyday practice in the Western World. Constant bacteriological checks on the water supply, and foods; inspections of cafés and restaurants; notification of infectious diseases; the construction of reservoirs and maintenance of sewers. In spite of all these precautions, there are some 4 million family doctor consultations for acute diarrhoea each year in Britain. Occasionally also, apparently careful food regulations fail to protect consumers, a point well illustrated in Aberdeen, Scotland, in 1964, where over 500 people suffered from typhoid fever. This was traced to tins of South American corned beef which appeared to be sound and edible: they had, however, been unknowingly cooled, after heat sterilisation, in contaminated river water, and typhoid bacilli had been sucked into the tins through minute pores in the seams.

The other major preventive measure against some of these infections is inoculation of the individual by vaccine to build up, over a space of weeks, active immunity. There was a higher mortality among British troops serving in the Boer war from enteric fevers than from wounds, and this prompted a search for a method of immunisation. Almroth Wright showed that injection of a suspension of virulent typhoid bacilli, killed by heating in a waterbath to 57°C for 2 hours, produced active immunity: this was boosted 10 days later by a further injection of double the dose. This vaccine was widely used in the British Army during the 1914–18 war, and even in Middle Eastern campaigns the incidence of typhoid was minimal. In the Second World War it was usual to combine vaccines of both typhoid and paratyphoid A and B, and also *Clostridium tetani,* with valuable results, especially to combat typhoid fever and tetanus.

Nowadays, when 400 million people travel by air each year, it is common for citizens of developed countries to visit those with less stringent standards of hygiene. They may acquire an infection abroad but complete the incubation period a week or two after returning home, when a serious but unfamiliar disease may go unrecognised. Advice to travellers on precautions when visiting subtropical and tropical countries is of great practical importance (p. 348).

PRINCIPLES OF DIAGNOSIS OF ALIMENTARY INFECTION

It may be difficult to distinguish between alimentary infections and other causes of abdominal pain, fever, and diarrhoea, e.g. neoplasms or inflammatory bowel disease. Blood and mucus may be present in the stool in both 'infective' and non-infective illness, and their presence does not help in differentiation. It is therefore of considerable therapeutic and 'public health' importance that all patients who present with this syndrome should be investigated for the possibility of alimentary infection. Depending on the clinical circumstances, specific search for alimentary infection will often proceed simultaneously with other alimentary investigations, including radiology: plain abdominal x-rays may provide important information (p. 229).

The Clinical History

This is of paramount importance, not only in the detection of alimentary infection but also in establishing potential routes of spread. Specific enquiry should always be made into the possibility of recent exposure, at home or at work, to diarrhoeal illness; recent 'dining out'; recent travel abroad; possession of pets or other animals; and occupation (e.g. farmers, abattoir workers, sewage workers, cooks). The clinical history very often gives the first warning that referral of the patient to an infectious diseases or isolation unit is desirable. Careful enquiry at this stage will greatly facilitate tracing contacts (and so define the possible extent, and help to contain an outbreak of alimentary infection).

A careful drug history will avoid confusion between an alimentary infection and the gastrointestinal upset which can be induced by drugs such as laxatives, and antibiotics (and others which cause diarrhoea less frequently, e.g. mefenamic acid).

Information should also be obtained on the timing of any vaccinations (e.g. against typhoid) previously administered to the patient, as this may avoid confusion in the subsequent interpretation of specific blood agglutination reactions.

Clinical Examination

This may differentiate alimentary infection from other diagnoses (e.g. colonic neoplasm) but will not usually help in defining the infecting organism. It is important to remember that the macroscopic appearances at sigmoidoscopy, and histological findings on biopsy, of the rectal mucosa may be identical in inflammatory bowel disease and in many alimentrary infections.

Laboratory Specimens

Where vomiting has been part of the clinical presentation it is important to send a sample of vomitus, as well as stool, to the laboratory at an early stage. All specimens should be sent in suitable water-tight containers, taking care not to contaminate the outside of the container. Such specimen containers are a major potential health hazard to nursing staff, porters, and laboratory workers; to minimise the risk of cross-infection, they are usually transferred to the laboratory in polythene bags.

In children and in the elderly, where stool collection may not be practical, rectal swabs may provide the diagnostic specimen. Usually stool culture will allow a diagnosis to be reached but sometimes, in the early stages of alimentary infections such as typhoid, blood culture and, later, urine culture, are necessary to establish the diagnosis. Culture of ascitic fluid or liver biopsy material may be necessary to establish the diagnosis in patients with alimentary tuberculosis; and examination of jejunal aspirate may be the only method of confirming the diagnosis of giardiasis (see p. 339).

In the later stages of alimentary infection, the diagnosis may be confirmed by demonstration of high or rising titres of specific agglutinins, or by complement fixation tests (see p. 336).

Routine Laboratory Investigation of Alimentary Infection

Naked-eye inspection of the stool specimen will usually reveal the presence of blood, pus or mucus. If these are present, and if other causes are excluded, this usually denotes serious alimentary infection.

Wet microscopic preparations are used for the detection of *Entamoeba histolytica* and other protozoa, as well as worms, ova and larvae. Cholera vibrios can be recognised, on microscopy of fluid stool, as characteristic rods with darting motility, but this is not a reliable method (see p. 334). Gram-staining the stool may detect staphylococci or candida. Aerobic culture on appropriate media is used to detect *Escherichia coli, Staph. aureus, Salmonella* and *Shigella*. Selective culture is necessary for campylobacters; *Clostridium difficile* and its toxin can be detected in the stool by special techniques.

IMPORTANT GENERAL CONSIDERATIONS IN THE MANAGEMENT OF ALIMENTARY INFECTION

When the diagnosis is suspected, great care must be taken in the handling of all excreta. The highest standards of personal hygiene must prevail for both patients and their attendants. Seriously ill patients should be admitted early to isolation facilities with fully trained medical and nursing staff. Rehydration is a very important part of medical treatment in all alimentary infections, and the specific measures appropriate to each disorder are discussed below.

The Management of Acute Diarrhoeal Illnesses

In the vast majority of patients, acute diarrhoea is a mild (though unpleasant) illness of short duration. In the initial phase the sufferer may need to be away from work for a day or two and should eat little or nothing but drink freely. Because most attacks are self-limiting, there is no need to undertake stool culture unless symptoms continue.

However, it is vital to remember that diarrhoea and vomiting can be early symptoms of other serious disease, e.g. acute appendicitis, and there are other patients who need special attention:

- patients with diarrhoea severe enough to cause dehydration and prostration
- patients with bloody diarrhoea
- the young and also the old and frail: babies in particular can become seriously dehydrated very quickly
- patients in hospital wards and institutions where spread to others can easily occur
- patients on immunosuppressive drugs
- travellers recently returned from abroad.

Whenever the oral route of rehydration is clearly failing, and especially in the young and the old, hospital admission should not be delayed. The combination of diarrhoea and vomiting with acute abdominal pain should always raise the suspicion of a 'surgical' cause. After admission, investigation will follow the lines already outlined.

The most important aspect of management is fluid replacement. This may be achieved orally using a glucose-electrolyte solution, but intravenous therapy is sometimes required because of vomiting or severe dehydration. In the latter situation central venous pressure monitoring may be advisable. It is important to promote the concept that acute diarrhoea is usually a beneficent mechanism tending to wash the pathogens out of the gut: therefore, commonly prescribed anti-diarrhoeal remedies, e.g. anticholinergics or codeine, are not logical and there is evidence that they impair mechanical clearance of the gut, increase the risk of bacterial invasion, and thus prolong and intensify the illness. The combination of diphenoxylate and atropine is effective, but overdosage is dangerous, especially in children, because it can produce an acute obstructive syndrome. Loperamide seems to be the safest of the anti-diarrhoeal agents. There is no evidence that antimicrobial chemotherapy curtails the illness, and it may indeed pose additional problems, including promoting bacterial resistance and chronic carrier states.

Fluid replacement

Although sodium and potassium may be lost in considerable amounts, hyponatraemia and hypokalaemia are not common because of accompanying water loss. In severe cases, bicarbonate is actively secreted along with sodium and this, together with reduced renal hydrogen ion excretion, may lead to a metabolic acidosis. Whilst these dramatic fluid and electrolyte movements are taking place, the serum potassium may be spuriously high, despite considerable and dangerous depletion of the predominantly intracellular total body potassium.

Studies of the pathogenesis and treatment of cholera in recent years have led to increasing understanding of basic mechanisms, and to the development of logical oral fluid and electolyte replacement. Balanced glucose-electolyte solution exploits the facilitated sodium/glucose symport mechanism of absorption (p. 117) and allows more efficient oral fluid replacement, even in severely ill patients. The relative concentrations are critical. In temperate climates, such a balanced mixture is:

sodium 35 mmoles
potassium 20 mmoles
chloride 37 mmoles
bicarbonate 18 mmoles
dextrose 200 mmoles
water to 1 litre.

This is available in some commercial preparations (e.g. Dioralyte). It can be prepared *de novo* by adding 20 g glucose (dextrose), 3.5 g sodium chloride, 2.5 g sodium bicarbonate, and 1.5 g potassium chloride to a litre of drinking water. In underdeveloped countries, sucrose (40 g) has been used with some success in the absence of dextrose supplies. About 1.5 volumes of fluid should be given for each volume of stool. The great majority of patients with acute diarrhoea respond well to this regime.

Intravenous replacement is sometimes necessary where dehydration is severe, and either Hartmann's solution (B.P.) can be used, or a solution of 4 g sodium chloride, 6.5 g sodium acetate and 1 g potassium chloride to a litre.

Notification of alimentary infection

There are three forms of acute diarrhoea notifiable by law in Britain:

cholera
food poisoning
dysentery, both bacterial and amoebic.

INFECTIONS OF THE ALIMENTARY TRACT

Viral Infections

Infections by many viruses, such as adenovirus, Coxsackie and ECHO viruses, may produce alimentary symptoms. Work over the last 10 year has revealed the importance of rotavirus, parvovirus-like agents, and 'Norwalk' virus.

Rotavirus

The name derives from the wheel-like appearance (Fig. 15.3). In temperate climates, this virus is now recognised as being the most important single cause of acute diarrhoea in infants between 6 months and 2 years. Respiratory and quite severe gastrointestinal symptoms develop. It is important to recognise that the rotavirus attacks the brush border on the tips and sides of the small bowel villi: consequently, function may be impaired, including the digestion of milk, and so the rational treatment is to stop milk feeds for a day or two and give glucose-electrolyte solution by mouth.

The diagnosis may be confirmed both serologically and by isolating the virus from the stool.

Parvovirus-like agents

This group comprises many different agents. Winter outbreaks occur affecting children and adults alike. Following an incubation period of 24–48 hours, symptoms of fever, myalgia, nausea, vomiting and diarrhoea develop and persist for two to three days. There is associated broadening and blunting of the intestinal villi.

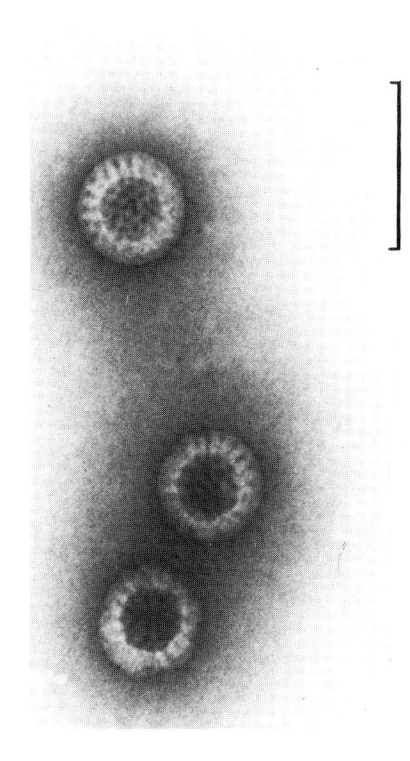

Fig. 15.3 *Electron micrograph of rotavirus; typical appearance in faeces. Barline = 100 nm.*

Treatment: There is no specific treatment for these viral infections, which are fortunately self-limiting. Dehydration, however, is common and may require vigorous intravenous fluid replacement.

Bacterial Infections

Bacterial pathogens can be divided into four groups by their effect upon the intestinal mucosa:

Exotoxin-producing organisms (e.g. *Vibrio cholerae*, enteropathogenic *Escherichia coli*): The exotoxin is produced by proliferating organisms after ingestion. Its action is to inhibit sodium and chloride absorption and increase bicarbonate excretion, with consequent increased fluid losses. This active secretory mechanism is mediated through the cyclic AMP mechanism (p. 23).

Endotoxin-producing organisms (e.g. *staphylo-*

cocci): In this group the toxin is produced within contaminated food which is kept, before ingestion, in warm conditions (10–50°C). Proliferation of the organism produces large quantities of toxin, which may act (after ingestion) as a neurotoxin, through ill-understood humoral mechanisms. These toxins are resistant to cooking.

Invasive and mucosa-destroying organisms (e.g. *Shigella*): Generally the small bowel is affected first and the colon may be involved later, sometimes producing a picture similar to idopathic proctocolitis.

Diffuse inflammation-producing organisms (e.g. *Salmonella, Campylobacter*): In this group the lamina propria is diffusely infiltrated.

Specific infections

Campylobacter infections. Infection with *Campylobacter jejuni* has recently been recognised as a common cause of diarrhoea. Large outbreaks have followed milk-borne infections, and infection has also been transmitted directly from chickens and dogs. The organism invades the mucosa and may elaborate an enterotoxin.

Following an incubation period of 3–5 days, the illness is heralded by rigors, headache, and myalgia. Abdominal pain may be so severe as to precipitate admission to a surgical unit. Diarrhoea may occur one or two days later; it is initially watery and subsequently may contain blood. Some patients develop a reactive arthritis. Colitis may also occur, when the sigmoidoscopic and histological appearance of the rectal mucosa can resemble that seen in patients with idiopathic inflammatory bowel disease, from which it may be difficult to distinguish this infection. The diagnosis is made by stool culture and serology. A high antibody titre is present as early as the fifth day of illness, which may explain why blood cultures, unless taken early, are often negative.

Treatment is by fluid replacement. Although usually self-limiting, erythromycin may be indicated if the symptoms are severe. Relapses occur in approximately 10% of cases.

Cholera. From a reservoir in the Ganges delta, pandemics of cholera have radiated across the developing world (Fig. 15.4). In 1961 a new pandemic caused by the El Tor biotype spread through SE Asia, parts of Africa, and the Middle East. It remains endemic in many areas today and, in contrast to the classical biotype, is hardier, is excreted for a longer period, and produces a lower incidence of clinical disease.

The organism is transmitted by the faecal–oral route (p. 340), and the symptoms are caused by the elaboration of a toxin in the gut. This is not associated with mucosal damage but exerts its effect by activation of adenylate cyclase (and thereby the cyclic AMP system), with the production of a secretory diarrhoea (Chapter 2, p. 23).

Cholera vibrios will grow rapidly in alkaline peptone water (pH 8.0 or greater), and will form yellow colonies on TCBS (thiosulphate, citrate, bile salts, sucrose) agar. Their identity is confirmed by agglutination with specific OI antiserum, and their subtypes are established by a series of other tests.

After an incubation period of 1–5 days, the patient develops symptoms of vomiting and profuse watery diarrhoea, and the stool soon acquires the colourless, odourless features characteristic of the so-called 'rice water' stool. Rapid dehydration with consequent hypovolaemia may result in renal failure, metabolic acidosis and, eventually, death.

Rehydration is the most important aspect of management. Absorptive mechanisms are unimpaired and oral isotonic glucose–electrolyte solution (e.g. Dioralyte) may reduce net fluid excretion by 'solvent drag' (p. 117). Intravenous rehydration will still be needed in severe cases. The use of tetracycline (given orally where possible) will reduce the severity and duration of illness. Recent interest has focused on the use of chlorpromazine which, by blocking adenylate cyclase activity, exhibits an antisecretory effect. Unfortunately, because it also has alpha-blocking properties, its use in dehydrated subjects may induce profound hypotension.

Clostridium difficile infection. It has recently been recognised that many cases of pseudo-

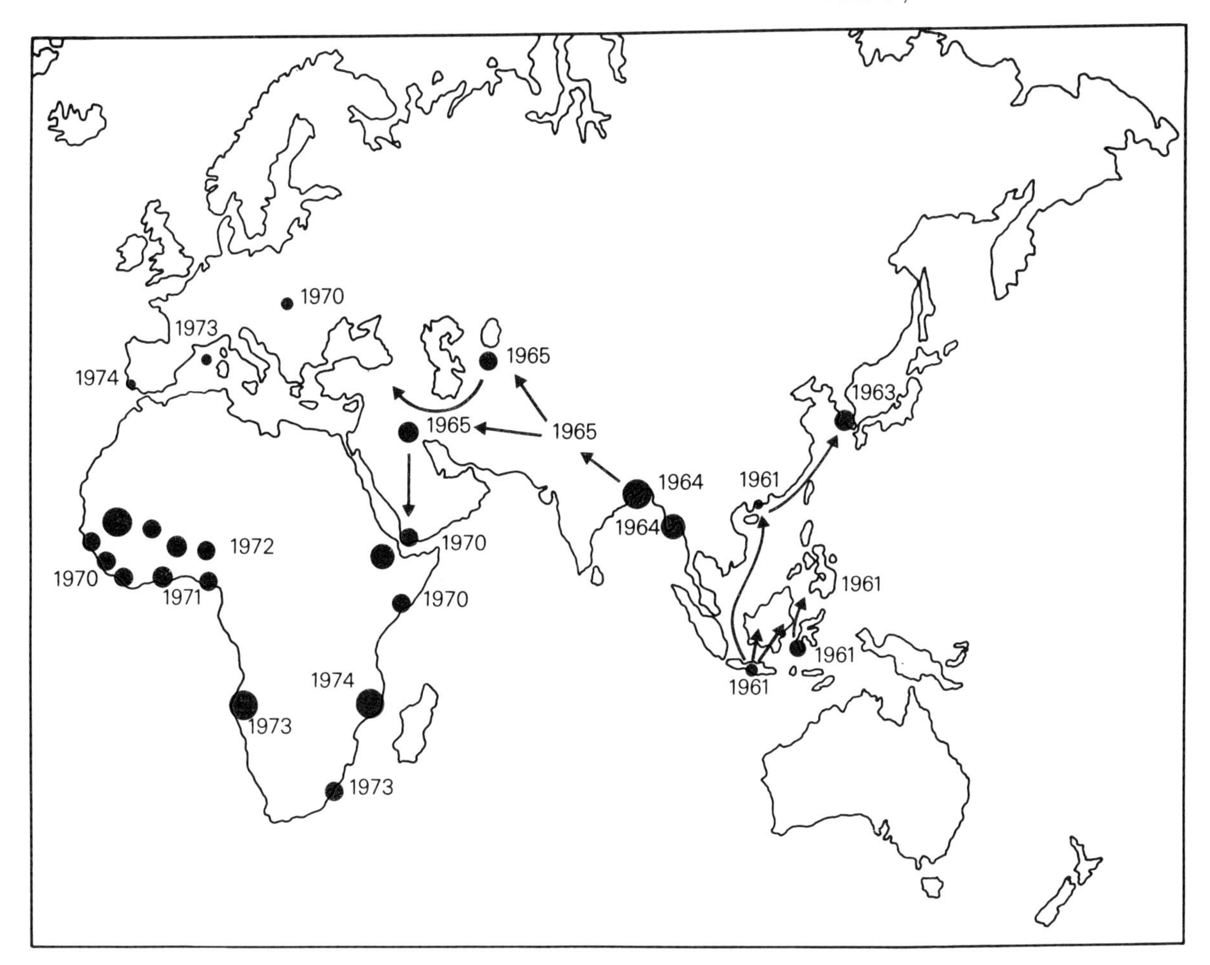

Fig. 15.4 *Map showing the spread of the El-Tor cholera pandemic of 1961–74. Main areas are shaded in red, with date of outbreak. Sporadic cases were found in air travellers to Europe and Australasia.*

membraneous colitis (PMC) are caused by the toxin which is elaborated by certain strains of *Cl. difficile* (see Chapter 10). This organism is responsible for a spectrum of disease, from post-antibiotic diarrhoea to PMC. Toxigenic *Cl. difficile* is not commonly found in the bowel flora, but is acquired in a similar manner as other enteric pathogens, so it is not surprising that case clustering has been observed. Patients most at risk of developing the syndrome of PMC are those in whom the normal bowel flora has been disturbed, most commonly by antibiotics but also following surgery, ischaemia, or bowel obstruction.

The features, diagnosis and treatment of PMC are dealt with in Chapter 10 (p. 243).

Escherichia coli infections. Three groups of pathogenic *E. coli* are recognised:

Enteropathogenic strains are responsible for some cases of infantile gastroenteritis (p. 345).
Enterotoxigenic strains produce heat-labile and heat-stable toxins which promote a secretory diarrhoea. These are an important cause of traveller's diarrhoea (p. 348), the resulting illness being usually mild and self-limiting.
Enteroinvasive strains invade the colonic

mucosa and produce a dysentery-like illness, with diarrhoea, which contains blood and mucus.

Salmonella infections: The numerous serotypes fall into two categories:

1. Pathogens exclusive to humans (e.g. *S. typhi* and *S. paratyphi*) which are associated with the syndrome of enteric fever, which is primarily a bacteraemic illness.
2. Pathogens which primarily affect animals (e.g *S. typhimurium, S. enteritidis and S. heidelberg*) produce a form of food poisoning which, when contaminated food or water is ingested, is a gastroenteritis confined to the bowel mucosa. Patients who are ill or pyrexial, however, may have a bacteraemia, and blood cultures should be taken. Occasionally there is an associated colitis, and toxic dilatation has been reported, though it usually settles with medical management. With bacteraemia, metastatic infections, e.g. osteomyelitis, arthritis or endocarditis, may be seen.

Typhoid and paratyphoid fevers. These conditions are commonly grouped under the term 'enteric fever'. The only reservoir of *S. typhi* and *S. paratyphi* is man, and patients can only contract the infection from human excreta containing the salmonellae. Faecal carriers are therefore of great importance in the spread of the disease. Outbreaks may be water-borne (as when a carrier cleans out a well), shellfish may be taken from seawater contaminated by sewage, and milk and dairy products are much at risk if cooks and handlers are carriers.

Although a systemic disease, the most serious complications affect the gut. The portal of entry is the mouth. Typhoid bacilli multiply in the small bowel and penetrate the lymphoid tissue (Peyer's patches) in the submucosa, where they multiply. Blood-borne dissemination then occurs, reaching the reticuloendothelial cells of liver and spleen. At the end of the incubation period of 10–14 days (sometimes up to 21 days), the organisms re-emerge into the blood stream, and there is heavy recolonisation of the gut via infected bile. This leads to severe ulceration of the surface of the Peyer's patches, especially in the lower ileum, and it is this deep ulceration which can cause severe melaena or free perforation of ileum into the peritoneal cavity.

The patient complains of headache, malaise, anorexia, cough and fever and tends to the constipated. If untreated, the patient may become severely ill by the end of the first week. Headache and confusion are prominent (typhoid derives from a Greek word meaning stupor) and the abdomen is somewhat distended and doughy. At this time the spleen should become palpable and the classical rose spots are seen – these are small macules which fade with pressure. Untreated, the severely affected patient sinks further into stupor, runs a high fever, and may pass loose green stools. Haemorrhage and perforation are major risks in the third week (Fig. 15.5).

With the advent of diagnostic methods and effective treatment, this picture is unlikely to be seen except in places far from medical assistance. Blood culture is usually positive during the first week, and faeces and urine cultures are positive during the second and third weeks.

Serological tests (Widal reaction) have a limited place in diagnosis, but may help if enteric fever seems likely even though the cultures are negative. An elevated (more than 1:80) and, especially, a rising titre of antibodies to H (flagellar) and O (somatic) antigen is very suggestive from about the tenth day, but titres will also be high in those previously infected and in the vaccinated. The Widal reaction may be negative in the early stages and it is then that a positive blood culture may establish the diagnosis.

Management. General management has already been discussed (p. 331). Chloramphenicol is the antibiotic of choice, 500 mg four-hourly until defervescence and then 500 mg 6-hourly for a total of 10 days. Some resistant strains of *S. typhi* have emerged, and co-trimoxazole is then helpful.

Stool cultures should become negative before the end of 3 months. If persistently positive, the carrier state must be treated, using amoxycillin and mecillinam, or co-trimoxazole. Chloramphenicol is not then helpful.

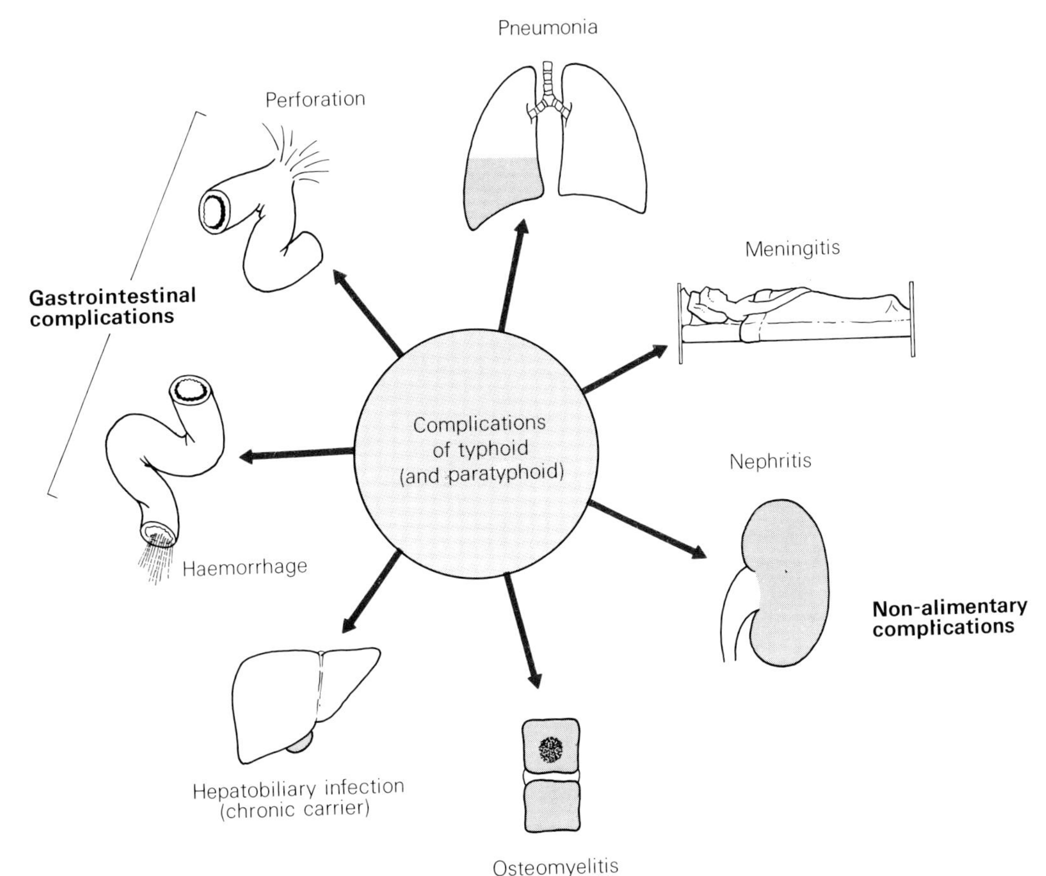

Fig. 15.5 *The complications of enteric fever.*

Continuation of the carrier state may need treatment by cholecystectomy, because infection can lie dormant in gall-bladder mucosa for years, especially if gallstones are present.

Shigella infections (bacillary dysenteries). The four groups of shigella, *Sh. sonnei, Sh. flexneri, Sh. boydei, Sh. dysenteriae* are exclusive human pathogens and they are responsible for the syndrome of bacillary dysentery. These organisms spread rapidly under poor social conditions. Although uncommon in the UK, they are common in underdeveloped countries. After an incubation period of 24–72 hours, a secretory diarrhoea may be followed by bloody stool associated with colonic invasion. The diarrhoea may be accompanied by cramping and lower abdominal pain, and the patient is frequently febrile. Extra-intestinal manifestations of the disease include meningism and seizures, haemolytic uraemic syndrome, reactive arthritis, and Reiter's syndrome. The diagnosis may be suggested by the clinical presentation and is confirmed by stool culture.

Most cases in the UK are due to infection with *Sh. sonnei*, which is associated with a mild illness. Antimicrobials are usually only required for more severe infections.

Tuberculosis. Abdominal tuberculosis was a common condition in Western countries when pulmonary tuberculosis was rife and there was wide use of unpasteurised milk from herds infected with bovine tuberculosis. Because these hazards have now largely disappeared, abdominal tuberculosis is now a rarity in most Western countries, but it is still likely to be seen in immigrants from less developed regions.

Infection occurs through swallowing tubercle

bacilli in infected milk (bovine), or sputum (human bacillus). The lymphoid tissue in the wall of the bowel (especially in the ileocaecal region) becomes infected, and then the mesenteric lymph nodes are involved. The Peyer's patches ulcerate and, later, infection spreads through the bowel wall producing thickening and fibrosis which bears a strong naked-eye resemblance to Crohn's disease. The mesenteric nodes tend to caseate and may break down, with the development of tuberculous peritonitis.

Symptoms of tuberculous enteritis are initially vague, with some abdominal pain, distension and diarrhoea, but it should be remembered that about 50% of patients also have pulmonary tuberculosis. Later, weight loss is noticeable as partial obstruction develops. It is often possible to feel a fixed mass in the right iliac fossa, and a faecal fistula may form. If tuberculosis affects the rectum and anal canal it is even more difficult to distinguish from Crohn's disease, and then the presence of pulmonary tuberculosis gives an important hint of the diagnosis: a strongly positive Mantoux test may also help, and tubercle bacilli may be seen in a biopsy treated by Ziehl–Nielsen stain.

Tuberculous enteritis may yield to specific drug treatment (rifampicin, isoniazid and ethambutol in standard dosage). Often surgery is needed because of obstruction.

Tuberculous peritonitis presents as gradually accumulating ascites. In the tropics it may account for 25% of patients with ascites but in temperate climates it is rare, and diagnosis may depend on withdrawing a milky fluid containing excess protein and many lymphocytes: acid-fast bacilli are not often seen. Sometimes matted omental masses can be felt after tapping. Peritoneal biopsy, with guinea pig innoculation, may be needed to confirm the diagnosis.

Yersiniosis. Infection with two organisms, *Yersinia pseudotuberculosis* and *Y. enterocolitica,* have been increasingly recognised over the past 15 years in man, mammals and birds. Though not common, these infections produce effects which closely resemble other familiar conditions, so it is important to recognise them because they are self-limiting.

Upwards of 3000 cases have now been described and the clinical picture shows two major forms:

1. *Right iliac fossa syndrome*.

About 90% of patients, mostly boys and youths, with a *Y. pseudotuberculosis* infection present with pain in the right lower quadrant, vomiting, and fever. Local tenderness and guarding understandably leads to a number of the patients being operated on for acute appendicitis. The appendix is normal but there is a very marked degree of ileocaecal mesenteric lymphadenitis, and the terminal ileum looks swollen and hyperaemic. *Y. pseudotuberculosis* can readily be grown from a biopsy of the nodes, though rarely from stool culture. These patients recover and there is no evidence that the ileitis is a precursor of Crohn's disease.

2. *Enteritis*.

As its name implies, *Y. enterocolitica* produces an acute illness with diarrhoea, vomiting, abdominal pain and fever.

It mainly affects young children and is now the commonest manifestation of yersiniosis. Occasionally this organism produces the right iliac fossa syndrome.

Septicaemia, erythema nodosum and arthritis are occasional complications.

The laboratory diagnosis of *Y. pseudotuberculosis* is made either by culture of blood or a lymph node biopsy, or by demonstrating a rising serum antibody titre. *Y. enterocolitica* is identified in a similar way, although there is a better chance of growing the organism from the stools.

Y. pseudotuberculosis is widely distributed among mammals and birds, and humans probably acquire infection by direct contact with animals. *Y. enterocolitica* may be spread through contaminated food. Both types produce outbreaks in families and schools.

Infection with unidentified bacteria: Whipple's disease (see Chapter 7) is associated with rod-shaped bacteria within foamy macrophages of the intestinal tract and lymph nodes. Diagnosis may be made by PAS staining of jejunal biopsy. Males are more commonly affected, and the clinical features include diarrhoea with malabsorption, polyarthralgia, and lymphadenopathy. Treatment is discussed in Chapter 7.

Tropical sprue (see Chapter 7) is a malabsorption syndrome which is prevalent in underdeveloped and tropical countries and is sometimes discovered in people who have recently visited the tropics. The cause is uncertain but bacterial colonisation would appear to be important and jejunal histology shows partial villous atrophy. The condition responds best to tetracycline and nutritional replacement therapy, e.g. folic acid.

Protozoal Infections

Giardiasis

Thus is usually acquired by ingestion of contaminated food or water, but may also be transmitted by male homosexuals. The *Giardia lamblia* trophozoite (Fig. 15.6) inhabits the proximal small intestine, where it multiplies and forms cysts. The infection is frequently asymptomatic but some people develop diarrhoea with associated nausea and abdominal pain. Occasionally the diarrhoea persists for many weeks. Rarely there is associated malabsorption of fat, when it is necessary to consider other conditions, such as intestinal colonisation and hypogammaglobulinaemia (especially IgA deficiency), which may coexist with giardiasis. The diagnosis is made by identifying cysts in the stool or, more predictably, trophozoites in fresh duodenal aspirate. Metronidazole in a single daily dose of 2 g for 3 days, or tinidazole in a single dose of 2 g, are effective treatment.

Amoebiasis

Infestation with *Entamoeba histolytica* appears to be confined to man and is of world-wide distribution, though much commoner in warm climates with poor sanitation: it is said to affect 5% of non-travelled residents of the USA.

Infection occurs by swallowing mature cysts in contaminated water or food (Fig. 15.7): boiling the

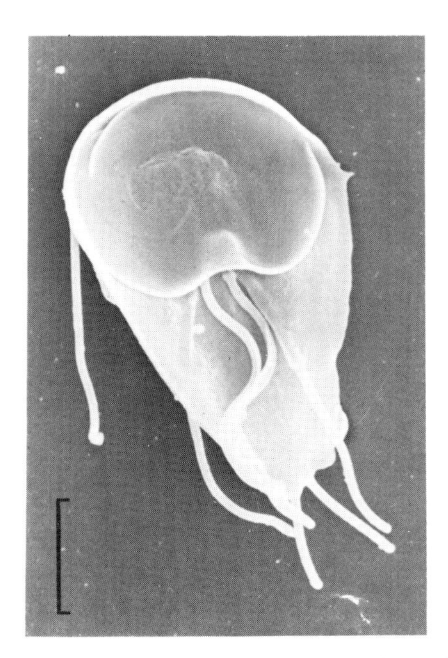

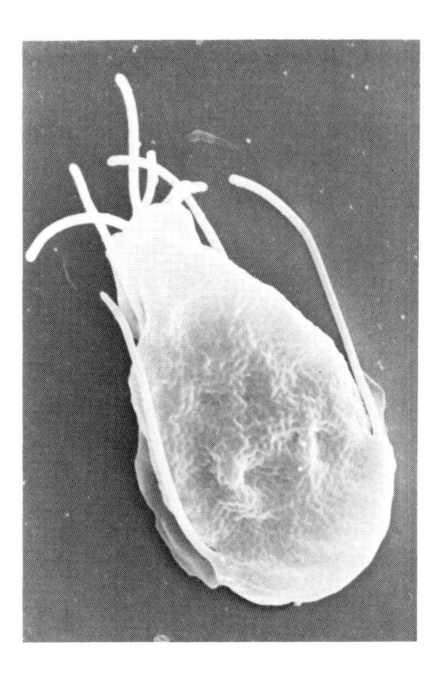

Fig. 15.6 *Electron micrograph of* Giardia lamblia *trophozoite. Ventral view (left) shows sucker area, by which it attaches to mucosa. Barline = 3 μm.*

water kills cysts, but acceptable levels of chlorination do not. In the distal ileum or colon, the cyst develops into the trophozoite – a four-nucleated amoeba – which divides into four single-nucleated entamoebae. If the patient has diarrhoea, these amoebae, containing ingested red cells, can be seen in the stools, but if there is no diarrhoea there is time for the amoebae to encyst: it is these mature cysts in the faeces which are the infective form of *E. histolytica*. Children seem to be more susceptible to infection than adults and some races, e.g. the Bantu of South Africa, are liable to particularly severe forms of amoebiasis.

As the amoebae develop they penetrate the colonic mucosa and, by a process of invasion and destruction, produce typically flask-shaped ulcers, which may or may not penetrate the muscularis mucosae. The secondary infection which accompanies repeated ulceration can lead to oedema, granulation tissue and fibrosis, forming an inflammatory mass – an amoeboma: these may be found anywhere in the colon, more often in the proximal part.

Metastatic spread can occur, especially to the liver (p. 189), and may be facilitated by inappropriate corticosteroid therapy.

The clinical picture of amoebiasis can be misleadingly similar to both inflammatory bowel disease and colorectal cancer. Even though amoebiasis is comparatively rare in temperate climates, the possibility of this diagnosis should be considered before a major colonic resection is

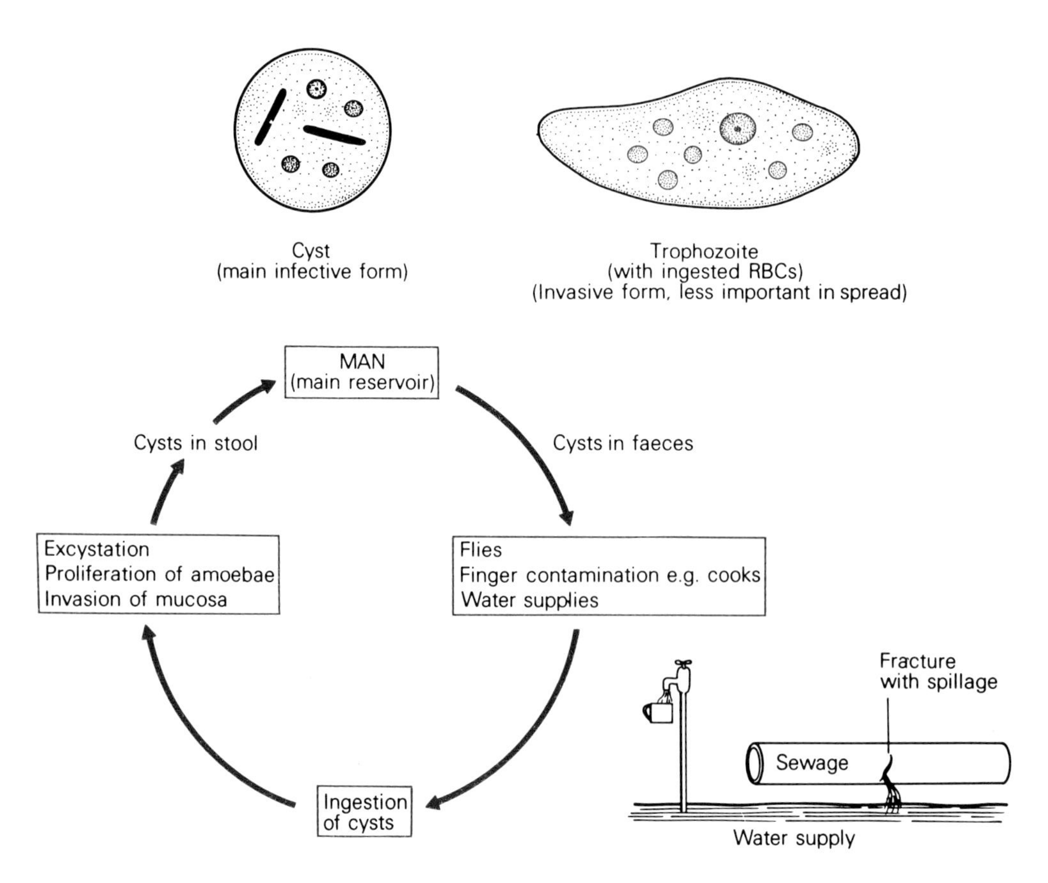

Fig. 15.7 *Amoebiasis, showing a cyst (the main infective form), and the trophozoite or amoeba, which invades colonic mucosa. The epidemiological cycle is shown.*

undertaken. The need for positive histology, before excising the rectum for cancer, is an obvious corollary of this.

Typically, amoebiasis precipitates dysentery-like illness of days or weeks which, if untreated, is followed by a quiescent period during which the patient tends to be constipated. Some patients have a chronic form of amoebic colitis, with irregularity of the stools and some intestinal discomfort. If an amoeboma forms, this gives a palpable mass which is very difficult to distinguish from a carcinoma or Crohn's disease. Serology (amoebic complement fixation test) is useful in non-endemic areas for the diagnosis of amoebiasis and amoebic abscess.

Treatment with a combination of metronidazole, 400 mg 8-hourly for 5 days, with diloxanide furoate, 500 mg 8-hourly for 10 days, gives the best results.

Worm Infestations

Three categories of worm infestation are recognised:

nematodes (roundworms)
cestodes (tapeworms)
trematodes (flukes)

Nematode infestations

Hookworm (Ancylostoma duodenale and Necator americanus): Human infection with the two species of hookworm is estimated to affect up to one quarter of the world's population, and is found in tropical and subtropical regions.

Eggs pass out with the stools and, under suitable conditions, hatch into larvae which may penetrate the skin (Fig. 15.8). The larvae are carried in the circulation to the lungs and, after penetration of the alveolar wall, make their way to the small intestine via the trachea, and swallowed sputum.

Clinical manifestations include an itch at the site of penetration, transient chest symptoms with radiological opacities, and eosinophilia during the stage of migration. Abdominal discomfort and diarrhoea occur during the phase of worm attachment, and ultimately iron deficiency anaemia develops due to blood loss. The diagnosis is established by finding eggs in the stool. Heavy infestations require treatment with mebendazole and ferrous sulphate.

Roundworm (ascariasis). Infestation with *Ascaris lumbricoides* is extremely common throughout the tropics and subtropics. These are larger white worms, males being about 15 cm long and females over 20 cm. Consequently a major infestation can be a serious matter, with the lumen of the small bowel being occupied by a mass of worms, causing some degree of obstruction and malnutrition: they may also migrate into the biliary tree.

Infection occurs in poor hygienic conditions from ingestion of ova from the stools of a patient. These ova can survive for a long time, even in dust, so acquisition of infection, especially in children, is easy. When the ova are swallowed they develop in the small bowel into larvae, which burrow through the intestinal wall and are carried in the portal blood to the liver and on into the lungs. Cough, dyspnoea and eosinophilia may occur at this stage. The larvae migrate through the alveolar wall, up the bronchial tree to reach the pharynx, and are swallowed with food and saliva. In the small bowel they develop into adult worms: fertilised eggs from the females pass in the stools and are ready to repeat the cycle in another individual.

Heavy roundworm infestations provide striking pictures in plain abdominal x-rays. Diagnosis can also be made by finding ova in the stools.

Piperazine is the treatment of choice.

Threadworm (Enterobiasis). Otherwise known as pinworms, infestation with *Enterobius vermicularis* is extremely common world-wide. These are very small white highly motile worms, about 1 cm long, which can quite often be seen in the rectosigmoid at sigmoidoscopy, wriggling over the mucosal surface. The females migrate out onto perianal skin, where they deposit their ova, and this migration sets up considerable irritation.

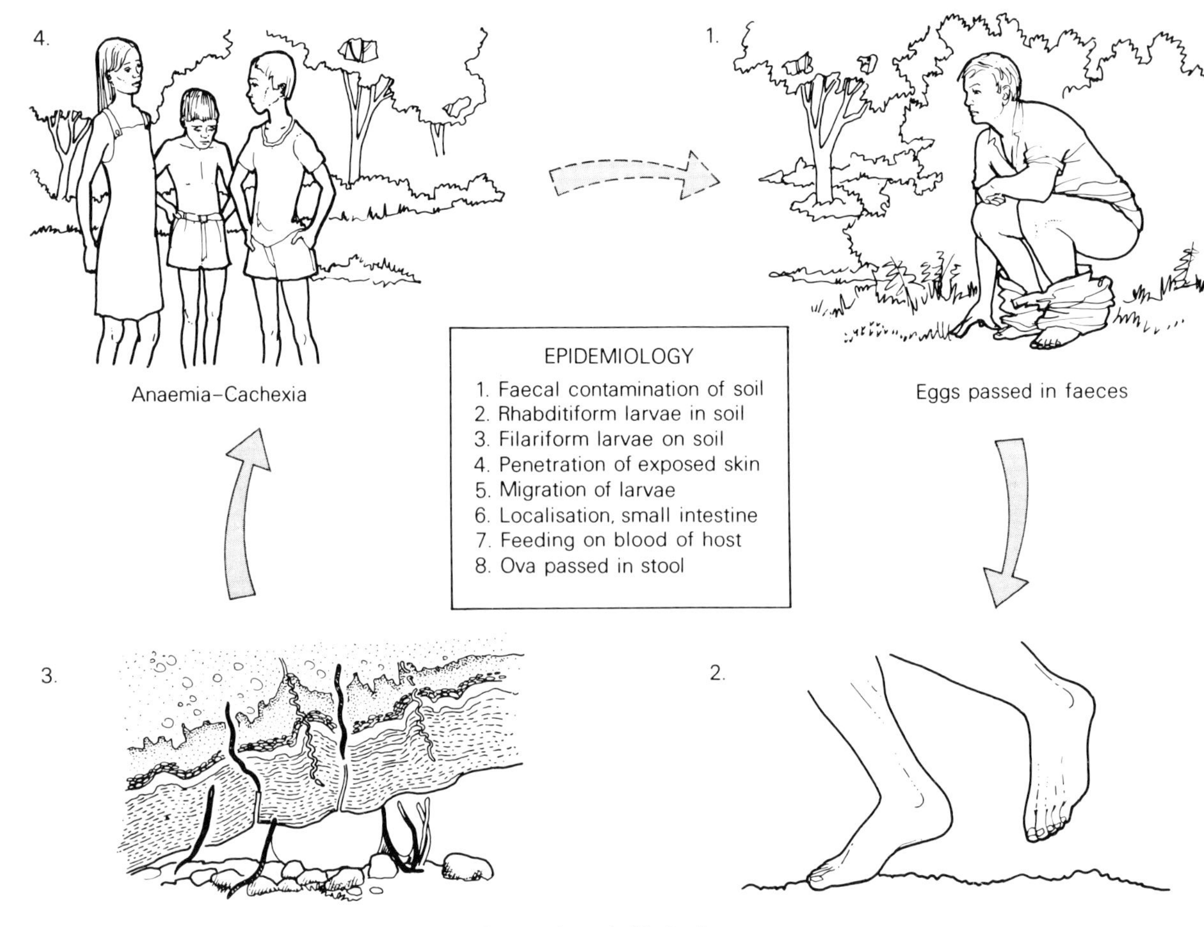

Fig. 15.8 *Epidemiology of hookworm disease.*

Patients naturally tend to scratch, contaminate their fingers with ova and readily re-infect themselves. Cross-infection through use of contaminated family linen and towels can easily occur, so when one case is identified the rest of the family must be checked. Ova may be identified on adhesive paper applied to the perianal area and suitable stained.

Piperazine compounds are non-toxic and effective and often the opportunity is taken to treat the whole family.

Whipworm (trichuriasis). Infestation with *Trichuris trichiuria* is very common in tropical countries. Larvae from swallowed eggs attach to the mucosa of the distal small bowel, where they mature into adult worms, 3–5 cm long. Light infestations are asymptomatic, but heavy infestations may cause diarrhoea with bleeding. Diagnosis is confirmed by finding eggs in the stools and mebendazole is the treatment of choice.

Toxocariasis. Toxocara canis is commonly found in the intestine of dogs, and children are particularly likely to ingest ova. Larvae are liberated in the stomach and may migrate through the body, producing allergic reactions. Granulomata may develop around dead larvae, especially in the eye and the liver.

Treatment is unsatisfactory, but prevention by

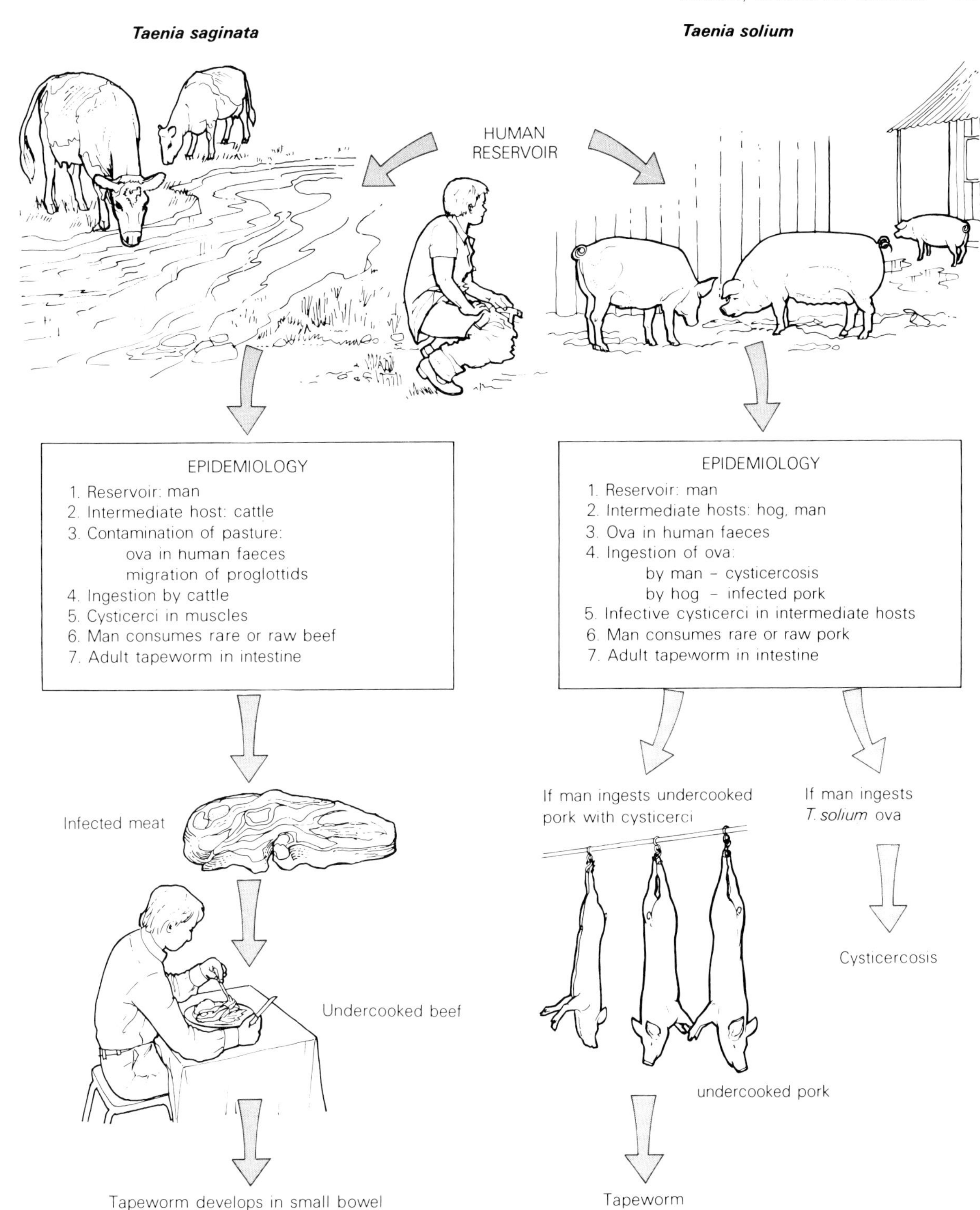

Fig. 15.9 *Epidemiology of the taeniases – tapeworm diseases.*

the regular worming of pet animals, and careful hygiene, is very effective.

Many parasites gain access to the body through the intestinal tract. A number with primarily non-intestinal clinical features may sometimes produce alimentary symptoms, including malabsorption. These include strongyloidiasis, capillariasis, and trichinosis.

Cestode infestations

Cestodes (tapeworms) are widely distributed, especially in tropical and subtropical countries. Infection is acquired by the patient eating the encysted larva (cysticercus) in the undercooked flesh of *Taenia saginata* (in beef) or *T. solium* (in pork) (Fig. 15.9).

In the case of *T. saginata,* the cysticercus is digested and liberated in the upper small bowel and the head of the worm attaches itself to the mucosa; the adult develops by proliferating thousands of segments, and can measure up to 12 metres. There are few symptoms and patients usually only realise they have a worm infestation when segments are seen in the faeces. If the ova in faeces are ingested by the intermediate host – beef cattle – the embryo is liberated, enters the bloodstream and settles in the animal's tissues and becomes a cysticercus. If eaten, undercooked, by man this completes the cycle of development (Fig. 15.9).

The life cycle of *T. solium* has one important, and unfortunate, difference. Whereas the larval cysticercoid stage usually occurs in the flesh of the pig, it can (unlike *T. saginata*) also occur in the tissues of the sufferer because, if man swallows the eggs of a gravid segment of a worm (either his own by the faecal – oral route, or by the liberation of many eggs within the intestine, or from another worm) the larvae liberated from these eggs in the small bowel can penetrate the bowel wall and circulate to encyst in the tissues. When the cysticerci settle in connective tissue or voluntary muscle they gradually calcify and can be seen in plain radiographs. However, in the other site of lodgement, the central nervous system, the cisticerci tend to swell as they age and can give rise to pressure effects, e.g. epileptic fits. The prognosis of this complication is serious.

Infection with the fish tapeworm, *Diphyllobothrium latum,* may cause a macrocytic anaemia due to vitamin B_{12} deficiency.

All cestode infestations are diagnosed by recovery of segments of worm from the stools, and all respond to treatment with niclosamide.

The smallest tapeworm of importance is *Echinococcus granulosus,* for which man is one of the intemediate hosts as a carrier of hydatid cysts (p. 352).

Trematode infestations

Important examples include schistosomiasis (blood flukes), clonorchiasis (liver flukes) and paragonimiasis (lung flukes): only schistosomiasis will be discussed. It is estimated that there are 200 million sufferers from this disease, which is found in parts of Africa, South America and the Far East (Fig. 15.10). The three main species are *S. haematobium, S. mansoni,* and *S. japonicum,* and they share a similar life-cycle (Fig. 15.11). When the life-cycle is considered, it is easy to understand how widespread infection becomes in these countries.

Infection is acquired when the skin is penetrated by cercariae, or by drinking water contaminated with cercariae. These lose their tails and migrate to the liver, where they develop over three months in the portal venous system into adult worms. The worms then migrate to their final habitat: *S. haematobium* to the bladder and uterine plexus; *S. mansoni* to the tributaries of the inferior mesenteric veins; and *S. japonicum* to the superior and inferior mesenteric veins. Numerous eggs are laid, and some reach the exterior via the urine (*S. haematobium*) or stool (*S. mansoni and S. japonicum*), and hatch in water to liberate miracidia. These penetrate the intermediate host, a snail, in which cercariae develop. Many eggs remain in the tissues and provoke a fibrotic reaction in the bladder or intestinal wall, and some are swept up the portal vein and provoke periportal hepatic fibrosis. The consequent presinusoidal hypertension results in portal systemic shunting, which is

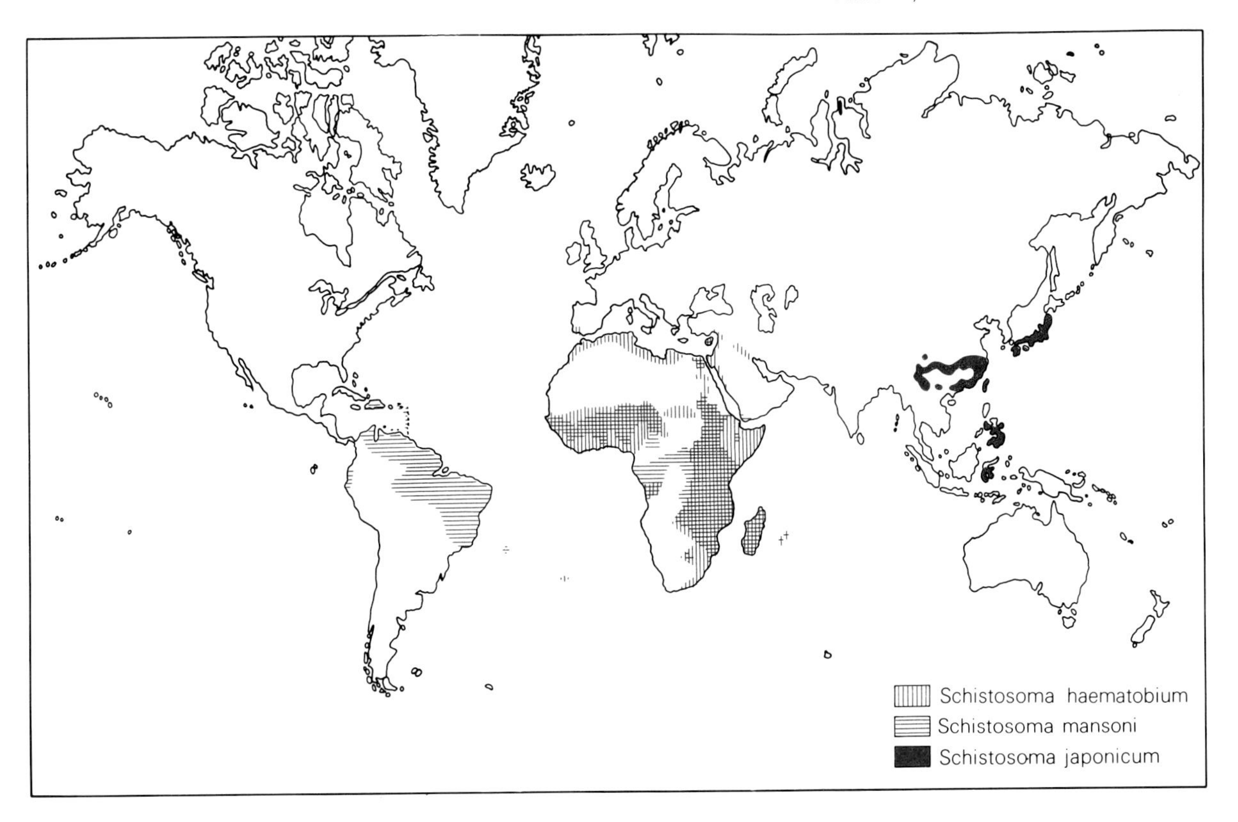

Fig. 15.10 *Schistosomiasis; geographical distribution.*

how some eggs are carried into the lungs and other organs.

Three clinical phases are recognised. Pruritus at the site of penetration may be followed by a systemic illness, with fever and eosinophilia, which corresponds to the onset of egg-laying, and finally chronic schistosomiasis ensues, in which symptoms relate to egg deposition in different organs. Thus, with intestinal infection, abdominal pain and diarrhoea with blood in the stool are frequent features, and hepatosplenomegaly may subsequently develop.

Diagnosis depends on the identification of eggs in the stool or terminal urine (Fig. 15.11): mucosal biopsy at sigmoidoscopy (or cystoscopy) is a more reliable diagnostic technique. Serological methods may be useful in following response to therapy. Treatment with niridazole is appropriate for urinary and uncomplicated intestinal disease, but severe neuropsychiatric reactions preclude its use in the presence of portal hypertension or hypoalbuminaemia. Under these circumstances there is a choice of praziquantel (active against all species) or oxamniquine, which is the treatment of choice for *S. mansoni* infection.

SPECIAL ASPECTS OF ALIMENTARY INFECTIONS

Infantile Gastroenteritis

This is a common disorder which affects 5% of infants in temperate climates during their first year; 10% of those affected require admission to hospital. The incidence is increased in poor socioeconomic conditions, so it is even more important in developing nations. In the UK, most cases are caused by viral infections, of which the recently-

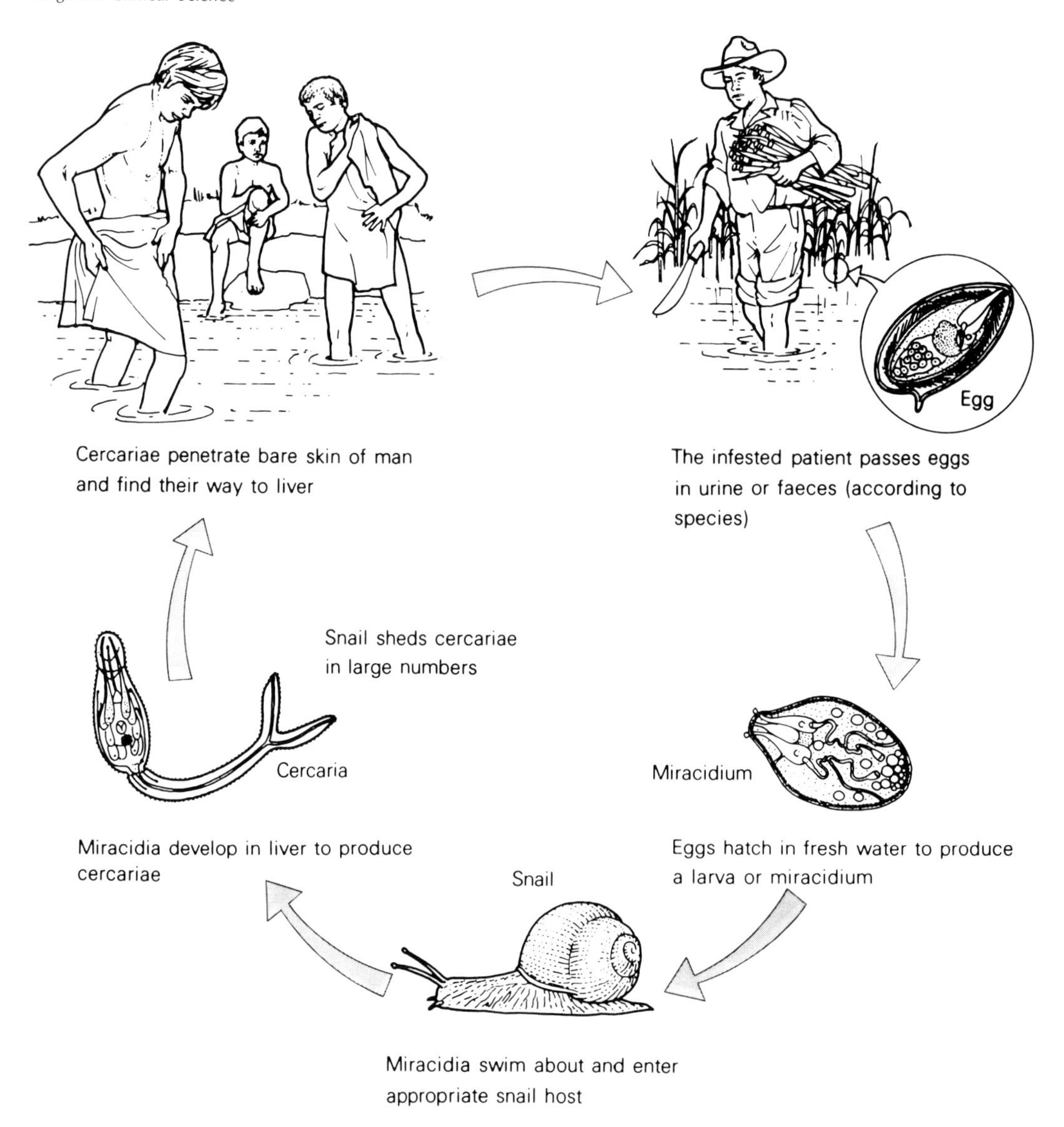

Fig. 15.11 *Schistosomiasis; epidemiology.*

recognised rotavirus is the most important example. Other viral pathogens include adeno, ECHO, and astroviruses. Bacterial pathogens such as enteropathogenic *Esch. coli, Salmonella* or *Shigella* are less common, but can cause serious infections. Giardiasis should not be overlooked, but is uncommon in this age-group.

Diarrhoea and vomiting are the presenting symptoms. The condition is usually readily differentiated from coeliac disease and cows-milk intolerance (which have a more protracted course), pyloric stenosis (in which diarrhoea is not a feature), and intussusception (with the characteristic abdominal mass and 'redcurrant jelly' stool). It is also vital to remember that many systemic illnesses in infancy, e.g. urinary tract infection, tend to present with refusal of feeds, listlessness, vomiting and loose stools.

Recognition of the degree of dehydration is most important. Mild dehydration (loss of less than 5%

of the body-weight) is not easy to detect. With moderate dehydration (when 5–10% of the body-weight has been lost) the fontanelle is depressed, the eyes appear sunken, and there is loss of skin turgor. With more severe degrees of dehydration there develop signs of peripheral vasoconstriction and a rapid weak pulse.

Rehydration is the mainstay of treatment and the great majority can be successfully treated by drinking glucose–electrolyte solution. About 10% of babies are sufficiently ill to require intravenous replacement, but considerable skill must be exercised in the choice of fluid and speed of infusion. Hypernatraemic dehydration is corrected slowly over 48 hours, to minimise the risk of cerebral oedema.

Milk is withdrawn for 48 hours because of temporary lactose intolerance (p. 118). Persistent diarrhoea may be caused by a prolonged phase of lactose intolerance (check the pH of stools, and test for reducing sugars), or cow's-milk-protein intolerance. These problems require the temporary use of special diets.

Bacterial Food Poisoning

Food is an excellent culture medium at kitchen temperatures: some organisms cause obvious putrefaction, when the food will not be eaten, but there are many bacteria which can make food dangerous while it is not unpleasant to eat. Broadly, they produce their effects in two distinct ways.

1. Salmonella

These bacteria can contaminate food quite heavily. Poultry of all kinds and their eggs, pigs, cattle and oysters can all carry salmonellae. The risk occurs when, for instance, large batches of egg powder are dried and used in creams or custards without proper heating, or when a large bird, e.g. turkey, is not given the length of time in the oven necessary for thorough heat sterilisation of the centre of the carcass.

In these circumstances, ingestion can carry a large dose of salmonellae into the intestine, mucosal invasion occurs, and within 12–24 hours the patient suffers from diarrhoea and vomiting, which may last several days.

Campylobacter jejuni behaves similarly (p. 334).

Clostridium perfringens (Cl. welchii) produces spores which resist boiling. A large stew is simmered for some hours and then left to cool: in the anaerobic centre, the clostridia can easily grow. On ingestion they sporulate and, when the spores are lysed in the intestine, an enterotoxin is released which causes abdominal pain and diarrhoea.

2. Staphylococcus aureus

This causes food poisoning in a completely different way – by the formation of toxin outside the body: the illness is due to the ingestion of toxin, not the organisms themselves. Outbreaks have occurred in the past due to milk being contaminated from staphylococcal sepsis on the cow's udder or the milker's hands, but refrigeration and pasteurisation have made this rare. A cook with a staphylococcal pustule on the hand is a great danger if suitable culture media such as cream cakes and meats are contaminated and stand about at temperatures over 10°C and under 40°C: efficient refrigeration should therefore be a sufficient protection, but toxin may be elaborated during the warming up of a meal. The toxin itself is heat-stable and, when swallowed, produces very quickly (in 2–3 hours) violent vomiting, abdominal pain and diarrhoea.

Clostridium botulinum can survive much boiling and, if processing is inadequate, can survive in vegetables (especially beans), where the spores produce a neurotoxin: the important point is that the toxin is destroyed by boiling for 10 minutes. If toxin is ingested, 12–36 hours later a flaccid paralysis comes on with prolonged respiratory failure. Botulism is rare but nearly always fatal.

Bacillus cereus. Fried rice is the food most frequently contaminated by this organism, which survives preliminary boiling, multiplies at room temperatures, and may not be killed by rapid frying. Ingestion of the preformed enterotoxin induces vomiting in one to six hours.

Vibrio parahaemolyticus. This contaminates raw fish and is ingested with seafood. An enterotoxin produces vomiting, pain and diarrhoea within 12–24 hours.

Travellers' Diarrhoea

Gut disturbances are so common among visitors to many parts of the world – especially hot climates where sanitation is poor – that they are almost accepted as the norm. Such charming local varieties as 'Delhi belly', 'Gyppy tummy' (Egypt) and 'Montezuma's revenge' illustrate the world-wide nature of the disease. They are commonly due to enterotoxigenic strains of *Esch. coli*, but other organisms to be considered include:

salmonellae,
shigellae,
Vibrio cholerae,
Campylobacter jejuni,
Amoebae, and
Giardia.

The illness is usually mild and transient, and merely causes social inconvenience. However, there may be more serious implications for the very young and elderly, who are particularly susceptible to dehydration. Most laboratories do not possess the facilities for confirmatory diagnosis based on stool examination for *Esch. coli* and toxins, but the stool should be examined for more important pathogens, e.g. *Salmonella*, if the symptoms persist. The prophylactic use of antibiotics such as doxycycline and nalidixic acid and also sulphonamides is not now recommended because of the risk of drug resistance and, in some disorders, the development of a carrier state.

Advice to travellers going abroad to countries of low sanitary standards is as follows:

1. Obtain pre-travel vaccination against typhoid, paratyphoid and cholera sufficiently early to give protection, as well as any other prophylaxis such as polio, yellow fever, hepatitis, etc., where appropriate.
2. Use the utmost care in selecting drinks – no tap water – and avoid washed salads or fruits and ice. Water-sterilising tablets may be used in emergency.
3. Take a supply of loperamide (Imodium), but use *only* if necessary.
4. Glucose–electrolyte is ideal, but not very practical for the average traveller to include in his luggage.
5. If diarrhoea persists more than three days, seek medical attention.

A logical treatment for severe travellers' diarrhoea (after stool microscopy and culture if possible) would be: metronidazole 400 mg three times daily for 7 days, *plus* co-trimoxazole or doxycycline 100 mg daily for 7 days.

INFECTIONS OF THE LIVER

Viral Hepatitis (see also p. 157).

Although hepatic involvement occurs in many viral infections, e.g. yellow fever, infectious mononucleosis, CMV and rubella among others, the term viral hepatitis is applied to infection with the primary hepatitis viruses, of which more than three are currently recognised. These are classified as type A, type B and type non-A, non-B.

Viral agents: type A virus

This is transmitted primarily by the faecal–oral route, it is excreted in the faeces for approximately two weeks after the onset of the illness, and may be responsible for epidemics in areas with poor sanitation. The infection, which develops after an incubation period of two to six weeks, is commonly subclinical, and the majority of clinical infections are anicteric, particularly in children. Fulminant hepatitis may occasionally occur, but there is no evidence that chronic viraemia and chronic hepatitis are associated with this virus.

The type B virus

This has a complex structure (Fig. 15.12). The surface protein coat, detected in serum as the surface antigen (HBsAg, 'Australia antigen') covers the viral core to form the large spheres (Dane particles), but may also be found in excess as small spheres and tubules. The viral core contains the viral DNA and DNA polymerase. The activity of this enzyme relates to the presence of the 'e' antigen, the detection of which implies active viral replication and hence infectivity. The core antigen is not detected in serum because of the surface coat, but the core antibody may be the most sensitive marker of hepatitis B virus (HBV) infection. The appearance of the HBV markers during an episode of type B hepatitis is illustrated in Chapter 8, Fig. 8.24. HBV is transmitted parenterally (by contaminated needles or blood and by oral or sexual contact). Illness develops after an incubation period of 2–6 months and is usually more prolonged and severe than HAV infection. Fulminant hepatitis, chronic viraemia, and chronic liver disease may follow, and chronic viraemia is associated with the development of hepatoma.

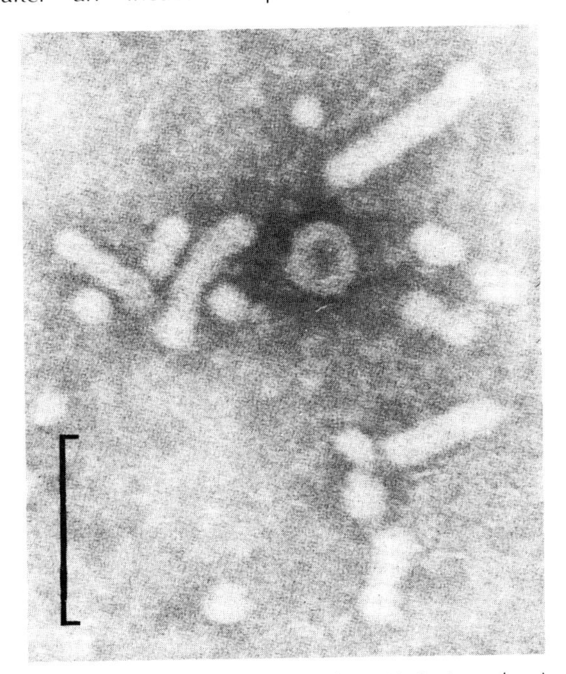

Fig. 15.12 *Electron micrograph of hepatitis B virus, showing 45 nm Dane particle, and 22 nm small particle HBs antigen; rod is same in elongated form. Barline = 100 nm*

So far, little is known of the third viral agent, which has been labelled non-A non-B. Epidemiological evidence suggests that three viruses are involved. One is similar to type A virus, and one to type B virus, but with an intermediate incubation period. Chronic hepatitis and persistent viraemia frequently develop.

Clinical features: see p. 158.

Diagnosis. The diagnosis of acute viral hepatitis is supported by typical biochemical changes (very high serum aspartate aminotransferase, normal or only moderately elevated alkaline phosphatase), and the identification of viral markers (HBsAg or IgM antibodies to type A virus). At present no serological markers are available for non-A non-B infections.

The differential diagnosis includes:

1. Other infections e.g. cytomegalovirus, rubella, the Epstein-Barr viruses, and leptospirosis.
   Drug-induced liver disease, e.g. with isoniazid, sulphonamides, methyldopa, and halothane.
3. Alcoholic liver disease.
4. An acute presentation of chronic active hepatitis.
5. Extrahepatic biliary obstruction.

The presence of other clinical features, such as lymphadenopathy in infectious mononucleosis, and nephritis in leptospirosis, help to identify these infections. A careful drug history is most imporant; drug hepatitis may be difficult to distinguish from viral hepatitis although occasionally eosinophilia is a useful pointer to drug-sensitivity. Alcoholic hepatitis may be associated with abdominal pain, a leucocytosis (in contrast to viral hepatitis), and marked elevation of the serum γGT. An acute presentation of chronic active hepatitis may also be difficult to distinguish from viral hepatitis.

Clinical stigmata of chronic liver disease and elevated gamma globulins are more frequently associated with chronic liver disease. A liver biopsy is sometimes required for accurate diagnosis. Ultrasonography is useful in identifying dilatation of bile ducts due to extrahepatic biliary obstruction.

Chronic carrier state: HBV markers persist in up to 10% of patients following HBV infection. Approximately 0.1% of the UK population are HBV carriers, HBV carriage is much commoner in other populations, e.g. from the Mediterranean area. In males, HBV carriage appears to be associated with an increased risk of subsequent hepatoma. Epidemiological evidence suggests that chronic carriage occurs after non-A non-B hepatitis, but more precise information awaits the development of serological markers.

Prevention and treatment: Gamma globulin will provide a degree of protection against type A hepatitis for suceptible subjects who are travelling in endemic areas. Passive protection against HBV requires specific hyperimmune globulin. This reduces the risk of developing infection, from six to one per cent, when given within 7 days of accidental exposure. Personnel who have been clearly contaminated by the blood or body fluids of a patient with a positive test for HBV antigen should receive hyperimmune globulin, assuming they themselves are antigen (HBsAg) negative.

Active immunisation against HBV infections, using a vaccine derived from the surface antigen, is now available for high-risk groups: these would include medical and nursing staff working in infectious disease and renal dialysis units, and laboratory staff handling blood from hepatitis patients. While supplies of vaccine remain limited, difficult decisions over priorities have to be made.

Patients who develop acute liver failure need intensive care (p. 198).

The detection of ensuing chronic liver disease in patients with type B and non-A non-B infections can only be achieved by careful follow-up, which may include liver biopsy. However the management of such patients is not clearly established and the role of corticosteroids is uncertain.

Leptospirosis

These diseases are caused by spirochaetes of the complex *Leptospira interrogans,* of which the best known is *L. icterohaemorrhagiae,* the causative organism of icteric leptospirosis or Weil's disease.

Rats are the best known hosts (*L. icterohaemorrhagiae*), but dogs (*L. canicola*) and other animals can be infected: in all, the leptospires survive in the renal tubules of the host and are therefore shed in the urine. In days gone by, farm and sewer workers, fish cleaners and miners all worked in places where rats were numerous and chance abrasions allowed easy entry of spirochaetes to the body; infection can also enter through the mucosae of the eyes, nose, mouth and throat. Nowadays, preventive measures have made this a rare condition in Western countries.

Ninety per cent of infections are anicteric and many are subclinical. In these patients, the septicaemic phase develops after 7–10 days, with myalgia, pyrexia, abdominal pain and proteinuria. The temperature settles after 3–7 days, but the second immune phase develops 3 days later, with a recurrent temperature. Skin rashes, uveitis and meningitis may develop. In the icteric form (Weil's syndrome) the two phases merge, and these patients are frequently very ill with jaundice, renal failure and circulatory collapse. Organisms can be isolated from blood or cerebrospinal fluid only during the first week of illness. Subsequently the diagnosis depends on serology. Antibiotic therapy in the form of benzyl penicillin or tetracycline is only helpful when administered early in the illness.

Liver Abscess

Pyogenic abscess

It is important to recognise this uncommon condition because, when undiagnosed, it carries a high mortality. The most important cause now is ascending cholangitis, associated with stones in the bile duct. Other forms of abdominal sepsis, e.g. acute diverticulitis of the colon, may cause an abscess by spread through the portal vein, but it has become very rare after appendicitis. Liver abscess may be a major late complication of hepatic injury.

These patients are generally ill, often from the original cause of the abscess, and usually complain of aching pain in the hepatic area. Fever, rigors, anorexia and weight loss are usual and, if the diaphragm is involved, there may be shoulder tip pain. The liver may be enlarged and tender. Some patients run a very chronic course, when diagnosis is especially difficult.

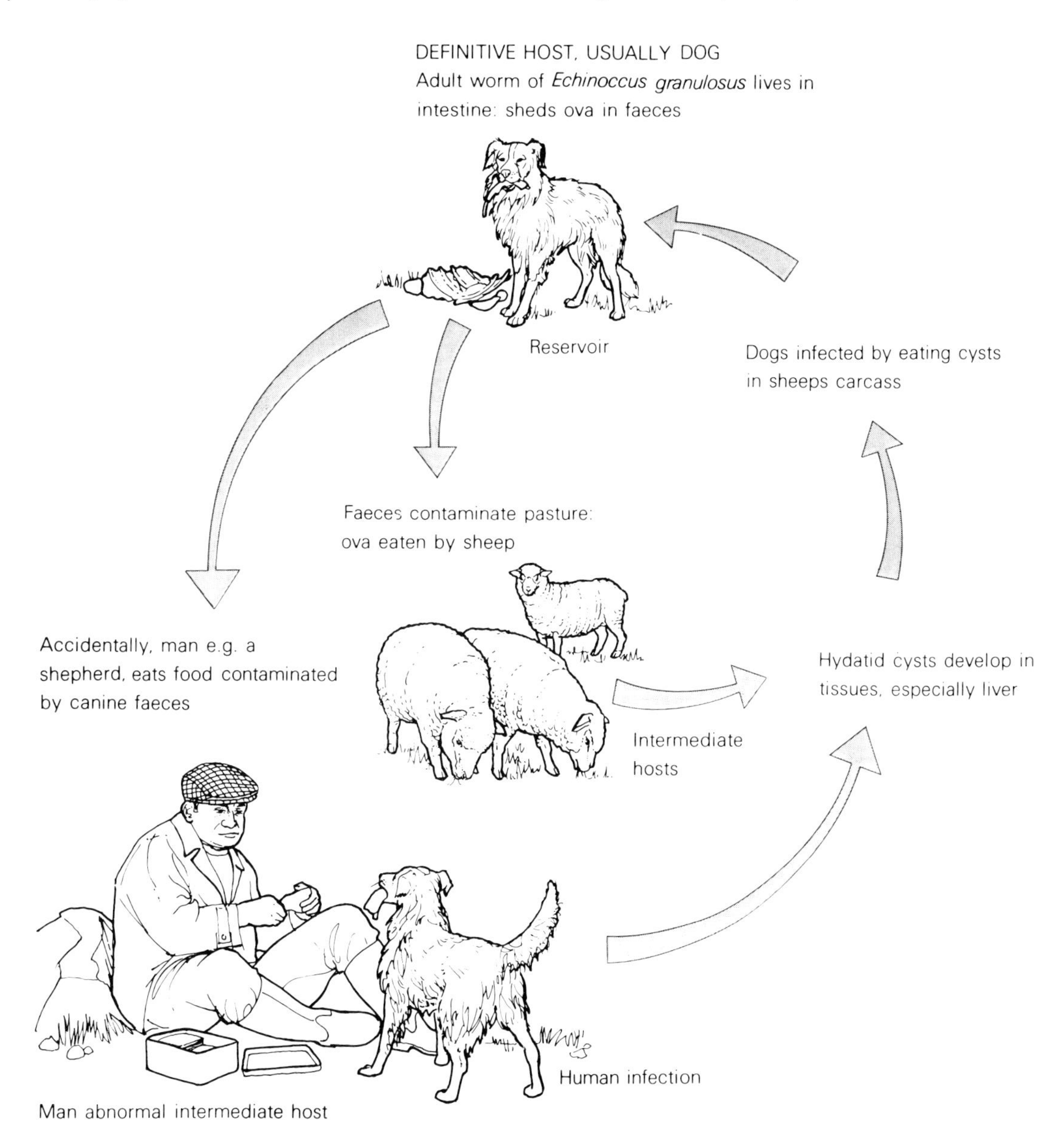

Fig. 15.13 *Epidemiology of hydatid disease.*

Once the diagnosis is considered, it can be speedily confirmed by ultrasonic scanning. Some of these patients have a severe endogenous bacterial illness (p. 327) and need intensive treatment: if at all possible, the abscess should be drained and the original cause (e.g. stones in the bile duct) dealt with.

Amoebic abscess

Amoebic infections have been discussed in the first section of this chapter. Amoebic abscesses usually develop in the right lobe of the liver and are frequently painful and tender. Serology may be useful in diagnosis. Treatment is with metronidazole, and larger abscesses may require aspiration.

Hydatid disease

The adult worm of *Echinococcus granulosus* lives in the small intestine of the definitive host – the dog. Eggs are passed in the faeces and are eaten by the intermediate hosts – sheep and cattle. Hydatid cysts (which are the larval stage) develop in the tissues of these herbivores and, if that flesh is eaten by a dog, the cycle is completed with the development of further worms, which will pass ova in the canine faeces (Fig. 15.13).

The disease is endemic in some parts of the world and it is clearly difficult for some humans, e.g. shepherds, who are living rough, to avoid accidental contamination of their food by ova from canine faeces. Hydatid disease is now a rarity in Britain apart from some cases from the northern and western isles of Scotland.

Man therefore becomes affected by sharing with herbivores the role of intermediate host. When ova from canine faeces reach the small bowel the embryo is liberated, gains access to the bloodstream, and may lodge in liver, lung, brain or other tissues. Each cyst grows slowly, having an inner germinal layer secreted by the cyst with a fibrous capsule developed from the tissues of the host: new cysts develop within the germinal layer.

As the cyst grows it causes swelling and pain, but liver function is usually normal. An x-ray may show characteristic calcification of the capsule. The Casoni test is sensitive but not very specific, and the diagnosis is confirmed by specific complement fixation tests.

Careful surgical removal of the cyst may be required to relieve pressure effects, but great care must be exercised because any accidental spillage of cyst fluid into the tissues may cause a fatal anaphylactic reaction, and there is also a risk of the spread of daughter cysts. For the same reasons, percutaneous liver biopsy or aspiration is dangerous and should not be performed.

Specific treatment with mebendazole is as yet at an early stage, but it may prove valuable and diminish the risks of surgery.

Further Reading

Allan R.N., Keighley M.R.B., Alexander-Williams J., Hawkins C. (1983). *(Inflammatory Bowel Diseases.* Edinburgh:Churchill Livingstone.

Bouchier I.A.D. ed. *Recent Advances in Gastroenterology.* Edinburgh: Churchill Livingstone. (Series publication with new edition about every two years.)

Clinics in Gastroenterology. Published three times a year by W.B. Saunders. Each issue reviews a topic in Gastroenterology.

Dickerson J.W.T., Lee H.A. (1978). *Nutrition in the Clinical Management of Disease.* London: Arnold.

Duthie H.L., Wormsley K.G., eds. (1979). *Scientific Basis of Gastroenterology.* Edinburgh: Churchill Livingstone.

Morson B.C., Dawson I.M.P. (1979). *Gastrointestinal Pathology,* 2nd edn. Oxford: Blackwell Scientific.

*Shearman D.J.C., Finlayson N.D.C. (1982). *Diseases of the Gastrointestinal Tract and Liver.* Edinburgh:Churchill Livingstone.

*Sherlock S. (1981). *Diseases of the Liver and Biliary System,* 6th edn. Oxford:Blackwell Scientific.

*Sleisenger M.H., Fordtran J.S. (1983), *Gastrointestinal Disease,* 3rd edn. Philadelphia:Saunders.

Thomson J.P.S., Nicholls R.J., Williams C.B. (1981). *Colorectal Disease: An Introduction for Surgeons and Physicians.* London:Heinemann Medical Books.

**These three books are currently the principal reference works.*

Index